Drugs
ACROSS THE SPECTRUM

SIXTH EDITION

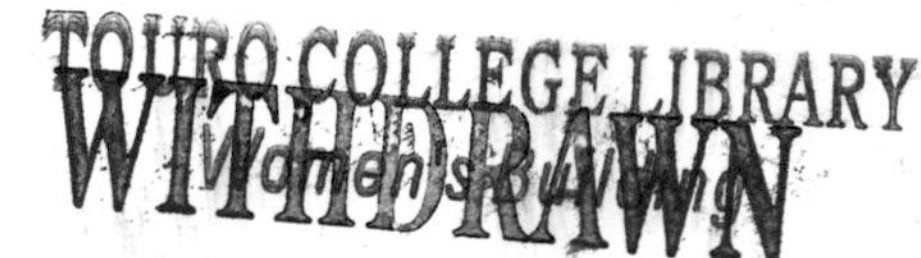

Raymond Goldberg, Ph.D.

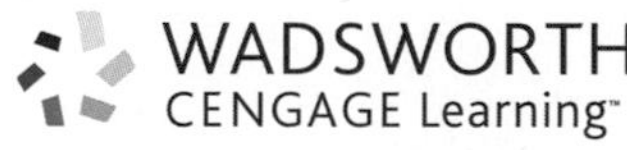

Australia • Brazil • Japan • Korea • Mexico • Singapore • Spain • United Kingdom • United States

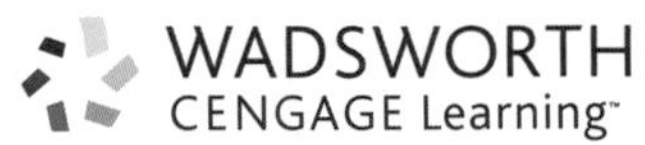

Drugs Across the Spectrum, Sixth Edition
Raymond Goldberg

Publisher: Yolanda Cossio
Senior Acquisitions Editor: Laura Pople
Developmental Editor: Elesha Feldman
Assistant Editor: Samantha Arvin
Editorial Assistant: Jenny Hoang
Media Editor: Lauren Tarson
Senior Marketing Manager: Laura McGinn
Marketing Assistant: Elizabeth Wong
Marketing Communications Manager: Belinda Krohmer
Content Project Management: Pre-Press PMG
Creative Director: Rob Hugel
Art Director: John Walker
Print Buyer: Linda Hsu
Rights Acquisitions Account Manager, Text: Margaret Chamberlain-Gaston
Rights Acquisitions Account Manager, Image: Leitha Etheridge-Sims
Production Service: Pre-Press PMG
Text Designer: Pre-Press PMG
Photo Researcher: Bill Smith Group
Copy Editor: Pre-Press PMG
Cover Designer: Jeanne Calabrese
Cover Images: © Reed Kaestner/Corbis; © image100/Corbis; © Luca Da Ros/Grand Tour/Corbis; © Fred de Noyelle/Godong/Corbis; Tek Image/Photo Researchers, Inc.
Compositor: Pre-Press PMG

Library of Congress Control Number: 2009924501

ISBN-13: 978-0-495-55793-7

ISBN-10: 0-495-55793-5

Wadsworth
10 Davis Drive
Belmont, CA 94002-3098
USA

Cengage Learning is a leading provider of customized learning solutions with office locations around the globe, including Singapore, the United Kingdom, Australia, Mexico, Brazil, and Japan. Locate your local office at **www.cengage.com/global**

Cengage Learning products are represented in Canada by Nelson Education, Ltd.

To learn more about Wadsworth visit **www.cengage.com/wadsworth**

Purchase any of our products at your local college store or at our preferred online store **www.ichapters.com**

Printed in the United States of America
1 2 3 4 5 6 7 8 9 12 11 10 09

CONTENTS

PREFACE

Mind-altering substances have had a profound effect on society ever since humans first roamed the planet. The goal of this book is to impart an understanding of drugs and their impact on individuals, families, communities, and society. In addition to providing a thorough review of illicit drugs, the book devotes much attention to licit, or legal, drugs. This focus is pertinent because drugs such as tobacco and alcohol account for far more deaths and disabilities than do illicit drugs. Also, millions of people use prescribed and over-the-counter drugs that are potentially harmful. The book also covers performance-enhancing drugs such as anabolic steroids because of their increased use in the past decade.

Unlike some texts, *Drugs Across the Spectrum* goes beyond the presentation of abstract concepts and impersonal information to examine issues that warrant personal reflection. One goal of *Drugs Across the Spectrum* is to make the information relevant to the reader. It is understood that no one is immune from the effects of drug use. People face decisions about their own drug use and drug use by family members and friends. Societal effects and public policy are also areas that require knowledge on which to base responsible decisions.

Organization

Drugs Across the Spectrum is divided into three parts. The first provides an overall view, including a historical perspective, the motivations for drug use, social implications of drug use, legal ramifications, and factors affecting how drugs interact with the human body. Part II focuses on specific categories of drugs, exploring their psychological and physiological effects. The last part critically examines treatment and prevention, including various modes of drug treatment, the effectiveness of drug treatment, and the impact of education and prevention in addressing problems caused by drug use, misuse, and abuse.

New in the Sixth Edition

Chapter 1 Drugs in Perspective

- Emphasis on drug use throughout the lifespan with special emphasis on drugs and the elderly
- Updated research on the history of drugs

Chapter 2 Drugs in Contemporary Society

- A current view of the U.S. government's budget for dealing with drug abuse
- An international perspective on drug use
- The most recent data on the "Monitoring the Future" study and the "National Survey on Drug Use and Health"
- The most recent data on drug-related mortalities and emergency room episodes

Chapter 3 Motivations for Drug Use

- Updated research on the effects of advertising on drug use, especially alcohol and tobacco
- An expanded section on "Performance-Enhancing Drugs"
- Cutting-edge research on THG (tetrahydrogestrinone)

Chapter 4 Drugs and the Law

- A new section on early drug regulations
- Updated statistics on federal drug control spending
- An expanded discussion on the pros and cons of drug legalization
- A new section on the effects of drug convictions on college students

Chapter 5 The Pharmacology and Physiology of Drug Use

- Updated information on the effects of drugs on older people
- Current data on the purity levels of various drugs
- Expanded information about the effects of drugs on the brain and various systems of the body
- Current statistics on HIV infection and various behaviors, especially injection drug use

Chapter 6 Alcohol

- Updated data on historical trends in alcohol consumption
- Current information on factors that affect drinking levels
- A section devoted to binge drinking
- Current information regarding drinking and ethnicity

- Additional information on adolescents and "alcopops"
- New data on alcohol and its effects on driving

Chapter 7 Tobacco

- Updated data on trends in tobacco use
- A new section of the effects of light cigarettes
- An expanded section on tobacco use in various countries
- New tables and graphs showing the trends in the use of various tobacco products
- New information regarding smoking cessation techniques

Chapter 8 Narcotics

- Revised statistics on the use of narcotics
- Greater emphasis on drugs from a global perspective
- New section on "Fentanyl, Methadone, and Other Synthetic Opiates"

Chapter 9 Sedative-Hypnotic Drugs

- A new section on adolescents and prescription drugs
- Updated discussion on inhalants and young people

Chapter 10 Psychotherapeutic Drugs

- A new section addressing mental illness and special populations
- Dual diagnosis (co-occurring disorders) was added to this chapter
- A new section on Wellbutrin

Chapter 11 Stimulants: Cocaine, Amphetamines, Methamphetamines, and Caffeine

- Revised statistics on cocaine use, including crack cocaine and emergency room episodes
- New section on the adverse effects of methamphetamines
- Information regarding clandestine methamphetamine laboratories was added
- New section on high energy caffeinated beverages

Chapter 12 Marijuana

- Updated information on indoor cultivation of marijuana
- Revised data on trends in marijuana and hashish use
- Expanded section on the legalization of medical marijuana

Chapter 13 Hallucinogens

- Revised data on rates of LSD and other hallucinogen use
- New research on the effects of salvinorin A
- An update on legal issues related to salvinorin A
- Information on the medical benefits of hallucinogens

Chapter 14 Over-the-Counter Drugs

- New section on generic versus brand name drugs
- New information regarding gastric reflux medications
- Expanded section on herbal drugs
- Information about over-the-counter drugs used to make methamphetamines
- New section on the weight-loss drug orlistat

Chapter 15 Substance Abuse Treatment

- Updated research on the benefits of treatment
- New section on drug courts
- New section on acamprosate, a pharmacologic treatment for alcoholism
- New section on Narcotics Anonymous

Chapter 16 Drug Prevention and Education

- Updated research on drug abuse prevention
- Expanded research on identifying youths at high risk for drug abuse
- Current research on drug education programs

Features

- Chapter objectives at the beginning of each chapter put the content into a meaningful framework.
- Color photos, illustrations, and tables reflect the latest drug statistics and trends.
- "Thinking Critically" questions at the end of each chapter promote critical thinking and stimulate classroom discussion.
- "On Campus" boxes in each chapter focus on facts and statistics that are relevant to college students.
- Each chapter includes "Fact or Fiction?" questions that enable readers to examine their beliefs and possible misconceptions about various drugs.
- Key terms are highlighted and defined as they are discussed in the text to give readers easy access to the meaning of vocabulary essential to their understanding.
- A brief summary concludes each chapter.
- Web resources at the end of each chapter have been thoroughly updated and include brief descriptions to direct readers to specific information related to chapter topics.

Ancillaries

The following ancillaries are available without charge to qualified adopters:

- **Instructor's Manual and Test Bank:** Contains chapter outlines, InfoTrac© College Edition activities, and multiple-choice, matching, true/false, and essay questions.

- **Power Lecture CD-ROM:** Includes the Instructor's Manual, Test Bank, JoinIn on TurningPoint questions, and a PowerPoint presentation for customization and use in the classroom.

Acknowledgments

This book has benefited from the assistance of many people. Developmental editor Elesha Feldman was especially important to the quality of this text. Elesha spent numerous hours helping me to clarify and update information. Other individuals who were instrumental in seeing this project come to fruition include Yolanda Cossio, publisher; Melissa Sacco, senior project manager from Pre-Press PMG; Matthew Ballantyne, senior content project manager; Samantha Arvin, assistant editor; Lauren Tarson, senior media editor; and Jenny Hoang, editorial assistant. Their expertise and support throughout this endeavor are greatly appreciated.

I would like to give special thanks to the reviewers, whose input has been very valuable for this revision:

Jewel Carter, William Paterson University
Catherine Marrone, SUNY Stony Brook
Blair Allyn Thornton, University of Kansas
Robin Lee Weeks, Onondaga Community College

I would also like to thank Kerry Redican for his thorough work on the Instructor's Manual and Test Bank.

Last, I would like to thank my daughters, Tara and Greta, for their continuing love and support.

—Raymond Goldberg

ABOUT THE AUTHOR

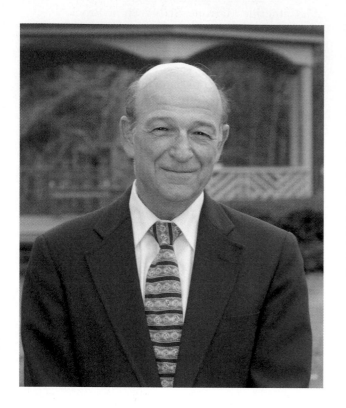

Raymond Goldberg is the Dean of Health Sciences at Vance-Granville Community College in North Carolina. Previously, he was a professor of health education and associate dean at the State University of New York at Cortland. Over the course of his professional life, Ray has taught a variety of drug-related courses, authored numerous articles on health- and drug-related topics, and received several significant research grants for his work in health and drug education. Ray is the author of *Taking Sides: Clashing Views on Controversial Issues in Drugs and Society*, eighth edition (McGraw-Hill/Dushkin). He received his undergraduate degree from the University of North Carolina at Pembroke, his master's degree from the University of South Carolina, and his Ph.D. from the University of Toledo.

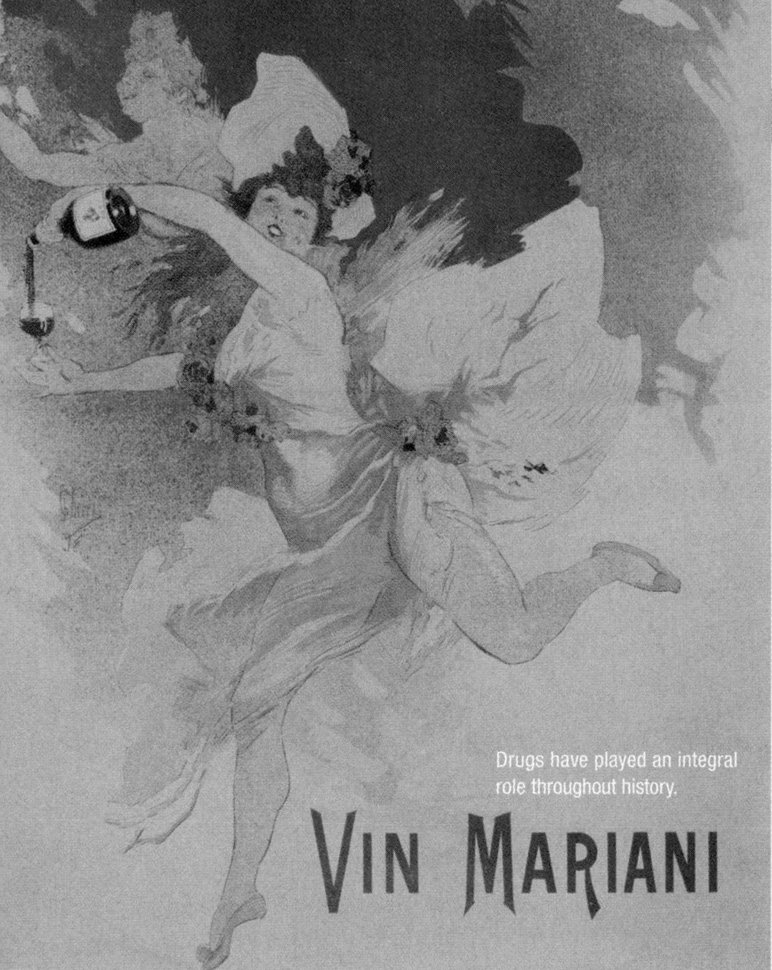

Drugs have played an integral role throughout history.

FACT OR FICTION?

1. The federal government estimates that there are more than 1.5 million Americans age 50 or older who are addicted to drugs.
2. The early settlers in Colonial America were strongly opposed to alcohol use.
3. Marijuana was first cultivated for people to use to get high.
4. At one time opium was given to children to relieve sore gums.
5. Sigmund Freud was praised for advocating cocaine use for various medical conditions.
6. When first developed, barbiturates were believed to be nonaddictive.
7. A known way that methamphetamine abusers obtain money is through identity theft. The state with the highest rate of identity theft is Arizona.
8. LSD was originally developed to cure heroin addicts.
9. Profits from the sale of tobacco were used by early Colonialists to defeat the British.
10. Cowboys in the American West in the 1800s preferred chewing tobacco to smoking cigarettes.

Turn the page to check your answers

1 Drugs in Perspective

Chapter Objectives

After completing this chapter, the reader should be able to describe:

- How historical events affect our perception of drugs
- How drug use, misuse, and abuse differ
- The role of opium in wars between the Chinese and British governments
- The economic effect of the rum trade in New England
- Attitudes toward alcohol in Colonial America
- Factors leading to the increase in alcohol consumption in the United States in the early 1800s
- Factors leading to the increase in morphine abuse in the United States in the 19th century
- The development of minor tranquilizers and other mind-altering drugs in the United States in the 1950s
- The importance of tobacco to the economic viability of the New World

FACT OR FICTION?

1. **Fact:** The official estimate from the federal government is 1.7 million.
2. **Fiction:** The fact is—Settlers in Colonial America drank more alcohol proportionately than Americans today.
3. **Fiction:** The fact is—Marijuana was first cultivated for fiber and for medicinal purposes.
4. **Fact:** The Egyptians gave opium to children to relieve pain.
5. **Fiction:** The fact is—Freud was severely criticized for advocating the medical use of cocaine.
6. **Fact:** When first developed, barbiturates were considered safe drugs.
7. **Fact:** Arizona leads the country in identity thefts with a rate of 147.8 per 100,000 people.
8. **Fiction:** The fact is—LSD was originally developed to ease respiratory problems.
9. **Fact:** The French bought tobacco from early Americans, and this enabled the early settlers to buy armaments to defeat the British.
10. **Fact:** For cowboys riding horses, it was much easier to chew tobacco than to smoke it.

When listening to the news or reading accounts of drug use, one may get the impression that drug use and abuse is a new phenomenon. Certainly, the use and abuse of drugs is prevalent in society. After all, it is estimated that one-third of adolescents consumed alcohol in the past 12 months, that one out of five have used an illegal drug, and that one out of six have smoked cigarettes.[1] Teenage girls are more likely than teenage boys to misuse prescription drugs.[2] Moreover, rates of drug abuse among the elderly have increased. To better understand the present, it is helpful to look back at drug history.

A historical perspective on drugs provides insight into the role that drugs have played over time. We also can benefit from a common understanding of what the terms **drug**, **drug misuse**, and **drug abuse** mean. Many factors affect how these words are defined. Is a substance defined as a drug according to its behavioral effects, pharmacological effects, effects on society, or chemical makeup? If drugs are viewed as only illegal or menacing substances, we may not acknowledge substances such as caffeine and tobacco as drugs. If caffeine and tobacco are not considered drugs, one may think they cannot be misused or abused because only illegal drugs are misused or abused. Or a person may grow up thinking that any drug use, from aspirin to nasal decongestants, is unacceptable. If someone takes three aspirins a day, is he or she misusing or abusing drugs? What if a person has a glass of beer with dinner and a glass of wine each night before going to bed?

Living with a diabetic, asthmatic, or alcoholic person may alter one's perception of drugs. Religious groups and their rituals play a crucial role in how drug use is defined. For example, the Native American Church uses the hallucinogen peyote in a spiritual context but not recreationally.[3] If college students were to experiment with hallucinogens to enhance their spirituality, however, this drug use would be perceived differently. Communion wine is part of the service in the Catholic Church and in some Protestant denominations. Drugs used within a religious framework are not likely to be abused.[4] In addition, adults who attend religious services regularly are less likely to use legal and illegal drugs.[5] The point is that any definition is limited and is influenced by one's experiences and background. Moreover, definitions are arbitrary.

Definitions

Although definitions for the word drug abound, there is no legal definition. One definition of **psychoactive drugs** is "substances that act to alter mood, thought processes, or behavior, or that are used to manage neuropsychological illness."[6] When a substance affects one's ability to get along with others, to work, to cope, or to think rationally, it can be classified as a drug. Based on this definition, many substances could be designated as drugs. Drugs encompass illegal substances, prescription medicines, and over-the-counter medications.

Could foods be included as drugs? Many people crave ice cream and chocolate to cope with unpleasant experiences or simply to raise their spirits. Should these be considered drugs? Are they used differently from many substances identified as drugs? How would chocolate and ice cream connoisseurs react to the idea that they are drug users? No doubt, support groups for ice cream users would spring up!

Drug Misuse

Drug misuse refers to the unintentional or inappropriate use of prescribed or over-the-counter drugs. One group especially vulnerable to drug misuse is the elderly.[7] Although elderly people comprise a small proportion of the population, this group accounts for one quarter of the prescription drugs sold in the United States.[8] About 3% of Americans undergoing drug treatment are age 55 or older. More people seeking treatment for alcohol abuse are older than age 55.[9] Even aspirin can be fatal when used improperly.

drug Any substance that alters one's ability to function emotionally, physically, intellectually, financially, or socially

drug misuse The unintentional or inappropriate use of prescribed or over-the-counter drugs

drug abuse The intentional and inappropriate use of a drug resulting in physical, emotional, financial, intellectual, or social consequences for the user

psychoactive drug Any substance that has the capability of altering mood, perception, or behavior

Drug misuse arises from not understanding a drug's effects. For example, if a student studies for a test and drinks alcohol to improve his or her study skills, the student is misusing alcohol because it does not improve learning. Misuse may arise from deluding oneself about one's purpose for using drugs. This is illustrated by a person who consumes five glasses of wine daily and says it is for spiritual purposes. Examples of drug misuse are the following:

- Discontinuing prescribed medicines against the physician's recommendation (some people, for example, stop taking blood pressure medication once their blood pressure is under control)
- Mixing drugs (some drugs, particularly depressants, can be fatal when consumed together)
- Consuming more of a drug than prescribed (if one pill or tablespoon is good, five are not five times as good!)
- Using more than one prescription at a time without informing the physician who wrote the prescription
- Saving or using old medications (the properties of drugs and their effectiveness change over time)
- Not following the directions for a drug; some drugs are ineffective when taken at certain times, such as after eating

Drug Abuse

Drug abuse is the intentional and inappropriate use of a drug resulting in physical, emotional, financial, social, or intellectual consequences. The National Institute of Drug Abuse defines *addiction* as "a chronic, and for many people, reoccurring disease characterized by compulsive drug seeking and use in spite of negative consequences that result from the prolonged effects of drugs on the brain."[10] Any substance, if used by the wrong person, in the wrong dosage, or at the wrong time or place, can be abused. Some drug abuse perhaps results from emotional problems. A lifetime of major depression, for example, has been linked to the abuse of alcohol and other drugs.[11] People who exhibit anxiety disorders self-medicate with alcohol and other drugs.[12]

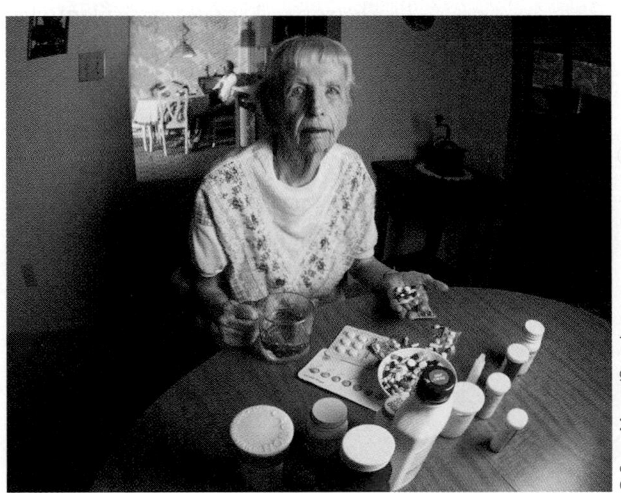

The elderly use more prescription and over-the-counter drugs than people in other age groups.

Two factors associated with drug abuse are dependency and chronic use. Whether chronic use is relevant to drug abuse is a pertinent question. For example, if a person drinks alcohol or uses heroin only on weekends and becomes disoriented from taking either drug, is that person abusing drugs? How does the illegal status of heroin and the legal status of alcohol affect our view of drug abuse? Millions of people smoke or chew tobacco daily or hourly. Are tobacco users drug abusers?

In a recent year, more than 1.7 million Americans were treated in emergency rooms because of a drug-related episode.[13] Over one-fourth of those individuals were treated for problems stemming from pharmaceutical drugs.[14]

Drug addiction is pervasive in society. As indicated, addictions are not limited to substances. The following list identifies substances and behaviors to which people are addicted along with the number of people in the United States for whom these substances or behaviors are a problem:[15]

- Alcohol—18.7 million people; 7.7% of the population
- Drugs—3.6 million people; marijuana, cocaine, and pain relievers are leading drugs
- Tobacco—71.5 million tobacco users; more males use tobacco than females
- Caffeine—80% to 90% of Americans consume caffeine through coffee or soda
- Food—about 15% of mildly obese people eat compulsively
- Gambling—an estimated 2 million Americans are compulsive gamblers
- Shopping—5% of the population are believed to be compulsive shoppers
- Sex—16 million Americans engage in compulsive sexual behavior

On Campus

One study found that first-year college students who exercised vigorously and frequently were less likely to smoke cigarettes but were more likely to drink significantly more alcohol than infrequent exercisers.

Source: M. J. Moore and C. Werch, "Relationship Between Vigorous Exercise Frequency and Substance Use Among First-Year Drinking College Students," *Journal of American College Health*, 56 (2008): 686–690.

The concept of drug abuse may not relate to whether a drug alters consciousness or is used frequently but, rather, whether the drug is socially acceptable. Alcohol, tobacco, and caffeine use is not considered deviant. Heroin use, in contrast, is not socially accepted. To many people, therefore, heroin use is abusive regardless of its effects or frequency of use. Most people who use drugs do not abuse drugs. Also, predicting which drug users will become abusers is difficult.[16]

A Historical Perspective of Drug Use

Many drugs used today, such as opium and marijuana, have long histories. Other drugs—such as designer drugs (drugs altered molecularly in the laboratory), major and minor tranquilizers, amphetamines, herbal ecstasy, Rohypnol, and LSD—have relatively short histories. In any case, every culture sanctions the use of some drugs and strongly disapproves of others. Figure 1.1 illustrates some societal problems associated with drug use.

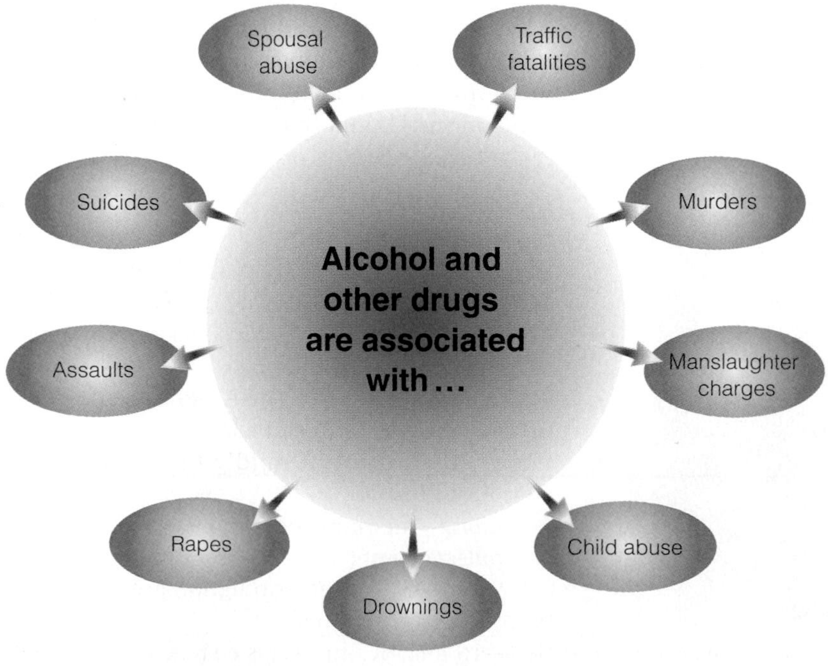

Figure 1.1 America's Problem with Alcohol and Other Drugs

Alcohol

Beverages might have been fermented intentionally as early as the Neolithic period, about 10,000 B.C.[17] Wine made from berries and beer has existed since 6400 B.C. The Bible includes several references to wine, including passages warning against immoderate consumption.[18] The early Egyptians revered wine and beer, attributing spiritual qualities to them; they also cautioned others about spending too much time in taverns.[19]

The early Hebrews were fond of alcoholic beverages, as were the ancient Chinese, Greeks, and Romans.[20] Bacchus was the Roman god of wine, and Dionysius was the Greek god of wine; Dionysius was credited with celebrating the harvest and the origins of life. The early Greeks considered wine essential to a civilized society. The word *wine* comes from the Greek word "oin."[21] Hippocrates, the Greek father of medicine, recommended wine for therapeutic purposes.[22] Plato praised moderate wine consumption for its healthful benefits and for the happiness it brought.[23]

The Egyptians developed the process of **distillation**, which produces a higher alcohol content than fermentation. Consuming distilled spirits was the privilege of nobility. The word *alcohol* originated from the Arabic **alkuhl,** meaning "the essence."

By the end of the 13th century, after alcohol was introduced to Europe, Arnauld de Villenueve, a University of Montpelier medical professor, called alcohol **aqua vitae,** the "water of life." In 16th-century England, *aqua vitae* was associated with increased criminal activity. The Irish referred to alcohol as "whiskey." Not surprisingly, it was the Scots who came up with *scotch,* made by drying fermented barley in kilns fired with burning peat, a process that gives scotch its distinctive taste.

Brandy, made by fermenting fruit juice, is derived from the Dutch expression "burnt wine." Gin comes from the Dutch *junever,* a term derived from the juniper berries contained in the distillation. In the 1600s the Russians made vodka by adding water to fermented potatoes or grain; *vodka* means "little water." By the 17th century, France was producing champagne.

Alcohol played a significant role in the early history of the United States. One reason advanced for the Pilgrims landing at Plymouth rather than traveling farther south was that they ran out of beer.[24] The early settlers did not drink to excess, nor were they puritanical about alcohol—they objected to drunkenness, not drinking.[25] As far back as 1619, the Virginia Colony imposed penalties for drunkenness, but, ironically, the Virginia Assembly introduced legislation promoting the production of distilled spirits and wine. The Massachusetts Bay Colony disciplined—with fines, whippings, and confinement in the stocks—those who drank to excess.

In the early settlement days sanitation was nonexistent, drinking wells were contaminated, and cows' milk transmitted tuberculosis. Alcohol is an effective preservative. Also, the yeast left in the settlers' homemade beer and wine supplied many important vitamins and minerals.[26] During the Civil War beer was often called "liquid bread" because of the nutrients it provided.[27]

One type of alcohol integral to the economic vitality of New England was Jamaican rum, made from molasses.[28] The rum trade was highly profitable and unsavory. Rum was transported to the west coast of Africa, where it was traded for slaves. The slaves were then sent to the West Indies, where they were exchanged for molasses. Molasses then was shipped to New England and used in producing rum. New England distilleries made great profits from the slave trade until Congress prohibited the importation of slaves.

After the Revolutionary War, transportation became a significant issue. The cost to farmers in Virginia, Kentucky, Maryland, and western Pennsylvania of transporting grain to "eastern" markets was greater than the amount of money they received for selling the grain. Farmers increased their profits by converting the grain into whiskey.

Many distilleries came into existence; perhaps the best known was a distillery in Bourbon County, Kentucky. The Reverend Elijah Craig put whiskey into charred oak barrels and was credited with developing bourbon. The whiskey was exchanged for money, and the federal government imposed an excise tax on it.

In 1791, the farmers of southwestern Pennsylvania protested the tax. This action precipitated the **Whiskey Rebellion**, in which farmers not only refused to pay the tax but actually tarred and feathered the revenue officers. To squelch the protest, President George Washington sent in militia from several states.[29] This historical event established the federal government's authority to enact and enforce federal laws.

distillation A heating process that increases alcohol content

alkuhl An Arabic word meaning "the essence," from which the word alcohol is derived

aqua vitae Literally means "water of life"; another expression for alcohol

Whiskey Rebellion A protest by farmers in southwestern Pennsylvania against a tax on whiskey

temperance Moderate alcohol use, rather than abstinence

Alcohol consumption reached its peak in the early 1800s. Americans during that time probably consumed three times as much alcohol as do Americans today.[30] The average person drank 6 or more ounces of alcohol daily. During that period society was less stable because of a rising transient population and migration to the West. Concern over excessive drinking grew. One prominent group in the early 1800s consisted of reformed drinkers, the "Washingtonians," who preached the evils of alcohol.[31] This eventually led to the **temperance** movement that developed in the 1830s. Initially, the temperance movement strived to moderate alcohol consumption, but it eventually advocated total abstinence from alcohol.[32]

Leading the charge toward temperance was Dr. Benjamin Rush, who warned the public about the hazards of alcohol.[33] Rush was a leading medical authority in Colonial America and took stands on many social issues, including alcohol abuse. His interest in alcohol and alcohol abuse may have stemmed from having an alcoholic father.[34] Temperance advocates sought to reduce alcohol use, not eliminate it. Within a decade, alcohol use was curtailed by 75%.[35]

In 1851, Maine became the first state to ban alcohol. By 1855, 13 states had enacted prohibition legislation. Though several states repealed these laws, the National Prohibition Party was formed in 1874 and renewed the effort to ban alcohol. The impetus for prohibition grew, and between 1907 and 1919, 34 states passed laws favoring prohibition. The desire by many cultural groups to prohibit alcohol, especially around schools and churches, further strengthened the movement to forbid alcohol.[36]

Women in particular fought to ban alcohol with a major theme of "home protection." Women saw themselves as the protectors of home, children, and morality.[37] Eventually, national prohibition legislation went into effect in 1919 under the 18th Amendment to the Constitution. Although some argued that prohibition was beneficial because alcohol-related medical illnesses declined along with alcohol consumption,[38] the amendment was repealed in 1933 because the consequences of alcohol use generally were seen as less harmful than the ban on alcohol.

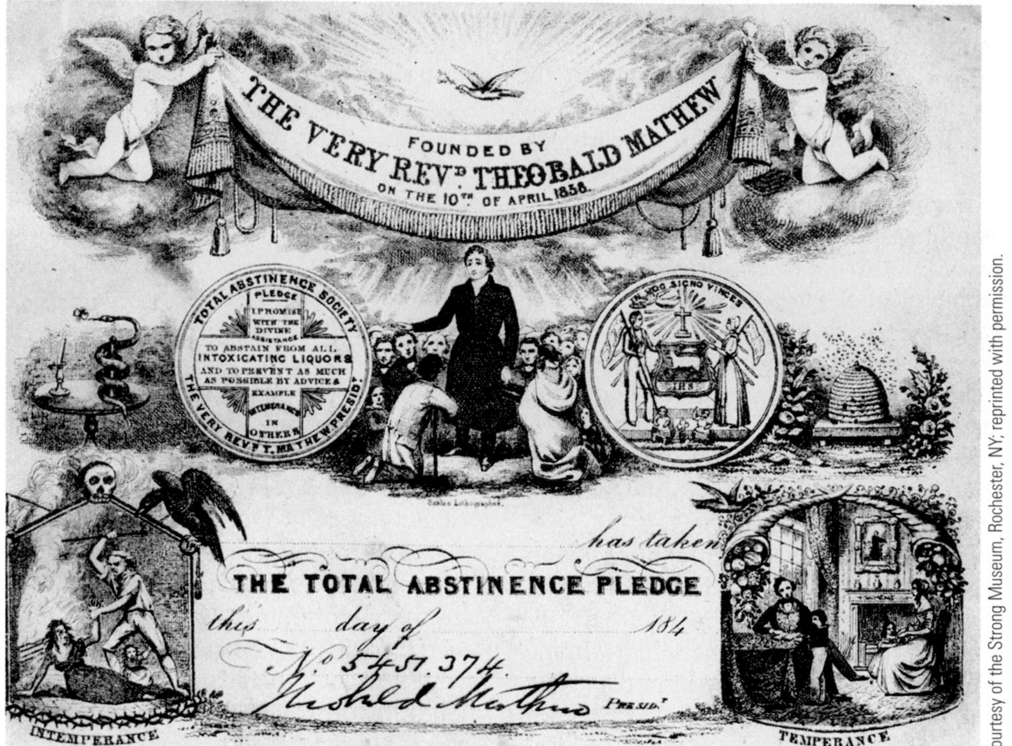
THE VERY REVD THEOBALD MATHEW
FOUNDED BY
ON THE 10TH OF APRIL 1838.
TOTAL ABSTINENCE SOCIETY
PLEDGE
I PROMISE WITH THE DIVINE ASSISTANCE TO ABSTAIN FROM ALL INTOXICATING LIQUORS AND TO PREVENT AS MUCH AS POSSIBLE BY ADVICE & EXAMPLE INTEMPERANCE IN OTHERS
THE VERY REVD T. MATHEW PRESIDT
IN HOC SIGNO VINCES
has taken
THE TOTAL ABSTINENCE PLEDGE
this day of 184
No 5,457,374
PRESIDT
INTEMPERANCE
TEMPERANCE

Courtesy of the Strong Museum, Rochester, NY; reprinted with permission.

This pledge card displays powerful and contrasting symbolism about temperance.

Marijuana

Marijuana is one of the oldest known psychoactive plants. It is believed that marijuana has been cultivated for its fiber since at least 8000 B.C.[39] As far back as 4,700 years ago, the Chinese Emperor Shen Nung prescribed it for ailments such as gout, malaria, gas pains, absentmindedness, and rheumatism.[40] Although one of marijuana's effects is impaired short-term memory, ironically Shen Nung recommended the drug as a cure for forgetfulness. The Chinese banned marijuana in 500 B.C., when they came to believe it would cause young people to disrespect the elderly.

In the 2nd century B.C., marijuana was mentioned in the Indian work *Atharva Veda.* Marijuana was used extensively in India for festive and religious purposes. Greek historian Herodotus noted that marijuana had the dual purposes of producing both cloth and an intoxicating effect. The Roman physician Galen described how marijuana seeds were eaten to stimulate appetite and bring about a sense of warmth. The Persians and Assyrians used marijuana to control muscle spasms, ameliorate pain, and treat indigestion.

During his travels in the 13th century, Marco Polo recounted how a group of men called **hashishiyya** terrorized and killed people while under the influence of hashish. From this legend the word *assassin* is derived from hashishiyya.

When marijuana was introduced to Western Europe is not known, but an urn containing marijuana seeds and leaves dating back to 500 B.C. was uncovered near Berlin, Germany.[41] Following their campaign in Egypt, Napoleon's troops returned to France with hashish. Shortly thereafter, other Europeans began using marijuana. In the mid-1800s, many writers and artists were said to be using opium and hashish. Alexander Dumas's classic novel *The Count of Monte Cristo* referred to hashish. English writers Thomas De Quincey and Samuel Taylor Coleridge were reported to have experimented with opium and hashish.

Use of marijuana was noted in the Americas as early as 1545.[42] English settlers grew marijuana, which they called hemp, to make clothing, rope, linens, and blankets. Even George Washington cultivated marijuana.[43]

A medical professor named W. B. O'Shaughnessy noted an early account of marijuana use in a report. In 1839, he wrote that a tincture of hemp (a solution of cannabis in alcohol) was an effective analgesic and muscle relaxant. He returned to England and provided cannabis to pharmacists.[44] Additional accounts of medical benefits of marijuana were described in the 1870 book *The Hasheesh Eater,* by Fitz Hugh Ludlow.

By the late 1800s numerous reports detailed cannabis use for many medical conditions. Because its potency varied and people responded erratically to the drug, however, other drugs replaced it. As a result, research into its medical benefits dwindled.

In the early 1900s, marijuana was used primarily by Hispanics in the Southwest and by Blacks in ghettos. As long as use was limited to these groups, middle-class White Americans were not disturbed. Concern about marijuana use increased with the immigration of a large number of Mexican laborers.[45] Negative sentiment against immigrants—and the drugs they used—escalated in the 1930s, when the country was in an economic depression and had a surplus of laborers.[46]

hashishiyya A group of men who, while under the influence of hashish, allegedly terrorized and killed people

narcotics Any of the opium-based central nervous system depressants used to relieve pain and diarrhea

opiate A class of drugs derived from opium

laudanum A drug derived from opium

Narcotics

The term **narcotics** is used interchangeably with the terms **opiates** or *opioids.* Opiate refers to opium and derivatives of opium, a naturally occurring substance that has effects similar to those of morphine.[47] The earliest reference to opium, derived from the opium poppy, *Papaver somniferum,* dates back to a 6,000-year-old Sumerian tablet that portrayed the poppy as a "joy plant." The Egyptians (c. 1500 B.C.) used opium for medical purposes, such as soothing children who cried excessively. Although the idea of providing opium to children may seem absurd today, in the past many parents gave children paregoric, an opium derivative, to relieve gum soreness resulting from teething and for stomachaches.

Opium was a staple in ancient Greece and Rome.[48] Hypnos, the Greek god of sleep, and Somnus, the Roman god of sleep, were depicted as carrying a container of opium pods. Homer's *Odyssey* referred to opium in about 1000 B.C. Though opium was primarily a medicinal drug in Rome, the Greeks used it for more than just medicine; Galen discussed the use of opium in candies and cakes. He described Roman Emperor Marcus Aurelius as being dependent on it. Even though opium use was believed to be extensive, probably few people actually became dependent on it.[49]

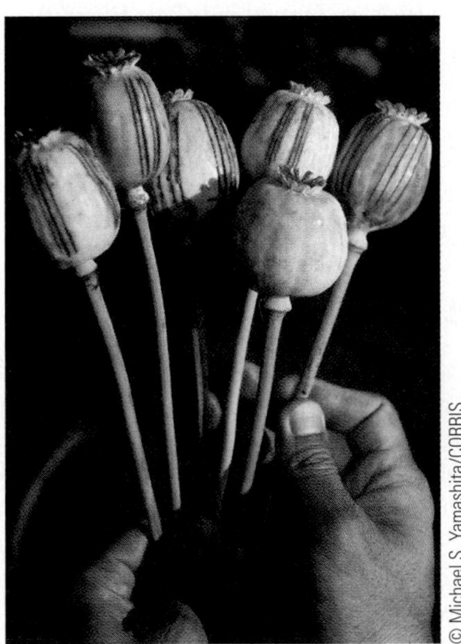

The poppy Papavar somniferum *in the main source of nonsynthetic narcotics.*

In the Arab world opium was used widely, perhaps because of the Koran's decree forbidding alcohol. The Arabs were introduced to opium through their trading in India and China. Arab physician Avicenna (c. A.D. 1000) wrote an exhaustive medical textbook describing the merits of opium. Ironically, he died from an overdose of opium mixed with wine.

Opium was the central factor in a war between China and the British government. Because Chinese citizens used opium excessively, which threatened the country's vitality, China passed a law in 1729 forbidding opium smoking. Despite the penalty of strangulation, opium smoking remained rampant. Opium was smuggled into China from India. Great Britain encouraged opium cultivation in India because it was a profitable enterprise to barter and maintain favorable trading practices.

In 1839, the Chinese emperor sent an official to Canton, India, to enforce its ban on importation of opium. The British turned over the opium, worth several million dollars, to the Chinese official, who proceeded to destroy it. Tension mounted, leading to the Opium War, which lasted from 1839 to 1842. Though the British sent only 10,000 soldiers, they defeated the Chinese because of superior naval strength. In a second Opium War, in 1856, the British again were victorious. Opium continued to be imported into China until the start of the 20th century.

Medical uses of opium became widespread in Europe in the 16th century, when English physician Thomas Sydenham developed the opiate preparation **laudanum**. He praised opium, stating, "Among the remedies which has pleased Almighty God to give to man to relieve his sufferings, none is so universal and so efficacious as opium."[50]

Laudanum was popular among White middle-class Americans during the 1700s and 1800s, and many writers in the early 1800s experimented with opium. In *Confessions of an English Opium Eater,* Thomas De Quincey praised opium for enhancing his creativity.[51] Samuel Taylor Coleridge wrote his classic work *Kubla Khan* while under the influence of opium. Among other literary figures who indulged in opium use were Edgar Allan Poe, Elizabeth Barrett Browning, Alexander Dumas, and Baudelaire.

In 1805, German pharmacist Frederick Serturner isolated the active ingredient in opium and called it **morphine**.[52] Named after Morpheus, the Greek god of dreams, morphine was hailed as a "wonder drug." A development in 1853, however, revolutionized drug use. Scottish physician Alexander Wood perfected the hypodermic syringe, which increased both the potency of the drug and the speed by which drugs take effect. Before the hypodermic was invented, opium was either ingested or smoked raw.[53] Morphine was believed, erroneously, to be nonaddicting and a cure for opium addiction.[54]

During the American Colonial period opium was used regularly, primarily to relieve pain.[55] Morphine abuse escalated in the United States during the Civil War, as soldiers injected themselves with morphine to relieve pain, dysentery, and fatigue. U.S. Army surgeons readily prescribed morphine.[56] By the end of the Civil War, morphine dependency was so common that it was called **soldier's disease**.[57] Morphine was readily available in patent medicines and through Chinese immigrants who brought their opium-smoking practices with them when they came to the United States. Tens of thousands of women were given narcotics to deal with a variety of medical ailments, especially gynecological problems.[58]

These factors contributed to the estimated 1 million Americans who were dependent on morphine and other narcotics by the end of the 19th century. Many patent medicines that were promoted in the late 1800s to cure narcotic addiction included opium and alcohol.[59] Eventually, drug laws were enacted to stem the use of narcotics, although those laws were racially motivated due to the link between opium and the Chinese and cocaine and African Americans.[60]

Dr. William Halsted, one of the founders of the Johns Hopkins Medical School and a skilled surgeon who became known as "the father of modern surgery,"[61] was one of the first physicians to give cocaine to patients during surgery. Unfortunately, Halsted himself became dependent on cocaine. To overcome his cocaine dependency, Halsted turned to morphine. It is noteworthy that Halsted's most brilliant work occurred while he was dependent on morphine. Around this same time, Bayer Laboratories in Germany developed a new drug to combat morphine dependency. This drug not only enabled a person to overcome morphine dependency but also was thought to be nonaddicting. Moreover, the drug was believed to be more effective than morphine for pain relief. This newest "wonder drug" was **heroin (diacetylmorphine)**, which has become the drug of choice for many people in the past several years. It is synthesized from morphine, and it was first developed in 1874.[62]

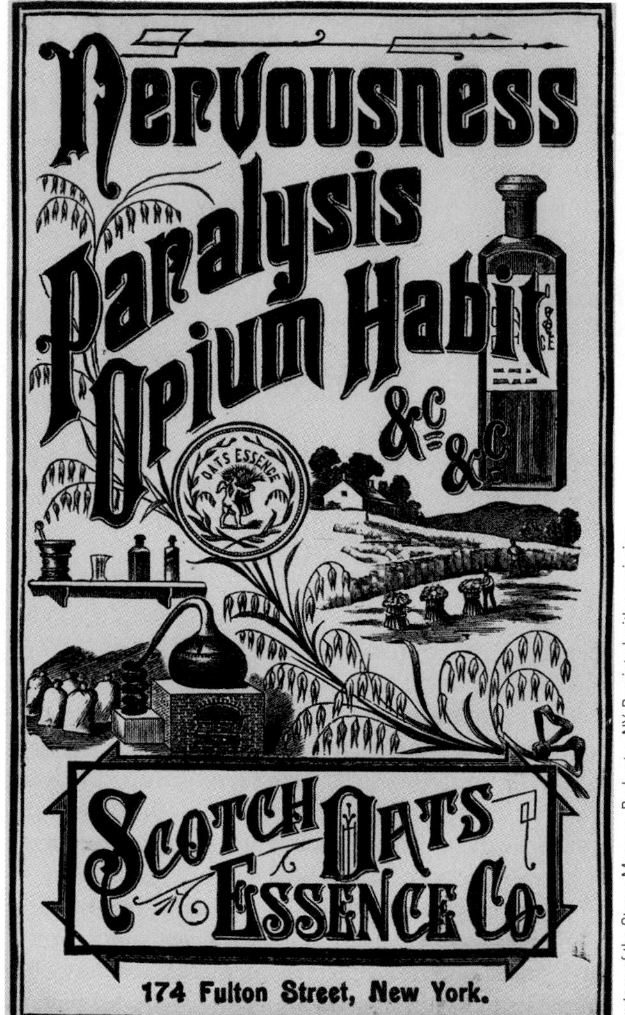

Courtesy of the Strong Museum, Rochester, NY. Reprinted with permission.

Some physicians and businessmen believed that natural substances such as Scotch and Oats Essence could cure chemical dependency.

Coffee

One of the earliest written references to coffee dates back to A.D. 900 in Arabia. The Chinese reportedly used **caffeine**, the principal ingredient in coffee, almost 5,000 years ago.[63] The Mohammedans used coffee to stay awake during lengthy religious vigils. This practice took shape after Mohammed heard about a goatherd named Kaldi who, along with his goats, stayed awake all night after eating the berries of a certain plant. The Koran, the holiest book of Islam, however, condemned coffee as an intoxicant and banned its use.[64] In the 16th century, when coffee was introduced into Egypt, it was forbidden there also.

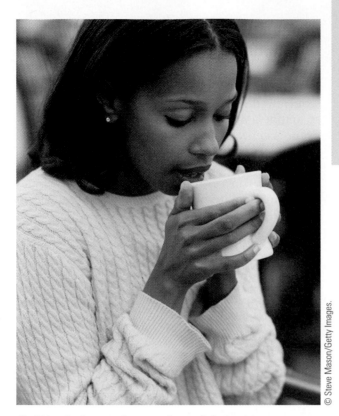
© Steve Mason/Getty Images.

Caffeine is the number one drug of choice for many Americans.

morphine An analgesic drug derived from opium; used medically as a painkiller

soldier's disease A name given to morphine dependency during the Civil War

heroin (diacetylmorphine) A potent drug that is a derivative of opium

caffeine A mild stimulant found in coffee, tea, soda pop, and chocolate

Coffee was associated with medicinal qualities despite attempts by England's King Charles II and English physicians to forbid its use. Consuming coffee was a popular pastime in 17th-century Europe.[65] Once coffee reached England and France in the mid-1600s, coffeehouses became centers for learning, conversation, relaxation, and business deals. For a cup of coffee, which cost one penny, one could listen to the most well-known literary and political leaders of the day.[66] One famous insurance company, Lloyd's of London, originated around 1700 from the coffeehouse of Edward Lloyd.[67]

These "penny universities," as they were called, were not popular with the wives of men who frequented them. In response to the long hours men spent in coffeehouses, a number of women published the pamphlet *The Women's Petition Against Coffee* in 1674. In the United States today, more than 90% of adults consume coffee or tea.[68]

Cocaine

Drawings found on pottery in South America suggest that people were chewing coca leaves prior to the rise of the Incan Empire, as early as 3000 B.C. Cocaine was believed to be in Egyptian mummies dating back 3,000 years. The coca plant was held in high esteem; it was seen as a present from the gods and was incorporated into religious rituals and burials.[69] Andean Indians used coca in their folk medicine.[70] Also, people chewed coca leaves for practical reasons: They improved endurance greatly despite high altitudes, and people who chewed coca leaves required less food and water.

The first verified use of coca has been traced to a gravesite in Peru from around A.D. 500, where a person was buried with a supply of coca leaves.[71] Grown in the Andes Mountains, coca plants were not cultivated until around A.D. 1000. Eventually the coca plant was incorporated into the spiritual and political structure of the early Incan Empire.[72]

When Pizarro and his fellow Spaniards conquered the Incas, they realized the importance of coca leaves to the natives. Coca leaves eventually were used to barter with the Incas for their gold and silver. Because of the reduced supply of food and the hardships endured under the Spaniards, the Incas chewed even more coca leaves. Also, chewing coca leaves helped to ward off fatigue.[73]

Even though the Europeans did not chew coca leaves, the extract from coca leaves figured prominently in Europe. In 1859, Italian neurologist Paolo Mantegazza described the medicinal virtues of coca leaves;[74] in 1860, Albert Niemann published a paper stating that he had successfully isolated cocaine from the coca leaf.[75] In the latter part of the 19th century, the French chemist Angelo Mariani developed a popular red Bordeaux wine called Mariani's coca wine, which included the active ingredients from coca leaves. In addition to Pope Leo XIII and Thomas Edison—who praised Mariani's wine and allowed their pictures to be used in advertisements for it—others approving of the wine included the kings of Sweden and Norway, the Prince of Wales, and the Russian czar.

An early proponent of cocaine was Sigmund Freud, who used it to relieve his own depression and indigestion. Freud advocated cocaine to help people overcome morphine addiction. He was so enthusiastic about cocaine that he recommended it to his fiancée, sister, colleagues, and friends. Freud became disillusioned with cocaine after giving it to his friend Ernst von Fleischl-Marxow, who was suffering from a painful disease of the nervous system. Marxow experienced cocaine psychosis and almost died.[76] Freud was criticized for promoting the "third scourge of humanity" (after alcohol and opium).

Cocaine was used in literary circles as well. Robert Louis Stevenson allegedly wrote *Dr. Jekyll and Mr. Hyde* while under the influence of cocaine. Sir Arthur Conan Doyle described the effects of cocaine in his accounts of Sherlock Holmes.[77]

At one time the popular soft drink Coca-Cola contained cocaine. The inventor of Coca-Cola, John Stith Pemberton, used extract from coca leaves and the **kola nut** to develop a new medicinal tonic to remedy a host of ills. People often used cocaine for colds, headaches, toothaches, asthma, and impotence. It was touted as a safe alternative to alcohol.[78] The following advertisement extols the virtues of this new beverage:

> This "Intellectual Beverage" and Temperance Drink contains the valuable Tonic and Nerve Stimulant properties of the Coca plant and Cola (or Kola) nuts, and makes not only a delicious, exhilarating, refreshing and invigorating Beverage . . . but a valuable Brain Tonic, and a cure for all nervous afflictions—Sick Headache, Neuralgia, Melancholy, etc.[79]

In the 1880s cocaine was used for eye, nose, and throat surgeries because of its anesthetic properties and because it limited blood flow by constricting the blood vessels.[80] Use of cocaine in the United States began in the mid-1880s and peaked between 1900 and 1915.[81] Its popularity dropped after the Harrison Narcotic Act of 1914 banned it from patent medicines and beverages.[82] Also contributing to the decline of cocaine was the abundant supply of heroin, the unavailability of cocaine, and its high cost.[83]

Cocaine reemerged as a popular drug in the 1970s, with many accounts of athletes, celebrities, and entertainers using it. Around the same time a variation of cocaine, called **freebase**, emerged. Freebase cocaine was different because users smoked it rather than snorted it. By the mid-1980s, **crack cocaine**, made by mixing cocaine with baking soda and so named because of the crackling sound it produces when smoked, came on the scene.[84] Contributing to its popularity were crack's low cost and easy production.[85]

Amphetamines

Amphetamines have a relatively brief history. They were first synthesized in Germany in 1887[86] but were not used medically for another 45 years. During World War II, German, British, Japanese, and American troops used amphetamines to overcome fatigue and increase their endurance.[87] One of their first strictly medical uses was to treat asthma and narcolepsy, a sleep disorder. Amphetamines enlarge the nasal and bronchial passages, raise blood pressure, and stimulate the central nervous system.

Benzedrine was available over-the-counter in 1932 for treating asthma and nasal congestion. Subsequently, there was widespread and unregulated use of amphetamines.[88] In the 1960s, **methamphetamines** appeared. Also called *crank*, *crystal*, and *ice*, these drugs are more powerful than amphetamines. Methamphetamines are often produced in covert laboratories in rural areas.[89] Amphetamines and methamphetamines are discussed more thoroughly in Chapter 11.

Sedative-Hypnotic Drugs

Drugs including **barbiturates**, nonbarbiturate sedatives, minor tranquilizers, and inhalants are classified as sedative-hypnotic drugs.

Barbiturates

Barbiturates were discovered in 1863 by Adolph von Baeyer. He synthesized his new discovery from uric acid and named it barbituric acid or barbiturates. The name was derived when, to celebrate his discovery, he went to a tavern, where he encountered army officers commemorating the Day of Saint Barbara, the patron saint of artillerymen. The drug was not used medically until 1903, when two German scientists, using von Baeyer's acid, developed **barbital**, which was used initially to treat anxiety and nervousness.

Nonbarbiturate Sedatives

Nonbarbiturate sedatives have a longer history than barbiturates.[90] Three types of nonbarbiturate sedatives are the following:

1. **Bromides** were introduced in the 1860s as a remedy for epileptic convulsions. They are no longer used because they accumulate in the body, causing bromide poisoning. Symptoms of bromide poisoning include delirium, constipation, acne, and coma.
2. **Chloral hydrate** was first synthesized in 1832.[91] Also known as "knockout drops," it was combined with alcohol to induce sleep. One of its side effects is severe gastric irritation.
3. **Paraldehyde**, used since 1882, is relatively safe and effective; however, it has a bitter taste and smell and leaves the user with bad breath.[92] The drug is used currently for treating children with seizures.[93]

Minor Tranquilizers

Minor tranquilizers, or antianxiety agents, were first marketed in the early 1950s. **Meprobamate**, under the trade names of Miltown and Equanil, was readily accepted. Sales of the drug escalated from $7,500 in May 1955 to $500,000 in December of the same year. Meprobamate, however, produced tolerance and physical and psychological dependence.[94] Interestingly, as is the case today, there were concerns regarding over-medication.[95]

Another group of antianxiety drugs that followed are the **benzodiazepines**. These drugs superseded barbiturates as the drugs of choice for anxiety and insomnia.[96] Benzodiazepines were supposed to relieve anxiety without producing sedation. It was believed, falsely, that they were nonaddicting.[97] Two well-known benzodiazepines are Librium and Valium, the latter of which is the most prescribed drug in the history of U.S. medicine.

Inhalants

Inhalants have the distinction of being taken in through the airways. In addition, inhalants—especially solvents, gases, and aerosols—are among the first drugs used by young children.[98] Individuals who initiate use as children do not tend to use inhalants when they reach adulthood; hence, adults who use inhalants typically initiated their inhalant use as adults.[99] They include paints, solvents, aerosol sprays, glues, petroleum products, and cleaning supplies. The use of inhaled drugs is recorded among the early Egyptians, Babylonians, Africans, and North and South American Indians.

kola nut A part of a plant originally used in Coca-Cola

freebase A variation of cocaine in which cocaine is separated from its hydrochloride salt by heating, using a volatile chemical such as ether

crack cocaine A variation of cocaine made by heating cocaine after mixing it with baking soda and water

amphetamines Powerful central nervous system stimulants

Benzedrine An amphetamine used to treat nasal congestion and asthma

methamphetamine A more potent form of amphetamine

barbiturate (barbituric acid) A member of a class of drugs that have depressant effects

barbital A sedative-hypnotic drug used to treat anxiety and nervousness; the original barbiturate

bromides Nonbarbiturate sedatives used to treat epileptic convulsions

chloral hydrate A nonbarbiturate sedative; also called "knockout drops" or Mickey Finns; induces sleep

paraldehyde A nonbarbiturate sedative-hypnotic drug used with severely disturbed mental patients

meprobamate A minor tranquilizer marketed under the trade names of Miltown and Equanil; also used for treating psychosomatic conditions

benzodiazepines A type of minor tranquilizer; examples are Librium and Valium

inhalants Drugs that are inhaled or "sniffed"

nitrous oxide An inhalant also known as laughing gas

ether An inhalant dating back to the late 1700s

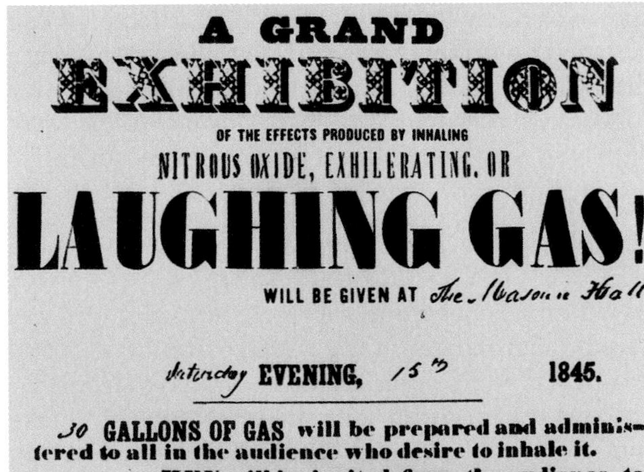

Americans' attitude concerning nitrous oxide was nonchalant in the first half of the 19th century.

Nitrous oxide, commonly called laughing gas, was synthesized in 1776 by the English chemist Sir Humphrey Davy. While working with the gas, Davy inhaled it with pleasurable effects and related this discovery to others. Use of nitrous oxide by Americans was first noted in the early 1800s. One enterprising individual, Gardner Quincy Colton, quit medical school and went into business demonstrating nitrous oxide.

Ether is an inhalant dating back to the late 1700s. Although this gas was developed for medical purposes, nonmedical use by English and American students quickly followed. Ether was popular in Ireland, especially after the British imposed a stiff tax on home-distilled Irish whiskey. Its use in England escalated in the 1790s when the government raised the tax on alcohol.[100] The benefits of ether were recognized in the mid-1800s. In 1866 a statue was erected in Boston Public Garden to celebrate ether.[101] As alcohol became cheaper and easier to obtain, the use of ether diminished, although it reappeared in the

United States during the years of prohibition. During the past three decades inhalant abuse has been recognized as a drug abuse problem.[102]

Hallucinogens

LSD, lysergic acid diethylamide, is the most widely publicized hallucinogen. Though LSD is relatively new—its discovery dates back only to 1938[103]—various cultures have used **hallucinogens** in rituals throughout history.[104] Of the estimated half-million species of plants, about 150 have been used for hallucinogenic purposes.[105]

The mushroom *Amanita muscaria* is believed to be the drug referred to in an Indian text dating back to 1500 B.C. Central American natives used mushrooms containing the hallucinogen **psilocybin** more than 2,000 years ago. The Aztecs incorporated these mushrooms, called "God's Flesh," into their spiritual rituals,[106] and statues of large mushrooms in Guatemala can be traced back to A.D. 1000. The Swiss chemist Albert Hofmann, best known for discovering LSD, extracted the psychoactive ingredient, psilocybin, in 1958. Unfortunately, mushrooms containing psilocybin closely resemble mushrooms that are highly toxic. Nonetheless, psilocybin was used in the 1950s and early 1960s to study how it affects one's psyche.[107]

Another drug utilized for spiritual purposes, **peyote**, may date back 7,000 years.[108] Peyote contains the psychoactive ingredient **mescaline**, which was isolated from the cactus in 1896.[109] Prehistoric Mexican tribes and the Aztecs used peyote, and the drug's spiritual or medicinal use is deduced from symbolic portrayals in rock art, ceramics, and textiles.[110] In the early 1800s, various Indian tribes used it for religious purposes.[111] Currently, members of the Native American Church use it ceremoniously;[112] after ingesting it, church members chant, drum, and pray.

A hallucinogen deriving its name from one of the first colonies settled in the United States is the **Jamestown weed**, commonly known as jimsonweed or locoweed. A member of the genus *Datura,* it was mentioned in early Chinese texts. Buddhists highly valued *Datura,* and it maintained a divine significance in ancient Greek temples.[113] One species of this plant, *Datura stramonium,* grows wild in the United States, and Algonquin Indians used it to help their adolescents establish their identity.[114]

LSD was originally synthesized in 1938 at the Sandoz Laboratories in Switzerland by Hofmann and Stoll. While working with the drug, Hofmann had taken it unwittingly. Because his experience from taking the drug was unusual, Hofmann repeated the experience and had his assistant record the effects. Hofmann's own account of his initial experience is interesting:

> Last Friday, April 16, 1943, I was forced to stop my work in the laboratory in the middle of the afternoon and to go home, as I was seized by a peculiar restlessness associated with a sensation of mild dizziness. Having reached home, I lay down and sank in a kind of drunkenness which was not unpleasant and which was characterized by extreme activity of imagination. As I lay in a dazed condition with my eyes closed (I experienced daylight as disagreeably bright), there surged upon me an uninterrupted stream of fantastic images of extraordinary plasticity and vividness and accompanied by an intense, kaleidoscope-like play of colors.... This condition gradually passed off after about two hours.[115]

On April 29, 2008, Albert Hofmann died after suffering from a heart attack at the age of 102.[116] LSD's popularity grew in the 1960s. Some people attribute its rise to Augustus Owsley Stanley, a sound engineer for the Grateful Dead, who developed a pure form of LSD.[117]

People experienced the effects of LSD-like substances long before LSD was actually developed. LSD originated from the ergot fungus, which grows on grain, especially rye, and causes the condition **ergotism**.[118] Symptoms of ergotism include muscle tremors, a burning sensation, mania, hallucinations, convulsions, delirium, and gangrene.

An outbreak of ergotism in the 12th century was known as Saint Anthony's fire. Those affected could be cured by making a pilgrimage to Saint Anthony's shrine in Egypt. Some speculate that girls and women condemned as witches in Salem, Massachusetts, were displaying symptoms similar to those of ergotism.[119]

Tobacco

Based on Mayan stone carvings, humans were believed to have first sampled tobacco around A.D. 600 to A.D. 900.[120] The word *tobacco* was derived from "tabaco," a two-pronged tube that natives used to take snuff. When Christopher Columbus arrived in San Salvador in 1492, the natives gave him tobacco leaves.

The Mayans believed that smoke from tobacco would bring rain during the dry season. The Aztecs used tobacco for medical and spiritual purposes.[121]

Shortly after Columbus came to the New World, tobacco was introduced into Europe. One of the first people to use tobacco there was a member of Columbus's crew, Rodrig de Jerez. He was arrested because smoke was coming out of his mouth and nose and his friends thought he was possessed by the Devil.[122] After several years he was released from jail only to find people doing the same thing for which he had been arrested. By 1575, smoking had become commonplace, and Mexico's Catholic Church forbade smoking in church.[123]

Tobacco originally was viewed with curiosity but soon was regarded as a valuable medicine.[124] One person who used tobacco medically was Catherine de Medici, queen of Henry II of France. In 1559, Jean Nicot, France's ambassador to Portugal, sent tobacco to the queen to treat her migraine headaches. Tobacco also was used to treat the Black Death, heart pains, snake bites, and fever.

The spread of tobacco can be attributed primarily to Portuguese sailors who established a tobacco trade with China, Japan, Brazil, India, Africa, and Arabia. Many questioned the desirability of tobacco as a drug. England's Sir Francis Bacon described the addictive quality of tobacco in this comment:

> The use of tobacco is growing greatly and conquers men with a certain secret pleasure, so that those who have once become accustomed thereto can later hardly be restrained therefrom.[125]

Despite Bacon's protestations, tobacco use was popular, as evidenced by the 7,000 tobacco shops in London. It was forbidden in many other places throughout Europe, such as Bavaria in 1652, Saxony in 1653, and Zurich in 1667. Pope Urban VIII, in 1642, threatened to excommunicate those using tobacco. In Constantinople in 1633, Sultan Murad IV decreed the death penalty for anyone smoking tobacco, and a year later Russian czar Michael Romanov imposed a law to have the noses of smokers slit. In China the penalty for anyone dealing tobacco was decapitation.[126] Although tobacco was forbidden and harsh penalties were imposed, tobacco use continued to flourish.

Tobacco figured prominently when the United States was colonized. Englishman John Rolfe was sent to Virginia in 1610 to develop a tobacco industry. Rolfe was unsuccessful at first because he planted a certain species, *Nicotiana rustica,* that did not grow well in Virginia soil. After obtaining some seeds of the Spanish tobacco species *Nicotiana tabacum,* Rolfe was successful.[127] Tobacco helped to make the commander of the Revolutionary Army, George Washington, a wealthy man. He saw the value of tobacco and was quoted as saying, "If you can't send money, send tobacco." Realizing that tobacco was important to the colonies (it was exported to France for money for the war effort), Britain's General Cornwallis tried to destroy the tobacco plantations. Despite the efforts of Cornwallis, tobacco crops flourished and hundreds of young Englishmen came to Virginia to seek their fortune.[128]

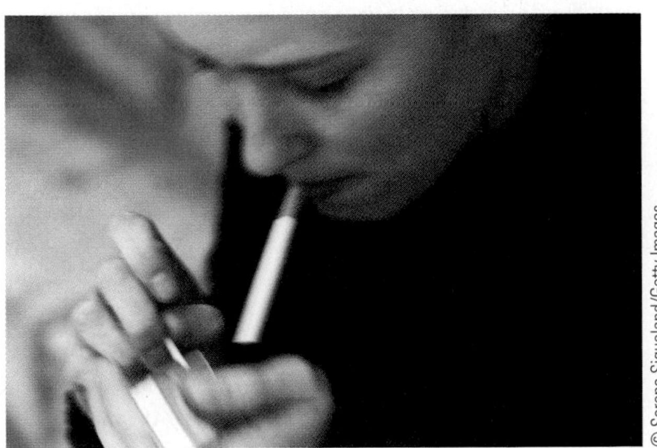
© Serena Siqueland/Getty Images.

Cigarette smoking is the single largest preventable cause of illness and premature death in the United States.

LSD (lysergic acid diethylamide) A powerful hallucinogen derived from a fungus

hallucinogens A class of drugs that induce perceived distortions in time and space

psilocybin A hallucinogen found in certain mushrooms in Central America

peyote A cactus containing the hallucinogen mescaline

mescaline A psychoactive agent, or hallucinogen, derived from the peyote cactus

Jamestown weed (jimsonweed) Any hallucinogen derived from the Datura plant; also known as "locoweed"

ergotism A condition resulting from ingesting a fungus that grows on grains; marked by muscle tremors, burning, mania, delirium, hallucinations, and eventual gangrene

In the early 1900s, smoking tobacco was less popular than chewing and snuffing it. Of all the tobacco used until 1897, half was for chewing. All public buildings were required to have spittoons until 1945. After the beginning of the 20th century, use of chewing tobacco declined steadily.

Cigars became popular in the early 1800s. Recognizing that cigarettes were a threat to their industry, cigar manufacturers made many false statements about cigarettes—that cigarettes were made with opium, that cigarette papers were made by Chinese lepers, and that arsenic was put in cigarette paper, for example.

Inventor Thomas Edison criticized cigarettes severely when he said:

> The injurious agent in Cigarettes comes principally from the burning paper wrapper. . . . It has a violent action in the nerve centers, producing degeneration of the cells of the brain, which is quite rapid among boys. Unlike most narcotics, this degeneration is permanent and uncontrollable. I employ no person who smokes cigarettes.[129]

The cigarette habit spread throughout Europe during the Crimean War. In 1856, a Crimean War veteran established the first British cigarette factory. Within a few years cigarettes were manufactured by an English tobacco merchant named Philip Morris.

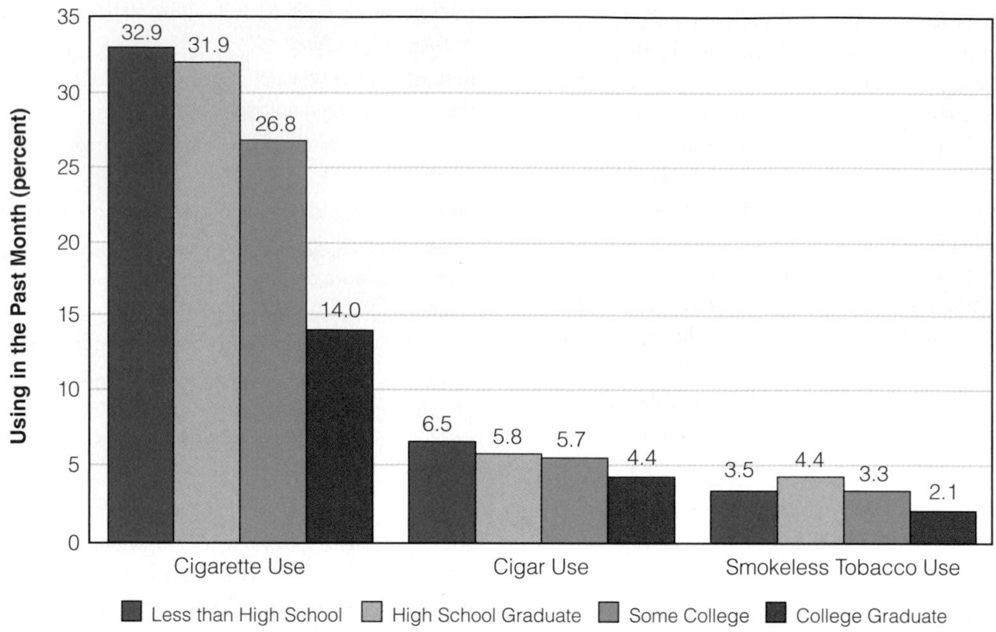

Figure 1.2 Past Month Tobacco Use among Adults

Cigarette use in the United States rose in the 1880s. It is hardly a coincidence that the cigarette-making machine was patented about the same time. Before that time, only four cigarettes could be rolled per minute. Cigarette smoking at that time was a man's activity, and smoking was illegal for women and young people in many states.

Determining how long cigars have been smoked is difficult. The Mayas of the Yucatan region are believed to have smoked cigars ritually as early as the 10th century.[130] Columbus and other early European settlers observed American Indians smoking cigars. Cigars have been prominent in the United States since the Colonial period.

In the late 1700s, most cigars were imported from the West Indies and Cuba. The first U.S. cigar factory was established in Connecticut in 1810, and other manufacturers throughout the country produced cigars as their popularity increased.[131] Since 1993, cigar sales, primarily of large cigars, have risen 50%. Figure 1.2 presents recent statistics regarding past-month cigar use among adults in the context of overall tobacco use.

Summary

Definitions related to drugs frequently reflect the biases of those who come up with the definition. What one person classifies as drug use, another may classify as misuse or abuse. Generally, misuse involves the unintentional or inappropriate use of a drug, whereas drug abuse typically entails chronic use of a drug that results in physical, intellectual, financial, social, or emotional problems. Even the word *drug* is subject to interpretation. One could argue that sugar and chocolate are forms of drugs.

Drug use is a valid concern because of its effects on individuals, families, and society. Abuse of prescription drugs by the elderly and abuse of inhalants by younger teenagers are growing concerns. Despite their potential harm, drugs have been used throughout history and continue to be used. The Bible records many accounts of drug use by early civilizations. The Egyptians, Hebrews, Greeks, and Romans used alcohol, and it figured prominently in the development of the United States. Even though Colonial settlers frowned on excessive alcohol use, the rate of consumption increased over time, resulting in the temperance movement and the Prohibition Era. The rum trade had a role in the economic expansion of the United States.

One of the earliest written accounts of marijuana use dates back to China, where people took it for medical problems. It was also used in ancient Persia and Assyria. Eventually marijuana spread to Western Europe and the United States, where it was used primarily by Hispanics in the Southwest and by Blacks in urban ghettos. Many early civilizations used opium, and it figured in clashes between China and Britain. After morphine was developed from opium, it played a significant role during the Civil War, when thousands of soldiers became dependent on it. To help people overcome morphine dependency, heroin was developed. South American natives regularly used cocaine even though Spanish conquistadors tried to halt its use. The popularity of cocaine rose after it was included in many products such as medicines, wine, and Coca-Cola. Freud's accounts of the medical benefits of cocaine contributed to its acceptance.

Naturally produced hallucinogens have a long history. In contrast are the synthetic drugs, including barbiturates, LSD, minor tranquilizers, and amphetamines, which are relatively new. One drug that grew out of exploration of the New World is tobacco. Tobacco sales were instrumental to the financial health of the colonies.

Thinking Critically

1. Consuming alcohol daily was common in the Colonial period, but drinking to excess was considered inappropriate. How would you characterize attitudes in society today regarding drinking and drunkenness?
2. In the past, illegal drug use was associated with socially and economically disadvantaged people, many of whom were immigrants. Early drug laws often were initiated as a form of prejudice against immigrants. Do you believe that current drugs laws would be different if illegal drug use had been associated with middle-class individuals?
3. When coffee was introduced in Europe, it met with resistance. Today, coffee is not viewed in the same way as illegal drugs. If caffeine were discovered this year, do you think our culture would accept or condemn it? Would coffee be viewed as a serious drug or an unhealthy substance?

Web Resources

National Institute on Drug Abuse (NIDA)
http://www.nida.nih.gov/
This site includes research reports on drug use and abuse.

National Institute on Drug Abuse—Club Drugs
http://www.clubdrugs.org
This site provides the most current information about club drugs such as Ecstasy, Rohypnol, methamphetamine, and LSD.

Notes

1. Office of Applied Studies, *The OAS Report: A Day in the Life of American Adolescents: Substance Use Facts* (Rockville, MD: Substance Abuse and Mental Health Services Administration, October 18, 2007).
2. Office of National Drug Control Policy, *Girls and Drugs* (Washington, DC: Government Printing Office, February 9, 2006).
3. J. M. Davis, "Hallucinogenic Plants and Their Use in Traditional Society: An Overview," *Cultural Survival Quarterly,* 9 (1985): 2–4.
4. D. M. Grilly, *Drugs and Human Behavior*, 4th ed. (Boston: Allyn & Bacon, 2005).
5. "Religious Involvement and Substance Use Among Adults," *The National Survey on Drug Use and Health Report* (Rockville, MD: U.S. Department of Health and Human Services, March 23, 2007).
6. R. M. Julien, *A Primer of Drug Action*, rev. ed. (New York: W. H. Freeman, 2007).
7. R. A. Clay, "Treatment for Older Adults: What Works Best?" *SAMHSA News* (Rockville, MD: U.S. Department of Health and Human Services, January/February, 2007).
8. J. W. Culbertson and M. Ziska, "Prescription Drug Misuse/Abuse in the Elderly," *Geriatrics*, 63 (September 2008): 22.
9. "Older Adults Numbers Increasing in Substance Abuse Treatment," *SAMHSA News* (Rockville, MD: U.S. Department of Health and Human Services, July/August, 2004).
10. "How Communities Can Strengthen Their Strategies to Fight Drug Abuse Using Research from the National Institute on Drug Abuse" (NIDA action kit) (Boston: Join Together, 2000).
11. A. Eriksen, N. S. Miller, M. S. Gold, and N. G. Hoffman, "Depression in Drug and Alcohol Dependency," in *Problems of Drug Dependence 1994,* edited by L. S. Harris (Proceedings of the 56th Annual Scientific Meeting, NIDA Research Monograph 153) (Rockville, MD: National Institute on Drug Abuse, 1995).
12. J. Bolton, B. Cox, I. Clara, and J. Sareen, "Use of Alcohol and Drugs to Self-Medicate Anxiety Disorders in a Nationally Representative Sample," *The Journal of Nervous and Mental Disease,* 194 (2006): 818–825.
13. Drug Abuse Warning Network, 2006: *National Estimates of Drug-Related Emergency Department Visits* (Rockville, MD: U.S. Department of Health and Human Services, August 2008).
14. Ibid.
15. "What Hooks Us," *Times South Pacific* (Australian/New Zealand edition), July 23, 2007.
16. J. Normand, R. O. Lempert, and C. P. O'Brien, *Under the Influence? Drugs and the American Work Force* (Washington, DC: National Academy Press, 1994).
17. D. J. Hanson, *Preventing Alcohol Abuse* (Westport, CT: Praeger, 1995).
18. J. Kinney, *Loosening the Grip: A Handbook of Alcohol Information* (New York: McGraw-Hill, 2007).
19. National Institute on Alcohol Abuse and Alcoholism, *Facts About Alcohol and Alcoholism* (Washington, DC: Government Printing Office, 1980).
20. J. D. Levin, *Introduction to Alcoholism Counseling: A Biosocial Approach* (Washington, DC: Taylor and Francis, 1995).
21. J. Yardley, "The Story of Booze, Hooch, Brew and the Veritas," *The Washington Post,* July 27, 2008.
22. J. Jung, *Under the Influence: Alcohol and Human Behavior* (Belmont, CA: Brooks/Cole, 1994).
23. Hanson, supra note 17.
24. H. Lee, *How Dry We Were: Prohibition Revisited* (Englewood Cliffs, NJ: Prentice-Hall, 1963).
25. W. L. White, *Slaying the Dragon: The History of Addiction Treatment in America* (Bloomington, IL: Chestnut Health

Systems/ Lighthouse Institute, 1998).
26. Hanson, supra note 17.
27. J. C. Burnham, *Bad Habits* (New York: New York University Press, 1993).
28. Kinney, supra note 18.
29. W. Hogeland, "Whiskey, Rebellion and the Religious Left," *Tikkun*, 22 (July/August 2007): 48–51.
30. R. L. Worsnop, "Alcohol Advertising," *CQ Researcher*, 7 (1997): 217–240.
31. G. D. Walter, *The Addiction Concept: Working Hypothesis or Self-Fulfilling Prophesy?* (Boston: Allyn and Bacon, 1999).
32. J. Warner, J. Riviere, and J. Carson, "On Wit, Irony, and Living with Imperfection," *American Journal of Public Health*, 98 (May 2008): 814–822.
33. B. S. Katcher, "Benjamin Rush's Educational Campaign Against Hard Drinking," *American Journal of Public Health*, 83 (1993): 273–281.
34. White, supra note 25.
35. W. Rorbaugh, *The Alcohol Republic: An American Tradition* (New York: Oxford University Press, 1979).
36. M. Lewis, "Cultural Norms and Political Mobilization: Accounting for Local and State-Level Liquor Laws, 1907–1919," *Journal of Cultural Geography*, 24 (2007): 31–52.
37. S. Ehlers, "Rep. Frank Offers Medical Marijuana Bill," *Drug Policy Letter* (Winter 1996): 5.
38. Burnham, supra note 27.
39. "Cannabits," *Forbes* (November 10, 2003): 146.
40. L. Guterman, "The Dope on Medical Marijuana," *Chronicle of Higher Education* (June 2000): A21–22.
41. R. P. Walton, *Marijuana, America's New Drug Problem* (Philadelphia: J. B. Lippincott, 1938).
42. B. Stimmel, *The Facts About Drug Use: Coping with Drugs and Alcohol in Your Family, at Work, in Your Community* (Yonkers, NY: Consumer Union of the United States, 1991).
43. Julien, supra note 6.
44. L. Grinspoon and J. B. Bakalar, *Marihuana: The Forbidden Medicine* (New Haven, CT: Yale University Press, 1997).
45. M. Cohen, "Jim Crow's Drug War: Coca Cola and the Southern Origins of Drug Prohibition," *Southern Cultures*, 12 (Fall 2006): 55–80.
46. D. F. Musto, "The History of Legislative Control Over Opium, Cocaine, and Their Derivatives," in *Dealing with Drugs: Consequences of Government Control*, edited by R. Hamowy (Lexington, MA: D. C. Heath, 1987).
47. J. F. Kauffman and G. E. Woody, *Matching Treatment to Patient Needs in Opioid Substitution Therapy* (Treatment Improvement Protocol Series 20) (Rockville, MD: U.S. Department of Health and Human Services, 1995).
48. Julien, supra note 6.
49. P. Nencini, "The Rules of Drug Taking: Wine and Poppy Derivatives in the Ancient World: VIII. Lack of Evidence of Opium Addiction," *Substance Use and Misuse*, 32 (1997): 1581–1586.
50. G. A. Austin, *Perspectives on the History of Psychoactive Substance Use* (Research Issues 24) (Washington, DC: National Institute on Drug Abuse, 1978).
51. S. B. Karch, *Karch's Pathology of Drug Abuse*, 4th ed. (Taylor and Francis, Inc., 2008).
52. Ibid.
53. A. Goldstein, *Addiction: From Biology to Drug Policy*, 2nd ed. (New York: Oxford University Press, 2001).
54. Center for Substance Abuse Treatment, *Alcohol, Tobacco, and Other Drug Abuse: Challenges and Responses for Faith Leaders* (Washington, DC: Substance Abuse and Mental Health Services Administration, 1995).
55. Musto, supra note 46.
56. "Morphine Daze," *Current Events*, 106 (March 5, 2007): 5.
57. Stimmel, supra note 42.
58. Emergency Department Trends, supra note 13.
59. White, supra note 25.
60. M. M. Cohen, "Jim Crow's Drug War: Race, Coca Cola, and the Southern Origins of Drug Prohibition," *Southern Cultures*, 12 (Fall 2006): 55–80.
61. E. M. Brecher, *Licit and Illicit Drugs* (Boston: Little, Brown, 1972).
62. "Heroin," *ONDCP Drug Policy Information Clearinghouse Fact Sheet* (Rockville, MD: Office of National Drug Control Policy, June 2003).
63. M. Ingall, "Caffeine: The (Mostly) Good News," *Ms* (September/October 1995): 26–29.
64. Brecher, supra note 61.
65. Goldstein, supra note 53.
66. H. Meyer, *Old English Coffee Houses* (Emmaus, PA: Rodale Press, 1954).
67. "The Story of Coffee," *Practice Nurse*, 28 (October 29, 2004): S4.
68. Karch, supra note 51.
69. P. G. Erickson, E. M. Adlaf, R. G. Smart, and G. F. Murray, *The Steel Drug: Cocaine and Crack in Perspective* (New York: Lexington Books, 1994).
70. A. Weil, "Letter from the Andes: The New Politics of Coca," *New Yorker*, 71 (January 1995): 70–80.
71. R. D. Weiss, S. T. Mirin, and R. B. Bartel, *Cocaine* (Washington, DC: American Psychiatric Press, 1994).
72. P. Vallely, "The History of Cocaine," *The Independent* (March 2, 2006).
73. "Cocaine," *ONDCP Drug Policy Information Clearinghouse Fact Sheet* (Rockville, MD: Office of National Drug Control Policy, November 2004).
74. Weil, supra note 70.
75. Erickson et al., supra note 69.
76. A. Daniels, "Freud on the Couch," *The Times* (London), May 5, 2006.
77. Grilly, supra note 4.
78. Musto, supra note 46.
79. C. L. Huisking, *Herbs to Hormones* (Essex, CT: Pequot Press, 1968).
80. "Cocaine," *ONDCP Drug Policy Information Clearinghouse Fact Sheet* (Rockville, MD: Office of National Drug Control Policy, 2008).
81. J. Spillane, "Did Drug Prohibition Work? Reflections on the End of the First Cocaine Experience in the United States, 1910–45," *Journal of Drug Issues*, 28 (1998): 517–538.
82. Julien, supra note 6.
83. Spillane, supra note 81.
84. J. A. Inciardi, D. Lockwood, and A. E. Pottieger, *Women and Crack-Cocaine* (New York: Macmillan, 1993).
85. "Crack," *ONDCP Drug Policy Information Fact Sheet* (Rockville, MD: Office of National Drug Control Policy, October 2006).
86. M. Ljungquist and S. Ostrander, "Doping in Sports Timeline," *Leading Issues Timeline* (Fall 2007).
87. H. E. Doweiko, *Concepts of Chemical Dependency*, 7th ed. (Cengage Learning, 2008).
88. N. Rasmussen, "America's First Amphetamine Epidemic 1929–1971," *American Journal of Public Health*, 98 (June 2008): 974–985.
89. Bourjally, P. "Watch Out for Meth Labs," *Field and Stream* (February 1, 2004).
90. Julien, supra note 6.
91. Stimmel, supra note 42.
92. Doweiko, supra note 87.
93. M. Goyal and M. Wiznitzer, "Emergency Management of Seizures in Children," *Lancet*, 367 (May 13, 2006): 1555–1556.
94. Julien, supra note 6.
95. "This Week 50 Years Ago," *New Scientist*, 195 (September 29, 2007): 39.
96. A. Chetley, *Problem Drugs* (Amsterdam, The Netherlands: Health Action International, 1995).
97. Doweiko, supra note 87.
98. "Inhalants," *ONDCP Drug Policy Information Clearinghouse Fact Sheet* (Rockville, MD: Office of National Drug Control Policy, February 2003).
99. L. Wu and C. L. Ringwalt, "Inhalant Use and Disorders among Adults in the United States," *Drug and Alcohol Dependence*, 85 (2006): 1–11.
100. Stimmel, supra note 42.
101. R. Fletcher, "The History of Ether, From Six Feet Under," *The Boston Globe* (June 17, 2007).

102. H. J. Harwood, "Inhalants: A Policy Analysis of the Problem in the United States," in *Epidemiology of Inhalant Abuse: An International Perspective,* edited by N. Kozel, Z. Sloboda, and M. De La Rosa (NIDA Research Monograph 148) (Rockville, MD: National Institute on Drug Abuse, 1995).
103. Karch, supra note 51.
104. Goldstein, supra note 53.
105. R. E. Schultes and A. Hofmann, *Plants of the Gods: Origins of Hallucinogenic Use* (New York: McGraw-Hill, 1979).
106. R. Waltz, *Psilocybin: De-mystifying the Magic Mushroom* (Tempe, AZ: D.I.N. Publications, 1996).
107. R. R. Griffith, W. A. Richards, U. McCann, and R. Jesse, "Psilocybin Can Occasion Mystical-Type Experiences Having Substantial and Sustained Personal Meaning and Spiritual Significance," *Psychopharmacology,* 187 (2006): 268–283.
108. Goldstein, supra note 53.
109. P. Jacob and A. T. Shulgin, "Structure Activity Relationships of Classic Hallucinogens and Their Analogs," in *Hallucinogens and Their Analogs: An Update,* edited by G. C. Lin and R. A. Glennon (NIDA Research Monograph 146) (Washington, DC: National Institute on Drug Abuse, 1994).
110. W. L. Bar, "New Evidence for the Antiquity of Peyote Use," *Current Anthropology,* 48 (February 2007): 1–5.
111. Karch, supra note 51.
112. Julien, supra note 6.
113. R. E. Schultes, "The Plant Kingdom and Hallucinogens, Part 3," *Bulletin on Narcotics,* 22 (1970): 43–46.
114. Schultes and Hofmann, supra note 105.
115. A. Hoffman, "Psychotomimetic Agents," in *Drugs Affecting the Central Nervous System,* edited by A. Burger (New York: Marcel Dekker, 1968).
116. C. S. Smith, "Albert Hofmann, the Father of LSD, Dies at 102," *New York Times,* April 30, 2008.
117. R. Greenfield, "The King of LSD," *Rolling Stone* (July 12, 2007): 115–122.
118. Grilly, supra note 4.
119. L. R. Caporael, "Ergotism: The Satan Loosed in Salem," *Science,* 192 (1976): 21–26.
120. C. E. Bartecchi, T. D. MacKenzie, and R. W. Schrier, "The Global Tobacco Epidemic," *Scientific American* (May 1995): 44–51.
121. Schultes, supra note 113.
122. Doweiko, supra note 87.
123. Center for Substance Abuse Treatment, supra note 54.
124. M. R. Digby, "Tobacco, Seduction and Puritanism," *Quadrant,* 51 (July/August 2007): 40–46.
125. A. Corti, *A History of Smoking* (London: George G. Harrup, 1931).
126. Austin, supra note 50.
127. C. Cottrell, "Journey to the New World: London and the New Colony," *History Today,* 57 (May 2007): 25.
128. P. C. Mancall, "What Began at Jamestown," *Chronicle of Higher Education,* 53 (May 18, 2007): 14–15.
129. J. E. Brooks, *The Mighty Leaf* (Boston: Little, Brown, 1952).
130. D. Hoffman and I. Hoffmann, "Chemistry and Toxicology," in *Cigars: Health Effects and Trends* (Smoking and Tobacco Control Monograph 9, National Cancer Institute) (Washington, DC: U.S. Department of Health and Human Services, 1998).
131. D. M. Burns, "Cigar Smoking: Overview and Current State of the Science," in *Cigars: Health Effects and Trends* (Smoking and Tobacco Control Monograph 9, National Cancer Institute) (Washington, DC: U.S. Department of Health and Human Services, 1998).

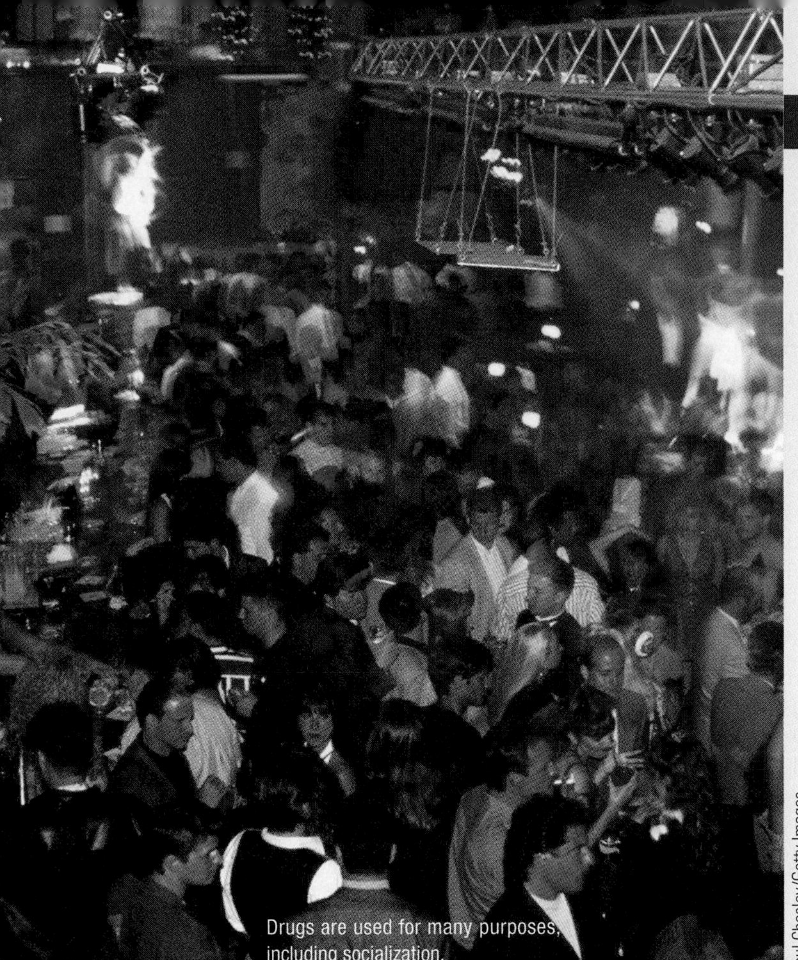
Drugs are used for many purposes, including socialization.

© Paul Chesley/Getty Images.

FACT OR FICTION?

1. The federal government spends more money on preventing drug use than on prosecuting drug users.
2. About 3 out of every 4 U.S. voters feel that the war on drugs has been a failure.
3. Every illegal drug in the United States was legal at one time.
4. Young people who use illegal drugs socially usually become dependent on drugs.
5. Individuals in the 12 to 17 age group are more likely to use illegal drugs on a monthly basis than individuals between ages 18 and 25.
6. The majority of high school seniors disapprove of people using marijuana occasionally.
7. All hospitals drug test women who have given birth to determine whether their babies may have drugs in their bloodstreams.
8. People who were abused as children have higher rates of alcoholism during adulthood compared with those people who were not abused as children.
9. More people fatally overdose from heroin than from cocaine.
10. Until 1985, it was legal to use Ecstasy.

Turn the page to check your answers

2 Drugs in Contemporary Society

Chapter Objectives

After completing this chapter, the reader should be able to describe:

- How the effects of drugs are affected by society's perception of drugs
- The impact that drugs have had on society
- Different reasons for experimental, social, and compulsive drug use
- Factors that have influenced the rate of drug use
- Changes in the incidence of drug use over the last 30 years
- Limitations of drug testing
- The effect of drugs on family, criminal activity, and academic achievement
- The differences among physiological, behavioral, acute, and chronic toxicity
- The risks associated with injecting, inhaling, and ingesting drugs
- Findings of the Drug Abuse Warning Network (DAWN)

FACT OR FICTION?

1. **Fiction:** The fact is—Far more money is allocated for prosecuting drug offenses than for preventing drug use.
2. **Fact:** According to Zogby International, 76% of U.S. voters feel that the war on drugs has been unsuccessful.
3. **Fact:** In the United States, a drug is legal until it is made illegal.
4. **Fiction:** The fact is—Social use of drugs does not usually lead to dependency. Drug use is more likely to result in dependency when drugs are used for personal reasons such as coping.
5. **Fiction:** The fact is—Individuals between the ages of 18 and 25 are almost twice as likely to have used an illegal drug in the previous month.
6. **Fact:** In the most recent survey of high school seniors, 58% disapproved of occasional marijuana use.
7. **Fiction:** The fact is—Some hospitals have tested pregnant women whom they suspected of having used drugs; however, most hospitals do not routinely test for drugs.
8. **Fact:** More people who were abused as children are likely to be alcoholics as adults, although most abused children do not become alcoholics.
9. **Fiction:** The fact is—For many years cocaine has been responsible for more drug fatalities than any other drug.
10. **Fact:** Many psychotherapists gave MDMA to their patients until the drug was made illegal in 1985.

Drugs pervade every facet of life. A fetus is affected by the mother's use of caffeine, tobacco, sedatives, and alcohol. Children are given stimulants to help them function more effectively in school. Adolescents use drugs to cope with daily stresses and to fit in with others. College students ingest amphetamines to stay awake and study late into the night. Club drugs such as Ecstasy and GHB are taken at nightclubs and rave parties to enhance the user's mood. Homemakers rely on tranquilizers such as Xanax to deal with life's problems. People living in poverty take drugs to mask the situations in which they find themselves. Affluent individuals use drugs out of boredom. Elderly people rely on drugs to manage ailments that accompany aging. Deeply imbedded in the human psyche is the tendency to use drugs to deal with pains, problems, frustrations, disappointments, and social interactions.

The Prevalence of Drug Use

Nearly every American has used a mind-altering substance by having a glass of wine, a cigarette, a cup of coffee, a soft drink, or a cup of hot chocolate. In the United States about 2 billion prescriptions are dispensed each year, and sales of prescription drugs totaled $286 billion in 2007.[1] American children consume 90% of all Ritalin produced worldwide.[2] In 2006, an estimated 741,425 people visited emergency rooms because of the nonmedical use of a prescribed drug, an OTC drug, or a nutritional supplement.[3] Pharmaceutical companies, meanwhile, are spending more money on marketing prescription drugs than on research and development of these drugs.[4]

A report from the World Health Organization noted that Americans ages 15 to 64 have higher rates of cocaine use and marijuana abuse than comparably aged individuals in Europe, Central America, and South America.[5]

Drug abuse is an expensive problem. The Office of National Drug Control Policy places the health and social cost of drug use at $181 billion annually.[6] Twenty-one million Americans who need treatment for illicit drug or alcohol use do not receive it.[7] An estimated 15% to 20% of all primary care and hospitalized patients are dependent on alcohol,[8] and the economic cost of alcohol abuse in the United States is estimated to be about $185 billion annually.[9]

More than 500,000 people are in American jails on any given day for violating a drug law. To address problems associated with drugs, the U.S. government is increasing its funding. By way of comparison, in 1980 the figure for combating drug abuse was $1 billion; in 2004, the United States government spent over $14 billion for drug control.[10] About two-thirds of that money was earmarked for domestic law enforcement and reducing the supply of drugs. Figure 2.1 shows the drug control budget for the 2009 fiscal year.[11]

The Impact of Drug Use and Abuse

Not only has binge drinking at American colleges been linked to student deaths, but it also has been associated with weak academic performance, injuries, vandalism, and property damage.[12] Female college students who drink alcohol are perceived as being more sexually interested.[13] Similarly, college women are more likely to experience verbal, sexual, and physical aggression on days they drink heavily.[14]

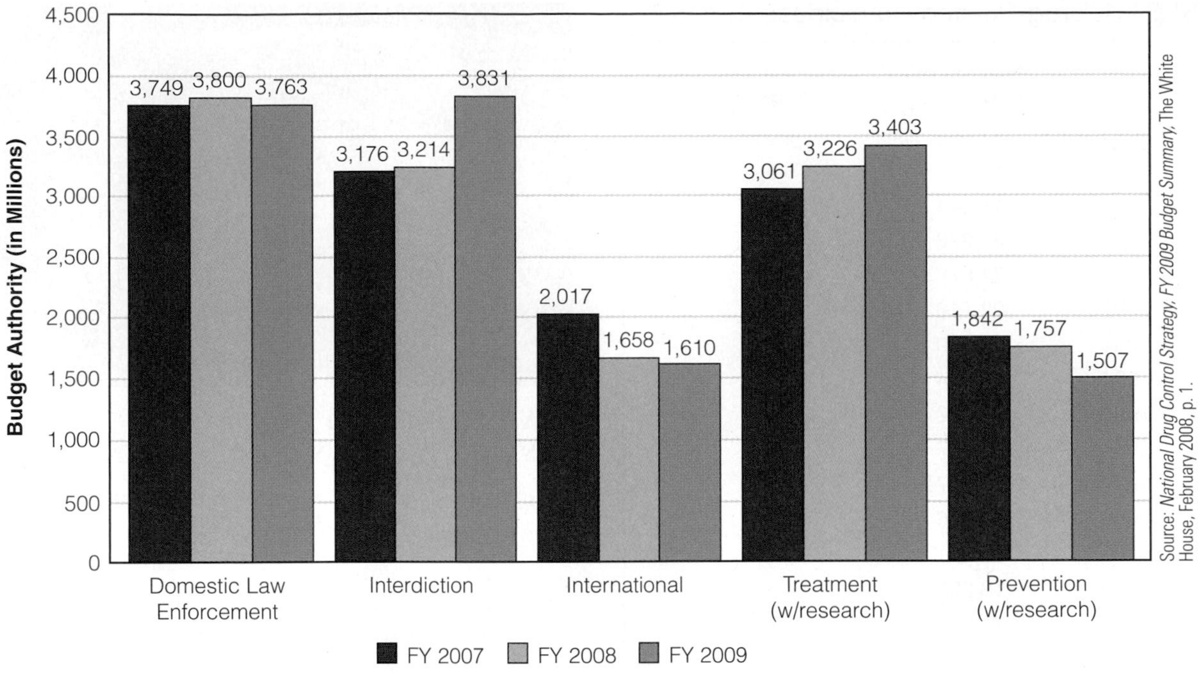

Figure 2.1 U.S. National Drug Control Budget for Fiscal Years (FY) 2007–2009

Alcohol is implicated in 30% to 90% of violent crime. Of crime victims, 37% indicated that alcohol was involved when crimes were committed against them. In nearly two-thirds of spousal abuse cases alcohol was a factor, and in 16% of child abuse incidents alcohol was a factor.[15]

Some people are concerned that drug use is destroying the fabric of society, that families and communities are undermined by drug use, and that moral decay will fester. In many instances, however, family and community problems might be the precursors to, rather than the effects of, drug abuse.[16] When addressing drug-related problems, there is a sense of frustration, that something must be done. A 2007 public opinion poll indicated that 73% of Americans considered drugs an extremely serious or very serious problem, although only 29% said that drugs were extremely serious or very serious where they live.[17]

In the 1990s Ecstasy was the drug of choice for many people. Heroin use also was rising. The cost of heroin was declining, purity was up, and more people were admitted to hospital emergency rooms or dying from heroin overdoses. At one time heroin was 7% pure. Today, its purity exceeds 30%.[18]

Nearly 500,000 Americans die each year from use of tobacco, alcohol, and illegal drugs. Nearly twice as many women die from lung cancer as from breast cancer.[19] In the United States, drug abuse–related health problems and resulting lost productivity cost more than $180 billion each year.[20]

Illegal drug use has a substantial connection to crime.[21] In 2006, there were 14,990 drug-related homicides.[22] More teenage males die from gunshot wounds than from all natural causes combined.[23] Being intoxicated increases the odds of being a victim of violence sixfold.[24] Thirty-two percent of state prisoners and 26% of federal prisoners indicate that they committed their current offense while under the influence of drugs.[25] Since 1972, the number of people incarcerated for drug-related crimes has increased fivefold, but despite this increase, drug use and crime have not declined.[26] Table 2.1 shows the number of drug-related homicides in the United States from 1987 to 2006.

Newspaper headlines recount stories of drug-crazed people perpetrating crimes on others, individuals whose drug use results in fatal diseases, males and females pawning their bodies for drugs, and women delivering drug-addicted and drug-impaired babies. The federal government estimates that over 4% of pregnant women used illicit drugs or binged on alcohol during the previous month.[27] Methamphetamine use during pregnancy results in slower intellectual, physical, emotional, and social development in children.[28] An estimated $500 million would be saved in the cost of obstetric and newborn care if cocaine abuse could be controlled.[29] At least one-third of all children in the child welfare system require those services because of parental drug abuse.[30] At the other end of the lifespan, an estimated 58,000 Americans age 55 and older are treated for substance abuse.[31]

The sixth-leading cause of death of Americans 25 to 44 years of age is acquired immunodeficiency syndrome (AIDS).[32] Those who used alcohol and

TABLE 2.1 Drug-Related Homicides

Year	Number of homicides	Percent drug related
1987	17,963	4.9%
1988	17,971	5.6
1989	18,954	7.4
1990	20,273	6.7
1991	21,676	6.2
1992	22,716	5.7
1993	23,180	5.5
1994	22,084	5.6
1995	20,232	5.1
1996	16,967	5.0
1997	15,837	5.1
1998	14,276	4.8
1999	13,011	4.5
2000	13,230	4.5
2001	14,061	4.1
2002	14,263	4.7
2003	14,465	4.7
2004	14,210	3.9
2005	14,965	4.0
2006	14,990	5.3

Note: The percentages are based on data from the Supplementary Homicide Reports (SHR) while the totals are from the Uniform Crime Reports (UCR). Not all homicides in the UCR result in reports in the SHR.

Source: Table constructed by ONDCP Drug Policy Information Clearinghouse staff from FBI, Uniform Crime Reports, Crime in the United States, annually.

other drugs while having sex were more likely to engage in high-risk sexual behaviors.[33] The impact of HIV is also greater on Blacks than other ethnic groups, with the rate seven times higher than among whites.[34] An encouraging fact is that the rate of HIV infection from injection drug use has declined in the last several years.[35] Needle exchange programs have been shown to reduce the transmission of HIV.[36]

Drugs are widely available, especially in the largest metropolitan areas where illegal drug use is more common. In the United States, 8.1% of people ages 12 and older used an illicit drug in the past month. However, in San Francisco that rate was 12.7%, and in Detroit, 9.5%.[37] In New York City, marijuana can be obtained at newsstands, record shops, video rental outlets, and so on. Some Manhattan nightclubs have resorted to hiring private ambulance companies to wait outside to take patrons who overdose to hospital emergency rooms. By doing this, they are able to bypass the 911 system and the attention of police.[38]

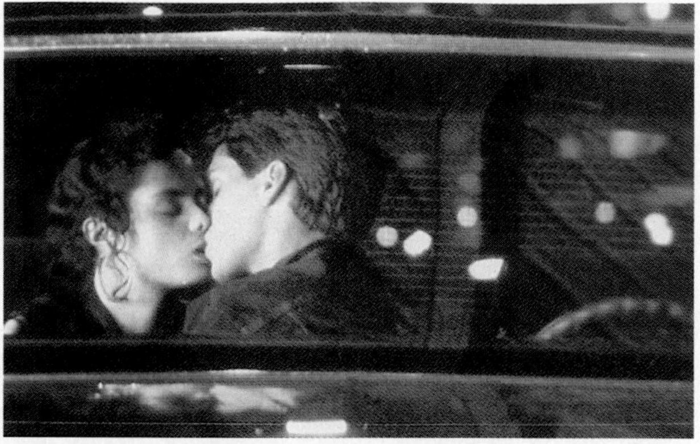

Photo courtesy of the National Institute on Drug Abuse, U.S. Department of Health and Human Services.

VANESSA WAS IN A FATAL CAR ACCIDENT LAST NIGHT. ONLY SHE DOESN'T KNOW IT YET.

Drug and alcohol use can make people more willing to have unplanned and unprotected sex.

To curb drug availability, billions of dollars are allocated for drug enforcement, prevention, and treatment. In 2009, the federal government's expenditures to interdict drugs will total $3.8 billion.[39] High schools and colleges conduct drug tests, especially with athletes. Passing a drug test is a condition of employment for most companies.

Drugs unquestionably can lead to violent behavior; dependency; mental and physical maladies; strained relationships among siblings, children, parents, and spouses; work-related problems; legal dilemmas; problems in school; financial difficulties; accidents and injuries; and death. Over the last several decades the United States has become much less tolerant of drug use. The sentiment of zero tolerance extends to other countries. For example, in Australia there is a movement away from minimizing the harm of drugs to zero tolerance.[40]

A report from the Brookings Institute suggested that the debate over how to address the drug problem is based on speculation, not on fact.[41] It is unclear how much of a drug a person has to take before problems arise and how often one has to use drugs before becoming dependent or developing a psychological or medical problem. No hard-and-fast rules are available for determining when drugs become a problem for an individual.[42]

Drugs from a Social Perspective

The effects that drugs produce are influenced greatly by society's perception of them.[43] For example, illegal drugs are condemned much more than legal drugs. Consequently, people who use legal drugs are not viewed in the same negative light as those who use illegal drugs. Tobacco use has been perceived more negatively in the 1990s and 2000s than in the 1980s, however. Society's reaction to an injection of morphine in a hospital is very different from that to an injection in one's home after obtaining morphine illegally. In addition to the pharmacological effects of drugs, social and psychological factors surrounding drug use play an important role.

Whether a given drug is defined as good or bad, socially acceptable or undesirable, conventional or "deviant," is not a simple outgrowth of the properties or objective characteristics of the drug itself, but is in no small measure a result of the history of its use, what social strata of society use it, for what purposes, the publicity surrounding its use, and so on. Whether the effects are experienced as pleasurable (euphoric) or unpleasant (dysphoric), weak or intense, hedonistic or depressing, hallucinatory or mundane, serene or exciting is largely a function of sociological factors.[44]

Risk factors that increase the potential for young people to use drugs include growing up in a chaotic household, having parents who abuse drugs, and lacking mutual attachment and nurturing. Parental drug use and poor family relations increase the likelihood of children using drugs.[45] (See Figure 2.2.)

Other risk factors include school failure, extreme shyness or aggressiveness in the classroom, poor coping skills, the perception that drug use is acceptable, and associating with peers who engage in drug use and other deviant behaviors.[46] In contrast, protective factors that reduce the likelihood of drug use are strong bonds with families, parents who take an active role in their children's lives, academic success, parents who monitor their children and provide clear rules for them, and children who adopt conventional norms regarding drug use.[47]

experimental drug use Infrequent drug use usually motivated by curiosity

social-recreational drug use Taking drugs in a social environment to share pleasurable experiences among friends

Patterns of Drug Taking

The National Commission on Marihuana and Drug Abuse devised a typology of five general patterns of drug-taking behavior: experimental, social-recreational, circumstantial-situational, intensified, and compulsive.[48]

Experimental Use

Individuals who use drugs infrequently and out of curiosity typify **experimental use**. This pattern involves short-term drug use. Experimental use is limited to 10 or fewer experiences with a given drug. Drug use usually does not go beyond the experimental phase, because the experimenter no longer has access to the drugs or simply does not find the drug experience enjoyable. If the person continues to use drugs, the drug use no longer is a matter of curiosity or experimentation.

Social-Recreational Use

Social-recreational use, the most common pattern, refers to taking drugs in a social environment to share pleasurable experiences among friends.

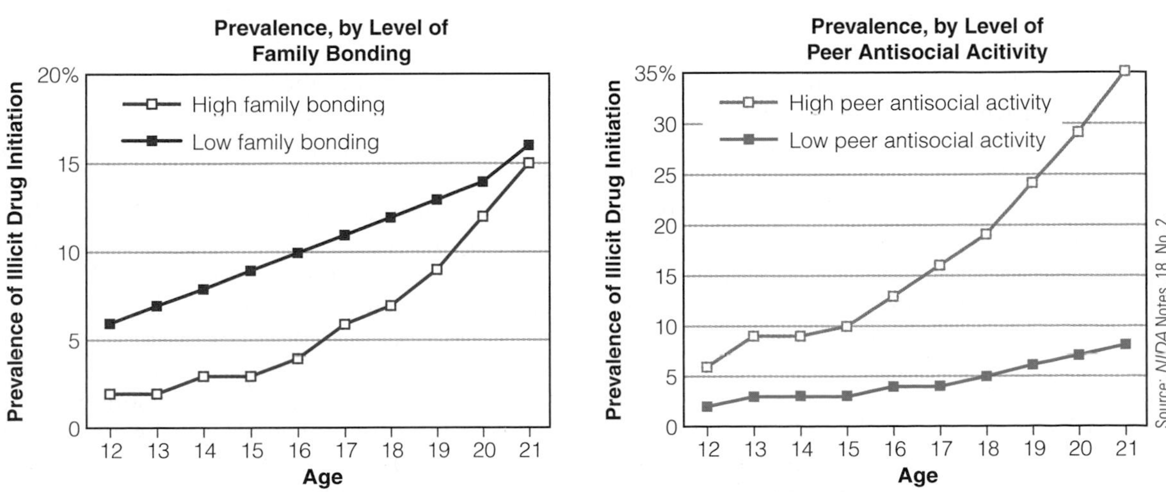

Figure 2.2 Family Bonding and Peer Antisocial Activity Impact Drug Initiation among Adolescents

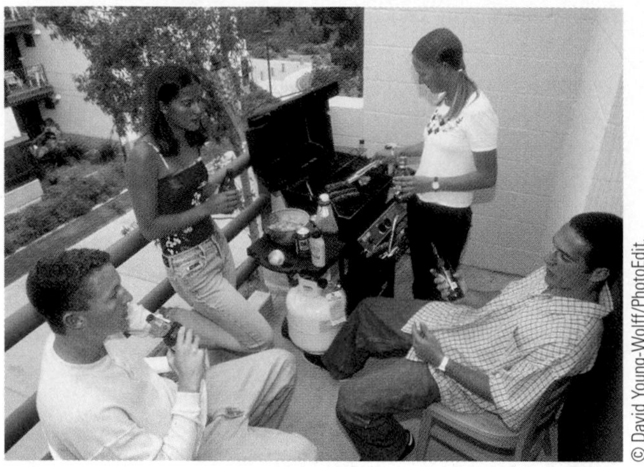

© David Young-Wolff/PhotoEdit.

Drugs such as alcohol are often used for social reasons.

On Campus

Beer drinking is not a rite of passage limited to college students. The Founding Fathers also had experiences with beer. Thomas Jefferson wrote much of the Declaration of Independence in Philadelphia's Indian Queen Tavern. Benjamin Franklin conducted business regularly in Philadelphia's taverns. One of George Washington's first acts as commander of the Continental Army was to allocate a quart of beer with daily rations to every one of his troops.

Social-recreational users do not tend to escalate their drug taking to the point of abuse. Many women who abuse drugs, however, were introduced to drugs through a male partner, which could be classified as a social-recreational situation.[49]

Circumstantial-Situational Use

Taking a drug on a short-term basis to contend with immediate distress or pressure characterizes **circumstantial-situational use**. Adolescents are more likely to use drugs when they are under stress, especially if their peers use drugs.[50] For instance, gay, lesbian, and bisexual youths, who are often under much stress, have significantly higher rates of substance use.[51] Also, easy access to drugs increases the likelihood of teenagers using drugs.[52] Likewise, easy accessibility for health care professionals can lead to drug abuse. In New York State, 2% of all practicing doctors are on the state's medical board so that they can be monitored for problems of substance abuse or mental health concerns.[53]

Joyous occasions such as weddings and holidays sometimes stimulate people to drink alcohol excessively. A student who has to write a 10-page paper that is due the next day might take amphetamines to stay up all night. This type of use can become a problem if the need to rely on drugs to cope with problems increases or if stressful events lead to consuming alcohol. Although some people use alcohol to reduce stress, alcohol use actually induces stress and leads to other self-destructive behaviors such as violence and suicide.[54]

Intensified Use

A person's drug-taking behavior is **intensified use** if he or she uses drugs on a steady, long-term basis to "achieve relief from a persistent problem or stressful situation or his [or her] desire to maintain a certain self-prescribed level of performance."[55] **Chronic drug use** indicates some extent of physical or psychological dependence. Unlike compulsive drug users, who tend to be alienated from society, chronic drug users maintain their place in society.

Compulsive Use

The person who consumes drugs compulsively and obsessively is not integrated into society. Acquiring and consuming drugs is the compulsive user's main focus. To a large extent, the media emphasize drug use by teenagers. A major problem, however, is compulsive drug use by hardcore users. There are an estimated 323,000 people dependent on heroin[56] and 1.67 million people dependent on cocaine in the United States.[57] These hardcore users also are responsible for most of the crime, child abuse, and fatal overdoses in the United States.

The compulsive user's lifestyle revolves around drugs. The compulsive user takes drugs to avoid discomfort, not to achieve pleasure. Unlike with other patterns of use, the social environment surrounding drug use does not dictate how and why drugs are used. In fact, the individual takes drugs despite the social situation. Society is justified in worrying about **compulsive drug use** because this pattern is destructive to the user and others. Compulsive drug users are likely to underestimate the extent of their drug use. Most people who use drugs, however, do not become compulsive users.

Extent of Drug Use

To determine precisely the extent of drug use is not easy because people might not answer questions about their personal behavior honestly, especially when illegal drugs are involved. Although obtaining information about the use of legal drugs, such as tobacco, alcohol, and prescription medicines, is easier, even that information may not be entirely accurate.

Even so, surveys repeated over time provide good data with respect to trends in drug use. Two comprehensive, large-scale studies are the National Survey on Drug Use and Health and the Monitoring the Future survey, which looks at drug use by 8th-grade, 10th-grade, and 12th-grade students.

National Survey on Drug Use and Health

Data regarding drug use have been collected periodically from U.S. households since 1971.[58] Those who participate represent a random cross section of people. The data received are grouped by respondents' ages (12–17, 18–25, and 26 or older), racial/ethnic groups, sex, and geographic regions. Table 2.2 shows monthly use of various drugs based on age groups.

Respondents were asked if they ever used drugs, if they had used them in the past year, and if they had used them in the past month. The group with the highest rate of illegal drug use during the past year and month was the 18 to 25 age group, and those 26 and older had the lowest annual and monthly rates. The most commonly used illicit drug was marijuana. It is used by approximately 8.0% of current users (*current* is defined as having used the drug within 30 days of the survey). The number of current cocaine users is estimated at 2.1 million Americans. About 1 million Americans currently use hallucinogens and 200,000 use heroin. In terms of overall drug use, males had higher rates of drug use than females. However, males and females have similar rates of using tranquilizers, stimulants, sedatives, and OxyContin. Among ethnic groups, the American Indian/Alaska Native population had the highest rate of current illicit drug use (12.6%), followed by people of two or more races (11.8%), Blacks (9.5%), Whites (8.2%), Hispanics (6.6%), and Asians (4.2%).

The highest rate of binge drinking (five or more drinks on one occasion within 30 days of the survey) and the highest rate of heavy drinking (consuming five or more drinks at least five times within 30 days of the survey) occurred among 18- to 25-year-olds. The binge alcohol rate for 12- to 17-year-olds was 9.7% and peaked at 45.9% for those ages 21 to 25.

Compared to 2006, lifetime drug use rates in 2007 did not differ significantly for all age groups. The number of people who used marijuana for the

circumstantial-situational drug use Short-term drug use to contend with immediate distress or pressure

intensified drug use Taking drugs on a steady, long-term basis to relieve a persistent problem or stressful situation

chronic drug use The habitual use of drugs

compulsive drug use Obsessive drug use without regard for society

TABLE 2.2 National Survey on Drug Use and Health: Percentages Reporting Past Month Use of Illicit Drugs, Tobacco, and Alcohol Aged 12 and Older, 2007

Past Month Use	Total	12–17	18–25	26 or Older
Any illicit drug	8.0	9.5	19.7	5.8
Marijuana and hashish	5.8	6.7	16.4	3.9
Cocaine	0.8	0.4	1.7	0.7
Crack	0.2	0.1	0.2	0.3
Heroin	0.1	0.0	0.1	0.1
Hallucinogens	0.4	0.7	1.5	0.2
LSD	0.1	0.1	0.2	0.0
Phencyclidine (PCP)	0.0	0.0	0.0	0.0
Ecstasy	0.2	0.3	0.7	0.1
Inhalants	0.2	1.2	0.4	0.1
Nonmedical Use of				
Psychotherapeutics[1]	2.8	3.3	6.0	2.2
Pain relievers	2.1	2.7	4.6	1.6
Tranquilizers	0.7	0.7	1.7	0.6
Stimulants	0.4	0.5	1.1	0.3
Methamphetamine	0.2	0.1	0.4	0.2
Sedatives	0.1	0.1	0.2	0.1
Cigarettes	24.2	12.4	36.2	24.1
Cigar	5.4	4.2	11.8	4.4
Smokeless tobacco	3.2	2.4	5.3	3.0
Alcohol	51.1	15.9	61.2	54.1
Binge alcohol use[2]	23.3	9.7	41.8	21.9
Heavy alcohol use[3]	6.9	2.3	14.7	6.1

[1]Nonmedical use of any prescription-type pain reliever, tranquilizer, stimulant or sedative; does not include over-the-counter products.
[2]Binge alcohol use is defined as drinking five or more drinks on the same occasion (within a few hours of each other) on at least 1 day in the past 30 days.
[3]Heavy alcohol use is defined as drinking five or more drinks on the same occasion on each of 5 or more days in the past 30 days.

Source: Substance Abuse and Mental Health Services Administration, Office of Applied Studies, *Results from the 2007 National Survey on Drug Use and Health: National Findings* (Rockville, MD: U.S. Department of Health and Human Services, 2008).

first time in 2007 was estimated at 2.1 million. One change in recent years is the number of people using pain relievers and tranquilizers for nonmedical purposes. Overall, the number of new users has not fluctuated much since 1995. New heroin users declined from 189,000 in 1997 to 106,000 in 2007. One difference among heroin users is that they were more likely to smoke, sniff, or snort heroin rather than inject it. The number of respondents who identified themselves as dependent was estimated at 3.7 million. An important corollary was that the younger one was when initiating drug use, the more likely one was to become dependent. Overall, more males are drug dependent than females, although males and females ages 12 to 17 have comparable dependency rates. Highlights of the 2007 survey are as follows:

- Some 19.8 million Americans were current illicit drug users.
- Almost 6.9 million Americans used psychotherapeutic drugs nonmedically. These include pain relievers (4.6 million), tranquilizers (1.8 million), stimulants (1.2 million), and sedatives (294,000).
- About 2.1 million Americans were current cocaine users. Current crack users were estimated at 610,000.
- The powerful painkiller OxyContin was used at least one time by almost 4.3 million people ages 12 or older.
- The number of people who have driven a car while under the influence of an illegal drug is 9.9 million.
- There are about 500,000 current Ecstasy users and 500,000 methamphetamine users.
- Among pregnant women ages 15 to 44, 5.2% reported using illicit drugs in the month before the survey. This figure is lower than among nonpregnant women ages 15 to 44.
- Inhalants are more likely to be used by those ages 12 to 17 than those in the 18 to 25 and 26 or older groups.
- About 57.8 million Americans ages 12 and older engaged in binge drinking (defined as five or more drinks on one occasion within 30 days of the survey). Some 17 million were heavy drinkers, meaning they had five or more drinks on five or more days during the past 30 days.
- The peak ages for current alcohol use, binge drinking, and heavy drinking are 21 to 25.
- About 1 in 8 Americans ages 12 or older had driven under the influence of alcohol in the previous 12 months. Males were nearly twice as likely to drive under the influence of alcohol.
- Approximately 60 million Americans reported smoking cigarettes (24.2%), 13.3 million smoked cigars, and 8.1 million used smokeless tobacco in the past month.
- Among 12- to 17-year-olds, 9.8% smoked cigarettes. There was no statistical difference between males and females. The age group with the highest rate of cigarette smoking, 38.5%, was 21 to 25.
- Among pregnant women ages 15 to 44, 16.4% had smoked cigarettes in the previous 30 days, compared to 28.4% of nonpregnant women.

Monitoring the Future: National Results on Adolescent Drug Use, 2008[59]

Beginning in 1975, the National Institute on Drug Abuse funded research examining the extent of legal and illegal drug use by high school seniors throughout the United States. The research, titled *Monitoring the Future*, expanded in 1991 to include 8th- and 10th-grade students. Besides drug usage, data were collected regarding attitudes about drugs, age at which drug use was initiated, and the availability of drugs. Although this annual survey excludes students who drop out of school and those who are absent from school on the day the survey is administered (suggesting that actual figures are underreported), it provides an excellent barometer of trends concerning drug use by 8th-, 10th-, and 12th-grade students.

The year 2008 data, which included nearly 50,000 students nationwide, showed a decline in illicit drug use among 8th-, 10th-, and 12th-grade students since the mid-1990s. Drugs that declined include marijuana, amphetamines, Ritalin, methamphetamines, and crystal methamphetamine. Also, alcohol and tobacco use showed significant decreases. Since 1999, cigarette smoking declined significantly for all three age groups. Smokeless tobacco use also declined. Ecstasy use increased from the mid-1990s to 2000 and then declined until 2007 when it increased slightly. The use of anabolic steroids peaked in 2000 and has declined since then.

Key variables in the increase or decrease in drug use are the perceived benefits and perceived risks of drugs. As the perceived benefits go up and as the perceived risks go down for a particular drug, the greater the likelihood that the drug will be used. Conversely, as perceived benefits decline and the perceived risks increase, there is less likelihood that a particular drug will be used. Another factor that affects drug use is peer disapproval: Peer disapproval results in a decline of drug use, whereas peer approval corresponds with an increase in drug use.

Other data revealed in the survey include the following:

- Since the mid-1990s, marijuana use has decreased for all three grade levels. In 2008, 5.8% of 8th graders had used marijuana within 30 days of the survey. In 1996, that figure was 11.3%. Tenth graders who had used marijuana within 30 days of the survey went from 20.4% in 1996 to 13.8%

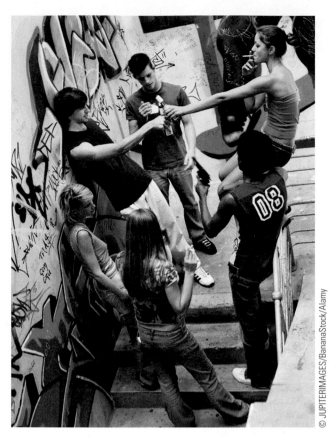

Peers are an important influence in drug use.

in 2008. Twelfth-grade students' monthly marijuana use went from 21.9% in 1996 to 19.4% in 2008. In the same year, 5.1% of high school seniors used marijuana daily.

- Annual cocaine use among 12th graders dropped from 6.2% in 1999 to 4.4% in 2008. Crack use by seniors declined from 2.7% in 1999 to 1.6% in 2008. Annual cocaine use for 8th- and 10th-grade students was 1.8% and 3.0%, respectively.
- Use of Ecstasy peaked among 8th-grade students with a rate of 3.5% in 2001. In 2008, the rate of Ecstasy use was 1.7%. For 10th-grade students the annual percentage went from 6.2% in 2001 to 2.9% in 2008. Annual use of Ecstasy for 12th-grade students decreased from 9.2% in 2001 to 4.3% in 2008.
- Steroid use within 12 months of the survey ranged from 0.9% of 8th-grade students to 0.9% of 10th graders to 1.5% of 12th graders.
- The one type of drug used more by 8th graders than by 10th or 12th graders was inhalants. The number of 8th-grade students who had used inhalants in the previous month was 4.1%, compared to 2.1% of 10th-grade students and 1.4% of 12th-grade students.
- Club drugs such as GHB and ketamine are not drugs of choice. The percentages of 8th-, 10th-, and 12th-grade students who used GHB in the past 12 months were 1.1, 0.5, and 1.2. Ketamine (Special K) was used by 1.2% of 8th graders, 1.0% of 10th graders, and 1.5% of 12th graders.
- Cigarette use on a daily basis for 10th graders dropped from 15.9% in 1999 to 5.9% in 2008. For high school seniors, daily cigarette smoking went from 23.1% in 1999 to 11.4% in 2008. The use of smokeless tobacco peaked in 1994 to 1995 and has declined steadily since then. In 1995, 12.2% of 12th graders had used smokeless tobacco within the previous month, but in 2008 usage had dropped to 6.5%. For 8th graders the rate in 2008 was 3.5%, and for 10th graders it was 5.0%. Like steroids, smokeless tobacco is used primarily by males.
- Binge drinking (five or more drinks on one occasion within two weeks of the survey) in 2008 was estimated at 24.6% for 12th graders, 16.0% for 10th graders, and 8.1% for eighth graders. The use of alcohol on a daily basis declined slightly for all three grade levels. Nonetheless, 27.6% of 12th graders and 5.4% of 8th graders reported being drunk at least once in the past month.

Previous surveys of high school students revealed that boys were more likely than girls to use drugs, that boys used drugs in greater amounts, that high school seniors in the Northeast used more drugs than seniors in other parts of the country, that non-college-bound seniors were more likely to use drugs than college-bound seniors, and that seniors in large cities were more likely to use drugs than seniors in smaller cities and rural areas. Table 2.3 shows prevalence of various drugs used by 8th-, 10th-, and 12th-grade students.

Drug Abuse by Older Adults

Drug abuse by Americans 60 years of age and older is an invisible epidemic. In the United States in 2005, more than 28,000 people ages 55 and older went to an emergency room as a result of an adverse reaction to an illicit drug, and more than 87,000 went to an emergency room due to the nonmedical use of a pharmaceutical drug.[60] Another 20,000 people ages 55 and older went to an emergency room after experiencing an adverse reaction from alcohol in combination with another drug.[61] Approximately 2.5 million older Americans have problems related to alcohol. It is estimated that 6% to 11% of elderly patients admitted to hospitals exhibit symptoms of alcoholism, as do 20% of elderly patients in psychiatric wards. Some older adults misuse over-the-counter drugs that have

TABLE 2.3 *Monitoring the Future* Study, 2008: Prevalence of Various Drugs for 8th Graders, 10th Graders, and 12th Graders

	8th Graders	10th Graders	12th Graders
Any illicit drug			
Annual	14.1%	26.9%	36.6%
30-day	7.6	15.8	22.3
Marijuana/hashish			
Annual	10.9	23.9	32.4
30-day	5.8	13.8	19.4
Inhalants			
Annual	8.9	5.9	3.8
30-day	4.1	2.1	1.4
LSD			
Annual	1.3	1.8	2.7
30-day	0.5	0.7	1.1
MDMA (Ecstasy)			
Annual	1.7	2.9	4.3
30-day	0.8	1.1	1.8
Cocaine			
Annual	1.8	3.0	4.4
30-day	0.8	1.2	1.9
Crack			
Annual	1.1	1.3	1.6
30-day	0.5	0.5	0.8
OxyContin			
Annual	2.1	3.6	4.7
Ritalin			
Annual	1.6	2.9	3.4
Methamphetamines			
Annual	1.2	1.5	1.2
30-day	0.7	0.7	0.6
Rohypnol (Roofies)			
Annual	0.5	0.4	1.3
GHB			
Annual	1.1	0.5	1.2
Ketamine (Special K)			
Annual	1.2	1.0	1.5
Steroids			
Annual	0.9	0.9	1.5
30-day	0.5	0.5	1.0
Alcohol			
5+ drinks in a row in last 2 weeks	8.1	16.0	24.6
Been drunk within last 30 days	5.4	14.4	27.6
Cigarettes			
30-day	6.8	12.3	20.4
$\frac{1}{2}$ pack + daily	1.2	2.0	5.4
Smokeless tobacco			
30-day	3.5	5.0	6.5
Daily	0.8	1.4	2.7

Source: *The Monitoring the Future Study: National Results on Adolescent Drug Use* (Rockville, MD: National Institute for Drug Abuse, 2008).

a high alcohol content, such as cough suppressants. The majority of older people engaging in substance misuse are men, even though women outnumber men. The small percentage of older adults who abuse illicit drugs usually are aging criminals and long-term heroin addicts.

Substance abuse by older adults accelerates the normal decline in physiological functioning that accompanies aging. Also, because older people are more affected by drugs, they are at higher risk for accidents and illness. Further, the percentage of older adults in the general population is projected to increase, so substance abuse problems are expected to become more apparent. A clear relationship exists between alcohol problems early in life and alcohol problems later in life. Also, there is an association between separated, divorced, and widowed adults and alcohol abuse.

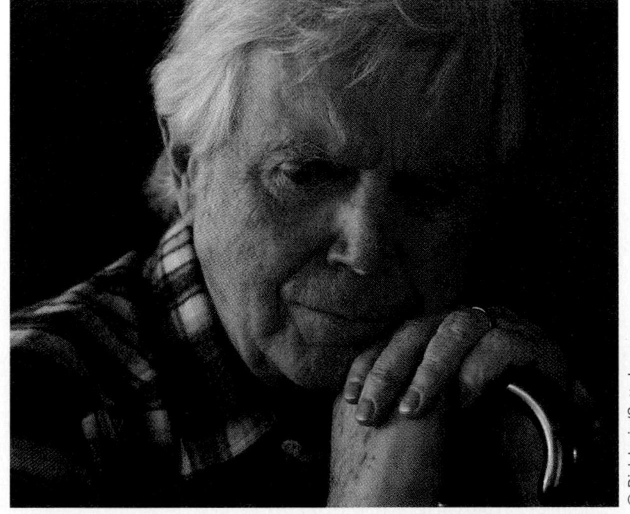

Many older people use drugs to deal with loneliness.

Problems with substance abuse by elderly people may be more common than believed, because health care providers underestimate, underidentify, underdiagnose, and undertreat the problem. Diagnosing symptoms of substance abuse in older adults is difficult, though, because many symptoms mimic symptoms of medical and behavioral disorders common to this population.

Contributing to substance abuse problems of older adults are shame and *ageism*. Many older adults feel shamed if they have a substance abuse problem; consequently, they are reluctant to seek treatment. Moreover, adult children of older individuals feel shamed if their parents have a substance abuse problem, and therefore choose not to address the problem.

Too often substance abuse by older adults is ignored because of the unspoken but pervasive attitude that treating older adults is not worth the trouble. Some people think that older people will not be around that much longer anyway, so why interfere with their lives if they are enjoying themselves? Unfortunately, older adults who self-medicate with alcohol or prescription drugs are more likely to characterize themselves as lonely, and they report lower life satisfaction.

Drugs in the Workplace

Substance abuse has a profoundly negative effect in the workplace, resulting in lessened productivity and increased accidents, absenteeism, and health-care costs. Workplace accidents cost employers $12,000 to $16,000 per incident.[62] People who are unemployed are more likely to use drugs than people who are employed; however, most substance users and those with substance abuse disorders work full time.[63] Part-time workers also have higher rates of drug use than full-time workers. The industries with the highest rates of drug use are food service workers and construction workers.[64] The latter have the highest rates of occupational injuries among the major industries.[65]

In 2007, the number of workers testing positive for cocaine and methamphetamines declined significantly from the previous year.[66] Most surveys figured that fewer than 10% of workers used alcohol or other drugs—excluding tobacco and caffeine—on the job. Nonetheless, alcoholism results in 500 million lost workdays each year. Chemically dependent workers are 3.6 times more likely to have on-the-job accidents.[67]

Workers who drink on the job have more performance problems than those who do not drink on the job.[68] Also, moderately heavy and heavy drinkers have more job-related accidents than very light, light, or moderate drinkers. Heavy beer consumption, rather than wine or liquor use, is strongly related to fatal accidents.[69] Also, the rate of alcohol-related accidents varies with the type of job.[70] Illicit drug users and heavy alcohol consumers were more likely to be involved in workplace accidents, miss work because of illness or injury, and have unexcused absences from work.[71] Ironically, teens who work more than 10 hours per week drink more heavily than teens who work less than 10 hours per week.[72]

Identifying drug problems in top-level managers is more of a dilemma than recognizing drug problems in other workers, because upper-level managers have less supervision and corporations often deny that their executives abuse drugs. To address drug abuse, most Fortune 500 companies use some type of drug testing and undercover surveillance. It is believed that drug testing has greatly reduced drug use among American workers. The percentage of individuals testing positive for drugs declined from 13.6 in 1988 to 3.8 in 2006.[73]

An interesting question involves whether employers can fire workers who test positive for marijuana even though the marijuana was used for medical purposes. The California State Supreme Court ruled by a margin of 5 to 2 that employers do have the right to fire workers who test positive for marijuana.[74]

employee assistance programs (EAPs) Company-sponsored programs to help employers deal with their employees who have problems, including drug use

Employee Assistance Programs

Many corporations have devised **employee assistance programs (EAPs)** to help workers deal with legal, family, health, or other problems that affect job performance.[75] Some EAPs are offered on a voluntary basis, and others require that employees attend. Many workers benefit from EAPs, especially those who are given the choice of attending a program or being fired. Employers benefit because absenteeism declines, productivity increases, job-related problems decrease, and employee morale improves. Moreover, the cost of health care to the employer declines greatly.

A worksite program designed to prevent alcohol misuse by working adults found that alcohol consumption and problems related to alcohol use can be reduced.[76] It was reported that among workers who went to an EAP for alcohol or drug problems, mental health improved in 66%, physical health improved in 56%, and absenteeism showed an 80% improvement.[77] The Hazelden Foundation indicated that alcohol addiction improved in 89% of people treated through their employers.[78] Unfortunately, more employers are choosing to terminate addicted employees rather than treat them.[79]

Drug Testing

In the 1986 classic, *America's Habit: Drug Abuse, Drug Trafficking, and Organized Crime,* the President's Commission on Organized Crime advocated that all federal workers be drug tested and that federal contracts be withheld from private employers who do not initiate drug testing programs. In 2008, the federal government earmarked $17.9 million for testing of high school students.[80] Random workplace drug testing has effectively identified frequent users of illicit drugs.[81] It is important to note that 20% of workers between ages 18 and 25 have used drugs while at work.[82] An estimated 70% of illegal drug users and 77% of all heavy drinkers are employed full-time.[83]

Drugs inevitably affect an individual's ability to work. Companies that test employees for performance, however, found that fatigue, stress, and illness are the most common factors leading to poor job performance.[84]

Among full-time workers ages 18 to 49, 35% reported that their workplace tested for drugs at the time of hiring, 20% reported random drug testing, 28% reported drug testing if the supervisor had reasonable suspicion, and 23% reported that testing was conducted after a work-related accident.[85] The federal government recently passed legislation to assist small businesses to initiate workplace drug testing because drug users are absent from work an average of 5 days per month.[86]

Not all critics support drug testing, some arguing that it represents a billion-dollar business for the private sector. Who should be drug tested? For example, should teachers be drug tested? When school superintendents were asked about drug testing teachers, the majority felt they had the right to drug test teachers but most would not because they felt the problem of drug use by teachers is too small to warrant testing. The superintendents were more comfortable drug testing as a condition for hiring teachers.[87] In Hawaii, the governor proposed that teachers be drug tested, but because she allocated no money for the testing, whether teachers in Hawaii will be tested remains unclear. Previous court cases involving drug testing teachers have been struck down by one court and upheld by another.[88]

Most Americans view drug testing as degrading and dehumanizing.[89] A group especially subjected to drug testing is pregnant women. In addition, Black women are 1.5 times more likely to be tested for illicit drugs than non-Black women.[90] In many jurisdictions physicians are required to report women who use

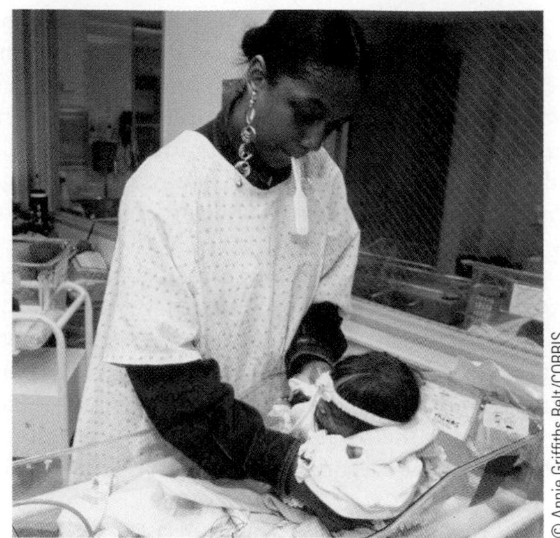

Having low-birthweight babies is a side effect of drug use by pregnant women.

drugs during pregnancy or infants who test positive for drug use by their mothers. However, the Supreme Court indicated that pregnant patients cannot be tested for illegal drugs if the purpose is to alert police to crime. Rather, drug testing is permissible if the purpose is to help the pregnant woman receive better health care.[91] Drug testing with the intent of punishing the pregnant woman is opposed by the American Medical Association, the American College of Obstetrics and Gynecology, and the American Academy of Pediatrics.[92]

Women whose babies test positive for drugs such as cocaine are subject to losing custody of their children because they are viewed as unfit parents. As a result, women may not receive adequate prenatal care for fear of losing their children. And, even though cocaine use during pregnancy is unhealthy, alcohol use and cigarette smoking during pregnancy have been shown to cause worse problems.

Testing of Athletes

Drug testing is a concern in many professional and amateur athletic programs. To increase alertness, competitiveness, and aggression, some competitors use stimulants. Others use beta-blockers to reduce anxiety. Still others use steroids to augment muscle development.[93] Beta-blockers are especially beneficial in sports requiring steadiness, such as putting in golf.[94] One unfortunate side effect is that they interfere with sexual performance.

Almost all high schools randomly drug tested athletes, while 65% randomly drug tested students participating in extracurricular activities and 14% randomly drug tested all students.[95] Court rulings have been mixed as to whether drug testing violates the privacy of high school and college athletes. The United States Supreme Court said that drug testing does not violate a student-athlete's right to privacy[96] and confirmed a school district's decision to drug test all students involved in extracurricular activities. In a 2001 ruling, the Supreme Court upheld lower court rulings that prevent school districts from drug testing nonatheletes.[97] However, steroids are used by nonathletes because friends use them, to enhance physical appearance, and to improve physical performance.[98] The effectiveness of drug testing is questionable. In Texas, $6 million was allocated for testing student athletes for steroids. Of 10,000 students, only two tested positive.[99]

Some people argue that drug testing of athletes should be abandoned for several reasons, among them questions regarding the validity of the tests and whether the levels that are considered inappropriate are arbitrary.[100] Another concern is that drug testing has not kept up with new ways to avoid detection; thus, there is inconsistency in which athletes are caught doping.[101]

immunoassay A drug-testing procedure that tests for metabolites of drugs

gas chromatography A drug-testing procedure that is more specific, sensitive, and expensive than the immunologic assay

thin-layer chromatography A simple, inexpensive, urine-based drug test

gas chromatography/mass spectrometry A type of drug test, highly sophisticated and sensitive, but time-consuming and expensive

false positive A test that is positive for drugs even though no drugs are present in the urine

false negative A test that is negative for drugs even though drugs are present in the urine

Methods of Drug Testing

Testing for drugs can be done by examining urine, saliva, hair, blood, or breath. The ability to detect drugs depends on the type of test, the dose, and the sensitivity of the test. A new test for detecting drugs developed by University of Illinois researchers involves a litmus-like paper strip that examines molecules in saliva, urine, or blood.[102] Urine testing is the most common method and has been shown to be accurate and reliable. The methods used to test urine for drugs are immunoassay, gas chromatography, thin-layer chromatography, and gas chromatography/mass spectrometry.

1. **Immunoassay** is fast and less expensive than other methods but may give false-positive readings.
2. **Gas chromatography** is more expensive and time-consuming than other methods.
3. **Thin-layer chromatography** is simple and inexpensive, but it requires expert interpretation, and it is less sensitive than the immunoassay procedure.
4. **Gas chromatography/mass spectrometry** is highly sophisticated and sensitive but is time-consuming and expensive.

The detectability of drugs in urine or hair varies with the drug. Although amphetamines and methamphetamines are detectable in urine 4 to 5 days after use, a hair test can detect their presence up to 90 days after use. Phencyclidine (PCP) is detectable in urine 2 to 10 days after use and is detectable through hair analysis up to 90 days after use. Urine tests can detect cocaine 4 to 5 days after use, and hair tests can detect cocaine 90 days after use. A person can test positive for heroin one to two days after use via urine and 90 days after use via a hair sample. Marijuana can be detected from 3 to 30 days after use by a urine test and up to 90 days later through a hair test. In one county in Iowa, Child Protective Services is hair-testing children soon after they are born to determine whether they have been exposed to smoked drugs, especially crack.[103] Table 2.4 compares the detectability of drugs through urine and through hair.

Two problems with drug testing are false positives and false negatives:

1. A **false positive** means that a person tests positive for a drug even though no drug is present in the person's urine. For example, ibuprofen, the active ingredient in Motrin and Advil, may cause a false positive test for marijuana. A person may test positive for opiates after consuming poppy seeds or cough syrups containing codeine. It has been shown that individuals who lack the enzyme UGT2B17 may test positive for excessive testosterone.[104]
2. A **false negative** means that a person tests negative even though drugs are present in the person's urine.

TABLE 2.4 Detectability of Drugs in Urine

Drug	Urine Detection Period	Hair Detection Period
Alcohol	6–12 hours	Not detectable
Amphetamines/ methamphetamines	4–5 days	Up to 90 days
Barbiturates	2–12 days	Not assayed
Cocaine	4–5 days	Up to 90 days
Marijuana	3–30 days	Up to 90 days
PCP	2–10 days	Up to 90 days

Questions Regarding Drug Testing

- Should a person have the right to refuse to take a drug test?
- Who sees the results of a drug test? How is confidentiality assured?
- Are standards applied to minors in drug testing different from those for adults?
- If a person tests positive, is there an appeal process?
- Are consequences different for testing positive for legal drugs as opposed to illegal drugs?
- Does a positive drug test constitute a medical, legal, or educational problem?
- If students have to pass a drug test to be on athletic teams, should students also have to pass similar tests to be in school plays or in the band?
- How accurate are drug tests?
- Should a person be penalized for a positive drug test that is a result of passive marijuana smoke?

Some people employ inventive ways to test negative: by obtaining someone else's urine, by drinking vast amounts of water before testing, or by placing salt and detergent in the urine sample. Another potential problem with drug testing is that one's medical condition may be revealed to the employer. For example, a drug test may indicate whether a person is taking certain medications for certain medical conditions or is genetically predisposed to other conditions such as heart disease or cancer. It may cause an employer to forgo hiring a prospective employee to avoid potential health insurance costs.

Legality of Drug Testing

The legality of drug testing was debated in two cases that came before the U.S. Supreme Court: *Skinner* v. *Railway Labor Executive Association* and *National Treasury Employees Union* v. *von Raab*. The *Skinner* case dealt with the constitutionality of random drug testing of employees and applicants of private railways. In 1985, the Federal Railroad Administration (FRA) adopted regulations that prohibited employees from possessing or using alcohol or any controlled substance while at work or from reporting to work while under the influence of alcohol or a controlled substance. These regulations were implemented because a number of employees had come to work impaired by alcohol or had become drunk while at work.

In 21 or more railway accidents between 1972 and 1983 that involved fatalities, serious injuries, and millions of dollars of damage to property, alcohol or other drugs were the probable or contributing cause.[105] By a 7–2 vote, the U.S. Supreme Court upheld the FRA's plan to test railway workers. While recognizing the need to protect individuals' rights, the Supreme Court noted that the safety considerations of certain jobs override those rights. Because the impairment of railway workers posed a considerable threat to the public, the Supreme Court ruled that drug testing is warranted.

The second case before the Supreme Court, *National Treasury Employees Union* v. *von Raab*, dealt with whether applicants for the U.S. Customs Service must pass a drug test. Individuals testing positive would not have to turn over the results for prosecution. The purpose was to prevent individuals from getting the jobs in the first place. The Customs Service argued that drug users were subject to bribery and blackmail, that drug users may be unsympathetic to their task of interdicting narcotics, and that drugs might impair employees who carry firearms.

Even though only five employees of 3,600 had tested positive for drugs, the Supreme Court narrowly (5–4) agreed with the Customs Service. Because the testing program was designed to prevent drug use and the integrity of the Customs Service had to be maintained, the Court ruled that the testing program was justified.

Consequences of Drug Use

Drug use is a factor in family stability, social behavior, education and career aspirations, and personal and social maturation. A relationship has been reported between adolescents' substance use, depression, and suicidal thoughts and attempts. It could be argued that drugs are not *the* problem, but just one piece of a much larger puzzle in which drug use is simply another component. An important question is whether drugs are a problem or whether they are symptomatic of other problems.

Drugs and the Family

Although drug use has not been *proved* to increase marital separation and divorce, an association exists between drug use and the likelihood that a couple will separate or divorce. Women with alcohol-dependent partners have significantly more family and marital problems. Also, women subjected to violence have higher rates of alcohol dependence and other drug abuse problems.[106] Family life may reduce drug involvement. Family interventions into adolescent alcohol use reduce the initiation and frequency of alcohol use.[107] Teaching adults how to improve their parenting skills has been shown to reduce the use of alcohol and other drugs among children and adolescents.[108] Moreover, children who are closely monitored by parents are less likely to drink alcohol.[109] Parental divorce, however, increases the likelihood that children will be prescribed Ritalin.[110] In a study of Finnish twins, intoxication by the father was shown to increase the likelihood of marijuana smoking, although cigarette use was a stronger predictor of marijuana use.[111]

In a study of marriage, it was found that individuals' illicit drug use declined after they married. Both husband and wife reduced their illicit drug use, but husbands were slightly more likely than wives to use drugs.[112] When couples cohabitate, licit and illicit drug use declines, although marriage produces a greater decline.[113] In a study of divorced couples, researchers noted that frequent alcohol intoxication was strongly related to divorce. Frequency of marijuana use was not a strong predictor of divorce.[114]

A number of studies have shown that parental substance abuse is a factor for between one-third and two-thirds of all children involved with the child welfare system.[115] Also, children with drug-using mothers were more likely to be placed in child protection services.[116] The likelihood of adolescents experiencing major depressive disorders increases when parents are alcohol dependent.[117]

Substance abuse is a prominent factor in many cases of child abuse and domestic abuse. For instance, in a study of United States soldiers, it was noted that 13% of those involved in child maltreatment were under the influence of alcohol or an illicit drug at the time of the incident.[118] Moreover, many of those individuals who were abused as children or abused by their intimate partners end up in substance abuse treatment. It was found that women in treatment who were abused as children were about 2.5 times more likely to be victims of intimate partner violence.[119] Although alcohol is implicated with child and domestic abuse, alcohol is also linked to other drugs. For example, it has been shown that there is a strong relationship between binge drinking and cocaine use.[120]

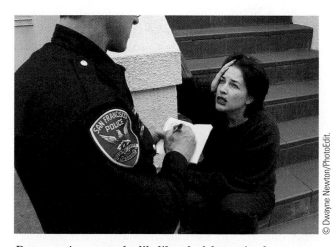

Drug use increases the likelihood of domestic abuse.

A study in Brazil reported that alcohol use or abuse was associated with the perpetration of sexual aggression, especially toward boys.[121] Adolescents who were sexually abusive and engaged in criminal sexual conduct were more likely to have caregivers who had histories of substance use and abuse.[122] Conversely, women who were sexually abused by age 13 have a greater incidence of alcohol dependence and abuse.[123] Sexually abused children are more likely to suffer from other forms of self-harm, eating disorders, sexual dysfunction, and attempted suicide.[124] Children of problem drinkers report much family disharmony.[125]

Substance abuse does not figure into every incident of maltreatment; however, caseworkers often cite it as a major factor. One study found that individuals who were abused or neglected as children do not necessarily grow up abusing alcohol, but have a greater risk of abusing alcohol.[126]

Drugs and Deviant Behavior

Drug use and deviant attitudes and behavior are closely associated.[127] The most important distinction between drug users and nonusers is their extent of *conventionality*.[128] Whether drug use provokes deviant attitudes and behaviors or whether deviant behaviors and attitudes provoke drug use is unclear. In any case, drug users display more independence, rebelliousness, acceptance of deviant behavior, and rejection of moral and social norms than nonusers.[129] Children of parents who use drugs are more likely to engage in delinquent behaviors than their peers whose parents do not use drugs.[130] The significance of this association is revealed by one recent study reporting that almost 5 million alcohol-dependent or alcohol-abusing parents have at least one child living with them.[131]

Some drugs are more likely to produce violent behavior whereas others, such as marijuana and heroin, are more likely to produce a passive response. (Heroin is linked to criminal behavior but not to violent behavior.) Stimulants such as methamphetamines and cocaine are associated with violence. The combination of hyperactivity and increased suspiciousness may cause sudden, unwarranted aggressiveness. The factor relating to violence may not be the amphetamine but, rather, the paranoia the drug causes.

The drug involved with the most violent incidents is alcohol. Wells, Graham, and West found that alcohol intoxication, and not mere alcohol consumption, was associated with physical aggression.[132] Binge drinking by college students is clearly linked to violence.[133]

The person using alcohol may perpetrate the violence or be the victim of another alcohol user. Among many victims of violence, it was believed that the perpetrator was under the influence of alcohol at the time; for example, of individuals who were victimized at work, 35% believe that the offender was under the influence of alcohol or other drugs.[134] In a study of 20,274 adolescents, 16% report being victims of dating violence. Most cases of dating violence occurred in the South, and in many instances, alcohol was implicated.[135] Some speculate that the pharmacological effect of alcohol, not simply one's expectations when drinking, is the link to aggressiveness.[136]

Drugs, Education, and Employment

There is a higher dropout rate from school for those who used alcohol, illicit drugs, and cigarettes.[137] In a study of African American students, it was found that the desire to do well academically was related to less marijuana use, parental substance use norms, and family financial concerns.[138] In their review of numerous studies, Lynskey and Hall speculate that the type of person who uses marijuana does poorly in school. Thus, poor school performance may reflect on the individual who uses marijuana, not on the drug itself.[139] In terms of cocaine use, those individuals with high education levels are less likely to use cocaine persistently than those people with low levels of educational achievement.[140]

Drug use is assumed to be a predictor of welfare dependency. In 1997 the federal government passed a law stipulating that all welfare recipients be denied Social Security income and disability insurance if alcohol and drug addiction were exclusively responsible for their disabilities. The relationship between drug use and welfare dependency is not limited to the United States. In New Zealand, marijuana use among adolescents and young adults negatively affected educational achievement, reduced employment, and increased welfare dependency.[141]

The Higher Education Act stipulates that college students who are convicted of a drug offense are denied federal financial aid. Legislation has been introduced to have federal financial aid restored to college students if they enroll in treatment and pass two drug tests.[142] Since 2000, more than 180,000 students were denied federal financial aid due to a drug conviction.[143]

Employed drug users have less stable job histories than nonusers. Whether job instability results in drug use or drug use causes job instability is unclear. Alcohol abusers earn significantly less money than moderate drinkers and abstainers.[144] Finally, drug use is associated with higher accident rates on the job and lower productivity.

Drug Toxicity

At a certain dose, many drugs are beneficial. At higher doses, the same drugs may be poisonous, or *toxic*. The difference between a safe level and a dangerous level, the **margin of safety**, can be slight. Even if one does not overdose, drug use can be fatal. In a study of U.S. veterans, it was found that substance use increased the risk of premature death significantly.[145] An Australian study reported that substance use was highly correlated to suicide attempts.[146]

Toxicity can be physiological, behavioral, acute, or chronic:

1. *Physiological toxicity* refers to the danger to the body as a result of taking the drug. An example is taking an excessive amount of barbiturates, causing breathing to cease.
2. *Behavioral toxicity* means that a drug interferes with one's ability to function. Behavioral toxicity is illustrated by drowning or getting into an automobile accident after consuming alcohol.
3. *Acute toxicity* alludes to the danger from a single experience with a drug, such as getting drunk.
4. *Chronic toxicity* is the danger posed by repeated exposure to a drug. An example is cardiac or pulmonary damage resulting from long-term cigarette use.

Toxicity does not reflect the legal status of a drug. The drug causing the highest death rate in the United States is tobacco, which is responsible for more than 400,000 deaths per year even though its production is subsidized by the federal government! The notion that if a drug is legal, it is safe—or at least safer than illegal drugs—must be dispelled.

Drug Abuse Warning Network

To get a better grasp of the magnitude of drug-related problems, the federal government monitors emergency room visits in many metropolitan areas through a system called the Drug Abuse Warning Network (DAWN). DAWN collects information on the number of times drugs are implicated in nonlethal visits to emergency rooms and in fatalities.

The drug responsible for the most fatalities is cocaine, although alcohol in combination with other drugs and narcotic-analgesics also accounts for many deaths. Opiates are the drugs most linked to suicide.[147] The majority of people dying from drug abuse are males. Males are 2.4 times more likely to die from drug misuse or abuse. The age group with the highest mortality rate is 35 to 54. The cities with the most drug-related fatalities are Baltimore and Albuquerque.[148]

TABLE 2.5 Drug-Related Emergency Room Visits, 2006

Illicit drugs only	31%
Pharmaceuticals only	28%
Alcohol only in patients under age 21	7%
Illicit drugs with alcohol	13%
Alcohol with pharmaceuticals	10%
Illicit drugs with pharmaceuticals & alcohol	3%
Illicit drugs with pharmaceuticals	8%

Source: Substance Abuse and Mental Health Services Administration, *Drug Abuse Warning Network, 2006: National Estimates of Drug-Related Emergency Room Visits* (Rockville, MD: U.S. Department of Health and Human Services, 2008).

In 2006, drug misuse or abuse accounted for 1.7 million visits to hospital emergency rooms. Table 2.5 shows the percentage of people who visited an emergency room because of various types of drugs. Illicit drugs were responsible for the most emergency room visits, followed by pharmaceutical drugs. Among illicit drugs, cocaine was the most commonly reported drug.

Emergency room visits arise from adverse emotional or physical reactions to drugs. The user may hallucinate or become irrational, overly anxious, or suicidal. The medical examiner determines whether death is caused by drugs. When a person visits an emergency room or has a fatal overdose, more than one drug usually is involved. Table 2.6 shows the number of drug-related deaths due to misuse and suicide in selected cities.

Many factors play a role in drug overdoses. Injected drugs pose a greater health threat than ingested drugs, and mixing drugs augments their potency significantly. Also, drug dosage, drug purity, and frequency of use figure into the potential risks. Adverse effects increase when larger amounts are consumed or when the drugs are taken at more frequent intervals. The DAWN data reflect **acute** drug-related problems, not chronic drug use.

If it were categorized by itself, alcohol would head the lists for both lethal and nonlethal incidents. One study found that among individuals reporting an emergency room visit, 245 had engaged in "risky drinking," which was defined as 14 or more drinks per week for men and 7 or more drinks per week for women. Eight percent reported being problem drinkers and 3% were alcohol dependent.[149]

It should be noted that drug mortality figures only represent a small percentage of drug overdoses. It is estimated that only 20% of all deaths are reviewed by a medical examiner or coroner.

margin of safety The difference between a beneficial level and a harmful level of a drug

toxicity A drug's ability to disturb or nullify homeostasis

acute Describes a condition that arises abruptly and is not long lasting

designer drugs Synthetic substances that are chemically similar to existing drugs

analog A synthetic derivative of an existing drug

TABLE 2.6 Drug-Related Deaths per 1,000,000 Population in Selected Cities, 2003

	Drug Misuse Deaths	Drug-Related Suicide Deaths
Atlanta	204.0	23.5
Baltimore	205.6	4.6
Boston	109.5	14.2
Chicago	57.0	14.0
Cleveland	130.5	15.4
Denver	102.0	24.9
Detroit	129.4	12.6
Kansas City	113.6	16.1
Miami	67.9	8.1
Minneapolis/St. Paul	53.3	15.9
New Orleans	188.3	18.6
New York	93.4	5.5
Philadelphia	103.8	28.1
Phoenix	114.8	30.1
St. Louis	84.8	25.7
Salt Lake City	183.0	32.8
San Diego	120.1	29.3
San Francisco	96.4	18.0
Seattle	91.2	17.9
Washington, DC	63.5	7.5

Source: Substance Abuse Mental Health Services Administration, *Drug Abuse Warning Network, 2003: Area Profiles of Drug-Related Mortality* (Rockville, MD: U.S. Department of Health and Human Services, 2005).

Designer Drugs

Someone with knowledge of chemistry may alter the chemical structure of a compound and produce a new drug that not only is psychoactive but also is legal.[150] The effects of **designer drugs** often mimic those of opium, morphine, and heroin.[151] In 1986, the U.S. Congress passed legislation curbing the manufacture of these **analogs**. Nevertheless, the business of designer drugs, according to the Drug Enforcement Administration (DEA), exceeds a billion dollars a year. The concept of designer drugs also applies to pharmaceutical drugs. There are recent developments in drugs that are similar to Viagra and Levitra, drugs used for erectile dysfunction.[152] Among the better known designer drugs are fentanyl, meperidine, and MDMA.

Fentanyl

Fentanyl is the generic name for Sublimaze, a synthetic narcotic developed for its anesthetic properties. It is estimated to be 50 to 100 times more potent than morphine.[153] When used in surgery, it is administered by injection. People who use fentanyl illegally either smoke or snort it. It usually is not taken orally, although it is absorbed readily through the tissues under the tongue.[154] Fentanyl depresses the respiratory system, decreases the heart rate and blood pressure, and causes constipation. It can be fatal. Death is so swift that needles have been found in people who apparently died while injecting themselves. Whether death is attributable to the drug or to its contaminants is unclear.

When fentanyl is used clinically, side effects include nausea, dizziness, delirium, decreased blood pressure, vomiting, blurred vision, and possible cardiac and respiratory arrest.[155] The anesthetic effects last 1 to 2 hours, although the effects on respiration last longer. Unfortunately, some patients given a fentanyl patch to moderate pain have used the patch to commit suicide.[156]

The euphoria that fentanyl produces is briefer than the high from heroin. In many instances, fentanyl is combined with other drugs, especially heroin.[157] If one is unaware that fentanyl is mixed into other drugs, there is a greater potential for an adverse reaction. The potential for rapid addiction is strong. In California, an estimated 20% of people already dependent on opiates use a powerful derivative of fentanyl nicknamed **China white**. In 2005, more than 9,100 people went to emergency rooms because of fentanyl,[158] and between April 2005 and March 2007, 984 people died from nonpharmaceutical fentanyl. The vast majority of deaths occurred among males.[159]

Meperidine

A dangerous designer drug derived from **meperidine** (Demerol), MPTP is a synthetic derivative of morphine that produces powerful and unfortunate results. Although meperidine has only one-sixth the analgesic potency of morphine, it is highly toxic. Toxicity is marked by muscle twitching and convulsions. According to government statistics, 1,440 people were treated in emergency rooms because of meperidine in 2006.[160]

MPTP causes a Parkinson's-like condition that results in paralysis to the brain and nervous system. Symptoms of this condition can be improved, but not cured, through traditional treatment for Parkinson's disease.

Another analog derived from meperidine is **MPPP**. MPPP has the potential to be extremely toxic and leads to the synthesis of MPTP within the body.

MDMA

Also called Ecstasy, E, XTC, and Adam, **MDMA (methylenedioxymethamphetamine)** is a hallucinogen with amphetamine-like properties.[161] MDMA has been called a "psychedelic amphetamine."[162] First developed in 1914, MDMA is akin to the hallucinogen **MDA**. Intended originally as an appetite suppressant, it received little attention until it resurfaced in the 1960s. LSD and MDMA were available at the same time. LSD, however, did not evoke nausea and vomiting as MDMA did. After being promoted by illicit manufacturers, MDMA became more popular by the mid-1970s. By 1985, production had grown to about 500,000 doses.

Subsequently, MDMA became illegal. Punishment for trafficking could mean a 15-year imprisonment and a substantial fine. Despite its illegality and the substantial penalties associated with it, the demand and cost of MDMA increased throughout the 1990s (see Figure 2.3). However, its use is now declining.[163] One factor cited by college students for abstaining from MDMA use is the perceived lack of enjoyment from the drug.[164] As with other drugs,

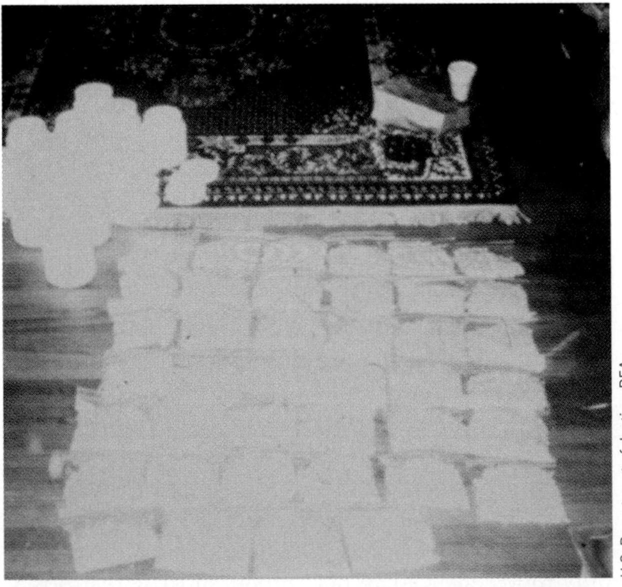

U.S. Department of Justice, DEA.

These batches of MDMA had been packaged for bulk distribution.

peers are influential in the use of or abstinence from MDMA.[165]

Today, MDMA is popular in many dance clubs, especially in Europe,[166] although recent studies found that its use at rave parties in the United States may have decreased.[167] Users claim that it "creates a loving presence and an improved orientation toward intimate relationships. And it deepens meditative calmness."[168] The percentage of students using MDMA is depicted in Table 2.7.

The side effects of MDMA include nausea, sleeplessness, loss of appetite, depression, headache, hangover, jaw clenching, teeth grinding, and panic. A serious immediate effect is heatstroke, because it can trigger convulsions or seizures and widespread blood clotting followed by collapse and coma. Death can result from MDMA use as well.[169] The drug accounted for 10,752 emergency room visits in 2005. In England and Wales, the number of deaths attributed to MDMA went from 20 in 1994 to 48 in 2006.[170]

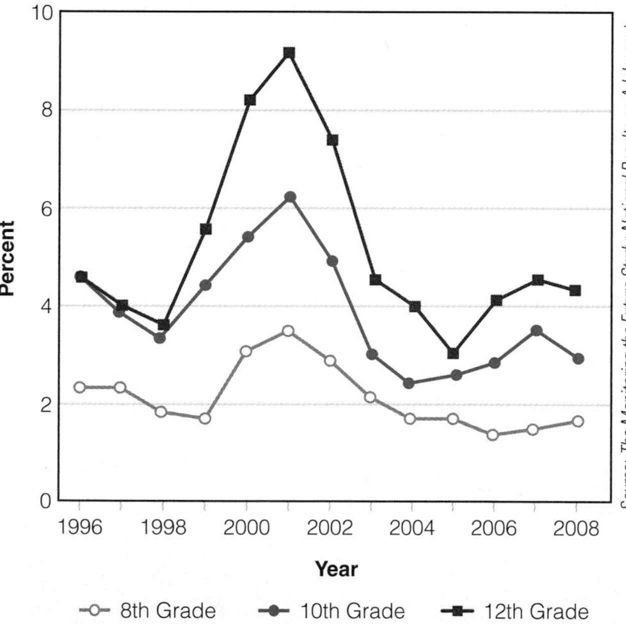

Figure 2.3 Ecstasy (MDMA): Trends in Annual Use, Grades 8, 10, and 12

TABLE 2.7 MDMA Use by Students: *Monitoring the Future* Survey, 2008

	8th Grade	10th Grade	12th Grade
Lifetime	2.4%	4.3%	6.2%
Past Year	1.7%	2.9%	4.3%
Past Month	0.8%	1.1%	1.8%

fentanyl A synthetic narcotic that is 1,000 times more potent than heroin

China white A synthetic analgesic drug, derived from fentanyl, that mimics heroin but is considerably more potent

meperidine A synthetic derivative of morphine

MPPP A synthetic drug that is similar to meperidine

MDMA (methylenedioxymethamphetamine) A synthetic hallucinogen related to amphetamines; also called Ecstasy

MDA A hallucinogen that is structurally similar to amphetamines

look-alike drugs Substances that appear similar to illegal or pharmaceutical drugs

sound-alike drugs Substances with names that sound similar to those of illegal or prescription drugs

A British study found that MDMA can result in depression,[171] whereas an Australian study noted that MDMA use may lead to Alzheimer's disease.[172]

In the 1970s, psychotherapists gave MDMA to their clients to reduce anxiety and facilitate communication. They believed the drug effectively elicited feelings of empathy and improved insight, attitudes, and interpersonal relationships.[173] The Food and Drug Administration (FDA) has approved studies to determine whether MDMA relieves physical pain and psychological trauma in dying cancer patients, chronic pain, and arthritis. In addition, there is research into whether MDMA is effective for treating post-traumatic stress disorder.[174] MDMA is erroneously believed to allow men to prolong sexual intercourse without ejaculating. Although it is labeled an aphrodisiac, MDMA actually hinders erection and inhibits orgasm in men and women. It has been implicated as a cause of decreased sexual desire.[175]

Current research shows that MDMA may affect the brain, although there is much controversy regarding the validity of the research demonstrating brain damage. Nonetheless, users experience problems with learning and memory, especially frequent users.[176] There is evidence that some women who used MDMA during pregnancy had babies with higher rates of congenital abnormalities.[177]

Look-Alike and Sound-Alike Drugs

Another contemporary phenomenon is the proliferation of **look-alike** and **sound-alike drugs**. Typically, they include over-the-counter preparations such as decongestants and antihistamines. These drugs commonly resemble legal drugs such as **biphetamine**, also known as "black widow." Another popular look-alike drug is referred to as "peashooter." An example of a sound-alike drug is herbal ecstasy. Some people confuse this stimulant, which often is purchased through mail-order catalogs, with MDMA.

In a study of medication errors due to sound-alike and look-alike drugs, it was found that 1.4% resulted in harm to patients, including seven patients who died. This same study noted 3,170 pairs of names that sounded or looked similar.[178] An example of two drugs that are mistaken is Januvia and Enjuvia. Januvia is used for treating type 2 diabetes, whereas Enjuvia is used to treat moderate symptoms associated with menopause.[179] Besides increasing the risk of exposure to undesirable side effects, this dilemma leads to an increase in cost.[180]

One factor leading to the increase of bogus drugs was a decline in prescriptions for diet pills. Much concern then arose over look-alike drugs containing caffeine, ephedra, and phenylpropanolamine, because many people using these drugs developed convulsions and fell into comas. In 1982, the FDA banned these products when used together. The FDA eventually banned all nonprescription stimulants containing products other than caffeine. Over-the-counter drugs for weight loss and relief of cold symptoms are still legal.

In 2000, the FDA requested that phenylpropanolamine (PPA) be removed from the hundreds of over-the-counter weight-loss products that contained it. Ephedra, which was implicated in the deaths of several professional athletes, was removed from the marketplace.[181]

The Drug Business

The drug trade is big business with no imminent signs of slowing down. In the 2008 budget, the federal government has allocated $2.18 billion to the DEA as well as $1.49 billion to the Department of State to deal with the drug trade.[182] Despite this vast sum of money, tactics for stopping the flow of drugs into the United States—using military force, reducing aid to countries where drugs are produced, and promoting crop substitution—have proved ineffective. Contributing to the difficulty in stopping the flow of drugs is the increased production of drugs in countries such as Colombia and Afghanistan.[183] According to the World Drug Report, there were 1.6 million drug seizure cases in 2006. Marijuana represented 65% of the seizure cases.[184] In the United States in 2007, 96,713 kilograms of cocaine were seized, 625 kilograms of heroin, 356,472 kilograms of marijuana, and 1.086 kilograms of methamphetamines.[185] Illegal drug profits are so high that a drug-trafficking organization could lose 90% of its product and still make money.[186] Most people may not realize the long-reaching tentacles of the drug trade.

Like ordinary consumers of ketchup or toothpaste, millions of Americans smoke marijuana, snort cocaine, or shoot up heroin without considering the long chain of manufacturers and middlemen who bring to their communities the quality products they demand. The supply lines are tortuous, threading from foreign fields, across seas and through fissures in the wall of domestic law enforcement. But the drugs do get through, despite the herculean efforts of

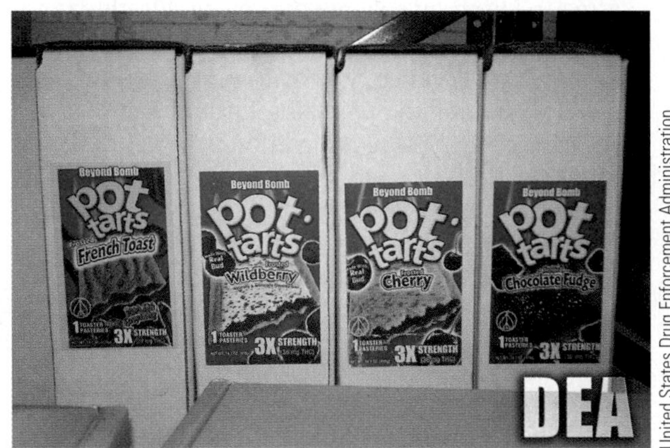

United States Drug Enforcement Administration

These "Pot-Tarts," seized by law enforcement in 2006, demonstrate the ingenuity of some illicit drug distributors. Upon raiding this facility, investigators found hundreds of marijuana-laced candies and soft drinks, including "Stoney Ranchers," "Munchy Way," "Rasta Reece's," and "Buddafingers."

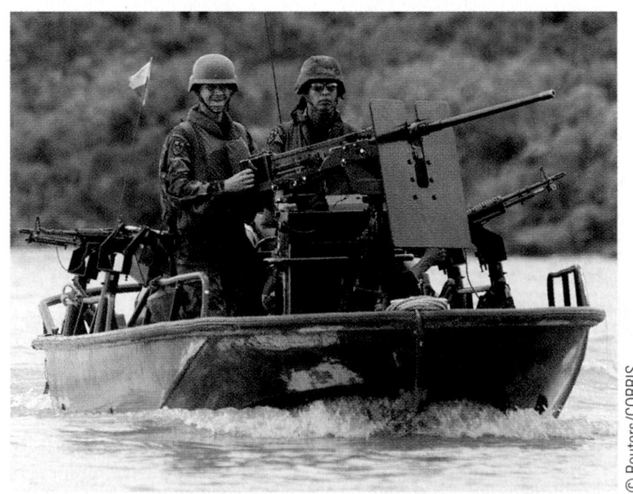

The federal government has steadily increased funding to interdict drugs.

the police, courts, and prisons to deter the traffic in mood-altering chemicals.[187]

Heroin and cocaine produced in South America has proliferated since the early 1990s. The United States has been successful in suppressing the drug trade along Colombia's Caribbean coast and by aerial spraying of coca crops. However, the Drug Enforcement Agency estimates that three-fourths of the cocaine coming into the United States departs from camps along the coastlines of Panama and Ecuador.[188] Domestic production of methamphetamines has declined, but that void was filled by Mexican drug organizations.[189]

The demise of the Soviet Union resulted in excessive poverty there, and with it renewed interest in the drug trade.[190] Thus, the drug trade expanded in former Soviet bloc countries.[191]

With American financing, Thailand is exporting marijuana it has processed. Lebanon is exporting heroin. The drug trade has destabilized some Latin American countries through bribery and intimidation. High-ranking government officials in the Bahamas, Mexico, Jamaica, and Honduras reportedly have been on the take.[192]

The economic clout of the drug trade is felt around the world. The increase in the narcotics trade in Eurasia and elsewhere is fueled by its tremendous profitability. In parts of Asia, drug money is used for lawlessness and bribery. In northern Burma, drug barons finance private armies to protect the fields of opium poppies. Officials in South Korea maintain that Internet use has contributed greatly to international drug trafficking.[193]

A country inundated with money obtained through the sale of illegal drugs is Colombia. After billions of dollars were spent, coca growth by farmers in Colombia rose 27%.[194] The former foreign minister described the enormity of Colombia's drug trade this way: "The size of this business overwhelms our economy. Just imagine if the United States had a Mafia richer than the federal budget." Colombian drug lords seldom go to jail in their country. Judges often face the choice of receiving a payoff or having their families killed. Colombians who fight the cocaine trade are tortured and killed.[195]

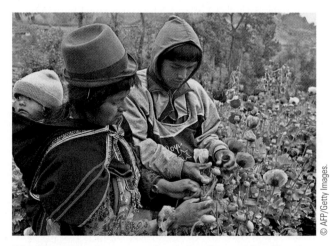

© AFP/Getty Images.

The benefits to farmers makes it hard to combat illegal drug production.

biphetamine A powerful stimulant

Halting the flow of drugs is difficult because cocaine sales result in extreme wealth for drug barons, banks' coffers are filled with money from the sale of drugs, and drug money reduces unemployment in Latin American countries. In an ironic twist, when counter-narcotics programs are effective, the cost of cocaine increases.[196] In essence, successful interdiction does not decrease profits.

Despite extradition of several top men of the cocaine cartel, cocaine continues to cross into the United States unabated. In recent years Colombian drug suppliers have used small, semi-submersible watercraft to smuggle cocaine into the United States.[197]

In addition to domestic production, marijuana is grown in Asia, the Caribbean, and Mexico, although Colombia is the largest exporter. Stopping the drug trade is like sticking a finger in a dike. No sooner is one hole plugged than another hole leaks. A number of leaders of antidrug campaigns in Europe and Russia feel that stemming the illegal drug trade is futile. They recommend that drugs such as cocaine be legalized in order to better regulate their use.[198] One author writes: "The war on illegal drugs engenders corruption, terrorism, and family breakdown, weakening America while strengthening our enemies."[199]

Preventing drugs from entering the United States or reducing the amount of drugs grown in the country is a matter of demand, not supply. Of the billions of dollars allocated to address drug-related problems, a minority of the money goes to demand reduction and the majority to supply reduction. Until demand decreases, drugs will always be abundantly available. Moreover, the resources of drug dealers for distributing drugs are greater than the resources aimed at interdicting drugs. In a 2008 poll, three-fourths of Americans indicated that the United States is losing the war on drugs. Although 25% thought that stopping drugs at the border was the best strategy for the war on drugs, slightly more felt that legalization of some drugs was best. Figure 2.4 shows how people responded when asked for their opinion about the best way to deal with the war on drugs.[200]

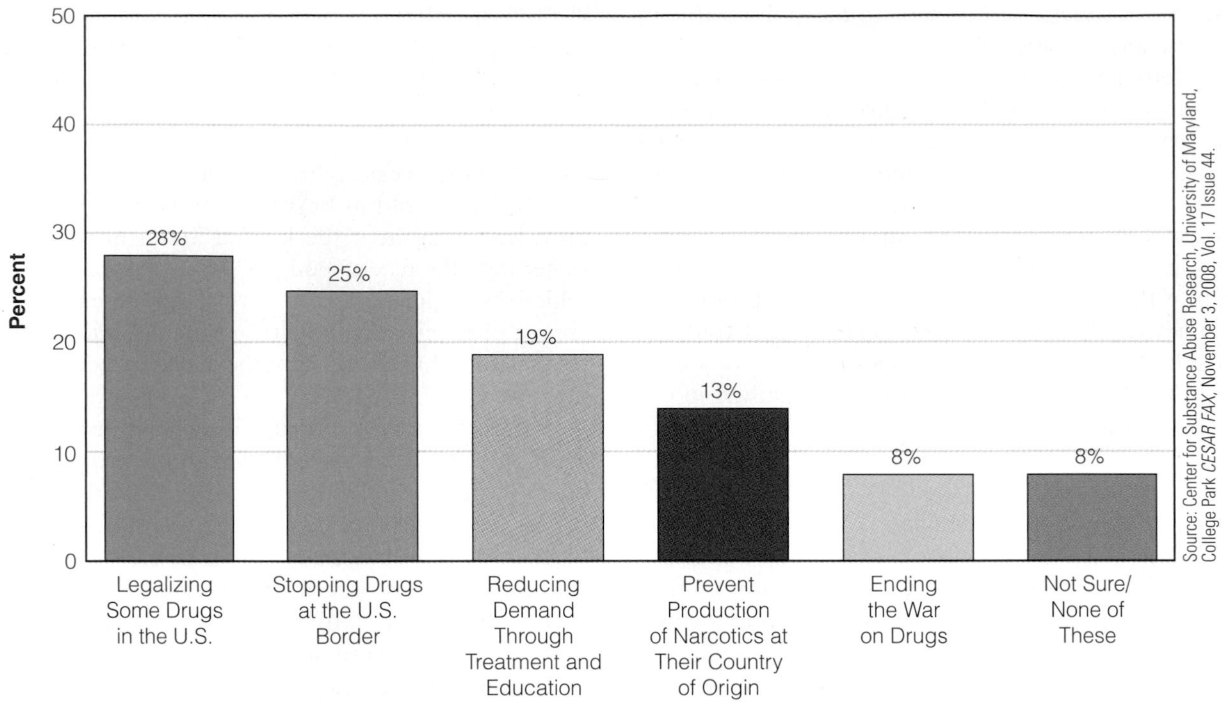

Figure 2.4 Poll Responses to the Question: "Which of the Following Do You Feel is the Single Best Way to Handle the War on Drugs?" (*n* = 4,730)

Summary

Drugs affect people throughout life, from the fetus to the elderly. Drug-use patterns vary considerably—from experimental use motivated by curiosity, to social-recreational use, to circumstantial-situational use, to intensified use, to compulsive use dictated by a psychic or physical need for drugs. The age group most likely to use illegal drugs is 18 to 25. National surveys pointed to an upward trend in the early 1990s, although modest declines are now occurring. As people perceive drugs to be harmful, the rate of use tends to go down.

To address drug use in the workplace, many companies have developed employee assistance programs (EAPs), designed to help employees deal with personal problems, including those that are drug related. The purpose of these drug programs is to help employees, not to punish them. Companies benefit from EAPs because they are able to retain already trained employees rather than having to replace them. As a condition of employment, many companies require applicants to take drug tests. The constitutionality of drug testing remains to be answered definitively.

Drug use has been linked to family instability and deviant behavior, including violence, although it is still uncertain whether the tie between drugs and violence reflects the type of person using the drugs or the effects of the drugs themselves. Alcohol is the drug most commonly related to violence. Drug use also correlates with crime. As the cost of drugs increases, the rate of criminal activity increases. Drug use also interferes with educational goals and career advancement.

One danger posed by drugs is their toxicity. Although many illegal drugs are toxic, the chronic use of cigarettes is the leading drug-related cause of death. Fatal and nonfatal drug incidents are monitored in the United States by the Drug Abuse Warning Network (DAWN).

Synthetic drugs, also termed designer drugs, present great potential for harm. Examples are fentanyl, meperidine, and MDMA. Many substances that look like and sound like current drugs can be purchased over the counter or by mail order.

One reason illegal drugs will continue to abound is that the drug trade is big business. In some instances money derived from growing and trading drugs helps to finance governments. In other cases the drug trade has destabilized countries. About half of all marijuana consumed illegally in the United States is grown domestically. Perhaps the most important factors contributing to the enormity of the drug trade are that drug traffickers have access to many financial, human, and sometimes political resources and that the demand for drugs continues to be high.

Thinking Critically

1. Are drugs really a problem in society, or is the concern excessive? The drawbacks to using drugs are numerous. In the attempt to reduce drug use and abuse, what is the best approach? Should drug policy focus on reducing the supply of drugs or the demand for drugs? Which approach would result in the least harm?
2. Drug testing, many argue, invades an individual's right to privacy. But employers contend that drugs cost their businesses, and therefore consumers, a great deal of money. How can the rights of the individual be balanced against the rights of the employer? Should regulations regarding testing be determined by the type of job—for example, airline pilot, sales clerk, nurse, carpenter? If so, which jobs would you include?
3. Do you believe that over-the-counter weight-reducing products should be more closely regulated? If so, how would this be accomplished?

Web Resources

National Clearinghouse for Alcohol and Drug Information
http://ncadi.samhsa.gov/
This site contains up-to-date developments and research in drug use.

The Weiner Nusim Foundation
http://www.weinernusim.com
Drug education materials are available through this Web site.

Notes

1. K. Musante, "Prescription Drug Sales Rate Hits 47-Year Low," *CnnMoney.com*, March 12, 2008.
2. R. Goldberg, *Taking Sides: Clashing Views on Controversial Issues in Drugs and Society,* 6th ed. (Guilford, CT: McGraw-Hill/Dushkin, 2004).
3. Office of Applied Studies, *Drug Abuse Warning Network, 2006: National Estimates of Drug-Related Emergency Room Visits* (Rockville, MD: U.S. Department of Health and Human Services, 2008).
4. A. McQueen, "Study: Drug Makers Pay More for Marketing Than Research," *Cortland Standard,* July 18, 2001.
5. United Nations Office on Drugs and Crimc, *World Drug Report 2008* (Geneva: The United Nations, 2008).
6. Office of National Drug Control Policy, *The Economic Costs of Drug Abuse in the United States* (Washington, DC: Government Printing Office, December 2004).
7. Office of National Drug Control Policy, *Current State of Drug Policy: Successes and Challenges* (Washington, DC: Government Printing Office, March 2008).
8. A. Kelly and J. Saucier, "Is Your Patient Suffering from Alcohol Withdrawal?" *RN,* 67 (February 2004): 27–33.
9. National Institute on Alcohol Abuse and Alcoholism, *Five Year Strategic Plan: FY08-13* (Bethesda, MD: NIAAA, 2008).
10. Office of National Drug Control Policy, *National Drug Control Strategy, 2009 Budget Summary* (Washington, DC: Government Printing Office, February 2008).
11. Ibid.
12. V. B. Faden and M. L. Baskin, "An Evaluation of College Online Alcohol-Policy Information," *Journal of American College Health,* 51 (November 2002): 18–36.
13. T. W. Maurer and D. W. Robinson, "Effects of Attire, Alcohol, and Gender on Perceptions of Date Rape," *Sex Roles,* 58 (2008): 423–434.
14. K. A. Parks, Y. P. Hsieh, C.M. Bradizza, and A. M. Romosz, "Factors Influencing the Temporal Relationship between Alcohol Consumption and Experiences with Aggression among College Women," *Psychology of Addictive Behaviors,* 22 (2008): 210–218.
15. G. Gmel and J. Rehm, *Harmful Alcohol Use* (Rockville, MD: National Institute on Alcohol Abuse and Alcoholism, 2003).
16. M. D. Stanton, "The Role of Family and Significant Others in the Engagement and Retention of Drug-Dependent Individuals," in *Beyond the Therapeutic Alliance: Keeping the Drug-Dependent Individual in Treatment,* edited by L. S. Onken, J. D. Blaine, and J. J. Boren (NIDA Research Monograph 165) (Washington, DC: U.S. Department of Health and Human Services, 1997).
17. J. Carroll, "Little Change in Public's View of the U.S. Drug Problem," *Gallup News Service,* October 19, 2007.
18. National Drug Intelligence Center, *National Drug Threat Assessment 2008* (Johnstown, PA: National Drug Intelligence Center, 2007).
19. American Cancer Society, *Cancer Facts & Figures 2008* (Atlanta: American Cancer Society, 2008).
20. Office of National Drug Control Policy, *The Economic Costs of Drug Abuse in the United States* (Washington, DC: Government Printing Office, December 2004).
21. R. L. DuPont, "Violence and Drugs," *Journal of Psychoactive Drugs,* 29 (1997): 303–305.
22. Bureau of Justice Statistics, *Drugs and Crime Facts* (Washington, DC: U.S. Department of Justice, 2008).
23. P. J. Goldstein, "The Drugs/Violence Nexus," in *The American Drug Scene,* edited by J. A. Inciardi and K. McElrath (Los Angeles: Roxbury Publishing Company, 2004).
24. I. Leshner, "Addressing the Medical Consequences of Drug Abuse," *NIDA Notes,* 15 (March 2000): 3–4.
25. Bureau of Justice Statistics, supra note 22.
26. L. D. Moore and A. Elkavich, "Who's Using and Who's Doing Time," *American Journal of Public Health,* 98 (September 2008): 176–180.
27. The NSDUH Report, *Substance Use During Pregnancy: 2002 and 2003 Update* (Rockville, MD: Office of Applied Studies, June 2, 2005).
28. L. M. Smith, et al., "Prenatal Methamphetamine Use and Neonatal Neurobehavioral Outcome," *Neurotoxicology and Teratology,* 30 (2008): 20–28.

29. J. R. Woods, "Clinical Management of Drug Dependency in Pregnancy," in *Medications Development for the Treatment of Pregnant Addicts and Their Infants,* edited by C. N. Chiang and L. P. Finnegan (NIDA Research Monograph 149) (Washington, DC: Government Printing Office, 1995).
30. J. Howard, *Substance Abuse Treatment for Persons with Child Abuse and Neglect Issues* (Rockville, MD; Center for Substance Abuse Treatment, 2000).
31. *SAMHSA News* (Rockville, MD: U.S. Department of Health and Human Services, July/August 2004).
32. M. P. Heron, D. L. Hoyert, J. Xu, Chester Scott, and B. Tejada-Vera, "Deaths: Preliminary Data for 2006," *National Vital Statistics Reports*, 56 (2008): 1–52.
33. W. J. Woods, A. L. Avins, C. P. Lindan, E. S. Hudes, J. A. Boscarino, and W. W. Clark, "Predictors of HIV-Related Behaviors Among Heterosexuals in Alcoholism Treatment," *Journal of Studies on Alcohol,* 486–493.
34. *The Centers for Disease Control and Prevention Announces New HIV Incidence Estimates for the United States* (Atlanta: Centers for Disease Control, 2008).
35. Ibid.
36. *Sterile Syringe Access* (Needle Exchange), Drug Policy Alliance Network, 2006.
37. The NSDUH Report, *Substance Use in the 15 Largest Metropolitan Statistical Areas: 2002–2005* (Rockville, MD: Office of Applied Studies, January 5, 2007.
38. J. Steinhauer, "Nightclubs Hire Ambulances for Overdoses, Skipping 911," *New York Times,* April 20, 2001.
39. Office of National Drug Control Policy, supra note 10.
40. P. Mendes, "Zero Tolerance or International Conspiracy: A Critical Analysis of the House of Representatives Inquiry into Illicit Drugs," *Social Alternatives*, 27 (2008): 51–55.
41. P. B. Stares, "Drug Legalization: Time for a Real Debate," *Brookings Review,* 14 (1996): 18–20.
42. R. G. Smart, "What I Would Most Like to Know: What Are the Rules of Thumb for Avoiding Problem Drug Use?" *Addiction,* 88 (1993): 179–181.
43. E. Goode, *Drugs in American Society,* 7th ed. (New York: McGraw-Hill, 2007).
44. Ibid.
45. A. Mann, "Relationships Matter: Impact of Parental, Peer Factors on Teen, Young Adult Substance Abuse," *NIDA Notes,* 18 (August 2003): 11–13.
46. D. Wright and M. Pemberton, *Risk and Protective Factors for Adolescent Drug Use: Findings from the National Household Survey on Drug Abuse* (Rockville, MD: Office of Applied Studies, Substance Abuse and Mental Health Services Administration, 2004).
47. Ibid.
48. National Commission on Marihuana and Drug Abuse, *Drug Use in America: Problem in Perspective* (Washington, DC: Government Printing Office, 1973).
49. B. Powis, P. Griffiths, M. Gossop, and J. Strang, "The Differences Between Male and Female Drug Users: Community Samples of Heroin and Cocaine Users Compared," *Substance Use and Misuse,* 31 (1996): 529–543.
50. Mann, supra note 45.
51. M. P. Marshal, et al., "Sexual Orientation and Adolescent Substance Use: A Meta-analysis and Methodological Review," *Addiction*, 103 (April 2008): 546.
52. H. Wyatt, "Teens Cite Ease of Access to Drugs," *The Washington Post,* August 14, 2008: A2.
53. D. Hakim, "State Watch for 2 Percent of Doctors," *The New York Times*, May 7, 2008: B1.
54. H. A. Siegal and J. A. Inciardi, "A Brief History of Alcohol," in *The American Drug Scene,* edited by J. A. Inciardi and K. McElroth (Los Angeles: Roxbury Publishing Company, 2004).
55. National Commission, supra note 48.
56. Substance Abuse and Mental Health Services Administration, *Results from the 2006 National Survey on Drug Use and Health: National Findings* (Rockville, MD: Office of Applied Studies, Substance Abuse and Mental Health Services Administration, September 2007).
57. Ibid.
58. Substance Abuse and Mental Health Services Administration, *Results from the 2007 National Survey on Drug Use and Health: National Findings* (Rockville, MD: Office of Applied Statistics, 2008).
59. L. D. Johnston, P. M. O'Malley, J. G. Bachman, and J. E. Schulenberg, *Monitoring the Future: National Results on Adolescent Drug Use* (Bethesda, MD: National Institute on Drug Use, 2009).
60. Substance Abuse and Mental Health Services Administration, *Drug Abuse Warning Network, 2006: National Estimates of Drug-Related Emergency Department Visits* (Rockville, MD: U.S. Department of Health and Human Services, 2008).
61. Ibid.
62. T. Nighswonger, "Just Say Yes to Preventing Substance Abuse," *Occupational Hazards,* 13 (April 2000).
63. S. L. Larson, J. Eyerman, M. S. Foster, and J. C. Gfroerer, *Worker Substance Use and Workplace Policies and Programs* (Rockville, MD: Substance Abuse and Mental Health Services Administration, Office of Applied Studies, 2007).
64. Ibid.
65. M. M. Lehtola, et al., "The Effectiveness of Interventions for Preventing Injuries in the Construction Industry: A Systematic Review," *American Journal of Preventive Medicine*, 35 (July 2008): 77–85.
66. Office of National Drug Control Policy, "Methamphetamine, Cocaine Use Plummet: New Workplace Drug Testing Data Show Effects of Supply Crunch," Press Release, March 12, 2008.
67. M. Prince, "Battling Workplace Drug Use: Employers Confronting the Costs of Chemical Dependency," *Business Insurance*, 35 (January 29, 2001): 20–23.
68. T. W. Mangione, J. Howland, B. Amick, J. Cote, M. Lee, N. Bell, and S. Levine, "Employee Drinking Practices and Work Performance," *Journal of Studies on Alcohol,* 60 (1999): 261–270.
69. J. P. Leigh, "Alcohol Abuse and Job Hazards," *Journal of Safety Research,* 27 (1996): 17–32.
70. *Alcohol and Health, Tenth Special Report to the U.S. Congress* (Rockville, MD: U.S. Department of Health and Human Services, 2000).
71. Nighswonger, supra note 62.
72. "Working Teens May Drink More Alcohol," *Alcoholism and Drug Abuse Weekly,* 16 (January 26, 2004): 8.
73. K. Gurchiek, "Employer Testing Credited for Lower Drug-Use," *HR Magazine*, 52 (June 2007): 36–41.
74. J. McKinley, "Ruling Puts Workplace Limits on California Marijuana Law," *The New York Times*, January 25, 2008: 16.
75. H. Tramer, "EAPs Help Companies Cope with Substance Abuse," *Crain's Cleveland Business*, 29 (February 11, 2008): 19.
76. R. Selvik, D. Stephenson, C. Plaza, and B. Sugden, "EAP Outcome on Work, Relationships, and Health Outcomes," *The Journal of Employee Assistance,* 12 (April 2004): 18–22.
77. Ibid.
78. "Hazelden Launches Campaign to Change Employer Attitudes," *Alcoholism and Drug Abuse*

Weekly, 15 (December 15, 2003): 1–4.
79. Ibid.
80. G. Beato, "The Golden Age," *Reason,* 39 (March 2008): 14–15.
81. "Debate Over Controversial Workplace Drug Test," *Drug Policy Alliance Newsletter* (July 22, 2004): 6.
82. R. L. DuPont, D. W. Griffin, B. R. Siskin, S. Shirake, and E. Katze, "Random Drug Tests at Work: The Probability of Identifying Frequent and Infrequent Users of Illicit Drugs," *Journal of Addictive Diseases,* 14 (1995): 1–17.
83. "Workplace Bill Reauthorization Would Boost Anti-Drug Coalition," *Alcoholism and Drug Abuse Weekly,* 16 (June 28, 2004): 1–2.
84. T. L. Stanley, "Workplace Drug Testing and the Growing Problem of Methamphetamines," *Supervision,* 68 (August 2007): 3–5.
85. Nighswonger, supra note 62.
86. P. K. Hersch and R.F. Cook, "Workplace Substance Abuse Prevention," *Prevention Pipeline,* 13 (May/June 2000): 3–7.
87. T. A. DeMitchell, S. Kossakoski, and T. Baldasaro, "To Test or Not to Test? Drug Testing Teachers: The View of the Superintendent," *Teachers College Record,* 110 (June 2008): 1207–1240.
88. L. Jacobson, "Teacher Drug-Testing Program in Hawaii Stalls Over Who Will Pay," *Education Week,* 27 (July 30, 2008): 16–17.
89. P. K. Hersch and R.F. Cook, "Workplace Substance Abuse Prevention," *Prevention Pipeline,* 13 (May/June 2000): 3–7.
90. H. V. Kunins, C. Chazotte, E. Du, and J. H. Arnsten, "The Effect of Race on Provider Decisions to Test for Illicit Drug Use in the Peripartum Setting," *Journal of Women's Health,* 16 (March 2007): 245–255.
91. K. Pulatie, "The Legality of Drug-Testing Procedures for Pregnant Women," *Virtual Monitor,* 10 (January 2008): 41–44.
92. Ibid.
93. R. Goldberg, supra note 2.
94. E. Davis, R. Loiacono, and R. J. Summers, "The Rush to Adrenaline: Drugs in Sport Acting on the (Beta)-Adrenergic System," *British Journal of Pharmacology,* 154 (June 2008): 584–597.
95. C. Ringwalt, et al., "Random Drug Testing in US Public School Districts," *American Journal of Public Health,* 98 (May 2008): 826–828.
96. Office of National Drug Control Policy, *What We Need to Know About Drug Testing in Schools* (Washington, DC: Government Printing Office, 2002).
97. J. Wilgoren, "Court Rulings Signal a Shift on Random Drug Tests in Schools," *New York Times,* March 25, 2001.
98. J. M. Berning, K. J. Adams, M. DeBeliso, B. A. Stamford, and I. M. Newman, "Anabolic Androgenic Steroids: Use and Perceived Use in Nonathlete College Students," *Journal of American College Health,* 56 (2008): 499–504.
99. "Few Positive Tests in Texas," *The New York Times,* July 24, 2008: 7.
100. "A Level Playing Field," *Nature,* 454 (August 7, 2008): 667.
101. J. Tierney, "Let the Games Be Doped," *The New York Times,* August 12, 2008: F1.
102. E. Mika, "Drug Busters," *Popular Science,* 270 (February 2007): 34.
103. D. Lewis, C. Moore, P. Morrissey, and J. Leikin, "Determination of Drug Exposure Using Hair: Application to Child Protective Services," in *Problems of Drug Dependence,* edited by L. S. Harris (Proceedings of 58th Annual Scientific Meeting, NIDA Research Monograph 174) (Rockville, MD: National Institute on Drug Abuse, 1997).
104. T. H. Saey, "Genetics May Affect Athlete Doping Tests," *Science News,* 173 (March 29, 2008): 195.
105. L. H. Glantz, "A Nation of Suspects: Drug Testing and the Fourth Amendment," *American Journal of Public Health,* 79 (1989): 1427–1431.
106. D. G. Kilpatrick, "Victimization and Posttraumatic Stress Disorder," in *Drug Addiction Research and the Health of Women,* edited by C. L. Wetherington and A. B. Roman (Rockville, MD: National Institute of Drug Abuse, 1998).
107. E. Smit, J. Verdurmen, K. Monshouwer, and F. Smit, "Family Interventions and Their Effect on Adolescent Alcohol Use in General Populations; A Meta-analysis of Randomized Controlled Studies," *Drug and Alcohol Dependence,* 97 (October 2008): 195–206.
108. C. Orte, C. Touza, L. Ballester, and M. March, "Children of Drug-Dependent Parents: Prevention Programme Outcomes," *Educational Research,* 50 (September 2008): 249–260.
109. S. K. Kubetin, "Highly Monitored Teens Less Likely to Drink: Parental Engagement Matters," *Child Psychiatry News,* 31 (November 2003): 38.
110. L. A. Strohschein, "Prevalence of Methylphenidate Use Among Canadian Children Following Parental Divorce," *Canadian Medical Association Journal,* 176 (June 5, 2007): 1711–1714.
111. T. Korhonen, et al., "Role of Individual, Peer and Family Factors in the Use of Cannabis and Other Illicit Drugs: A Longitudinal Analysis Among Finnish Adolescent Twins," *Drug and Alcohol Dependence,* 97 (September 2008): 33–43.
112. G. G. Homish, K. E. Leonard, and J. R. Cornelius, "Illicit Drug Use and Marital Satisfaction," *Addictive Behaviors,* 33 (February 2008): 279–291.
113. G. J. Duncan, B. Wilkerson, and P. England, "Cleaning Up Their Act: The Effects of Marriage and Cohabitation on Licit and Illicit Drug Use," *Demography,* 43 (November 2006): 691–705.
114. R. Collins, P. L. Ellickson, and D. J. Klein, "The Role of Substance Use in Young Adult Divorce," *Addiction,* 102 (May 2007): 786–794.
115. "Successful Treatment for Adolescents: Multiple Needs Require Diverse and Special Services," *Substance Abuse in Brief* (January 2000): 1–3.
116. K. Street, et al., "Is Adequate Parenting Compatible with Maternal Drug Use? A 5-year Follow-up," *Child: Care, Health and Development,* 34 (March 2008): 204–206.
117. S. Y. Hill, et al., "Psychopathology in Offspring from Multiplex Alcohol Dependence Families with and without Parental Alcohol Dependence: A Prospective Study during Childhood and Adolescence," *Psychiatry Research,* 160 (August 2008): 155–166.
118. D. A. Gibbs, et al., "Child Maltreatment and Substance Abuse among U.S. Army Soldiers," *Child Maltreatment,* 13 (August 2008): 259–268.
119. M. Engstrom, N. El-Bassel, H. Go, and L. Gilbert, "Childhood Sexual Abuse and Intimate Partner Violence among Women in Methadone Treatment: A Direct or Mediated Relationship," *Journal of Family Violence,* 23 (October 2008): 605–617.
120. S. T. Chermak, et al., "Partner Aggression among Men and Women in Substance Use Disorder Treatment: Correlates of Psychological and Physical Aggression and Injury," *Drug and Alcohol Dependence,* 98 (November 2008): 35–44.
121. D. A. Baltieri and A. G. de Andrade, "Alcohol and Drug Consumption among Sexual Offenders," *Forensic Science International,* 175 (February 2008): 31–35.
122. I. Way and D. Urbaniak, "Delinquent Histories of Adolescents Adjudicated

for Criminal Sexual Conduct," *Journal of Interpersonal Violence,* 23 (September 2008): 1197–1212.
123. L. Spak, F. Spak, and P. Allebeck, "Sexual Abuse and Alcoholism in a Female Population," *Addiction,* 93 (1998): 1365–1373.
124. T. J. Jarvis and J. Copelend, "Child Sexual Abuse as a Predictor of Psychiatric Co-morbidity and Its Implications for Drug and Alcohol Treatment," *Drug and Alcohol Dependence,* 49 (1997): 61–69.
125. Gmel and Rehm, supra note 15.
126. C. S. Widom, T. Ireland, and P. J. Glynn, "Alcohol Abuse in Abused and Neglected Children Followed-up: Are They at Increased Risk?" *Journal of Studies on Alcohol,* 56: 207–217.
127. Wright and Pemberton, supra note 46.
128. R. Jessor and S. L. Jessor, "A Social-Psychological Framework for Studying Drug Use," in *Theories on Drug Abuse: Selected Contemporary Perspectives,* edited by D. J. Lettieri, M. Sayers, and H. W. Pearson (NIDA Research Monograph 30) (Washington, DC: U.S. Government Printing Office, 1980).
129. Goode, supra note 43.
130. L. A. Drapela and C. Mosher, "The Conditional Effect of Parental Attachment and Adolescent Drug Use: Social Control and Social Development Model Perspectives," *Journal of Child and Adolescent Substance Abuse,* 16 (2007): 63–87.
131. "Report: Five Million Parents Have Alcohol Problems," *Alcoholism and Drug Abuse Weekly,* 16 (February 23, 2004): 3–4.
132. S. Wells, K. Graham, and P. West, "Alcohol-Related Aggression in the General Population," *Journal of Studies on Alcohol,* 61 (2000): 626–632.
133. R. Delgado, "Alcohol Blamed for 1400 Student Deaths, 70,000 Sex Assaults a Year," *San Francisco Chronicle* (April 10, 2002): A1.
134. Bureau of Justice Statistics, *Drug Use and Crime* (Washington, D.C.: United States Department of Justice, 2008).
135. B. S. Marquart, D. K. Nanninni, R. W. Edwards, L. R. Stanley, and J. C. Wayman, "Prevalence of Dating Violence. And Victimization: Regional and Gender Differences," *Adolescence,* 42 (Winter 2007): 645–657.
136. S. T. Chermack and S. T. Taylor, "Alcohol and Human Physical Aggression: Pharmacological Versus Expectancy Effects," *Journal of Studies on Alcohol,* 56 (1995): 449–456.
137. "Substance Use Among School Dropouts," *The NSDUH Report* (November 2003): 1–4.
138. J. H. Williams, L. E. Davis, S. D. Johnson, and T. R. Williams, "Substance Use and Academic Performance among African American High School Students," *Social Work Research,* 31 (Sept 2007): 151–161.
139. M. Lynskey and W. Hall, "The Effects of Adolescent Cannabis Use on Educational Attainment: A Review," *Addiction,* 95 (2000): 1621–1630.
140. V. S. Harder and H. D. Chilcoat, "Cocaine Use and Educational Achievement: Understanding a Changing Association Over the Past 2 Decades," *American Journal of Public Health,* 97 (October 2007): 1790–1793.
141. D. M. Fergusson and J. M. Boden, "Cannabis Use and Later Life Outcomes," *Addiction,* 103 (June 2008): 969.
142. B. Curley, "Legislation to End Student Aid Penalty Stumbles," *Join Together* (December 17, 2007).
143. C. Mulligan, B. Dolber, K. Wibby, and D. Borden, *Falling Through the Cracks: Loss of State-Based Financial Aid Eligibility for Students Affected by the Federal Higher Education Act Drug Provision* (Washington, D.C.: Coalition for Higher Education Act Reform, 2006).
144. D. Heien, "The Relationship Between Alcohol Consumption and Earnings," *Journal of Studies on Alcohol,* 57 (1996): 536–542.
145. C. S. Rosen, E. Kuhn, M. A. Greenbaum, and K. D. Drescher, "Substance Abuse-Related Mortality among Middle-Aged Male Psychiatric Patients," *Psychiatric Services,* 59 (March 2008): 290–296.
146. E. Maloney, L. Degenhardt, S. Darke, R. P. Mattick, and E. Nelson, "Suicidal Behavior and Associated Risk Factors among Opioid-dependent Individuals: A Case-Control Study," *Addiction,* 102 (December 2007): 1933.
147. Substance Abuse Mental Health Service Services Administration, *Drug Abuse Warning Network, 2003: Area Profiles of Drug-Related Mortality* (Rockville, MD: Department of Health and Human Services, 2005).
148. Ibid.
149. C. J. Cherpitel and Y. Ye, "Drug Use and Problem Drinking Associated with Primary Care and Emergency Room Utilization in the US General Population: Data from the 2005 National Alcohol Survey," *Drug and Alcohol Dependence,* 97 (October 2008): 226–230.
150. S. Morrison, "The Dynamics of Illicit Drug Production: Future Sources and Threats," *Crime, Law and Social Change,* 27 (1997): 1121–1138.
151. D. M. Grilly, *Drugs and Human Behavior,* 5th ed. (Pearson, 2005).
152. B. Venhuis, L. Blok-Tip, and D. de Kaste, "Designer Drugs in Herbal Aphrodisiacs," *Forensic Science International,* 177 (May 2008): 25–27.
153. S. B. Karch, *Karch's Pathology of Drug Abuse,* 4th ed. (Taylor and Francis, 2008).
154. H. E. Doweiko, *Concepts of Chemical Dependency,* 7th ed. (Cengage Learning, 2008).
155. *PDR Family Guide to Prescription Drugs* (Montvale, NJ: Thomson Healthcare Company, 2003).
156. D. A. Lounsbury and D. J. George, "The Fentanyl Patch at the Crime Scene," *Journal of Forensic Identification,* 57 (July/August 2007): 512–521.
157. Office of Diversion Control. *National Forensic Laboratory Information System (NFLIS) Special Report: Fentanyl, 2003–2006* (Washington, D.C.: U. S. Drug Enforcement Agency, 2008).
158. Office of Applied Studies, supra note 60.
159. "Nonpharmaceutical Fentanyl-Related Deaths—Multiple States, April 2005–March 2007," *MMWR (Morbidity and Mortality Weekly Report),* 57 (July 25, 2008).
160. Office of Applied Studies, supra note 60.
161. *NIDA InfoFacts: MDMA (Ecstasy)* (Rockville, MD: National Institute on Drug Abuse, August 2008).
162. Doweiko, supra note 154
163. Johnston et al., supra note 59.
164. H. Rosenberg, et al., "Attributions for Abstinence from Illicit Drugs by University Students," *Drugs: Education, Prevention and Policy,* 15 (August 2008): 365–377.
165. H. K. Vervaeke, L. van Deursen, and D. J. Korf, "The Role of Peers in the Initiation and Continuation of Ecstasy Use," *Substance Use and Misuse,* 43 (2008): 633–646.
166. "Ecstasy, Amphetamine Use on the Rise Worldwide," *Alcoholism and Drug Abuse Weekly,* 15 (September 29, 2003): 7–8.
167. G. S. Yacoubian and R. J. Peters, "An Exploration of Recent Club Drug Use among Rave," *Journal of Drug Education,* 37 (2007): 145–161.
168. E. Taylor, "Psychedelics: The Second Coming," *Psychology Today* (July/Aug, 1996): 57–59.
169. A. Sauvageau, "Death from a Possible Anaphylactic Reaction to Ecstasy," *Clinical Toxicology,* 46 (2008): 156.
170. *Deaths Related to Drug Poisoning, England and*

Wales (Great Britain: Office of National Statistics, 2007).
171. "Ecstasy Could Increase Risk of Developing Depression," *Mental Health Weekly,* 13 (April 7, 2003): 7–8.
172. "Ecstasy Use Could Lead to Alzheimer's Disease," *Alcoholism and Drug Abuse Weekly,* 15 (August 11, 2003): 8.
173. Grilly, supra note 151.
174. A. Turner, "Ecstasy Is the Key to Treating PTSD," *The Sunday Times,* May 4, 2008.
175. S. de Sola Llopsis, et al., "Cognitive Performance in Recreational Ecstasy Polydrug Users: A Two-Year Follow-up Study," *Journal of Psychopharmacology,* 22 (July 2008): 498–510.
176. W. W. Finger, M. Lund, and M. A. Slagel, "Medications That May Contribute to Sexual Disorders: A Guide to Assessment and Treatment in Family Practice," *Journal of Family Practice,* 44 (1997): 33–44.
177. R. Wood and L. Synovitz, "Addressing the Threats of MDMA (Ecstasy): Implications for School Health Professionals," *Journal of School Health,* 71 (January 2001): 38–51.
178. M. Barbella, "USP Report Shows Drug Mix-ups on the Rise, Jeopardizing Patient Safety," *Drug Topics,* 152 (March 10, 2008): 1.
179. "Take Steps to Avoid Confusing These Two Sound-Alike Drugs," *RN,* 70 (January 2007): 62.
180. M. C. Joshi, et al., "A Prospective Study of Medication Errors Arising Out of Look-Alike and Sound-Alike Brand Name Confusion," *International Journal of Risk and Safety in Medicine,* 19 (2007): 195–201.
181. P. Solotaroff, "Ban Ephedra Now!" *Men's Journal* (May 2003): 39.
182. Office of National Drug Control Policy, *National Drug Control Strategy, 2009 Budget Summary* (Washington, DC: Government Printing Office, February 2008).
183. *World Drug Report 2008* (United Nations Office on Drugs and Crime, 2008).
184. Ibid.
185. *DEA Drug Seizures* (Washington, DC: U.S. Drug Enforcement Administration, 2007).
186. K. E. Sharpe, "Addicted to the Drug War," *Chronicle of Higher Education* (October 6, 2000).
187. J. Marshall, "Drugs and the United States Foreign Policy," in *Dealing with Drugs: Consequences of Government Control,* edited by R. Hamowy (Lexington, MA: D. C. Heath, 1987).
188. A. D. Russell, "Colombia Coast Becomes Drug-War Focus," *Narcotics Law Bulletin,* 34 (September 2007): 5.
189. "Mexican Traffickers Distributing More 'Ice' in U.S., Drug Agency Says," *Criminal Justice Newsletter* (November 1, 2007): 4.
190. S. Flynn, "Worldwide Drug Scourge: The Expanding Trade in Illicit Drugs," *Brookings Review* (Winter 1993): 6–11.
191. R. W. Lee and S. B. MacDonald, "Drugs in the East," *Foreign Policy,* 90 (1993): 89–107.
192. L. Kraar, "The Drug Trade," *Fortune* (June 20, 1998): 27–29.
193. "Drug Trade Through Internet Soaring, Says South Korean Prosecution Chief," *Yonhap News Agency,* September 24, 2008.
194. "A Hulking Drug Problem; After 8 Years and Billions Spent, Cocaine Production in South America Appears Bulletproof," *Los Angeles Times,* July 1, 2008.
195. R. Conniff, "Columbia's Dirty War, Washington's Dirty Hands," *Progressive* (May 1992): 20–27.
196. "US Claims Cocaine Prices Increase Due to Enforcement Successes," *Narcotics Law Bulletin,* 34 (December 2007): 3.
197. K. Ellingwood, "The World; 20,000 Kilos Under the Sea; Mexico Seems to Have a New Problem in Its Drug War; Homemade Mini-Subs That Are Hard to Spot on Radar," *Los Angeles Times,* July 18, 2008.
198. P. O. Coffin, "A Duty to Censor: U.N. Officials Want to Crack Down on Drug War Protesters," *Reason,* 30 (1999): 54–55.
199. R. Leeson, "Addicted to the Drug War," *Hoover Digest* (Winter 2007): 80–84.
200. Zogby International, "Zogby Interactive Likely Voters 9/23/08 Through 9/25/08," http://www.zogby.com/news/X-IAD.pdf.

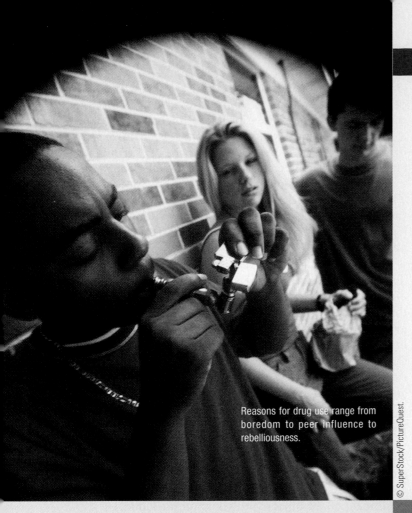

Reasons for drug use range from boredom to peer influence to rebelliousness.

FACT OR FICTION?

1. The most common reason for young people to try drugs is peer pressure.
2. Parents who abuse drugs are more likely to have children who abuse drugs.
3. Students who attend religious services regularly are less likely to use drugs.
4. It is more difficult to overcome physical dependency than to overcome psychological dependency.
5. After the attacks at the World Trade Center on September 11, 2001, there was an increase in drug use.
6. Most Americans support banning alcohol advertisements during college sports on television.
7. Even though cigarettes cannot be advertised on television, they can still be advertised on the radio.
8. The most common illegal drug portrayed in music videos is Ecstasy.
9. Steroids have no medical value.
10. Stimulants may increase cardiovascular endurance but may be lethal because they cause dehydration.

Turn the page to check your answers

3 Motivations for Drug Use

Chapter Objectives

After completing this chapter, the reader should be able to describe:

- How patterns of drug use reflect changes in society
- Reasons that motivate experimental, occasional, and chronic use of drugs
- The importance of peers and family on drug use
- The influence of society on the use of drugs
- The differences between drug addiction and drug dependency
- Personality traits associated with drug dependency
- How advertisers promote the use of alcohol, tobacco products, and prescription drugs
- The impact of the media on drug use
- How drugs affect athletic performance
- How drugs affect sexual performance

FACT OR FICTION?

1. **Fiction:** The fact is—Curiosity and experimentation are the most common reasons that young people try drugs.
2. **Fact:** Parents serve as strong role models for their children. Thus, if they abuse drugs, it is more likely that their children will abuse drugs.
3. **Fact:** More than two-thirds of students who attend religious services regularly report using drugs less frequently than students who do not attend religious services regularly.
4. **Fiction:** The fact is—It is easier to rid the body of the need for drugs than to get a person to no longer desire drugs.
5. **Fact:** There was a marked increase in drug use after the September 11, 2001, attacks.
6. **Fact:** Nearly three of four Americans support prohibiting alcohol advertisements during college sporting events.
7. **Fiction:** The fact is—The ban on advertising tobacco applies to radio as well as to television.
8. **Fiction:** The fact is—The most common illegal drug portrayed in music videos is marijuana, followed by cocaine.
9. **Fiction:** The fact is—Steroids have been prescribed to treat "wasting away" syndrome as well as to help undersized children develop.
10. **Fact:** Stimulants, including caffeine, increase endurance, but a number of athletes have died while competing after taking stimulants.

In many ways, drug use mirrors the broader society. Reasons for drug use and the needs that drugs fulfill are affected by societal changes. In our scientifically advanced, technological world, change occurs so rapidly that our ability to adapt cannot keep pace. Many inventions of the 20th century provide instant or immediate feedback: computers offer instant access to information; banks with automatic teller machines dispense money at any time of the day or night; fast-food restaurants and microwave ovens satisfy hunger speedily; pregnancy test kits let us know in a short time whether prenatal checkups are needed; communication with friends is instantaneous through our telephones. People adapt to a changing society by learning to cope, by withdrawing, or by escaping. Drugs are one means to that end.

Alternatives to using drugs include exercise programs, support groups, Internet games, watching television, listening to music, talking to friends, taking walks, and reading. In view of these alternatives, and others, why are drugs so popular?

Reasons for Drug Use

Drugs are easy to use, and they work quickly. If a person desires to alter consciousness, drugs can accomplish this relatively easily; little effort is required to inhale marijuana, swallow a pill, snort cocaine, or drink alcohol. Drugs are a quick fix. To overcome illness or to experience pleasure quickly, some people look to drugs because they fulfill immediate needs. This feature of modern society is called *immediacy,* the desire and expectation that things should be handled rapidly. It could well be the main reason that people use drugs.

People use drugs for many other reasons, too. The family structure and society have changed dramatically. Both parents working outside the home, the rising cost of living, the emphasis on immediate gratification, mass media, and the high degree of mobility—all have contributed to stresses on the family.[1] To deal with these stresses, some people experiment with drugs, others use drugs occasionally, and still others take drugs frequently or compulsively.

Experimentation

Curiosity is a common reason to try drugs. Especially among young people, curiosity is a natural phenomenon that easily leads to experimentation. Infants continually place objects in their mouths. Children cannot wait to open a package to find out its contents. Many schools inadvertently arouse interest and curiosity in drugs through "drug awareness programs," in which former addicts, police officers, pharmacists, judges, physicians, clergy, or drug therapists talk to students about the dangers of drugs. Newspapers and popular magazines contain articles about drugs, particularly drug use by well-known athletes, politicians,

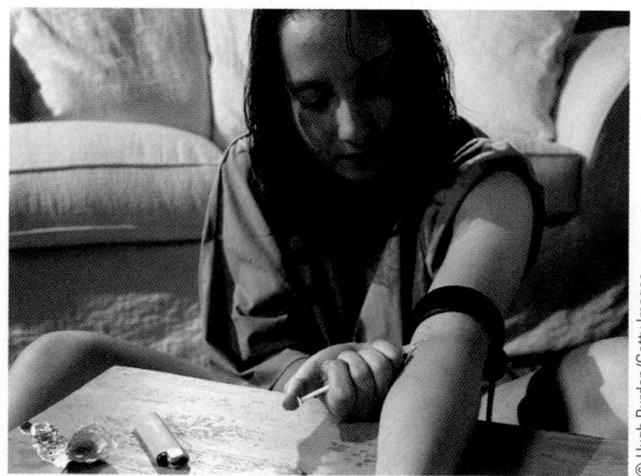

People who inject drugs are more likely to be compulsive drug users.

musicians, and actors. About 14.1% of 8th-grade students reported that they had experimented with an illegal drug in the previous year. About 7.6% had used an illegal drug in the previous 30 days.[2]

Adolescents are no exception. Among Norwegian girls, the mean age for the initiation of alcohol consumption is 14.8 years, and the younger they are when starting to use alcohol, the more likely they are to have problems with alcohol.[3] Girls who begin drinking at an older age have fewer alcohol-related problems. People who begin drinking before age 15 are four times more likely to develop alcohol dependence compared with those who begin drinking after age 20.[4] Similarly, the earlier children experiment with cigarettes, the more likely they are to become regular smokers.[5]

Some adolescents experiment with drugs due to poor impulse control or simply due to a lack of maturity.[6] Also, the use of one type of drug may lead to experimentation with another drug. For example, marijuana users who do not view marijuana use as having adverse effects are more likely to experiment with ecstasy.[7]

Pleasure/Escape from Boredom

Another reason for using drugs is pleasure. Many people simply like the feelings they receive from drugs. If drugs did not provide some type of perceived benefit, their use would be discontinued. Pleasure is the antithesis of boredom and an individual who is bored will engage in something pleasurable to relieve the boredom. Drugs become a source of reward.

In one survey of high school seniors, 49% indicated that they used drugs "to feel good or get high," 41% "because it tastes good," and 23% "because of boredom, nothing else to do."[8] To escape from feelings of stress many people use drugs.[9] One survey of college students revealed that many students took drugs to relieve stress, relax, have fun, and forget their problems.[10] Substance use among older people is not uncommon; many older people take drugs to escape from the psychological, social, and health problems they incur.[11]

Drugs that are used to increase pleasure or to reduce boredom are reinforcing, especially if the drugs are effective. The accompanying euphoria provides **positive reinforcement**, which encourages continued drug use. Conversely, drugs taken to alleviate discomfort can provide **negative reinforcement**. Distinguishing whether reinforcement for drug use arises from the urge for euphoria or the desire to eliminate dysphoria is sometimes difficult. Nevertheless, the drug user achieves some type of physical or social reward.

An interesting question pertains to whether drug use for the purpose of achieving pleasure should be viewed as acceptable. Some argue that drugs are part of society, most people can moderate their drug use, and drug use for pleasure should be accepted.[12] Others disagree, saying that people cannot easily control their drug use and that pleasure can turn into pain over time.[13]

positive reinforcement Pleasurable sensations associated with a behavior, motivating one to repeat the behavior

negative reinforcement Relief or avoidance of pain achieved by a behavior, motivating one to repeat the behavior

Peer Influence

Many young people use drugs to gain peer acceptance or approval. This point is illustrated in research on alcohol use by fraternity and sorority members.[14] Rates of alcohol consumption by fraternity and sorority members were found to be significantly higher than those of non-Greek-affiliated college students. Fraternity members had higher rates of alcohol use than sorority members. The researcher attributed this to peer norms and the perceived benefits of alcohol. These findings corroborate those of others, who also found that the leaders of fraternities and sororities had more problems than other Greek members.[15]

Just as drug use can be attributed to peer approval, drug abstinence can be associated with peer disapproval. The relationship between peer group affiliation and drug use is reciprocal.[16] It has been shown that teachers can set a climate in the school that promotes respect and healthy norms among students. Nondrug use becomes acceptable behavior.[17] Groups implicitly reinforce behaviors by showing acceptance and affection toward others who share their behaviors.[18] Parents, however, who explicitly tell their children that they do not tolerate drug use affect their children's use of drugs.[19]

Peer influence is affected by one's culture. European American and Chinese adolescents were found to be more affected by peers in their drug use than were Black adolescents.[20] In one Norwegian town adult guardians, such as social workers and volunteers, went to places where adolescents would gather. It was found that the presence of adults significantly reduced the use of alcohol and illegal drugs.[21] On the other hand, one study in Los Angeles found that neighborhood norms did not affect drug use.[22]

Starting in early adolescence, the influence of peers begins to exert a relatively greater role than the family as a socializing agent. Peers have more influence than parents on adolescent drinking behavior. Adolescent girls who develop early are more susceptible to

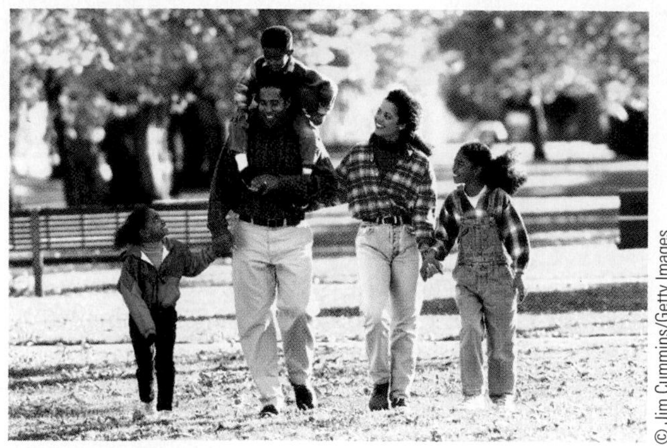

© Jim Cummins/Getty Images.

Strong family bonds are important to counter the influence of peers.

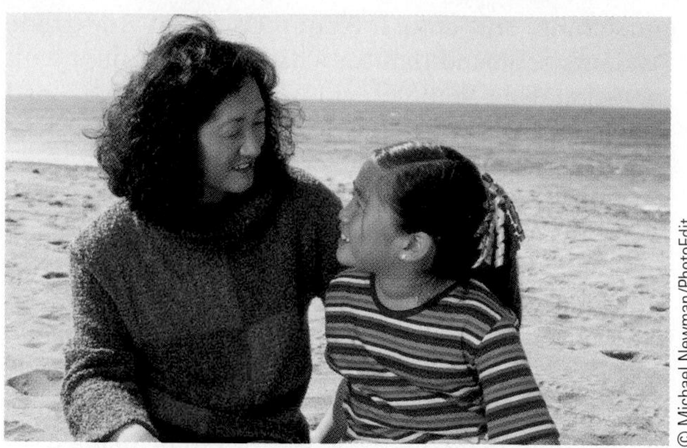

© Michael Newman/PhotoEdit.

Communicating with children reduces the risk of drug abuse.

pressure from older teens to use drugs and engage in other behaviors.[23] Yet, adolescents consistently overestimate the amount of drinking by their peers.[24]

At the same time, basic values, life goals, and aspirations still are influenced more by parents. Parents who communicate well with their children are able to pass on values discouraging drug use.[25] Positive family relationships deter drug use.[26] One study of 6th- to 8th-grade students found that although peers had a greater impact on cigarette smoking and alcohol use, students who had authoritative parents were likely to smoke and drink.[27] Parents indirectly alter their children's drug use by influencing their choice of friends and by emphasizing education.[28] Also, parental attitudes and reactions to the use of tobacco seem to have a greater effect on adolescent smoking than whether parents actually smoke.[29] In addition, children of mothers who smoked during pregnancy were more likely to be dependent on nicotine compared with children whose mothers did not smoke.[30]

The most likely common denominator within an adolescent's peer group, after age and sex, is drug use. Rather than peers exerting an influence on drug-taking behavior, those who use drugs could well seek out others who consume drugs. Young people choose to associate with those who share the same interests. If you are a parent or thinking of becoming a parent, what is the message? Either choose your child's friends carefully or make sure your child chooses friends who hold values similar to yours. One encouraging finding is that parents are becoming more aware of their children's use of drugs, especially cigarettes.[31]

Spiritual Purposes

Throughout history, people have used drugs to seek out or communicate with something or someone greater than themselves. A concept common to some world religions is that animals and plants acquire their special characteristics from a spirit contained within them. By consuming a plant with such a spirit, the person becomes endowed with the spirit. Hence, psychoactive plants have played a meaningful role in religious and spiritual practices of many societies around the world. Abuse is unlikely if drugs are restricted to religious rituals.[32] Ironically, spiritual/religious involvement with drugs might reduce substance abuse.[33]

One form of drug used for spiritual/religious purposes is hallucinogens. Many American Indian cultures use hallucinogens in a religious context. The Native American Church uses the hallucinogen peyote during religious ceremonies to treat alcoholism. Another drug used for spiritual purposes is bhang. Derived from cannabis, bhang is incorporated into Hindu religious rites. Holy men consume it to "center their thoughts on the eternal."[34] Moreover, it is used during Hindu festivals, marriages, and family celebrations. Timothy Leary promoted LSD in his religion, the League of Spiritual Discovery. Its motto was "Turn On, Tune In, and Drop Out." Unlike the Native American Church, which had been permitted to use peyote legally, members of the League of Spiritual Discovery were not legally sanctioned to use LSD.

Many religious rituals and ceremonies incorporate alcohol. In the Catholic Church and some Protestant sects, wine is used in communion. Conversely, many fundamentalist sects forbid alcohol.

Self-Discovery

Drugs sometimes are used to fill a void in one's life. In our hectic, consumer-oriented, impersonal world, people frequently question their purpose or role in life. Changes in modern times leave some people with a sense of uncertainty. The structure of the family has changed. Many jobs are eliminated or sent abroad. Religion is less important to many people. People move frequently. The concept of fair play has taken a backseat to a win-at-all-costs mentality. The emphasis on self equates to selfishness and a sense of not being connected to others. As our world becomes more complicated, understanding oneself becomes more difficult. The stress that many people experience may result in negative health and social consequences, including drug abuse.[35]

Trying to understand oneself is not a task limited to the young. Television programs, newspapers, and magazines have been replete with stories and articles about the midlife crisis. People living the good life—having an imported car, designer clothes, exotic vacations, bottled water with a label, a jacuzzi, or a gold credit card—question their purpose in life. In their quest, many people seek new partners, enter therapy, join support groups, or develop a new lifestyle. In some instances, drugs represent the good life. In other instances, drugs are used as a means of looking for answers to questions of self-fulfillment. They are seen at times as tools for self-exploration and self-discovery. Of course, people could take drugs to *not* understand themselves—to escape from reality and hide from life's problems. Thus, drug abuse can reflect inadequacies in one's life.

Social Interaction

As social beings, humans have a great need for interaction. These interactions range from working and dining together to being in the same organization to simply talking together. Drugs are used sometimes to facilitate interactions with others. In his research, Skager notes that young people use drugs because they feel that drug use is the social thing to do.[36] People often converse over a cocktail. In Japan, college students often mark the beginning of the academic year by drinking sake.[37] Increased use of alcohol by adolescents was found to be preceded by an increase in social activities.[38]

Illegal drugs are used in a social context also. Some people consider marijuana to be a drug that binds people together. As a sign of friendship, heroin addicts share drugs as well as hypodermic needles. For others cocaine is a social lubricant, included as part of a romantic evening and to attract a sexual partner.

On Campus

To stem the rise in binge drinking, some colleges such as the University of Nebraska and the University of Rhode Island have banned beer kegs, provide housing forbidding alcohol and tobacco, and offer courses on responsible drinking.

Source: "Colleges and Binge Drinking," *New York Times*, September 17, 2008 (page 8).

Rules and norms govern drug use in a social context. Even as alcohol use in a college dormitory might abound, there may be rules regarding when and where to drink. Parents who smoke marijuana might wait until their children go to bed. Certain social groups determine *how* a drug is used. For instance, it was found that social milieu of street life leads many young people to escalate their drug use, resulting in injecting drugs.[39] Many gay men, and to a lesser extent lesbians, use drugs to deal with homophobia.[40]

Drug use by soldiers in Vietnam provides an example of the moderating effect of social environment. At least 35% of enlisted men used heroin, and more than half of them became addicted while in Vietnam.[41] Contrary to dire expectations and warnings of government officials, only 10% of the addicts remained addicted after returning to the United States. One reason is that the social sanctions revolving around heroin use while in Vietnam were quite different from those found in the United States.

Rebelliousness

Another reason some people take drugs is that they are told not to. Rebelliousness is one of the best predictors of increased drug use among adolescents. A strong relationship has been found between drug use and recklessness and predelinquent behaviors such as aggression and poor emotional control. Young people rebel against the conventions of society, including warnings about drugs' dangers. Institutions such as religious groups, schools, and government identify rules by which people should behave. The more affiliated one is with these institutions, the less likely one is to use drugs.[42] On the other hand, antisocial behavior is a good predictor of drug abuse.[43]

From a young age, children are taught to conform. Parents and other adults impose rules when we visit relatives, attend school, walk through a shopping mall, get a haircut, pick out clothing, and so forth. Among the many ways to rebel against these proscriptions is to engage in behaviors that are deemed inappropriate. Adolescents who demonstrate oppositional behavior are more likely to engage in health risk behaviors including drug use.[44]

Other motivations for drug use range from relieving anger and tension to staying awake to feeling more energetic. Figure 3.1 highlights environmental factors, interpersonal and social factors, and individual factors contributing to the use of alcohol and other drugs.

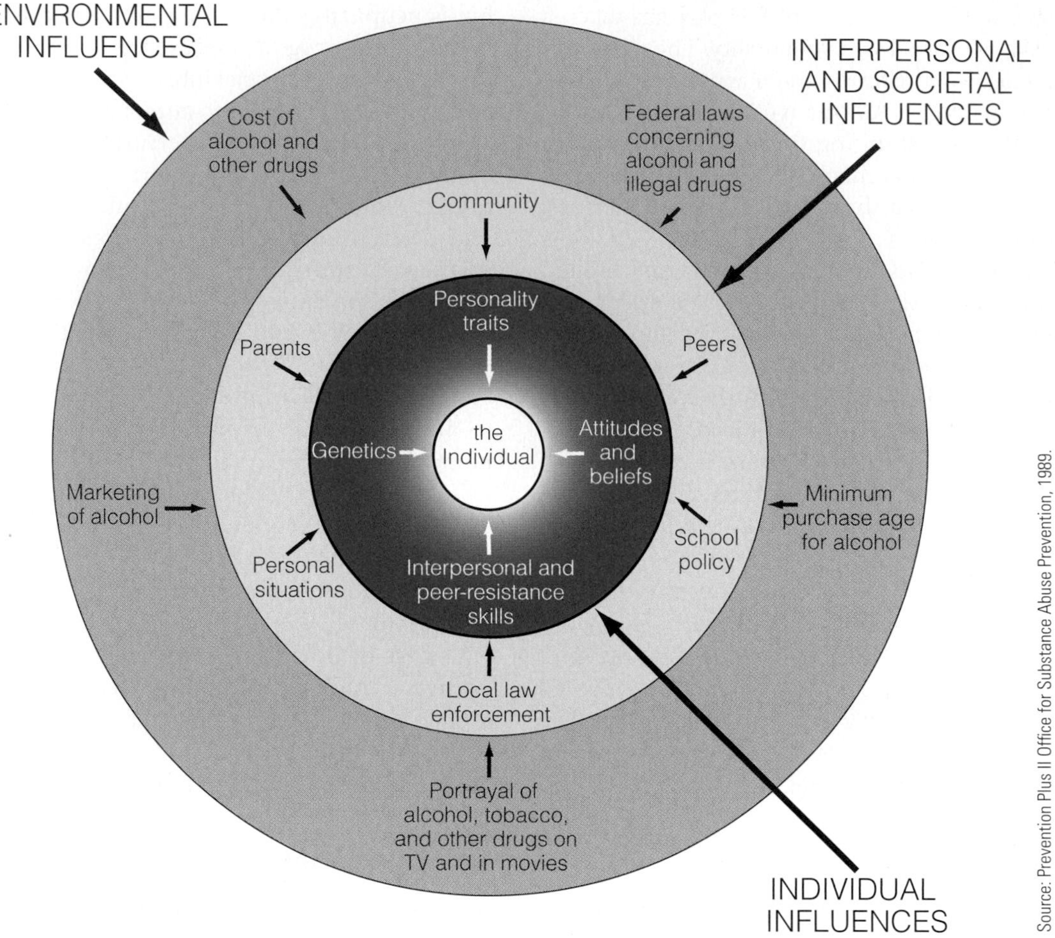

Figure 3.1 Factors That Influence the Use of Alcohol and Other Drugs

Drug Dependency versus Drug Addiction

Drug dependency can be physical or psychological. Before elaborating on the differences, we have to differentiate between the terms **drug dependency** and **drug addiction.** Both connote a compulsive need to use a drug and an inability to cease using it even if serious consequences ensue. Similarly, both *dependency* and *addiction* mean that drug use takes precedence over many other behaviors in one's life.

So how do these terms differ? Stereotypically, the term *drug dependent* conjures up an image of someone who is ill and in need of treatment and compassion. A *drug addict* might be perceived as a criminal and a degenerate who is best served by incarceration, not hospitalization. The terms *dependency* and *addiction* are applied to different drugs as well. For example, heavy smokers seldom are called nicotine addicts, whereas heroin users typically are called addicts.[45]

Because the notion of dependence evokes less condemnation than addiction does, the World Health Organization (WHO), four decades ago, proposed substituting the word "dependence" for "addiction."[46] Another reason for using *dependency* rather than *addiction* was that addiction was seen only in physical terms. The compulsive use of some drugs can be based on the psychic or perceived need for the drug, not only on physical need. Therefore, the term *drug addiction* is too limiting. Regardless of how compulsive drug use is defined, the National Institute on Drug Abuse views compulsive drug use as a treatable illness.[47]

1. *Physical dependency* is marked by **withdrawal symptoms**—the physical symptoms that appear after drug use ceases. People who are physically dependent on a drug need to take the drug to ward off withdrawal symptoms.
2. *Psychological dependency* refers to one's perceived need for a drug.

Some symptoms that show up after drug use ceases may be psychological rather than physical, and some drugs have more potential to cause addiction than others. Important factors in determining whether a drug results in addiction are how quickly it gets to the brain and its potency. Even though many withdrawal symptoms are psychological, they are quite real. Moreover, psychological dependency is harder to overcome than physical dependency, as illustrated in Figure 3.2. This lends credence to the idea that dependency reflects the inability to adapt to one's environment, or at least the inability to adapt in the absence of drugs.

In a nutshell, then, addiction is "an ingrained habit that undermines your health, your work, your relationships, your self-respect, but that you feel you cannot change."[48] According to the Weiner Nusim Foundation, addiction is defined as "a compulsive need for a substance (such as drugs, nicotine, food, or alcohol) or an action (such as gambling, shopping, work, sex, or exercise) that results in a loss of control and the continued use of that substance or action in spite of negative consequences."[49] Dependency is the need to take a drug for its pleasurable effects, the appearance of behavioral changes when drug use ceases, and the need to sustain a drug's initial effects by increasing either the dosage or the frequency.[50] Whether one uses the term *dependency* or *addiction,* long-term drug use is fraught with problems. A study in which narcotics addicts were followed up after 33 years found that there was a high rate of health problems, mental health problems, and involvement with the criminal justice system.[51] It has also been found that using drugs at an early age, including prescription drugs, can lead to dependency.[52]

drug dependency Recurring desire for drugs based on a psychic or a physical need

drug addiction Continuing desire for drugs based on a physical need

withdrawal symptoms Physical signs that appear when drug use is stopped

Is dependency a valid reason for legally prohibiting drugs? Scribner argues that antidrug laws do not protect against addiction and are counterproductive.[53] Volkow maintains that many addicts have no choice but to take drugs; however, she asserts that addicts are accountable for their behavior while on drugs.[54]

Dependency encompasses more than drugs. A person can become dependent on food, religion, love, exercise, or gambling. If one cannot exercise or sustain a romantic relationship, withdrawal symptoms, such as lethargy, irritability, difficulty concentrating, and interrupted sleep, may arise. An example of a new addiction is cyberaddiction.[55]

Theories of Drug Addiction

The U.S. Department of Health and Human Services states that addiction is a "chronic, life-threatening condition that has roots in genetic susceptibility, social

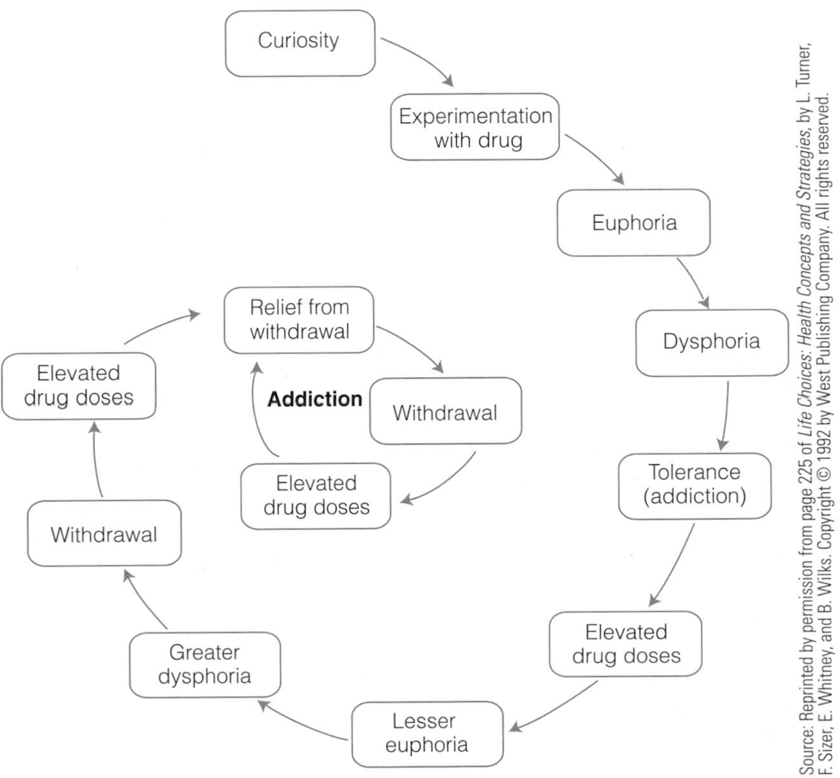

Figure 3.2 **Downward Spiral of Psychological Addiction**

circumstance and personal behavior."[56] Addiction is marked by "continued, compulsive use despite serious consequences—such as health problems and loss of job or family."[57] Many theories attempt to explain addiction. It has been attributed to poor self-control, ignorance, personality traits, bad genes, poverty, disease, and the absence of family values.[58]

When laypeople were surveyed to determine what they thought was the basis for heroin addiction, their political beliefs were a factor. Conservative voters tended to attribute addiction to low moral standards, and liberal voters attributed addiction to psychological and social reasons.[59] Although no single theory adequately covers every aspect of drug addiction, elements of various theories provide insight into drug addiction. A number of theories regarding drug abuse are examined here.

Personality Theories

Some specific personality traits have been related to drug dependence. What is difficult to know is whether certain personality traits lead to drug dependency or if drug dependency alters personality. It has been noted that substance abusers lack self-awareness.[60] Drug-dependent people tend to be negative, self-deprecating, depressed, and tense and have a sense of helplessness.[61] To deal with low self-esteem and accompanying tension, some people rely on drugs. In a study of Swiss adolescents, those who experimented or used drugs frequently were less optimistic and expressed more negative feelings than nonusers about the future.[62] Among adolescents, delayed behavioral or emotional development may be a factor in their substance abuse.[63]

Personality characteristics associated with drug abuse include the following:

- Low self-esteem
- Poor interpersonal skills
- Need for immediate gratification
- Defiant feelings toward authority
- Little tolerance for anxiety, frustration, and depression
- Impulsivity
- Risk taking
- Low regard for personal health

The problem with identifying personality characteristics is that drug abuse may have led to the change in personality rather than personality causing drug abuse.

Drug use can be a means of coping with anxiety. In reality, though, the person is probably exchanging one set of problems for another. "Addicts have problems with self-regulation and impulse control and tend to use drugs as a substitute for coping strategies."[64] To cope with feelings of anxiety and arousal by using drugs is one way to reduce negative aspects of one's life. Some people use narcotics to deal with internal feelings of aggression and rage. Traumatic events in a person's life often trigger substance abuse.[65] Figure 3.3 illustrates the cycle of psychological addiction.

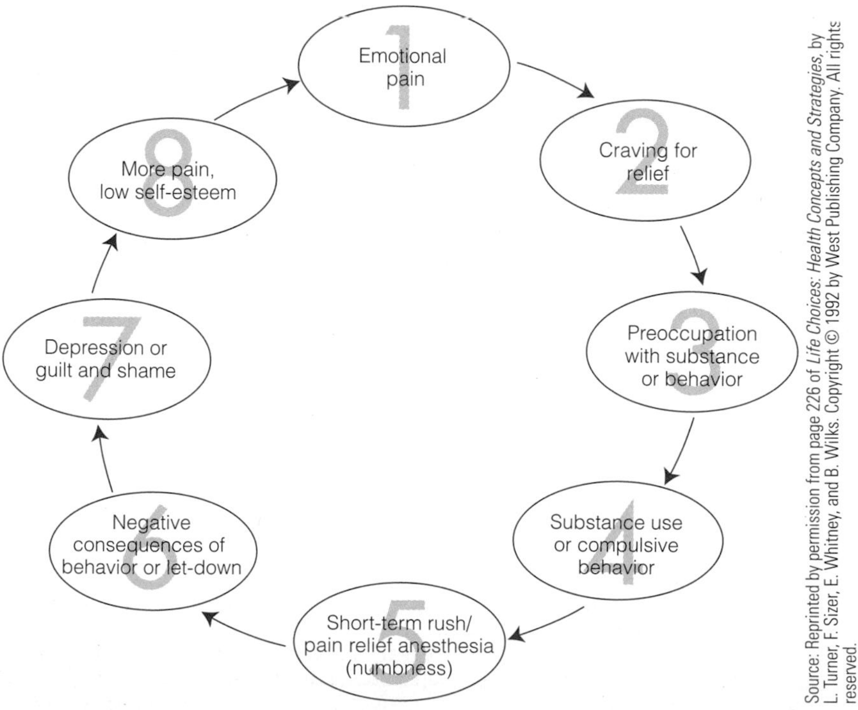

Figure 3.3 Cycle of Psychological Addiction

Source: Reprinted by permission from page 226 of *Life Choices: Health Concepts and Strategies*, by L. Turner, F. Sizer, E. Whitney, and B. Wilks. Copyright © 1992 by West Publishing Company. All rights reserved.

reinforcers Stimuli or events that lead to certain behaviors being repeated

primary reinforcers Stimuli that reduce physiological needs or are inherently pleasurable

secondary reinforcers Stimuli that signal the increased probability of obtaining primary reinforcers

Reinforcement Theory

All animals are believed to have pleasure and reward circuits in the brain that turn on when they are stimulated by addictive substances.[66] A behavior that results in stimulation of these circuits is reinforced—the animal is motivated to repeat that behavior. In some humans, addiction may arise from the reward system of the brain not functioning properly.[67]

Reinforcers are stimuli or events that increase the likelihood of a particular behavior. Reinforcers can be primary or secondary. **Primary reinforcers** reduce physiological needs or are inherently pleasurable; examples are food, water, and sex. **Secondary reinforcers** act as signals for the increased probability of obtaining primary reinforcers; money, for instance, is a secondary reinforcer because it does not provide immediate pleasure, but it can be used to secure a primary reinforcer.

Drugs can be primary or secondary reinforcers. People take drugs because of a payoff or benefit. The payoff might be acceptance from people with whom one wants to be associated, the pleasure derived from altering one's consciousness, or the relief accompanying elimination of withdrawal symptoms.

Reinforcement can be positive or negative. When a person is motivated to repeat behaviors because of the pleasurable sensations they bring, he or she is receiving positive reinforcement. Drugs produce a euphoria that many people seek to repeat. If behaviors provide relief from or avoidance of pain, the desire to repeat those behaviors is motivated by negative reinforcement. Examples of negative reinforcement are use of drugs to avoid the effects of withdrawal and the fear of losing status or approval among peers. A drug-dependent individual falls into one of two camps: the maintainers or the euphoria seekers. The maintainers seek to avoid pain. The euphoria seekers want to feel high.

Biological Theories

Theories focusing on the biological aspects of addiction deal primarily with genetic determination and metabolic imbalances.

Genetic Theory

The genetic theory postulates that a person is predisposed to drug addiction, including addiction to alcohol, by hereditary influence. Studies involving families, twins, and adoptees offer persuasive evidence that addiction is partly genetic and runs in families.[68] There is also research showing a link between compulsive eating and drug abuse, suggesting that both behaviors have a similar genetic component.[69] Although genetics may play an important role in addiction, it is also suggested that psychological and social factors are significant contributors.[70]

Because of biological differences, people become intoxicated at differing levels of consumption and metabolize drugs at different rates. Isolating biological or genetic factors from personality and environment is difficult, and most of the research linking genetics and drugs is limited to alcohol. Determining whether addiction is a result of heredity or environmental influences is also difficult. Nonetheless, Figure 3.4 assesses the genetic and environmental effects on twins.[71]

Metabolic Imbalance

Addiction to narcotics sometimes is attributable to a metabolic disorder.[72] Just as the diabetic person needs insulin, the narcotic user covets narcotics. Narcotics help addicts stabilize the metabolic deficiency caused by absence of the drug. Although this theory can be applied to narcotics users who take methadone

Genetic Versus Environmental Influences on Smoking and Drinking

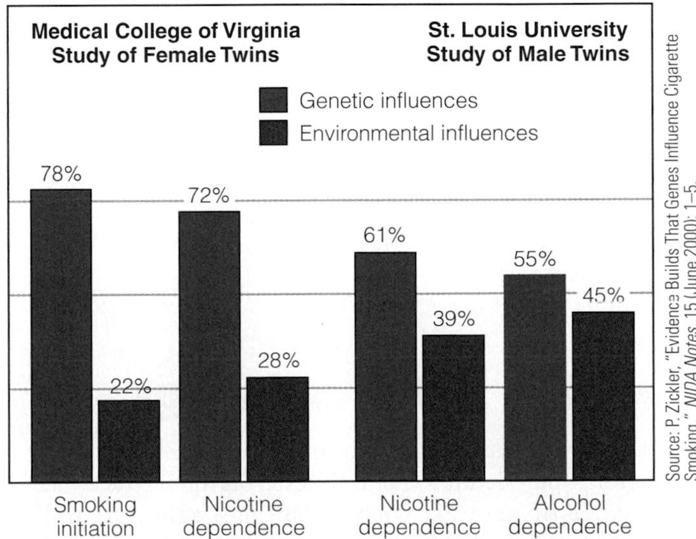

Figure 3.4 A Medical College of Virginia study involving 949 female twin pairs found genetic factors to be more influential than environmental factors in smoking initiation and nicotine dependence. Likewise, a St. Louis University study of 3,356 male twin pairs found genetic factors to be more influential for dependence on nicotine and alcohol

Summary of Drug Addiction Theories

- **Personality theory** is a view holding that addiction is related to low self-esteem, poor interpersonal skills, immediate gratification needs, defiance of authority, little tolerance for anxiety, frustration, depression, impulsivity, risk-taking, and low regard for personal health.
- **Reinforcement theory** is a perspective based on the idea that stimuli or events increase or decrease the likelihood of a behavior occurring.
- **Biological theory** is a view of addiction holding that it is based on genetics and metabolic imbalances.
- **Social theory** is the hypothesis that drug use is determined by cultural and social influences.

to stabilize their desire for narcotics, little evidence is available to support the metabolic deficiency theory.[73]

Social Theories

According to social theories, cultural and social influences contribute to drug abuse.[74] If individuals are rewarded for their behaviors, such as drug use, the risk of continuing those behaviors becomes greater. Rewards are derived from groups and others with whom we associate. Based on this premise, drug abuse is socially learned and benefits the individual by group acceptance.[75] An overlapping theory states that drug abuse arises from problem behavior,[76] although no one theory adequately determines drug addiction.[77]

Whether a behavior is categorized as a problem is a function of how society labels the behavior. In some instances, behaviors outside of social norms actually are considered desirable and are reinforced. In a convoluted way, "bad" is "good," and vice versa. In some social groups, drug abstinence is not valued, whereas drug use, although condemned by many people, is considered good.

Mass Media and Drugs

The impact of the media on drug use is hard to determine because it is only one factor in the total picture of parents, friends, siblings, religion, and schools. Nevertheless, one study reported that alcohol appeared in more than 93% of movies and that illicit drugs appeared in 22% of movies. Another study found that nearly half of G-rated animated films from 1937 to 2000 depicted characters using or abusing alcohol or tobacco.[78] Highlighted here are some forms of mass media that feature drugs—advertisements, billboards, television, music, and celebrities.

Advertisements

More than $2.5 billion was spent recently on advertising prescription drugs.[79] Between 2001 and 2005, alcohol companies spent $4.9 billion on television advertising.[80] The overriding message of advertisements for drugs is that drug-taking is acceptable and, in fact, the norm.

Whether antidrug messages such as those promoted by the Partnership for a Drug-Free America have any impact on reducing drug use is not known.[81] Despite this uncertainty, the U.S. government is proposing to allocate $100 million for the Youth Anti-Drug Media Campaign in 2009.[82] In addition, the federal government, in conjunction with several national organizations, initiated a multimedia campaign to inform young people and parents about the consequences of club drugs, including Ecstasy.[83] The federal government states that antidrug advertisements played a large role in the decline in drug use among secondary students.[84] Media campaigns have been effective in reducing the prevalence of smoking.[85]

In opposition to these government-sponsored advertisements are marketing campaigns for alcohol, cigarettes, and smokeless tobacco, which continue to encourage consumers to use these products.

Alcohol

The liquor industry voluntarily banned advertisements for hard liquor in 1936. Five decades later the Distilled Spirits Council of the United States announced that it was lifting its self-imposed ban on advertising for hard liquor. Two reasons for this shift in policy were the declining sales of distilled spirits at that time and the fact that beer and wine were advertised on television. Although hundreds of television stations carry commercials for distilled spirits, the four biggest broadcast networks in the United States have declined showing the commercials.[86]

Beer advertisements comprise the bulk of the TV commercials for liquor, usually in the context of a sports event. The ads convey stereotypical messages: Men are depicted drinking beer in groups, developing a sense of camaraderie, and becoming initiated into the male clan. In one study the appeal of beer advertisements to male adolescents increased if the advertisements included sports content.[87]

Seventy percent of Americans believe that beer advertisements during sporting events are geared to underage youths. College coaches are involved with a campaign to remove alcohol advertising from college sports. Almost three of four Americans support this ban.[88]

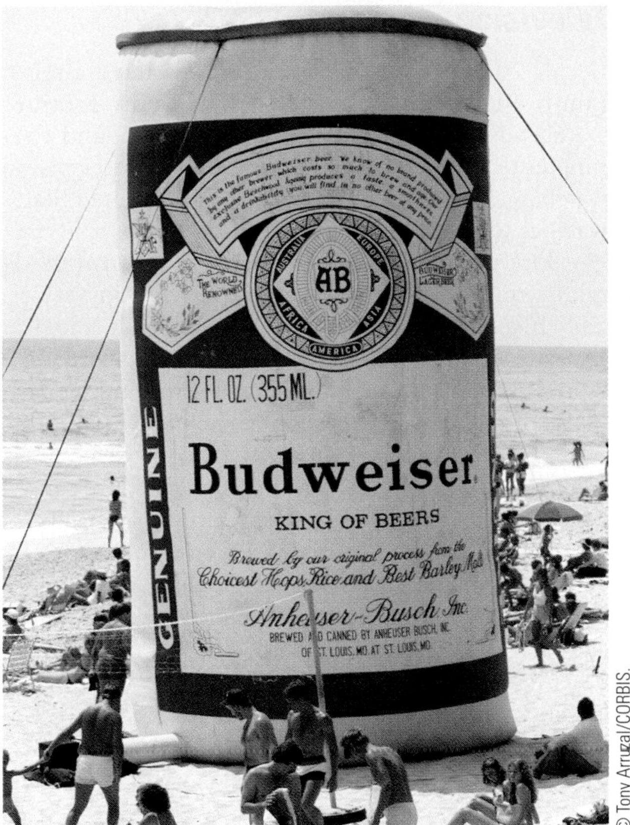

© Tony Arruzal/CORBIS.

Although beer is widely advertised, the effects of advertisement on behavior are hard to gauge.

Effects of alcohol advertisements on behavior are hard to gauge. Advertisers dismiss the importance of advertising on behavior, claiming that advertisements are designed to get viewers to try their products and promote brand loyalty. In one study, early adolescent exposure to alcohol advertising increased the likelihood of underage drinking,[89] while in another, inner-city students who were taught media resistance skills were less likely to drink alcohol.[90] Another author stated that prohibiting alcohol advertising has little effect on its use.[91] The state of Pennsylvania tried to enact a law banning alcohol advertisements in college newspapers. The federal appeals court considered the law unconstitutional.[92]

Cigarettes

In the 1920s, cigarette advertisements explicitly targeted women. Print advertisements associated cigarettes with being slim. The covert message was that cigarettes helped women control their weight. At one time, Lucky Strike advertisements stated that reaching for one of its cigarettes was better than eating dessert.

Today's advertisements for cigarettes play on many themes, particularly independence. In print ads, the Marlboro Man rides the wide open spaces on his horse. Virginia Slims cigarettes are "as free spirited as you." The idea of cigarettes representing independence is not new; in 1929, the American Tobacco Company organized women to smoke publicly and carry placards at the New York Easter Parade showing cigarettes as "torches of liberty." In essence, cigarettes were symbols of freedom.[93]

Through 2005, cigarette companies spent $46.4 million on print advertising. However, cigarette companies are reducing the amount of money being put into magazine and newspaper advertisements. Instead, they are promoting their products in stores, bars, and nightclubs, and through Web sites and direct mail.[94] The Internet, for instance, is used by cigarette manufacturers to promote cigarette sales. At this time, at least 39 states restrict the Internet sale of tobacco to minors, and some states have banned the Internet sale of tobacco products to everyone.[95] One difficulty is verifying the age of individuals purchasing products over the Internet.

The tobacco settlement (see Chapter 7) resulted in billions of dollars being paid by cigarette manufacturers to state governments. Presumably, much of that money was targeted for antismoking efforts. In recent years, however, the tobacco settlement money has been used for other purposes such as reducing taxes and building schools.[96]

Tobacco advertisements often target specific groups of people. For example, fashion magazines such as *Vogue* include advertisements for Camel No. 9, a cigarette geared toward young women. Despite the efforts of antitobacco groups and more than three dozen members of the House of Representatives, none of these magazines agreed to stop publishing the advertisements.[97] Camel No. 9s are enclosed in trendy black boxes and are described as "light and luscious."[98] Campaigns focus on certain ethnic groups as well: There is a greater concentration of pro-tobacco media messages in African American markets compared to Caucasian markets.[99]

Although not ostensibly targeted by tobacco advertising and promotions, adolescents who are receptive to them are more likely to smoke.[100] Likewise, teenagers who were exposed to cigarette advertising were more likely to smoke.

The Federal Communications Commission (FCC) prohibits television and radio advertisements for cigarettes. Despite this, cigarettes gain exposure on TV through various means. Not coincidentally, actors and actresses are prominently shown holding tobacco products. Another popular venue for promoting cigarettes is their appearance in movies. According to one researcher, movies have a greater impact on youth smoking than parenting role models or advertising.[101] Also, tobacco companies use coupons and value-added promotions by paying retailers for shelf space and by providing advertising allowances. The influence of mass media is subtle, but pervasive.

Smokeless Tobacco

After cigarette advertisements were prohibited from television in 1971, the void was filled with advertisements for smokeless tobacco. By 1986, smokeless tobacco advertisements were banned from electronic media, and warning labels were required on all packages. Nevertheless, sales of smokeless tobacco increased tremendously. The impetus for this increase stemmed from sports stars and country singers making pitches for smokeless tobacco products. The use of smokeless tobacco by baseball players rose to such an extent that Major League Baseball implemented a program to help players quit and reduce their public use of smokeless tobacco.[102] Tobacco firms promote smokeless tobacco as a safer alternative to cigarette smoking.[103]

Billboards

Alcohol and tobacco are heavily promoted through billboards and transit posters. More than $400 million is spent annually on outdoor advertising and transit posters. Many billboards are concentrated in poor urban neighborhoods, and it has been found that there are twice as many billboards advertising tobacco products in Black neighborhoods as in White neighborhoods.[104] In 1998, the advertising of Joe Camel (shown in the photo) via billboards was prohibited by law.

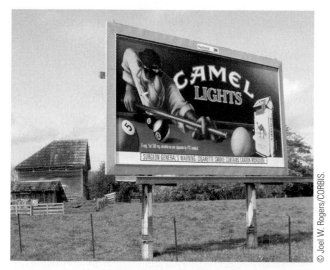

© Joel W. Rogers/CORBIS.

Billboards that advertise tobacco and alcohol are more likely to be found in poor urban neighborhoods than in this country setting.

Television

Of all 20th-century inventions, few have altered family life as much as television. Many families watch television programs during meals, and evening entertainment frequently centers on television watching. The average household in the United States watches television more than 7 hours a day.

The impact of this medium is enormous. If television influences our language, clothing styles, daily hygiene practices, and eating habits, it is logical that our views of drugs are affected by it as well. One study found that smoking behavior among teens is higher if they watch television while unsupervised.[105]

The drug shown on television most often is alcohol. During prime time, television programs are as likely to show teenagers drinking alcohol as adults.[106] In addition, alcoholic beverages are more likely to be consumed than nonalcoholic beverages.[107] About one-fourth of the time alcohol is consumed in television shows, it is paired with negative consequences. On the other hand, alcohol consumption is linked with humor in almost half of its television appearances.[108]

Music

Songs about alcohol and other drugs are not new. The connection between drugs and music in the United States dates back to the jazz musicians of the early 1900s in New Orleans, who advocated marijuana use. One of the earliest references to cocaine was Cole Porter's song, "I Get a Kick Out of You." During the 1940s, bebop jazz became popular, and the drug of choice for many musicians was heroin.

The 1950s saw the beginning of rock and roll, which young people listened to in a state of frenzy. This period in musical history marked the beginning of a period of rebellion by youth against authority and established values, including attitudes and behaviors surrounding drugs.

Antiwar, antiestablishment, and pro-drug messages were reflected in the music of the 1960s. Acid rock embodied the visual and auditory distortions associated with psychedelic drugs. Songs of that era included "Psychedelic Shack" by the Temptations, "She's a Rainbow" by the Rolling Stones, "Journey to the Center of Your Mind" by the Amboy Dukes, "A Girl Named Sandoz" by Eric Burdon and the Animals (LSD was manufactured by the Sandoz Laboratory), and "Lucy in the Sky with Diamonds" by the Beatles. LSD was readily available at Grateful Dead concerts.[109] In 1995, Jerry Garcia, the group's leader, died from a heart attack that may have been the result of years of heroin addiction. Despite Garcia's reputation as a drug user, his death was mourned by political leaders including former President Bill Clinton.

One group—the Doors—derived its name from the book *The Doors of Perception* by Aldous Huxley. In the book, Huxley wrote about his experiences with the drug mescaline. Two songs pertaining to the psychedelic genesis of the band's name are "When the Music's Over" and "Break on Through (to the Other Side)."

Many recording artists have overdosed, been arrested for drug use, or entered drug treatment programs. These singers include Anthony Kiedis and Dave Navarro of the Red Hot Chili Peppers, Steven Tyler of Aerosmith, Kurt Cobain of Nirvana (who eventually died from a self-inflicted gunshot wound), Snoop Dogg (real name Calvin Broadus), Scott Weiland of Stone Temple Pilots, David Gahan of Depeche Mode, Mick Jagger, Keith Richards, Iggy Pop, Little Richard, Paul McCartney, John Lennon, Ray Charles, James Taylor, and Eric Clapton. Musicians who have died from a drug overdose include Shannon Hoon of Blind Melon, Jonathon Melvoin of Smashing Pumpkins, and, earlier, Janis Joplin, Jimi Hendrix, and Elvis Presley.

An analysis of music videos revealed that displays of illicit drug, tobacco, and alcohol use are common. Figure 3.5 illustrates the types of drugs mentioned in music videos.[110] More than 30% of rap videos show people smoking, and alcohol use is included in more than 27%. More than 21% of rock videos show people smoking, and almost one-fourth include someone drinking alcohol—usually the lead singer. In the 1990s, rap music mentioned cocaine and crack in a positive way. In general, references in rap music promoting drug use have escalated.[111] Markert found that in the last decade heroin and cocaine have been portrayed negatively in songs, while marijuana is perceived as innocuous.[112]

Do lyrics influence drug-taking behavior? Though little evidence is available linking lyrics to drug use, the FCC has strongly advocated that broadcasters review music that exalts drugs. The inference is that lyrics and drug use are related and broadcasters should take responsibility for not encouraging drug use.

Celebrities

The presence of drugs within the entertainment industry is apparent. Movie stars including Heath Ledger, Robert Downey Jr., Dennis Quaid, and Melanie Griffith—and, longer ago, Judy Garland, Liza Minnelli, and Marilyn Monroe—have been adversely affected by drugs. Comedians in particular have a long legacy of drug-related problems. The role of alcohol in the lives of W. C. Fields, Buster Keaton, and Jackie Gleason is well documented. Comedian Lenny

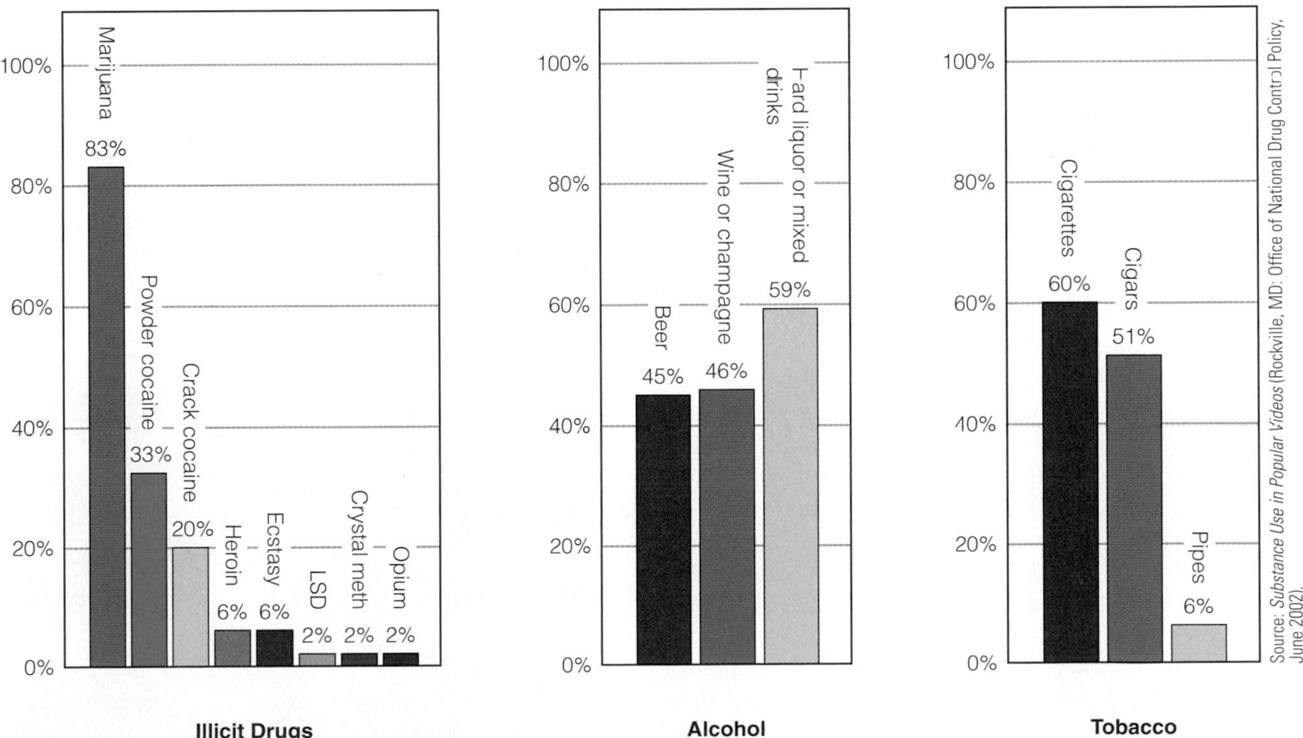

Figure 3.5 Based on the lyrics of 51 music videos in which illicit drugs were mentioned, on 95 music videos in which alcohol appeared, and on 53 music videos in which tobacco appeared. Categories sum to more than 100% because multiple substances appeared in the same music video

Bruce, known for his caustic and profane humor, died from a morphine overdose in 1966. Richard Pryor almost died from drug use. Less fortunate were Chris Farley and John Belushi. The latter died in 1982 from injecting a mixture of cocaine and heroin, called a **speedball.**

Performance-Enhancing Drugs

A strong motivation for many people to use drugs is the desire to enhance performance. Society's emphasis on competition could push people into taking drugs to gain an athletic or academic advantage. Likewise, because of the emphasis on sex appeal, some individuals look to drugs to enhance their sexual performance and experience. The effects of drugs, especially anabolic steroids, on performance will be examined here.

Performance-enhancing drugs, also known as **ergogenic aids,** are used to gain a competitive advantage. As early as the 3rd century B.C., Greek athletes ate mushrooms to enhance their performance.[113] In the 1800s, athletes took alcohol, opium, nitroglycerin, and strychnine to improve their performance. American Thomas Hicks won the 1904 Olympic Games marathon after reportedly taking strychnine and brandy, and he was not disqualified.[114] In the 1940s, some athletes and bodybuilders took anabolic steroids to increase their muscle mass and intensify their training regimens.[115]

Drug abuse in sports has become more publicized in the last few years. The media are replete with stories of drug use by athletes during the Olympic Games. Track and field stars such as Marion Jones have blemished careers due to drug use. Major League Baseball attracted much adverse attention due to its scandal with performance-enhancing drugs. Because athletes are seen as role models, their fall from grace touches a chord; moreover, drug use by athletes is antithetical to the idea that athletes represent a healthy lifestyle.

The type of sport and gender of the athlete have a bearing on the drug of choice. For example, athletes participating in contact sports showed preferences for cocaine, crack, and heroin, whereas athletes who engaged in noncontact sports preferred amphetamines.[116] The most preferred drug was marijuana regardless of whether the sport was contact or noncontact.[117] Male athletes prefer red alcohol, caffeine, anabolic steroids, marijuana, crank, heroin, LSD, and Ecstasy.[118] Female athletes preferred uppers/amphetamines and morphine. In regard to alcohol, women preferred wine and men preferred beer.[119]

Many individuals use sports supplements to enhance their performance or appearance. In Canada, over $1 billion is spent annually on sports supplements.[120] They can be purchased in gas stations as well as grocery and drug stores and over the Internet. Concerns regarding the use of sports supplements include their lack of regulation and absence of research into their long-term effects.

Anabolic Steroids

Prior to their use in athletics, **anabolic steroids** were used by German soldiers during World War II to increase their muscle strength and aggressiveness.[121] Reports of steroid use by male and female Soviet athletes appeared in 1954. Shortly thereafter, U.S. weightlifters began taking steroids, followed by football players and swimmers.

Anabolic steroids are synthetic substances related to the male sex hormones.[122] They mimic the action of testosterone. Steroids are only legally available through a prescription. They are believed to add bulk and strength if they are taken by motivated people who train intensively and follow a proper diet.[123] Taking testosterone during puberty augments muscle mass and strength, but steroid use later in adolescence stunts growth. Users experience a stimulant-like high and feelings of aggressiveness, and this may account for higher intensity while training and competing. Studies on their effects are conducted retrospectively, and factors such as diet, dosage, type of steroid, and level of training make it hard to answer the question conclusively. Further, users may engage in **stacking**—ingesting and injecting several steroids at the same time.

Athletes are not the only individuals using steroids. Many males use these drugs to improve their appearance. One study reported that college students took steroids to enhance appearance, because their friends took steroids, or to improve physical performance.[124]

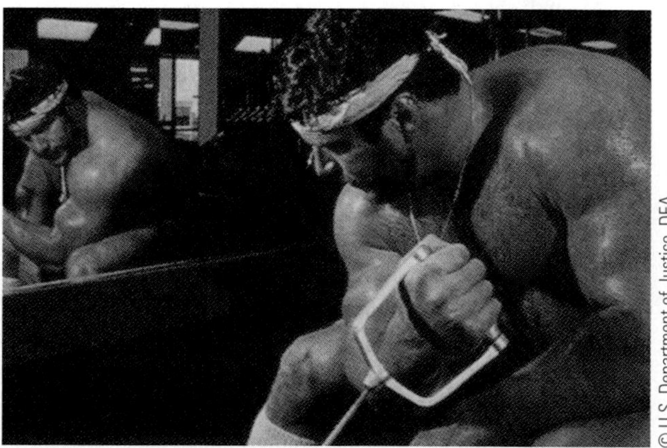

Steroid abuse often begins with an attempt to increase muscle size or to improve appearance.

Among college students, the rate of steroid use has not differed from the early 1990s to the present. Approximately 1% of college students have used steroids for nonmedical purposes.[125] Another study found that the average user is a 30-year-old, educated, White male who is not especially athletic.[126] Concern over teenage girls using steroids prompted the United States Congress to initiate hearings. However, due to the way survey questions are asked, it is difficult to get a good handle on the extent of steroid use by teenage girls.[127] It is believed that the use of steroids by college athletes is rampant. Some of these steroids are procured through friends, coaches, and the Internet.[128]

Liver and kidney tumors have been linked to steroids. Within 2 to 8 years, 1% to 3% of users develop liver cancer.[129] Other effects in men are low sperm count, testicular atrophy, high voice, gynecomastia (breast development), infertility, and baldness. These are reversible several months after stopping use of steroids.[130] Male bodybuilders have difficulty maintaining erections, according to some reports, but others say steroids enhance sexual desire.[131] There is a reported increase in steroid users who have sexual and reproductive disorders.[132]

Users display symptoms of depression, panic, anxiety, paranoia, mania, and suicidal behavior.[133] This mania has been called **roid rage**. Uncontrollable violence, which occurs for no apparent reason, also has been tied to steroid use. At one time anabolic steroids were not considered addictive. However, based on guidelines from the United States Sentencing Commission, steroids are now considered addictive.[134]

Anabolic steroids do have medical benefits when prescribed by physicians. Anabolic steroids were first developed in the late 1930s to treat hypogonadism, a condition in which the testes fail to produce enough testosterone.[135] They are still given to people who have some types of impotence and to AIDS patients to treat the body wasting often associated with that disease.[136]

speedball Injectable combination of heroin and cocaine

ergogenic aids Substances that provide an athletic advantage, also known as performance-enhancing drugs

anabolic steroids Substances used to increase muscle mass; related to male sex hormones

stacking Ingesting or injecting several steroids at the same time

roid rage Uncontrollable violence associated with use of anabolic steroids

human growth hormones Hormones that stimulate protein synthesis; used by athletes to enhance performance

erythropoietin Hormone that enhances cardiovascular endurance by increasing red blood cell production

Human Growth Hormones (HGH) and Erythropoietin (EPO)

Human growth hormones—which are naturally produced in the body and stimulate protein synthesis—and **erythropoietin** are other drugs used to enhance performance. Human growth hormones (HGH) were first isolated in the 1950s, although it was not until the 1980s that they were used as a doping agent.[137] One factor that has led to their use by athletes is that they are difficult to detect.[138] Human growth hormones are frequently used in conjunction with anabolic steroids because HGH is thought to increase the effects of steroids.[139]

Human growth hormones have been given to children who are especially small. Depending on the dosage, children will grow 1.5 to 4 inches,[140] and many of these children feel better about themselves after taking the hormones. In 2008 a bill was introduced into the U.S. Senate to ban human growth hormones for everyone, including children. However, that bill was defeated because of HGH's benefit to some children.[141] It is also believed that human growth hormones will counter the effects of aging.

Erythropoietin is a hormone that increases red blood cell production and improves endurance.

Known Effects of Steroids

Both Men and Women:

- acne
- increased susceptibility to infections
- abrupt mood changes
- hypertension
- decreased high-density lipoprotein levels (good cholesterol)
- effects on liver
- stunted growth

Men:

- increased penis size if used before puberty
- more frequent erections
- atrophied testicles
- enlarged breasts
- enlarged prostate
- infertility
- baldness

Women:

- baldness
- decreased breast size
- enlarged clitoris
- increased facial hair
- fluid retention
- deepened voice
- menstrual irregularities

A higher red blood cell count, however, can lead to blood clots, increasing the risk for heart attacks, stroke, and pulmonary embolism. Other side effects are increased bone growth of the jaw, forehead, feet, and hands; increased cholesterol levels; heart disease; impotence; and elevated blood sugar levels.

Creatine

An over-the-counter substance that has gained in popularity is the amino acid **creatine monohydrate**, referred to as a nutritional supplement. A number of professional athletes, coaches, and fitness researchers promote its use, although the physiological mechanisms by which it works are not well understood. Creatine is believed to increase water content in muscles, adding to their size and possibly their ability to function. Kutz and Gunter found that creatine provided a modest increase in total body weight, although the increase may have resulted from water retention.[142] A study of women between the ages of 58 and 71 who took creatine found that they had significant increases in muscle power and strength without experiencing adverse side effects.[143]

Some studies show that creatine is effective for improving an athlete's performance. One study of competitive female swimmers found that swimmers propelled themselves more quickly when using creatine, even though their body weight and body composition were unaffected.[144] Another study of creatine's effects on sprinting in hot, humid conditions revealed significant improvement.[145] In a separate study of young males, creatine was found to increase fat-free mass and muscle power.[146] No long-term benefits have been established.

Should its use be banned from athletic competition? Among Major League Baseball teams, 8 disapproved of creatine use, 7 took no position, and 1 approved it. In the National Basketball Association (NBA), 2 teams disapproved, 11 took no position, and 8 approved. In the National Football League (NFL), 8 teams disapproved, 4 took no position, and 5 approved. A higher percentage of football players are believed to use creatine than athletes in other sports.

A study of high school football players in Wisconsin found that 30% reported using creatine.[147] Among Wisconsin high school female athletes, 4% indicated having used creatine. The highest incidence was among swimmers.[148]

One benefit of creatine—in a roundabout way—is that it may prevent some people from using anabolic steroids. Another benefit, according to an Australian study, is that creatine may boost brain power in vegetarians.[149] A small study of ten people indicated that creatine may help relieve depression.[150] The physical benefits some people derive from creatine may be a result of their expectations of what the drug is capable of doing.[151]

Because creatine is a nutritional supplement and not a drug, the Food and Drug Administration (FDA) does not scrutinize it for safety. In essence, no regulations are in place regarding its sale and use.[152] Nonetheless, many people perceive creatine as a safe alternative to steroids. Reported side effects of creatine include muscle cramping, dehydration, water retention, and kidney problems. Other side effects are gastrointestinal distress, nausea, and seizures. Three college wrestlers who died in 1997 were believed to be taking creatine, although the relationship between creatine and their deaths could have been coincidental.

Tetrahydrogestrinone (THG)

Tetrahydrogestrinone (THG) is a new synthetic steroid that athletes are taking to improve athletic performance. THG is made by modifying another anabolic steroid. It is alleged that THG was designed and manufactured by a California company known as Bay Area Laboratory Cooperative (BALCO). BALCO's owner, Victor Conte, claims that THG is not a steroid but a nutritional supplement. Numerous athletes, such as baseball players Jason Giambi and Barry Bonds, football player Bill Romanowski, and track and field athletes including Marion Jones, are suspected of having used THG.[153]

The FDA has not approved THG for use. The FDA has warned individuals not to use THG because it has not undergone scientific scrutiny. Despite the lack of testing for THG, the FDA speculates that it may cause some of the same side effects as steroids.[154] Don Catlin, who heads a drug testing laboratory at the University of California in Los Angeles, fears that other designer drugs that can evade detection may be developed. When THG was first developed, the belief was that it could not be detected by conventional drug testing procedures because it deteriorates quickly. However, with improved drug testing it can now be detected. Nonetheless, it is difficult for testing to keep up with the changes in the variety of drugs that may be produced.[155]

Despite the stance of the U.S. Anti-Doping Agency (USADA), many athletes taking performance-enhancing drugs do not view themselves as cheaters. Rather, they consider the use of these drugs as a means of getting the edge over their competitors.[156] Though it is not known how extensively THG is used, its consumption is thought to be widespread. Moreover, the public expects to see athletes who are bigger, stronger, and faster. The era of the 250-pound professional lineman is over. Every 2 years when the Olympic Games are held, fans watch to see if world records are broken. Fans get excited when the home-run record is broken. Interestingly, the NBA and the National Hockey League (NHL) have not banned THG.[157]

Androstenedione (Andro)

Another muscle builder that has caught the attention of the public, primarily because it was used by home-run king Mark McGwire, is **androstenedione**. Major League Baseball did not forbid players from using androstenedione at that time, even though the National Collegiate Athletic Association (NCAA), the NFL, and the International Olympic Committee had banned it. Known as "andro," androstenedione, like creatine, is classified as a nutritional supplement, although it is no longer sold legally.

Androstenedione is a precursor molecule that is just one metabolic step away from testosterone. Its producers claim that androstenedione causes users to generate more testosterone for a few hours after a workout.[158] Androstenedione can be converted into the female sex hormone estrogen as well.

The effects of androstenedione are similar to those of anabolic steroids. For example, males may experience testicular atrophy, impotence, and breast enlargement. Women who take androstenedione may have increased facial hair, become bald, have deepened voices, and experience abnormal menstrual cycles. Women may also have an increased risk of breast and endometrial cancer.[159]

Stimulants

Cocaine use by collegiate and professional athletes is well documented. Cocaine impairs performance requiring hand-eye coordination and concentration. Most athletes use cocaine for social reasons, not to improve performance.

Amphetamines have been used in sports to reduce fatigue and sustain intense exercise. There were reports of amphetamine use in the 1952 and 1956 Olympic Games. By the 1960 Olympics, amphetamine use was rampant. On the first day of competition, a Danish cyclist died and three others collapsed from amphetamine use. This tragedy provided the impetus for drug testing of athletes.[160] In the 1996 Olympics, five athletes tested positive for a banned stimulant.

In 1968, the International Olympic Committee required athletes to submit to drug testing or face disqualification. The U.S. Olympic Committee publishes a list of drugs that result in disqualification. The list includes not only illegal drugs but prescribed and over-the-counter drugs as well.

Concerns over performance-enhancing drugs rose in the United States when professional football players reportedly used amphetamines during competition. The NFL officially banned these drugs in 1971. Although steroids were not seen as a problem at that time, the perception in the NFL has changed and steroids are now banned.

In 1995, the U.S. Supreme Court ruled that high schools have the right to drug-test athletes, that the interest of the school outweighs the privacy issues of its students. Also, in preparation for the 2002 Winter Olympics in Salt Lake City, the federal government allocated $3.3 million to support the anti-doping program. The drug-testing policies of professional sports are outlined in Table 3.1.

In a classic study, 75% of highly trained runners, swimmers, and throwers showed slight improvement after using amphetamines. Even though improvement

creatine monohydrate Natural substance used to increase strength and short-term speed

tetrahydrogestrinone A designer drug, closely related to the banned anabolic steroids gestrinone and trenbolone

androstenedione Food supplement used for muscle development

TABLE 3.1 Professional Sports and Drug Testing

Sport	Policy
National Football League	Players are tested during preseason and tested during season only for *reasonable cause.* Positive test results in outpatient counseling and 30-day probation or 30-day inpatient treatment. After three positive tests a player is banned from the NFL.
National Basketball Association	Testing is limited to cases of *reasonable cause* and random testing of first-year players during preseason. First-time violators who voluntarily seek help receive their salary and free treatment; the second time, they receive treatment but no salary. The third time, they are suspended for life but may petition for reinstatement after 2 years.
Major League Baseball	Players are tested only if they have known involvement with drugs or their contract has a clause. Penalties are handled on a case-by-case basis.
Boxing	World Boxing Council requires testing for world title fights; World Boxing Association does not require drug tests.
Tennis	Men's International Professional Tennis Council conducts drug tests at no more than two tournaments each year; a player testing positive must receive treatment or face a 1-year suspension; three positive tests result in a 1-year suspension.
National Hockey League	NHL has no drug-testing policy.

was slight, amphetamines could account for the margin of difference in highly trained athletes. Endurance improved, however, because symptoms of fatigue were masked, not because of improved physiology.[161] Research into whether amphetamines increase bulk strength is contradictory.

Caffeine is another stimulant that improves endurance, especially short-term endurance. In one study, the length of a bicycle ergometer ride was extended by nearly 20% after the subjects ingested 330 mg of caffeine, equivalent to three cups of coffee. The total energy output of individuals in a laboratory setting who rode for 2 hours was 7% greater after consuming 500 mg of caffeine.[162] Currently, the NCAA and International Olympic Committee ban caffeine at specified levels.

Depressants

Depressants such as barbiturates, benzodiazepines (minor tranquilizers), and alcohol are not perceived as ergogenic drugs, though they have been used to improve performance. Benzodiazepines and barbiturates reduce tremors, a quality important to hand-steadiness.[163] Weight throwers improved their performance, whereas swimmers were significantly impaired after taking a certain barbiturate. Benzodiazepines impair psychomotor performance, although this becomes less so as tolerance develops.

Alcohol significantly reduces psychomotor skills. Some endurance athletes drink beer before competition because they think it provides carbohydrates for energy. Calories from beer, however, are converted to heat and are not available as energy. Moreover, alcohol results in significant loss of fluid.[164] Alcohol also reduces aerobic capacity, and reaction time, fine and complex motor coordination, balance and steadiness, visual tracking, and information processing are impaired.[165] The only sport that formally bans alcohol is the modern pentathlon.[166] The pentathlon includes shooting events, and alcohol produces an anti-tremor effect at low doses.

Sexual Performance

Images of sex are used to sell products ranging from soft drinks to television shows to automobiles to alcohol. Sex denotes youthfulness and virility. Achieving or exuding a sexual image by making oneself look young and vital or by proving one's sexual prowess typifies society's preoccupation with sex.

A "sexual image" can be achieved in many ways: a beautiful tan, a well-toned body, the right clothes, a good mane of hair. The ability to perform sexually is important also. Many prescribed and over-the-counter drugs alter sexual functioning. On the other hand, drugs such as methamphetamines have been shown to lead to unsafe sexual practices.[167] One study of college students reported that alcohol use was associated with a reduced likelihood of contraceptive use.[168] It has also been found that women who voluntarily took drugs and then were sexually assaulted were more likely to be blamed for the assault.[169]

What effects do drugs have on sexual mood and performance? Alcohol is commonly believed to increase sexual desire. Similarly, although LSD often is viewed as sexually or romantically enhancing, it can have the opposite effect. Many drugs contribute to sexual dysfunction and interfere with the ability to enjoy sexual relations and to be intimate.

The unwarranted reputation of alcohol as an **aphrodisiac** was noted in *Macbeth,* when Shakespeare wrote: "Alcohol provokes the desire, but it takes away the performance." Nevertheless, because of its disinhibiting action at low dosages, alcohol can enhance sexual excitement. Chronic use of alcohol, however, reduces testosterone levels and, consequently, sexual desire.[170] Notably, the most frequently mentioned cause of impotence in middle-aged men is excessive use of alcohol.[171] It impedes performance, which leads to fear of failure and performance anxiety.

Females who drink alcohol have inhibited sexual desire because alcohol reduces vaginal vasocongestion. This may explain why many women who drink indicate decreased sexual pleasure. Women report difficulty achieving orgasm at moderate consumption levels. Despite the fact that drugs impair sexual performance, drugs are commonly used, especially in clubs, to make the user less sexually inhibited. One drug linked to lowered inhibitions is Ecstasy; however, the number of people at rave parties using Ecstasy has declined.[172]

Narcotics, too, adversely affect sexual desire, performance, and satisfaction. Males who use narcotics have difficulty achieving and maintaining an erection and are less likely to experience orgasm. Narcotics reduce the libido of men and women, although libido levels return to normal within 3 months of abstinence.[173] Alcohol, cocaine, opiates, and other commonly abused drugs interfere with the menstrual cycle, compromising a woman's reproductive ability.[174] Moreover, testosterone levels of male narcotics users were found to be lower than expected. Similarly, anabolic steroids lower testosterone levels and interfere with sexual functioning.[175]

In research on the effects of marijuana on sexual behavior, most people believed that its use before intercourse increased tactile awareness.[176] The researchers, however, found no physiological proof that this is true. It is difficult to determine whether the increased tactile sensitivity was attributable to the perceptions of marijuana's effects or to its disinhibiting effect. One-fifth of the males using marijuana daily had erectile problems. Women using marijuana reported painful intercourse because of vaginal dryness. Testosterone levels and sperm production of males using marijuana regularly were affected negatively, although these conditions were reversible.

Despite their reputation as aphrodisiacs, high levels of cocaine and amphetamines are detrimental to sexual behavior. The idea that stimulants act as aphrodisiacs can be attributed to their physical effects, which approximate sexual excitement. These drugs increase heart rate, blood pressure, and blood flow to the genitals. At moderate levels, cocaine and amphetamines impair a woman's ability to achieve orgasm. Men's problems focus on impotence and the inability to ejaculate. Also, use of methamphetamines may reduce one's immunity to sexually related diseases.[177]

To delay orgasm, some men place cocaine on the tip of the penis because it has an anesthetizing effect. Some women apply cocaine to the clitoris before intercourse to hasten sexual arousal and responsiveness. Unfortunately, street cocaine often contains contaminants, which cause infections. In extreme cases, gangrene can develop from these infections, necessitating amputation of the penis.

aphrodisiac Any substance that increases sexual desire and performance.

Summary

In our constantly changing society, people sometimes turn to drugs to cope. Drugs are easy to use, work quickly, and are transported easily. Other reasons for using drugs range from seeking pleasure to escaping boredom, to peer influence, spiritual purposes, self-discovery, social interaction, and rebellion. Others use drugs to cope with anxiety and depression.

The terms *drug dependency* and *drug addiction* are different. *Addiction* is a stronger term, implying an intense *physical* need. Today, the term *drug dependency* is favored because it has a psychological as well as a physical connotation. Drug dependency theories postulate that dependency is caused by personality characteristics, social and biological factors, and behavioral principles.

To determine the precise effects of mass media on drug-taking behavior is difficult. The federal government has increased funding for antidrug messages, although it is too early to know if these media messages will be effective. Advertisements tell us that drugs can remedy a host of ills. Drugs have figured prominently in the music world as well. Rock and roll and drugs became icons of rebelliousness, but more recently, many musicians and other celebrities have come out against drug use. Current studies show that public service announcements reduce drug use.

Drugs have been, and are, used to improve athletic and sexual performance. The most prominent of these are anabolic steroids—which are capable of producing fatal consequences. Other performance-enhancing substances include human growth hormone, creatine, and androstenedione. Drugs such as cocaine, barbiturates, and narcotics also have been used to improve athletic performance. In reality, the only drugs that have exhibited positive results on athletic performance are amphetamines and caffeine, though side effects have to be considered.

Drugs also are used with the expectation of heightened sexual experiences. Some people use drugs to enhance a romantic mood. Cocaine and other stimulants are thought to be aphrodisiacs. These perceptions are unjustified—drugs do not improve sexual performance, nor do they act as aphrodisiacs.

Thinking Critically

1. What drug-related norms or rules can you identify? How did you learn these norms? If you have lived in a different part of this country or in another country, how were drug-related norms different?
2. Look at the most popular songs for the past month. How many refer to drugs? Are drugs portrayed positively or negatively? Do the lyrics have any effect on your behavior or the behavior of those around you?
3. Because depressants such as barbiturates, alcohol, and minor tranquilizers affect sexual response negatively, should warning labels be put on medically prescribed depressants and alcoholic beverages? Why or why not?

Web Resources

The Substance Abuse and Mental Health Services Administration
http://www.drugabusestatistics.samhsa.gov
This site provides data on the incidence of drug use and other drug-related statistics.

National Institute on Drug Abuse (NIDA)
http://steroidabuse.org
Health risks associated with anabolic steroids and strategies for preventing steroid abuse can be accessed at this site.

Steroid Law
http://www.steroidlaw.com
This site provides numerous articles dealing with various aspects of anabolic steroid drug use. The articles range from legal issues to physical and psychological effects to trends in usage.

Notes

1. O. Curtis, *Chemical Dependence: A Family Affair* (Pacific Grove, CA: Brooks/Cole, 1999).
2. L. D. Johnston, P. M. O'Malley, J. G. Bachman, and J. E. Schulenberg, *Monitoring the Future, National Results on Adolescent Drug Use: Overview of Key Findings 2008* (Bethesda, MD: National Institute on Drug Abuse, 2008).
3. W. Pedersen and A. Skrondal, "Alcohol Consumption Debut: Predictors and Consequences," *Journal of Studies on Alcohol,* 59 (1998): 32–42.
4. "Underage Drinking: A Major Public Health Challenge," *Alcohol Alert,* 59 (April 2003): 2.
5. B. S. Lynch and R. J. Bonnie, *Growing Up Tobacco Free: Preventing Addiction in Children and Youths* (Washington, DC: National Academy Press, 1994).
6. B. J. Casey, S. Getz, and A. Galvan, "The Adolescent Brain," *Developmental Review,* 28 (March 2008): 62–77.
7. S. S. Martins, C. L. Storr, P. K. Alexandre, and H. D. Chilcoat, "Do Adolescent Ecstasy Users Have Different Attitudes Towards Drugs When Compared to Marijuana Users?" *Drug and Alcohol Dependence,* 94 (April 2008): 63–72.
8. L. D. Johnston and P. M. O'Malley, "Why Do the Nation's Students Use Drugs and Alcohol? Self-Reported Reasons from Nine National Surveys," *Journal of Drug Issues,* 16 (1986): 29–68.
9. "Stress and Drug Abuse," *New York Times Upfront,* 139 (February 5, 2007): 18–19.
10. J. A. Califano, "Wasting the Best and Brightest," *America,* 196 (May 28, 2007): 16–18.
11. "Substance Misuse among Older Adults: A Neglected but Treatable Problem," *Addiction,* 103 (March 2008): 347–348.
12. S. Hough, "The Moral Mirror of Pleasure: Considerations About the Recreational Use of Drugs," in *Drugs, Morality, and the Law,* edited by S. Luper-Foy and C. Brown (New York: Garland Publishing, 1994).
13. R. B. Edwards, "Why We Should Not Use Some Drugs for Pleasure," in *Drugs, Morality, and the Law,* edited by S. Luper-Foy and C. Brown (New York: Garland Publishing, 1994).
14. K. Steinman, "College Students' Early Cessation from Episodic Heavy Drinking: Prevalence and Correlates," *Journal of American College Health,* 51 (2003): 197–204.
15. J. R. Cashin, C. A. Presley, and P. W. Meilman, "Alcohol Use in the Greek System: Follow the Leader," *Journal of Studies on Alcohol,* 59 (1998): 63–70.
16. D. M. Gorman, "Etiological Theories and the Primary Prevention of Drug Use," *Journal of Drug Issues,* 26 (1996): 505–520.
17. M. LaRusso, D. Romer, and R. Selman, "Teachers as Builders of Respectful School Climates: Implications for Adolescent Drug Use Norms and Depressive Symptoms in High School," *Journal of Youth and Adolescence,* 37 (April 2008): 386–398.
18. D. Wright and M. Pemberton, *Risk and Protective Factors for Adolescent Drug Use: Findings from the 1999 National Household Survey on Drug Abuse* (Rockville, MD: Substance Abuse and Mental Health Services Administration, 2004).
19. M. Miller-Day, "Talking to Youth About Drugs: What Do Late Adolescents Say About Parental Strategies?" *Family Relations,* 57 (January 2008): 1–12.
20. C. Pilgrim, Q. Luo, K. A. Urberg, and X. Fang, "Influence of Peers, Parents, and Individual Characteristics on Adolescent Drug Use in Two Cultures," *Merrill-Palmer Quarterly,* 45 (1999): 85–107.
21. C. Bratt, "Guardians to Counter Adolescent Drug Use?" *Youth and Society,* 39 (March 2008): 385–405.
22. K. Musick, J. A. Seltzer, and C. R. Schwartz, "Neighborhood Norms and Substance Use Among Teens," *Social Science Research,* 37 (March 2008): 138–155.
23. "The Lingering Effects of Puberty," *Contexts: Understanding People in Their Social Worlds,* 7 (Winter 2008): 8.
24. *Alcohol and Health, Ninth Special Report to the U.S. Congress* (Rockville, MD: U.S. Department of Health and Human Services, 1997).
25. Wright and Pemberton, supra note 18.
26. L. A. Crawford and K. B. Novak, "Parent-Child Relations and Peer Associations as Mediators of the Family Structure—Substance Use Relationship," *Journal of Family Issues,* 29 (February 2008): 155–184.
27. B. Simons-Morton, D. L. Haynie, A. D. Crump, P. Eitel, and K. E. Saylor, "Peer and Parent Influences on Smoking and Drinking Among Early Adolescents," *Health Education and Behavior,* 28 (February 2001): 95–107.
28. S. J. Bahr, A. C. Marcos, and S. L. Maughan, "Family, Educational, and Peer Influences on the Alcohol Use of Female and Male Adolescents," *Journal of Studies on Alcohol,* 56 (1995): 457–469.
29. Lynch and Bonnie, supra note 5.
30. S. Perlstein, "Smoking Mothers, Smoking Children," *Pediatric News,* 38 (2004): 48.
31. The NSDUH Report, *Parent Awareness of Youth Use of Cigarettes, Alcohol, and Marijuana* (Rockville, MD: Substance Abuse and Mental Health Services Administration, April 24, 2008).
32. J. M. Davis, "Hallucinogenic Plants and Their Use in Traditional Society: An Overview," *Cultural Survival Quarterly,* 9 (1985): 2–4.
33. "Religious Beliefs and Substance Use among Youths," *The NSDUH Report.* (Rockville, MD: U.S. Department of Health and Human Services, January 30, 2004).
34. S. H. Snyder, "What Have We Forgotten About Pot?" *New York Times Magazine,* December 13, 1970.
35. J. N. Cleck and J. A. Blendy, "Making a Bad Thing Worse: Adverse Effects of Stress on Drug Addiction," *Journal of Clinical Investigation,* 118 (February 2008): 454–461.
36. R. Skager, "Reinventing Drug Education for Adolescents," *Drug Policy Letter,* 47 (July/August 2000): 17–19.
37. A. Brender, "Sake, Students, and Cherry Blossoms," *Chronicle for Higher Education* (March 2003): 4–5.
38. J. R. Vicary, E. Smith, L. Caldwell, and J. D. Swisher, "Relationship of Changes in Adolescents' Leisure Activities to Alcohol Use," *American Journal of Health Behavior,* 22 (1998): 276–282.
39. E. Roy, E. Nonn, and N. Haley, "Transition to Injection Drug Use among Street Youth—A Qualitative Analysis," *Drug and Alcohol Dependence,* 94 (April 2008): 19–29.
40. G. N. Weber, "Using to Numb the Pain: Substance Use and Abuse among Lesbian, Gay, and Bisexual Individuals," *Journal of Mental Health Counseling,* 30 (January 2008): 31–48.
41. L. N. Robins, D. H. Davis, and D. W. Goodwin, "Drug Use by U.S. Army Enlisted Men in Vietnam: A Follow-Up on Their Return Home," *American Journal of Epidemiology,* 99 (1974): 235–249.

42. Wright and Pemberton, supra note 18.
43. M. Fridell, M. Hesse, M. Meier, and E. Kuhlhorn, "Antisocial Personality Disorder as a Predictor of Criminal Behaviour in a Longitudinal Study of a Cohort of Abusers of Several Classes of Drugs: Relation to Type of Substance and Type of Crime," *Addictive Behaviors*, 33 (June 2008): 799–811.
44. M. Timmermans, P. A. van Lier, and H. M. Koot, "Which Forms of Child/Adolescent Externalizing Behaviors Account for Late Adolescent Risky Sexual Behavior and Substance Use?" *Journal of Child Psychology and Psychiatry*, 49 (April 2008): 386–394.
45. A. Goldstein, *Addiction: From Biology to Drug Policy,* 2nd ed. (New York: Oxford University Press, 2001).
46. N. B. Eddy, H. Halback, H. Isbell, and M. H. Seever, "Drug Dependence: Its Significance and Characteristics," *Bulletin of the World Health Organization,* 32 (1965): 721–733.
47. J. Interlandi and R. Kelley, "What Addicts Need," *Newsweek*, 151 (March 3, 2008): 36–42.
48. S. Peele, A. Brodsky, and M. Arnold, *The Truth About Addiction and Recovery* (New York: Simon and Schuster, 1991).
49. R. Nusim, *No Matter What the Consequences: A Guide to Help Teens Recognize and Understand Addiction* (Easton, CT: The Weiner Nusim Foundation, 2001).
50. B. Stimmel, *The Facts About Drug Use: Coping with Drugs and Alcohol in Your Family, at Work, in Your Community* (Yonkers, NY: Consumer Union of the United States, 1991).
51. Y. Hser, V. Hoffman, C. E. Grella, and M. D. Anglin, "A 33-Year Follow-Up of Narcotics Addicts," *Archives of General Psychiatry,* 58 (2001): 503–508.
52. S. E. McCabe, B. T. West, M. Morales, J. A. Cranford, and C. J. Boyd, "Does Early Onset of Non-medical Use of Prescription Drugs Predict Subsequent Prescription Drug Abuse and Dependence? Results from a National Study," *Addiction*, 102 (December 2007): 1920–1930.
53. P. Scribner, "Addiction and Free Will" in *New Frontiers in Drug Policy,* edited by A. S. Trebach and K. B. Zeese (Washington, DC: Drug Policy Foundation, 1991).
54. N. Volkow, "The Addicted Brain: Why Such Poor Decisions?" *NIDA Notes,* 18 (November 2003): 2–3.
55. M. J. Lawton, "A Great Prevention Program Gets Results and Attention," *Addiction Letter,* 11, no. 3 (1995).
56. U.S. Department of Health and Human Services, *White Paper: Effectiveness of Substance Abuse Treatment* (Washington, DC: Government Printing Office, 1995).
57. S. Satel, "The Human Factor," *The American* (July/August 2007): 92–102.
58. A. Mann and P. Zickler, "New Avenues of Research Explore Addiction's Disrupted and Destructive Decision-Making," *NIDA Notes,* 18 (November 2003): 1–6.
59. A. Furnham and L. Thomson, "Lay Theories of Heroin Addiction," *Social Science and Medicine,* 43 (1996): 29–40.
60. A. Verdejo-Garcia and M. Perez-Garcia, "Substance Abusers' Self-Awareness of the Neurobehavioral Consequences of Addiction," *Psychiatry Research,* 158 (March 15, 2008): 172–181.
61. M. M. Pearson and R. B. Little, "The Addictive Process in Unusual Addictions: A Further Elaboration of Etiology," *American Journal of Psychiatry,* 125 (1969): 1166–1171.
62. H. Schmid, "Swiss Adolescent Drug Users' and Nonusers' Optimism About Their Future," *Journal of Applied Social Psychology,* 28 (1998): 1889–1902.
63. K. S. Griswold, H. Aranoff, J. B. Kernan, and L. S. Kahn, "Adolescent Substance Use and Abuse: Recognition and Management," *American Family Physician,* 77 (February 1, 2008): 331.
64. J. R. Rodgers, "Addiction: A Whole New View," *Psychology Today,* 27 (1994):32–38.
65. R. Mathias, "Joint Treatment of PTSD and Cocaine Abuse May Reduce Severity of Both Disorders," *NIDA Notes,* 18 (June 2003): 1–6.
66. Mann and Zickler, supra note 58.
67. G. F. Koob and M. Le Moal, "Addiction and the Brain Antireward System," *Annual Review of Psychology,* 59 (2008): 29–53.
68. D. Ball, "Addiction Science and Its Genetics," *Addiction*, 103 (March 2008): 360–367.
69. K. L. Ozelli, "This Is Your Brain on Food," *Scientific American,* 297 (September 2007): 84–85.
70. M. S. Rosenthal, "Sadly, There Is No Magic Bullet," *Newsweek,* 151 (March 3, 2008).
71. P. Zickler, "Evidence Builds That Genes Influence Cigarette Smoking," *NIDA Notes,* 15 (June 2000): 1–5.
72. V. P. Dole and M. E. Nyswander, "Methadone Maintenance: A Theoretical Perspective," in *Theories on Drug Abuse: Selected Contemporary Perspectives,* edited by D. J. Lettieri, M. Sayers, and H. W. Pearson (NIDA Research Monograph 10) (Washington, DC: Government Printing Office, 1980).
73. E. Goode, *Drugs in American Society* (New York: McGraw-Hill, 2007).
74. M. D. Graham, R. A. Young, L. Valach, and R. A. Wood, "Addiction as a Complex Social Process: An Action Theoretical Perspective," *Addiction Research and Theory,* 16 (April 2008): 121–133.
75. Goldstein, supra note 45.
76. J. L. Goode, "Some Considerations on the Disease Concept of Addiction," in *The American Drug Scene,* edited by J. A. Inciardi and K. McElreth (Los Angeles: Roxbury Publishing Company, 2004).
77. E. A. Voth, "America's Longest War," *World and I,* 15 (2000): 24–31.
78. "Booze, Tobacco Prevalent in G-Rated Films, Study Suggests," *Cortland Standard,* June 7, 2001.
79. M. S. Roth, "Media and Message Effects on OTC Prescription Drug Print Advertising Awareness," *Journal of Advertising Research,* 43 (June 2003): 180–194.
80. The Center on Alcohol Marketing and Youth, *Drowned Out: Alcohol Industry "Responsibility" Advertising on Television, 2001–2005* (Washington, D.C.: Georgetown University, June 27, 2007).
81. D. Forbes, "This Is Your Ad Campaign Money. Any Questions?" *Drug Policy Letter,* (Summer 1998): 17–19.
82. Office of National Drug Controls Policy, *National Drug Control Strategy* (Washington, DC: Government Printing Office, 2008).
83. R. Wood and L. B. Synovitz, "Addressing the Threats of MDMA (Ecstasy): Implications for School Health Professionals, Parents, and Community Members," *Journal of School Health,* 71 (January 2001): 38–51.
84. "Student Drug Use," *The Education Digest*, 72 (March 2007): 73–74.
85. J. K. Ibrahim and S. A. Glantz, "The Rise and Fall of Tobacco Control Media Campaigns, 1967–2006," *American Journal of Public Health,* 97 (August 2007): 1383–1896.
86. S. Elliott, "New York Station Takes Chance on Liquor Ads," *The New York Times*, November 30, 2007.
87. M. D. Slater, D. Rouner, K. Murphy, F. Beauvais, J. Leuven, and D. Rodrigues, "Male

Adolescents' Reactions to TV Beer Advertisements: The Effects of Sports Content and Programming Context," *Journal of Studies on Alcohol,* 57 (1996): 425–433.

88. "Campaign Launched against Ads on College Sports TV," *Alcoholism and Drug Abuse Weekly,* 15 (November, 17, 2003): 8.
89. R. L. Collins, P. L. Ellickson, D. McCaffrey, and K. Hambarsoomians, "Early Exposure to Alcohol Advertising and Its Relationship to Underage Drinking," *Journal of Adolescent Health,* 40 (June 2007): 527–534.
90. J. A. Epstein and G. J. Botvin, "Media Resistance Skills and Drug Refusal Techniques: What Is Their Relationship with Alcohol Use among Inner-city Adolescents?" *Addictive Behaviors,* 33 (April 2008): 528–537.
91. E. Single, "The Impact of Social and Regulatory Policy on Drinking Behavior," in *The Development of Alcohol Problems: Exploring the Biopsychosocial Matrix of Risk,* edited by R. A. Zucker, G. M. Boyd, and J. Howard (NIAAA Research Monograph 26) (Rockville, MD: National Institute on Alcohol Abuse and Alcoholism, 1994).
92. "Court: Ban on Alcohol Ads in College Newspapers Unconstitutional," *Associated Press,* July 30, 2004.
93. U.S. Department of Health and Human Services, *Preventing Tobacco Use Among Young People: A Report of the Surgeon General* (Washington, DC: Government Printing Office, 1994).
94. S. Elliott, "Once a Mainstay of Magazines, Cigarette Makers Are Dropping Print Ads," *The New York Times,* November 29, 2007.
95. W. Richey, "Supreme Court Snuffs Maine's Internet Cigarette Sales Rule," *Christian Science Monitor,* February 21, 2008.
96. "States Spend Anti-Smoking Money on Everything But," *USA Today,* January 11, 2008.
97. A. Quindlen, "Killing the Consumer," *Newsweek,* October 1, 2007.
98. R. M. Cartoll-Johnson, "Fashionable Pink Camels," *Oncology Nursing Forum,* 34 (July/August 2007): 755.
99. B. A. Primack, J. E. Bost, and S. R. Land, "Volume of Tobacco Advertising in African American Markets: Systematic Review and Meta-Analysis," *Public Health Reports,* 122 (September/October 2007): 607–615.
100. E. A. Gilpin, M. M. White, K. Messer, and J. P. Pierce, "Receptivity to Tobacco Advertising and Promotions Among Young Adolescents as a Predictor of Established Smoking in Young Adulthood," *American Journal of Public Health,* 97 (August 2007): 1489–1495.
101. J. Wedekind, "The Smokescreen," *Multinational Monitor,* 28 (March/April 2007): 52.
102. G. N. Connolly, C. T. Orleans, and A. Blum, "Snuffing Tobacco Out of Sport," *American Journal of Public Health,* 82 (1992): 351–353.
103. S. Jay, "Tobacco Targets Youth," *The Saturday Evening Post,* January/February 2007.
104. N. Bakalar, "Vital Signs; Racial Disparity Affirmed in Tobacco Advertising," *New York Times,* August 28, 2007.
105. N. Seppa, "TV, Movies Linked to Adolescent Smoking," *Science News,* 171 (March 10, 2007): 149.
106. A. Mathios, R. Avery, C. Bisogni, and C. Shanahan, "Alcohol Portrayal on Prime-Time Television: Manifest and Latent Messages," *Journal of Studies on Alcohol,* 59 (1998): 305–310.
107. D. A. Roberts and P. G. Christenson, *"Here's Looking at You, Kid:" Alcohol, Drugs and Tobacco Entertainment Media* (New York: The National Center on Addiction and Substance Abuse, 2000).
108. Ibid.
109. C. Favret, "An LSD Distribution Network," in *LSD: Still with Us After All These Years,* edited by L. A. Henderson and W. J. Glass (New York: Lexington Books, 1994).
110. *Substance Use in Popular Music Videos* (Rockville, MD: Office of National Drug Control Policy, 2002).
111. D. Herd, "Changes in Drug Use Prevalence in Rap Music Songs, 1979–1997," *Addiction Research and Theory,* 16 (April 2008): 167–180.
112. J. Markert, "Sing a Song of Drug Use-Abuse: Four Decades of Drug Lyrics in Popular Music—From the Sixties to the Nineties," *Sociological Inquiry,* 71 (Spring 2001): 194–195.
113. T. Todd, "Anabolic Steroids: The Gremlins of Sport," in *Sport in America: From Wicked Amusement to National Obsession,* edited by D. W. Wiggins (Champaign, IL: Human Kinetics, 1995).
114. Ibid.
115. J. M. Hoberman and C. E. Yesalis, "The History of Synthetic Testosterone," *Scientific American,* 272 (1995): 76–91.
116. D. W. Pan and J. A. Baker, "Perceptual Mapping of Banned Substances in Athletics," *Journal of Sport and Social Issues,* 22 (1998): 170–182.
117. P. Issari and R. H. Coombs, "Women, Drug Use, and Drug Testing," *Journal of Sport and Social Issues,* 22 (1998): 153–169.
118. Pan and Baker, supra note 116.
119. Issari and Coombs, supra note 117.
120. M. Atkinson, "Playing with Fire: Masculinity, Health, and Sports Supplements," *Sociology of Sport Journal,* 24 (2007): 165–186.
121. Todd, supra note 113.
122. "Steroids (Anabolic-Androgenic)" *NIDA Info Facts,* March 3, 2004.
123. R. M. Julien, *A Primer of Drug Action,* 11th ed. (London: Worth Publishers, 2007).
124. J. M. Berning, K. J. Adams, M. DeBeliso, B. A. Stamford, and I. A. Newman, "Anabolic Androgenic Steroids: Use and Perceived Use in Nonathlete College Students," *Journal of American College Health,* 56 (March/April 2008): 499–504.
125. S. E. McCabe, K. J. Brower, B. T. West, T. F. Nelson, and H. Wechsler, "Trends in Non-medical Use of Anabolic Steroids: Results from Four National Surveys," *Drug and Alcohol Dependence,* 90 (October 8, 2007): 243–251.
126. J. Cohen, R. Collins, J. Darkes, and D. Gwartney, "A League of Their Own: Demographics, Motivations and Patterns of Use of 1,955 Male Adult Non-medical Anabolic Steroid Users in the United States," *Journal of the International Society of Sports Nutrition,* 4 (October 11, 2007): 12.
127. G. Kanayama, M. Boynes, J. I. Hudson, A. E. Field, and H. G. Pope, "Anabolic Steroid Abuse among Teenage Girls: An Illusory Problem?" *Drug and Alcohol Dependence,* 88 (May 11, 2007): 156–162.
128. W. Suggs, "Steroids Are Rampant among College Athletes, Senate Panel Is Told," *The Chronicle of Higher Education* (July 23, 2004): A33.
129. Julien, supra note 123.
130. "Steroids (Anabolic-Androgenic)," supra note 122.
131. H. B. Moss, G. L. Panzak,and R. E. Tarter, "Sexual Functioning of Male Anabolic Steroid Abusers," *Archives of Sexual Behavior,* 22 (193): 1–12.
132. *Steroid Abuse in Today's Society* (Washington, DC: Drug Enforcement Administration, 2004).
133. Hoberman and Yesalis, supra note 115.
134. "Big Changes from 1990 to 2006," *Occupational Health and Safety,* 76 (August 2007): 30.
135. *Anabolic Steroid Abuse, National Institute on Drug Abuse Report* (Rockville, MD:

National Institute on Drug Abuse, 2000).
136. "Anabolic Steroids," *NIDA Community Drug Abuse Bulletin* (Bethesda, MD: National Institute on Drug Abuse, 2000).
137. C. Ehrnborg and T. Rosen, "Physiological and Pharmacological Basis for the Ergogenic Effects of Growth Hormone in Elite Sports," *Asian Journal of Andrology*, 10 (May 2008): 373–383.
138. A. E. Nelson and K. K. Ho, "A Robust Test for Growth Hormone Doping—Present Status and Future Prospects," *Asian Journal of Andrology*, 10 (May 2008): 416–425.
139. D. Epstein, "The ABC's of HGH," *Sports Illustrated*, 108 (March 17, 2008): 32–33.
140. A. Underwood, "Will He Measure Up?" *Newsweek,* September 22, 2003.
141. A. J. Perez, "HGH Bill Altered After Protests," *USA Today*, April 16, 2008.
142. M. R. Kutz and M. J. Gunter, "Creatine Monohydrate Supplementation on Body Weight and Percent Body Fat," *Journal of Strength and Conditioning,* 17, (November 2003): 817–822.
143. L. Gotshalk, et al., "Creatine Supplementation Improves Muscular Performance in Older Women," *European Journal of Applied Physiology*, 102 (January 2008): 223–231.
144. A. J. Silva, et al., "Effect of Creatine on Swimming Velocity, Body Composition and Hydrodynamic Variables," *Journal of Sports Medicine and Physical Fitness*, 47 (March 2007): 58–64.
145. G. A. Wright, P. W. Grandjean, and D. D. Pascoe, "The Effect of Creatine Loading on Thermoregulation and Intermittent Sprint Exercise Performance in a Hot Humid Environment," *Journal of Strength and Conditioning Research*, 21 (August 2007): 655–660.
146. A. Safdar, "Global and Targeted Gene Expression and Protein Content in Skeletal Muscle of Young Men Following Short-Term Creatine Monohydrate. Supplementation," *Physiological Genomics*, 32 (January 2008): 219–228.
147. T. A. McGuine, J. C. Sullivan, and D. A. Bernhardt, "Creatine Supplementation in High School Football Players," *Journal of Athletic Training,* 36 (April–June 2001): 82.
148. J. L. Krzykowski, M. J. Streveler, T. A. McGuine, and J. C. Sullivan, "Creatine Supplementation in Wisconsin High School Female Athletes," *Journal of Athletic Training,* 36 (April–June 2001): 83.
149. E. Singer, "Sport Supplement Gives Vegetarians Brain Boost," *New Scientist,* 179 (August 16, 2003): 7.
150. S. Roitman, T. Green, Y. Osher, N. Karni, and J. Levine, "Creatine Monohydrate in Resistant Depression: A Preliminary Study," *Bipolar Disorders*, 9 (November 2007): 754–758.
151. D. M. Williams, E. S. Anderson, and R. A. Winett, "Social Cognitive Predictors of Creatine Use Versus Non-use Among Male, Undergraduate, Recreational Resistance Trainers," *Journal of Sport Behavior,* 27 (June 2004): 170–183.
152. C. Kilgore, "Creatine and Andro Popular Among High School Athletes," *Family Practice News,* 30 (June 1, 2000): 22–24.
153. W. Kondro, "Athletes' Designer Steroid Leads to Widening Scandal," *The Lancet,* 362 (November 2003): 1466.
154. D. Franklin, "FDA Warns About Dangers of THG: Banned Steroid," *Pediatric News,* 38 (January 2004): 44.
155. A. Weintraub, "Can Drug-Busters Beat New Steroids? It's Scientist vs Scientist as the Athens Olympics Approach," *Business Week,* (June 14, 2004): 82.
156. M. Emmons, "Risks of Doping Often Overlooked for Rewards," *San Jose Mercury News,* (November 12, 2003).
157. D. Patrick, "Thwarting Performance Enhancing Drugs Daunting," *USA Today,* (October 30, 2003).
158. C. A. Weber, H. M. Wood, and M. E. Ernst, "The Effects of Androstenedione Supplementation on Serum Gonadal Hormones," *Journal of Pharmacy Technology*, 23 (November/December 2007): 349–355.
159. J. R. Tynes, "Performance Enhancing Drugs: Effects, Regulations, and the Pervasive Efforts to Control Doping in Major League Baseball," *The Journal of Legal Medicine,* 27 (2006): 493–509.
160. D. Hain, *Drugs and AIDS: Deadly Combination* (Tempe, AZ: D.I.N. Publications, 1996).
161. M. Doherty, "The Effects of Caffeine on the Maximal Accumulated Oxygen Deficit and Short-Term Running Performance," *International Journal of Sports Medicine,* 8 (1998): 95–104.
162. G. M. Smith and H. K. Beecher, "Amphetamine Sulfate and Athletic Performance," *Journal of the American Medical Association,* 1970 (1959): 542–557.
163. J. Kinney, *Loosening the Grip: A Handbook of Alcohol Information,* 9th ed. (New York: McGraw-Hill, 2008).
164. C. P. O'Brien, "Alcohol and Sport: Impact of Social Drinking on Recreational and Competitive Sports Performance," *Sports Medicine,* 15 (1993): 71–77.
165. D. H. Catlin and T. H. Murray, "Performance-Enhancing Drugs, Fair Competition, and Olympic Sport," *Journal of the American Medical Association,* 276 (1996): 231–237.
166. C. M. Meston and B. B. Gorzalka, "Psychoactive Drugs and Human Sexual Behavior: The Role of Serotonergic Activity," *Journal of Psychoactive Drugs,* 24 (1992): 1–40.
167. D. Hollander, "Methamphetamine Use Is Linked to Risky Behavior in Heterosexual Encounters," *Perspectives on Sexual and Reproductive Health,* 40 (March 2008): 53–54.
168. A. Goldstein, N. P. Barnett, T. Pedlow, and J. G. Murphy, "Drinking in Conjunction with Sexual Experiences among At-Risk College Student Drinkers," *Journal of Studies on Alcohol and Drugs,* 68 (September 2007): 697–705.
169. A. L. Girard and C. Y. Senn, "The Role of the New 'Date Rape Drugs' in Attributions About Date Rape," *Journal of Interpersonal Violence*, 23 (January 2008): 3–20.
170. W. H. Masters and V. E. Johnson, *Human Sexual Response* (Boston: Little, Brown, 1996).
171. Ibid.
172. G. S. Yacoubian and R. J. Peters, "An Exploration of Recent Club Drug Use among Rave Attendees," *Journal of Drug Education*, 37 (2007): 145–161.
173. W. H. Masters, V. E. Johnson, and R. C. Kolodny, *Sex and Human Loving* (Boston: Little, Brown, 1986).
174. N. K. Mello, "Drug Abuse and Reproduction in Women," in *Drug Addiction Research and the Health of Women,* edited by C. L. Wetherington and A. B. Roman (Rockville, MD: National Institute on Drug Abuse, 1998).
175. *Anabolic Steroids: A Dangerous and Illegal Way to Seek Athletic Dominance and Better Appearance* (Washington, DC: Drug Enforcement Administration, March 2004).
176. R. D. Weiss, S. T. Mirin, and R. B. Bartel, *Cocaine* (Washington, DC: American Psychiatric Press, 1994).
177. J. Quittner, "Crystal's Destructive Path: Gay Men Continue to Be Systematically Ravaged by the Deadly Drug as Officials Try to Stop an Epidemic," *The Advocate* (March 16, 2004): 24–28.

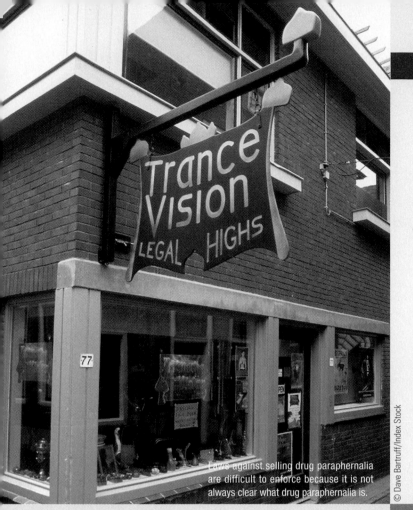

Laws against selling drug paraphernalia are difficult to enforce because it is not always clear what drug paraphernalia is.

FACT OR FICTION?

1. When Harvard University was started, students were prohibited from drinking alcohol.
2. At one time, any drug, including cocaine or heroin, could be bought in the United States without a doctor's prescription.
3. The Marijuana Tax Act of 1937 stated that individuals could use marijuana if they paid a federal tax.
4. The drug thalidomide, which caused thousands of babies to be born with deformities in the 1950s and 1960s, is prescribed today for numerous medical conditions.
5. In the United States, heroin, which is a Schedule I drug, can be used in extreme cases for pain relief.
6. In the last 5 years, the number of people incarcerated for drug offenses has decreased.
7. Students are more likely to commit drug law violations on school days than on nonschool days.
8. More people in the United States are arrested for offenses related to marijuana than to cocaine.
9. Marijuana use is lower in countries where marijuana is decriminalized, compared with the United States.
10. The penalties for powder cocaine are more severe than those for crack cocaine.

Turn the page to check your answers

4 Drugs and the Law

Chapter Objectives

After completing this chapter, the reader should be able to describe:

- How early drugs laws have affected drug-taking behavior
- The effects of the temperance movement on alcohol consumption
- Factors leading to the regulation of opium and other drugs in the United States
- How racism is a factor in drug legislation
- Reasons accounting for the high narcotic addiction rate in the United States in the early 1900s
- The purpose of the Harrison Act of 1914
- Events leading up to the Marijuana Tax Act of 1937
- Differences between the Food, Drug, and Cosmetic Act of 1938 and the Pure Food and Drug Act of 1906
- How the Anti-Drug Abuse Act differs from the Controlled Substances Act
- Whether drug enforcement policies are racist
- The differences between drug decriminalization, drug legalization, and harm reduction

FACT OR FICTION?

1. **Fiction:** The fact is—many original students at Harvard stored kegs of beer next to their supply of wine.
2. **Fact:** In the late 1800s and early 1900s, there were no federal laws prohibiting the purchase of cocaine or heroin.
3. **Fact:** If people paid a tax to the U.S. Treasury Department, they could use marijuana. The government refused to accept the tax payment.
4. **Fact:** Thalidomide is prescribed for numerous medical conditions, especially Hansen's disease (formerly called leprosy).
5. **Fiction:** The fact is—all Schedule I drugs are prohibited even for medical purposes.
6. **Fiction:** The fact is—the number of people incarcerated for drug offenses has climbed steadily over the last 5 years.
7. **Fact:** Due to several possible reasons, including access to other students, drug law violations are more likely to occur when school is in session rather than when it is not.
8. **Fact:** In recent years, marijuana has been implicated more frequently in arrests than cocaine. The opposite was true in the 1990s.
9. **Fact:** Decriminalization of marijuana has not increased its usage in countries that have adopted this policy.
10. **Fiction:** The fact is—current penalties for crack cocaine offenses are 100 times greater than those for powder cocaine offenses.

From the time the first settlers arrived in the New World, attempts have been made to regulate the use of mind-altering substances. The first substance subject to regulation was alcohol. Although moderate alcohol consumption was believed to be beneficial to the mind and body, excessive drinking was discouraged. In Massachusetts in 1645, taverns were fined for selling more than half a pint of wine to a person at one time.[1] Drunkenness resulted in fines for first-time offenders, whereas hard labor and whippings were punishments for chronic offenders.

The **temperance movement** was a prominent force in the United States in the late 1700s as a result of the work of eminent Philadelphia physician Benjamin Rush. Rather than promoting prohibition, Rush advocated that people become more educated about the hazards of alcohol.[2] Even though the temperance drive continued throughout the early 1800s, alcohol was not prohibited until 1851, when the governor of Maine, Neal Dow, enacted legislation to halt its use. Within 4 years, 11 states and 2 territories passed similar legislation. A complete description of the temperance movement and Prohibition is included in Chapter 6.

Early Drug Regulations

To generate much-needed income, Congress passed an excise tax on whiskey in 1791. Farmers in southwestern Pennsylvania violently objected to the excise tax because they considered whiskey an economic necessity. To squelch this insurrection, President George Washington sent in the militia from several states. This historical event, known as the *Whiskey Rebellion*, was important not only because the tax produced income for the federal government, but also because the government demonstrated that it had the power to enforce federal laws within a state.

Another drug that fell under government control was opium. The United States signed its first treaty to regulate the international opium trade in 1833. In 1842, the federal government imposed a tax on crude opium shipped to the United States. Taxing imported opium had very little impact on its use.

Fears regarding opium use increased with the importation of Chinese workers to work on the railroad.[3] It was reported that young men and women were being morally corrupted by visiting opium houses, or dens, although many brothels, where one easily found drugs, already existed.[4] In 1875, San Francisco passed an ordinance prohibiting opium smoking in opium dens. The legislation could have been motivated by racism because there was much anti-Chinese sentiment at the time.[5] In 1890 the federal government allowed only U.S. citizens to manufacture opium or import it. Opium poppies were legally grown in the United States until 1942.

Another drug-related problem looming in American society was the unregulated marketing and sale of proprietary (over-the-counter) substances. **Proprietary drugs** were sold for every possible problem ranging from colds to asthma to alcoholism to sexually transmitted diseases. Both heroin and cocaine were promoted as cures for morphine and alcohol addiction. Moreover, they were reportedly nonaddicting.[6] Because of the widespread abuse of these proprietary drugs, which often included drugs such as cocaine and opium, the *Pure Food and Drug Act of 1906* was enacted.

This law and other significant drug-related legislation are discussed in the following pages.

temperance movement A social trend that developed in the United States in the 1800s when groups sought to reduce alcohol use

proprietary drugs Drugs that can be purchased without a prescription; over-the-counter drugs

Significant Laws

Drug-related laws have had a great impact on society. Yet, the question remains: Do laws against drugs thwart drug-related problems or do they contribute to drug problems? Also, do drug laws affect whether people use drugs? Other questions regarding the goals of drug laws include the following:

- Should drug laws try to stop drug use, drug abuse, or drug dependency?
- Should drug laws be aimed at drug users, sellers, or traffickers?
- Should the role of government be to inform its citizens about drugs or to prevent its citizens from using drugs?
- Should a person be prevented from engaging in self-destructive behavior?

Pure Food and Drug Act of 1906

Before 1906, patent medicines were largely unregulated. The era between 1890 and 1906 was described as the "golden age of patent medicines." The United States was a free marketplace. Unlike authorities in European countries, the U.S. government had little control over physicians or pharmacists.

Concerns over patent medicines grew in the early 1900s. To regulate improperly labeled and contaminated foods, beverages, and drugs, President Theodore Roosevelt recommended legislation to prohibit the interstate commerce of adulterated and misbranded foods and drugs. Despite opposition from the patent medicine industry, the Pure Food and Drug Act of 1906 passed.

The Food and Drug Administration (FDA) was created to assess drug hazards and prohibit the sale of dangerous drugs. The law required drug manufacturers to report adverse reactions to their products.[7]

Shortly after Roosevelt's proposal, the putrid conditions of the meatpacking industry were recounted in the book *The Jungle* by Upton Sinclair. Sinclair's account provided further evidence for the need to regulate business.

Another concern was that morphine and other narcotics were being overused in patent medicines. Families were encouraged to avoid patent medicines containing opiates and other drugs. Magazines such as *Collier's* and *Ladies Home Journal* had articles warning of the dangers of patent medicines, especially those containing morphine and cocaine.[8]

The 1906 law allowed the government to enter the drug marketplace. The intent of the law was to regulate what was stated on the drug label. Drug producers were required to indicate whether opiates, cocaine, alcohol, or other psychoactive substances were in their products.[9] The law did not eliminate drugs such as cocaine, alcohol, heroin, and morphine from being included in products, but the amount or proportion of drugs in the medicine had to be listed on the label.[10] The law did not address how drugs were advertised. Nevertheless, the amount of morphine and cocaine in medicinal preparations was reduced.

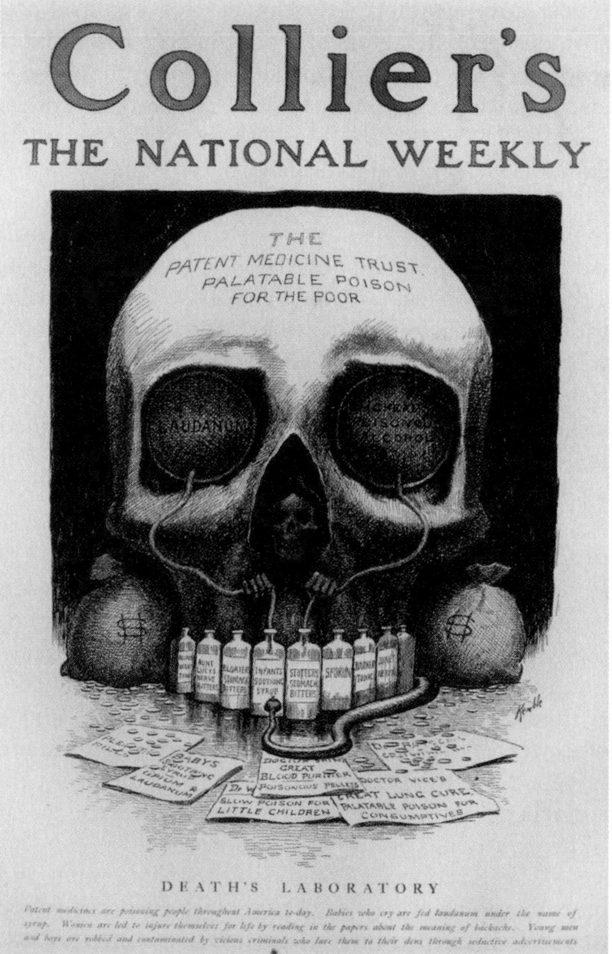

Magazine articles, such as this one in Collier's (June 3, 1905), were influential in the passage of the Pure Food and Drug Act of 1906.

Harrison Act of 1914

At the beginning of the 20th century, opiate dependency was believed to have reached its highest rate ever in the United States. With a population of 76 million, the United States had an estimated 250,000 narcotics addicts.[11] Contributing to this high rate of dependency were development of the hypodermic needle, the availability of narcotics via mail-order catalogs and over-the-counter medicines, and narcotic use by soldiers during the Civil War.[12] In 1912, the United States organized an international conference in The Hague, Netherlands, to control the opium trade. Several countries agreed to restrict international trade and domestic sale of narcotics.

The need to limit opiate use in the United States resulted in the passage of the Harrison Act. Before that, 29 states had passed laws to control opiate use, and 46 states had enacted laws regulating cocaine. The Harrison Act, written by Dr. Hamilton Wright, allowed a doctor to prescribe narcotics "in the course of his professional practice and for legitimate medical purposes." Doctors were required to register each year and pay a modest fee.[13] Doctors and pharmacists had to keep records of the prescriptions they wrote. Although cocaine is a stimulant, it was classified as a narcotic, and its nonmedical use became illegal. Thus, cocaine became a demonized drug, and its illegality became inevitable.[14]

The law's purported purpose was to govern the marketing and sale of narcotics. It regulated nonmedical narcotic use and made possession of narcotics without a prescription illegal.[15] One medical use was to prevent the withdrawal symptoms that addicts would otherwise have. Eventually, prescribing or taking narcotics to maintain addiction became illegal, and doctors who did this faced conviction. The adverse publicity ruined the careers of many doctors, even those who were not convicted.

The effects of the Harrison Act were counterproductive. Because people did not have legal access to narcotics, many became delirious from sudden withdrawal. Hospitals treated large numbers of people with drug problems. To obtain drugs, an increasing number of people resorted to criminal activity.[16] A medical problem became a legal problem. Those who were dependent on narcotics had no legitimate or safe place to obtain them. Moreover, medical personnel could not risk helping addicts, under the threat of prosecution.

A 1918 report to Congress noted that opium and other narcotics were still used extensively; that "dope peddlers" had formed a national organization, enabling drugs to be smuggled across U.S. borders; and that the wrongful use of narcotics had increased.[17] To thwart these problems, stiffer law enforcement was recommended. In 1924, heroin was totally prohibited, even for medical purposes. Ironically, after heroin was banned, its black market use increased greatly.[18]

Marijuana Tax Act of 1937

When the federal government passed the Marijuana Tax Act in 1937, 46 of the 48 states and the District of Columbia already had laws against marijuana. Some believe that passage of the federal law had racist overtones; just as the Harrison Act was motivated by anti-Chinese sentiment, the Marijuana Tax Act might have been linked to anti-Mexican feelings.[19] This law forbade recreational use but not medicinal or industrial uses. Anyone using marijuana was required to pay a tax, and failure to comply meant a large fine or prison term for tax evasion. In essence, using marijuana was not illegal if one paid the tax to use it. However, the federal government refused to accept the tax on marijuana; thus, by default its use is illegal. Recent data indicate that about 500,000 Americans are arrested annually for marijuana offenses.[20]

The person responsible for state and federal anti-marijuana laws was Henry J. Anslinger, commissioner of the Federal Bureau of Narcotics. Established in 1932, it later became the Drug Enforcement Administration (DEA).[21] Anslinger viewed drug addicts as immoral, vicious people who deserved swift, harsh punishment. State laws against marijuana were comparable to laws applied to heroin, morphine, and cocaine. Until 1971, the federal government labeled marijuana a narcotic.

Media reports sensationalized the hazards of marijuana use, particularly violent behavior, including rape.[22] *Scientific American* described marijuana users as sexually excitable and often vicious. The movie *Reefer Madness* depicted decent, clean-cut young men and women falling into a life of depravity and crime once they started using marijuana. A popular poster in the 1930s titled "The Assassination of Youth" illustrated the devastating effects of marijuana.

In testimony before Congress, Anslinger described how one young man, Victor Licata, became deranged after smoking one marijuana cigarette and hacked his family with an axe. Anslinger detailed how marijuana leads to addiction, violent crime, psychosis, and mental deterioration.[23] Not surprisingly, the Marijuana Tax Act passed through Congress with little debate.

During the congressional hearings about marijuana, no medical testimony describing its adverse effects was presented. However, the *Journal of the American Medical Association* (May 1, 1937) presented an editorial that was extremely critical of the proposed laws. The editorial stated that even though few physicians prescribed the drug, they should be able to prescribe it as they wished without incurring additional burdens of a tax, record keeping, and

elixir sulfanilamide An antibiotic that killed more than 100 people in the 1930s

diethyl glycol A chemical solvent

reporting. Moreover, the cost of this legislation would contribute to the rising cost of sickness. This same editorial expressed doubt that the law would have any effect on nonmedicinal use because antinarcotic legislation had little impact on narcotic and coca use.

The arguments against marijuana consisted largely of newspaper accounts. Dr. William Woodward, a physician-lawyer representing the American Medical Association (AMA), highlighted this point. He testified before Congress that the many horrific stories circulating about the effects of marijuana had no verifiable proof. Furthermore, Woodward said the law would be a nuisance for the medical profession. The AMA's arguments were disregarded.[24]

Woodward and the AMA were not alone in their opposition to marijuana legislation. Birdseed distributors protested that canaries would not sing as well, or at all, if marijuana seeds were removed from their diets. On this point Congress agreed, and the law was amended to allow the use of sterilized marijuana seeds.

The Marijuana Tax Act did not specifically prohibit marijuana. Physicians, dentists, and others could prescribe it by paying $1 per year for a license fee. Druggists were required to pay a license fee of $15 annually, marijuana growers paid $25 annually, and marijuana importers and manufacturers were assessed a $50 annual fee. Nonmedical use, possession, and sale of untaxed marijuana were illegal. In 1969 the Supreme Court declared that punishment for nonpayment was unconstitutional because payment of taxes would be self-incriminating.

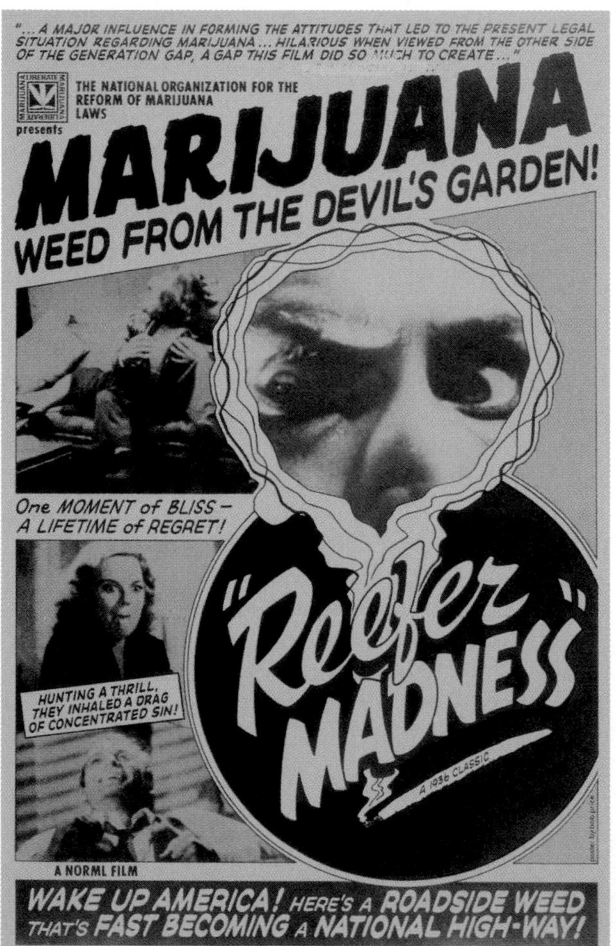

The 1930s movie Reefer Madness *distorted the effects caused by marijuana.*

Although the Marijuana Tax Act restricted the drug to medical uses, Commissioner Anslinger ultimately sought to have it banned altogether. Only a small percentage of physicians paid the tax. One could conclude that Anslinger succeeded, because the use of marijuana as a medical agent was in essence stopped. Because the federal government does not believe that marijuana has been proven to be medically beneficial, it continues to be illegal for medical purposes despite the fact that citizens in a number of states voted for its approval. Federal laws take precedence over state laws.

Food, Drug, and Cosmetic Act of 1938

Before World War II, all drugs except narcotics could be bought over the counter. Efforts to regulate nonnarcotic drugs were ineffective until a new antibiotic called **elixir sulfanilamide** reached the market. This product, made by dissolving a liquid form of a sulfa drug in the chemical solvent **diethyl glycol**, was extremely toxic. More than 100 people died from kidney poisoning. Under guidelines of the Pure Food and Drug Act of 1906, a drug manufacturer could not be prosecuted for these fatalities. When the need for some type of regulation became apparent, the 1938 federal Food, Drug, and Cosmetic Act was passed.

The 1938 law differed from the 1906 law in that

- Pharmaceutical companies were required to file applications with the federal government demonstrating that all *new* drugs were safe and properly labeled.
- Drug manufacturers had to submit a "new drug application" to the FDA, giving the FDA more authority and responsibility.

Besides listing all ingredients and their respective quantities on the label, instructions concerning proper use of the drug and warnings of the drug's dangers had to be included and written so that the average consumer could understand them.

Limitations of the 1938 Food, Drug, and Cosmetic Act included the following:

- It did not cover drugs that were previously marketed.
- Drugs had to be proven *safe,* but not proven *effective.*
- The federal government had little authority to enact penalties if the information on the labels was not written clearly.
- Drug manufacturers were given the responsibility for determining whether a drug would be sold as a prescription or an over-the-counter drug.
- Drug manufacturers conducted their own tests to determine a drug's effectiveness.

Passage of the 1938 law resulted in the creation of a class of drugs that could be bought only with a prescription. Whether a drug was accorded prescription or nonprescription status was determined by the manufacturer. Thus, a drug labeled as a prescription drug by one company could be marketed as an over-the-counter drug by another.

This quizzical situation existed until 1951, when the Humphrey-Durham Amendment was passed. However, neither the 1938 Food, Drug, and Cosmetic Act nor the Humphrey-Durham Amendment allowed for the federal government to oversee the clinical testing of drugs. The effectiveness of drugs was still determined by the drug manufacturers. In addition, it has only been since 2002 that the FDA required pediatric testing.[25] Previously, drug testing was only done with adults.

Kefauver-Harris Amendments

Efforts to get the federal government more involved in supervising drug testing were stymied until a sedative, used primarily in Europe, came to the United States. This drug, **thalidomide,** was first introduced in Germany in 1958 as an anticonvulsive agent[26] and later was used for treating hypertension, migraines, and morning sickness caused by pregnancy. Unfortunately, it altered the development of an embryo's arms and legs, resulting in about 8,000 deformed babies in Europe.[27] This resulted in the implementation of stronger regulations regarding drug testing. The Kefauver-Harris Amendments were passed in 1962, boosting the government's ability to regulate new and existing drugs.

It should be noted here that even though the effects of thalidomide on the fetus are acknowledged, research into its benefits in other areas has continued. The drug could be helpful in treating a myriad of conditions ranging from eye disease (macular degeneration) to rheumatoid arthritis, AIDS, ulcers of the mouth, diabetes, and cancers of the breast, brain,

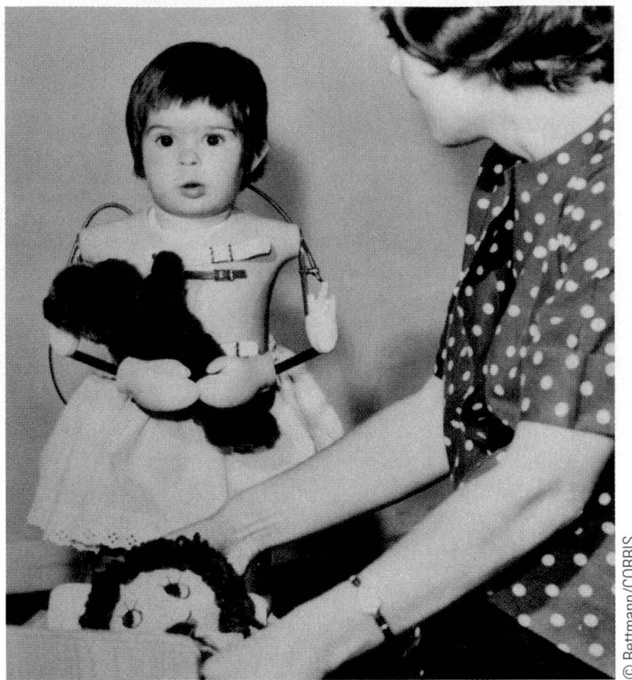

© Bettmann/CORBIS.

As a result of thalidomide's effects on the fetus, the United States strengthened its laws regarding the regulation of medicinal drugs.

and prostate. In 1998, the FDA approved thalidomide for treating Hansen's disease (formerly known as leprosy). One potential problem, however, is that once a drug is approved for any purpose, physicians can prescribe it for any other purpose. Thus, a concern is that the incidence of thalidomide-exposed babies will increase.

The Kefauver-Harris Amendments gave the FDA the authority to withdraw drugs from the marketplace. Also, drug advertisements directed to physicians were required to include the drug's side effects and its contraindicated uses. Although manufacturers still were responsible for drug testing, their testing procedures required prior approval from the FDA.

Extensive drug testing delays the introduction of beneficial drugs. Despite this, most people favor stringent drug-testing laws. At the same time, many politicians are putting pressure on the FDA to approve drugs more quickly. Another development is that pharmaceutical companies are now advertising prescription drugs directly to consumers.[28]

Between 1938 and 1962, several thousand prescription and over-the-counter drugs were introduced into the marketplace. To evaluate the effectiveness, safety, and claims of the manufacturers, the FDA asked the National Research Council to conduct a study of these drugs. The research project, undertaken in 1972, was called the *Drug Efficacy Study.* Because it would be especially onerous to evaluate each product, the researchers chose to evaluate the active ingredients in the products. The active ingredients were placed into one of three categories:

Category I drugs: those determined to be safe, effective, and properly labeled.

Category II drugs: those not generally recognized as safe and effective, or recognized as mislabeled; must be removed from medications within 6 months after the FDA issues its final regulations.

Category III drugs: those for which data are insufficient to determine general recognition of safety and effectiveness.

Due to several recent events, further drug safety reforms have been enacted. In 2004, Vioxx was removed from the marketplace because it was implicated with an increased risk of heart attacks and strokes. In addition, there are concerns over young people committing suicide while on antidepressant drugs. In July 2007, Congress enacted legislation (the FDA Revitalization Act) to give more authority to the U.S. FDA to track adverse effects from drugs and to fine companies that provide false or misleading information.[29]

Comprehensive Drug Abuse Prevention and Control Act of 1970

The Comprehensive Drug Abuse Prevention and Control Act, known as the Controlled Substances Act, had the effect of repealing, replacing, or updating all previous federal laws dealing with narcotics and dangerous drugs. Individual states still could impose their own regulations. The law, however, clearly stated that federal enforcement and prosecution take precedence if any illegal activity is involved. The original intent of this law, when presented before Congress, focused on rehabilitation, research, and education. The act expanded community health centers and Public Health Service hospitals for drug abusers. At its final passage, though, the bill emphasized enforcement because of the law-and-order sentiment that prevailed in Congress.

Several important components of this law are worth noting. A Commission on Marijuana and Drug Abuse was established to make recommendations subsequent to a 2-year study. Federal mandatory sentences for first-offense possession of an illegal drug were abolished, the possibility of parole was reimplemented, and public records of the conviction were erased. In essence, the record was restored to prearrest status and the violator was legally allowed to deny ever having been arrested on such a charge. Depending on the state, a violator still could receive a 1-year prison sentence or a $5,000 fine, or both, if convicted on a first-offense charge of possession of a controlled substance. Or the offender could receive a 1-year probation instead. The emphasis of the law was to punish the drug dealer, particularly organized dealers, rather than the drug user. A recent court decision questioned the application of the Controlled Substances Act to the possession of marijuana for medical purposes.[30]

The Controlled Substances Act of 1970 divided drugs into five categories called *schedules* (see Table 4.1). Penalties for distributing, manufacturing, and possessing psychoactive drugs depend on which of the five schedules includes the drug.[31] The Justice Department enforces the law, and the Department of Health and Human Services (DHHS) evaluates drugs to decide the appropriate schedule. The criteria for determining a drug's schedule are as follows:

- The drug's potential for abuse
- Scientific knowledge of the drug
- The drug's capacity to produce psychic or physiological dependence
- The drug's pharmacological effects
- The drug's risk to public health
- The drug's history, duration, scope, and current patterns of abuse
- Whether the drug is an immediate precursor of a substance already controlled under this title

thalidomide A sedative that was found in the 1960s to cause birth defects including missing or malformed limbs

Category I drugs Drugs determined to be safe, effective, and properly labeled

Category II drugs Drugs generally recognized as unsafe and ineffective or as mislabeled; must be removed from medications within 6 months after the FDA issues its final regulations

Category III drugs Drugs for which data are insufficient to determine general recognition of safety and effectiveness

Anti-Drug Abuse Act

The Anti-Drug Abuse Act was signed into law by President Ronald Reagan in 1988. Unlike the Controlled Substances Act, this legislation was directed at the drug user, not just the drug manufacturers or distributors. The point of this law was to reduce drug demand.

On Campus

Students convicted on drug charges become ineligible for federal financial aid and loans for up to 1 year after conviction. Repeat offenders can face permanent loss of financial assistance.

Source: Office of National Drug Control Policy, 2004.

Whereas previous legislation was directed to curtailing the *supply* of drugs, this law emphasizes stringent punishment of the user. Punishment could be waived if the user completes a drug rehabilitation program or makes an earnest effort to get into a rehabilitation program.

The law greatly increased the federal prison population and led to a new Cabinet position, Director of National Drug Control Policy, commonly known as the "drug czar."

The Anti-Drug Abuse Act stipulates that anyone who commits murder or orders someone's murder in conjunction with a drug-related felony can receive the death penalty. Other elements of this law include registration of the following:

- Chemicals used in the manufacture of drugs
- Sales of firearms to felons
- Airplanes

TABLE 4.1 Drug Schedules

	I	II	III	IV	V
Potential for abuse	High	High	Some, but not as much as drugs on Schedules I and II	Low, less than Schedule III drugs	Low, less than Schedule IV drugs
Medical use	None (marijuana is being used for medical purposes, but it is not authorized by the DEA as having medical application)	Yes	Yes	Yes	Yes
Maximum penalties for illegal manufacturing and distribution	*First offense (narcotics):* 15 years in prison, $25,000 fine, 3 years probation *Subsequent offenses:* 30 years in prison, $50,000 fine, 6 years probation *First offense (non-narcotics):* 5 years in prison, $15,000 fine, 2 years probation *Second offense:* 10 years in prison, $30,000 fine, 4 years probation	Same as Schedule I	*First offense:* 5 years in prison, $15,000 fine, 2 years probation *Second offense:* 10 years in prison, $30,000 fine, 4 years probation	*First offense:* 3 years in prison, $10,000 fine, 1 year probation *Second offense:* $20,000 fine, 6 years in prison, 2 years probation	*First offense:* 1 year in prison, $50,000 fine, *and* no probation period
Maximum penalties for illegal possession	*First offense:* 1 year in prison and $5,000 fine *Second offense:* 2 years in prison and $10,000 fine; probation may be granted for first offense	Same as Schedule I	Same as Schedule I	Same as Schedule I	Same as Schedule I
Production controlled	Yes	Yes	Yes	No	No
Examples	Heroin, LSD, mescaline, marijuana, methaqualone, peyote	Cocaine, methamphetamine, opium, morphine, methadone, codeine	Phencyclidine (PCP), stimulants (those not containing amphetamines), some narcotic preparations, some barbiturates	Diazepam (Valium), phenobarbital, barbital, meprobamate (Equanil, Miltown), some nonamphetamine stimulants not already included	Preparations with small amounts of narcotics, diluted opium and codeine compounds

Under this law, drug users are punished more stringently than rapists or robbers.[32] Also, the government can take anything in one's possession at the time of arrest. The effect has been that "in more than 80% of asset forfeiture cases, the owner is never charged with a crime, yet government officials can and usually do keep the seized property."[33] The penalties for drug possession are the following:

- Loss of all federal benefits, such as student loans and grants, for 1 year for a first offense and 2 years after a second offense
- Forfeiture of the car, boat, or airplane in which the drug is found (this may have implications if you lend your car, boat, or plane to someone caught with drugs)
- A civil fine of up to $10,000
- Removal of the individual and his or her family from public housing if that person engages in drug-related activity in or near public housing

College Students and Drug Convictions

The Anti-Drug Abuse Act has implications for college students. At the present time, college students who complete the federal financial aid form, also known as FAFSA, are asked if they have ever had a drug conviction. Students who were convicted of simple possession face a 1-year ban on financial aid. A second conviction of possession results in a 2-year ban on aid, and a third conviction means that one loses eligibility for financial aid indefinitely. A drug selling conviction means loss of eligibility for 2 years if that is one's first offense. An estimated 200,000 students have lost access to aid since this law went into effect. Some politicians are debating whether this law should continue because they feel it is discriminatory. Children of wealthy parents who are convicted of a drug charge do not need financial assistance to attend college.[34]

Legal Issues

Should the sale of drug paraphernalia be illegal? What effect would such a law have? Should people using small amounts of illegal drugs for personal enjoyment receive harsh criminal penalties? What are the advantages and disadvantages of decriminalizing or legalizing drugs? What impact has drug enforcement had on drug use? Should the vast amount of money spent on stopping drugs be used differently?

In trying to answer these questions, political forces take very different stances.[35] Cultural conservatives advocate more emphasis on enforcing drug laws but removing legal loopholes, technicalities, and restrictions. Free-market libertarians think that government is too intrusive, that people have the right to hurt themselves, and that individuals are ultimately responsible for their own behavior. Radical constructionists believe that drug abuse is symptomatic of greater problems in society and that we need to address the underlying social problems if drug abuse is to be curtailed. Nonetheless, the United States currently has more than 500,000 people in prison for drug-related offenses, which is more than 10 times as many as in 1980.[36]

drug paraphernalia Items that are aids to using drugs

Drug Paraphernalia

One way to reduce drug use, logically, would be to make **drug paraphernalia** illegal. Cigarette rolling papers, water pipes, razors, clay pipes, roach clips, spoons, mirrors, and other products in "head shops," novelty stores, and convenience stores have been used for illegal drugs. Prosecuting individuals for possessing drug paraphernalia is viewed as a deterrent for drug use.[37] Three decades ago, the federal government proposed the Model Drug Paraphernalia Act of 1979. Specifically, the bill attempted to halt the following items:

> all equipment, products, and materials of any kind which are used, intended for use, or designed for use, in planting, propagating, cultivating, growing, harvesting, manufacturing, compounding, converting, producing, processing, preparing, testing, analyzing, packaging, re-packaging, storing, containing, concealing, injecting, ingesting, inhaling, or otherwise introducing into the human body a controlled substance.

A flaw in this bill was that many household products could be construed as drug paraphernalia. The straws children use to drink milk can be used to snort cocaine, a small change purse could be used to conceal drugs, and some people use cigarette rolling papers to roll marijuana. Because this bill raised many constitutional questions, it was never adopted. More recently, the federal government has cracked down on the interstate sale of bongs and arrested legendary marijuana smoker Tommy Chong.[38]

The War on Drugs

In 1988 the U.S. Congress proclaimed that the country would be drug-free by 1995. This proclamation did not become a reality. Instead, political rhetoric has exacerbated the problem of drugs in the United States. Politicians rely on inflammatory speeches rather than on reasoned responses.[39] Despite vast amounts of money allotted for drug interdiction, the quantity of drugs interdicted while being smuggled into the United States is minimal. For the fiscal year 2008, the U.S. government proposed allocating $936.8 million to the Department of Defense, $3,493.7 million to the Department of Homeland Security, $2,797 million to the Justice Department, and $473.4 million to the Office of National Drug Control Policy.[40] The monetary expense and human resources employed to combat illicit drug use are enormous. Yet, the War on Drugs is being lost. In 1965, according to the Drug Enforcement Agency, fewer than 4 million Americans had ever used illegal drugs. Today, the number of Americans that have used illegal drugs has exceeded 110 million. In addition, the number of people who have used cocaine increased 700% in the last 35 years.[41]

People agree that drug abuse is undesirable. But should drug abuse be treated as a criminal problem or a public health problem? From a public health perspective, the consequences of U.S. drug policies are infection, violence, and criminal injustice. Tax dollars, some believe, are wrongly diverted from improving health care and education to fighting the drug war.

According to Ethan Nadelmann, a leading proponent of drug reform, government officials should stop wasting taxpayer money on ineffective criminal policies. They should stop arresting drug users and put more effort into reducing overdose deaths and reducing the number of nonviolent drug offenders behind bars.[42]

The government's assault on illicit drugs has resulted in social tension, ill health, violent crime, compromised civil liberties, and international conflict. Currently, drug offenders account for 60% of federal prisoners and 20% of state inmates. More than 2 million people are incarcerated for drug offenses.[43] Figure 4.1 shows the upward trend in the number of people arrested for drug abuse violations since 1970.

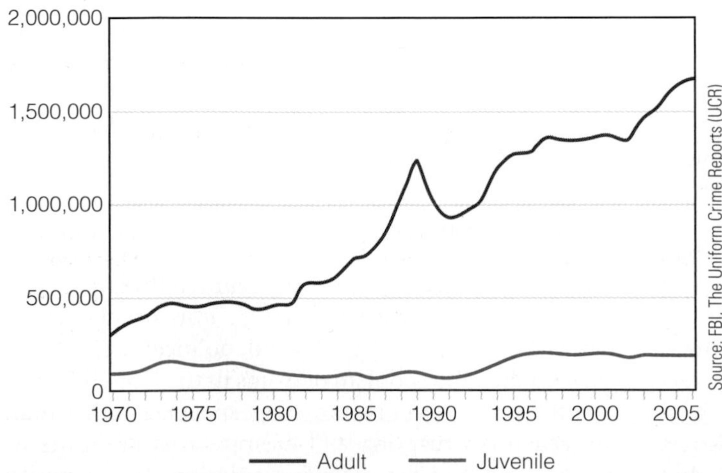

Figure 4.1 Drug Arrests, 1970–2006

Legislation

Con Arguments

Harmful and illegal drug use will never be totally stopped. Still, do drug laws help to prevent drug use, and would **decriminalization** reduce crime? Some argue that legalization would increase drug use, addiction, and drug-related deaths. Herbert Kleber, an adviser to President George H. W. Bush's administration, maintained that the main danger of legalization would be that the lower cost and availability would lead to more use and dependency.[44] And criminal activity would escalate because there would be more users and addicts.[45] Wilson contends that keeping drugs illegal prevents many people from abusing drugs.[46]

According to this line of reasoning, drug legalization would reduce the cost of drugs to somewhere between one-third and one-twentieth of the illegal price. Drug-related crimes might indeed fall, but the number of addicts would rise.[47] Consequently, legalization would result in more dysfunctional addicts who would be unable to support their lifestyles and drug use through legitimate means. And "more users would mean more of the violence associated with the ingestion of drugs."[48]

Pro Arguments

Half of all violence is drug-related.[49] Some argue that legalization would not eliminate the black market, while others maintain that there would not be enough treatment facilities for the larger number of addicts: Decriminalization is not a panacea. It will not stop the drug crisis, but it could substantially reduce the irrationality and inhumanity of our present punitive war on drugs. In addition, decriminalization could decrease law enforcement expenses, since it costs about $25,000 a year to keep a person in prison.[50] Another benefit of drug legalization, according to officials in the Netherlands, where marijuana use is allowed under certain circumstances, is that the quality of the drug can be assured.[51]

Many drugs have potentially destructive side effects. Intravenous drug use is a common source of new HIV/AIDS infections. However, since 1992, the number of people acquiring HIV from injecting drugs has decreased.[52] Figure 4.2 illustrates the number of AIDS cases from 1981 to 2004. Table 4.2 shows the estimated number of AIDS diagnoses, AIDS deaths, and persons living with AIDS, 2002–2006. By supplying users with access to clean needles and purer drugs, legalization may result in fewer HIV/AIDS deaths.

Many activities—for example, hang gliding, parachuting, or driving race cars—can cause harm. Yet, they are not banned. Could not the same argument apply to drug use? The fundamental question is: Should a person be coerced into abstaining from behaviors he or she finds desirable or necessary? If two people buy and sell drugs by mutual consent, is it criminal activity when neither the buyer nor the seller considers himself or herself a victim? The billions of dollars spent on drug enforcement, according to some drug experts, might be put to use more effectively if the money were directed toward education and treatment programs rather than enforcement.[53]

Drugs can be harmful, but so, too, can be the adverse consequences related to the drugs themselves or to their illegal status. "Prohibitions enhance the dangers not just of drugs but of the settings in which they are used."[54]

Does drug use cause criminal activity, or do people who engage in crime also use drugs? The answer is not clear. Some contend that, when drugs are made illegal, their costs increase and there is a corresponding rise in criminal activity.[55] Criminal behavior goes up, not down, when drugs become illegal, whereas their costs would decline if they were legalized.[56] The greater the risk associated with selling and trafficking drugs, coupled with scarcity of supplies, the more the cost of drugs rises.[57]

decriminalization The reduction or elimination of penalties for illegal activities

Twenty years of research showed that street-drug users in Miami were involved with criminal activity before using narcotics or cocaine and that drug use per se was not the root cause of criminality.[58] After looking into the link between narcotics and crime, however, the conclusion was that narcotics users are involved extensively with criminal activity, that their crimes against property and others are much greater when they use drugs, and that drug use extends the amount of time they engage in criminal activity.[59]

As the cost of drugs escalates, two possible scenarios can follow:

1. Some people stop or cut down on drug use.
2. Others engage in illegal conduct such as stealing or prostitution to afford drugs.

Hence, higher drug prices, because of drug laws, could generate criminal activity. A dilemma for drug users is that because they do business with the types of people who are willing to traffic in drugs, they themselves end up becoming victims of crime. Hence, dealing in the drug trade can be hazardous to one's health.[60] And drug users are liable to be victimized in another way, too. Drugs can be contaminated or more potent than expected because the quality and strength of illegal drugs are not regulated.

Ironically, if drug interdiction is successful and the supply of a given drug is reduced, other drugs fill the void. These replacements sometimes are

Figure 4.2 Number of Acquired Immunodeficiency Syndrome (AIDS) Cases, by Major Transmission Category and Year of Diagnosis—United States, 1981–2004*

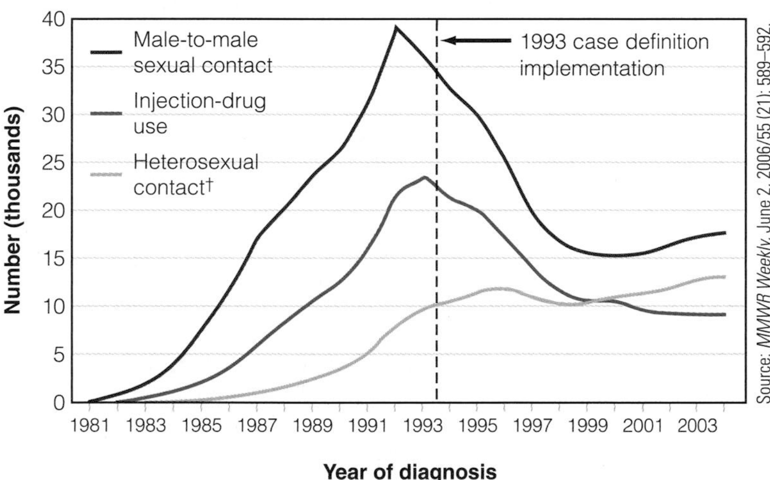

*Data adjusted for reporting delays. Cases without an assigned transmission category were redistributed on the basis of historical trends in risk factors.

†Defined as sexual contact with a person at high risk for or infected with HIV.

TABLE 4.2 Estimated Numbers of AIDS Diagnoses, Deaths, and Persons Living with AIDS, 2002–2006

	2002	2003	2004	2005	2006	Cumulative (1981–2006)
AIDS diagnoses	38,132	38,538	37,726	36,552	36,828	982,498
Deaths of persons with AIDS	16,948	16,690	16,395	16,268	14,016	545,805
Persons living with AIDS	350,419	372,267	393,598	413,882	436,693	NA*

*NA, not applicable (the values given for each year are cumulative). Based on data for the 50 states and the District of Columbia.

Source: *HIV/AIDS Surveillance Report*, U.S. Department of Health and Human Services, 2006.

TABLE 4.3 Arguments for and against Drug Decriminalization

For	Against
Quality of drugs is regulated	Drug use may increase
	More need for treatment
Less need for jails	Drug use could be perceived as acceptable
Crime might be reduced	
Profit motive is reduced	Drug dealers might target children
Drug users will be treated rather than incarcerated	Drug use is morally wrong
Protection of individual rights	Private drug use affects society
Money is directed to drug education instead of enforcement	Drug users are more likely to be arrested for serious offenses

more dangerous than the original drugs. If opiates are not available, enterprising chemists have been known to develop fentanyl or PCP (phencyclidine hydrochloride). Because the effects of PCP are less predictable than those of other drugs, it has greater potential for harm. Fentanyl and PCP can be made inexpensively and with less risk of detection by law enforcement.

Table 4.3 identifies the major arguments for and against decriminalizing drugs.

Drug Enforcement

Drug enforcement is designed to stem the flow of drugs coming into the United States and to punish the user. Approximately 254 metric tons of cocaine were interdicted by U.S. government officials in 2005.[61] Drugs manufactured in the United States include the powerful stimulant methamphetamines. Methamphetamine laboratories cause three main types of harm: physical injury from explosions, fires, chemical burns, and toxic fumes; environmental hazards; and child endangerment.[62] From 2004 to 2005, the number of seized clandestine methamphetamine labs declined 42% from 10,015 to 5,846. A factor that decreased the number of methamphetamine laboratories within U.S. borders is the implementation of laws at the state level restricting the sale of chemicals used to make methamphetamines.[63] However, some of the reduction in the domestic methamphetamine market has been negated by the increase in methamphetamines from Mexico.[64]

Table 4.4 shows the rate of drug-related arrests from 2001 to 2006 for various drugs.[65]

To stop drugs at their source, the State Department works with a number of foreign governments. In 2008, the U.S. State Department allocated $442.8 million for counternarcotics programs in the Andean region, $30 million dollars to Bolivia for interdiction and improving its law enforcement personnel, $367 million to Colombia for its Critical Flight Safety Program, $36.8 million to Peru for border control efforts, $9.8 million for operations in the Caribbean, and $13.2 million to Mexico for various drug enforcement and interdiction efforts.[66]

DEA agents are placed in countries to help block drugs from leaving those countries, to help eradicate crops, and to find and dismantle illegal laboratories. Crop eradication, however, is not a feasible strategy because if crops are eradicated in one location, other locations quickly fill the void. Nonetheless, the purity of cocaine has declined while the cost to purchase it has increased.[67] The reduced purity of cocaine is confirmed in various states where cocaine has been seized.[68] Andean Indians, who use and revere the coca plant, oppose efforts by the United States and the United Nations, pointing out that they have used coca for several thousand years, it is an integral part of their culture, and it enhances community, sociability, and communal spirit.[69] Moreover, the coca plant grows in soils that would not support other crops, it has few pests and predators, and it can be harvested several times a year. Peasant farmers in the Andes are asked to plant legal crops in place of coca, but the peasant farmers make more money from coca crops than legal crops.[70]

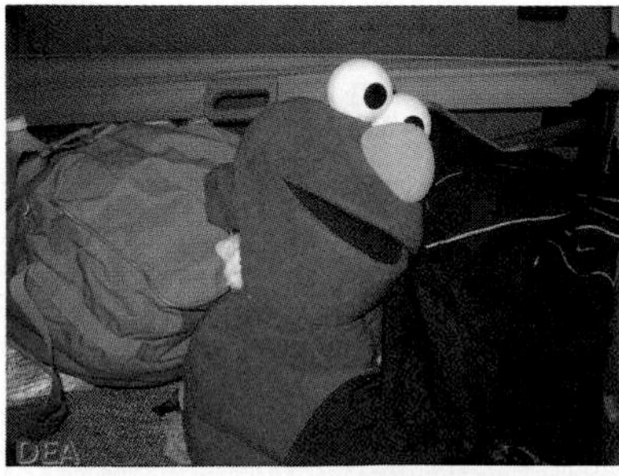

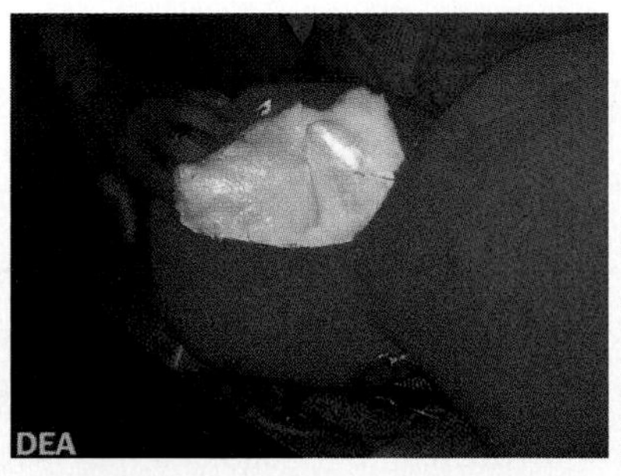

United States Drug Enforcement Administration

The DEA intercepted this shipment of four pounds of high-purity methamphetamine concealed inside a children's toy, which was being transported from California to Colorado for distribution in the Greeley area.

Almost 20% of the foreign-assistance money sent by the United States to Latin America has gone toward antidrug programs.[71] On a global scale, less than 10% of illegal crops are consistently eradicated.[72] An emerging trouble spot is the former Soviet Union and Eastern Bloc countries. Farmers in these countries receive 20 times more income for growing opium than cotton.

Actions of the U.S. government have resulted in some interesting twists. Without realizing it, the

TABLE 4.4 Drug-Related Arrests, United States, 2001–2006

	Drug	2001	2002	2003	2004	2005	2006*
Major Drugs	Cocaine	13,351	12,226	10,951	12,222	12,114	3,557
	Marijuana	6,461	5,509	6,216	6,252	5,599	1,667
	Heroin	3,106	2,578	2,169	2,534	2,141	519
	Methamphetamine	7,363	6,231	6,055	5,893	6,090	1,504
Other Dangerous Drugs	MDMA	1,974	1,506	1,023	937	764	167
	GHB	2	0	10	20	19	0
	LSD	93	27	21	25	8	13
	PCP	87	49	117	67	57	19
	Steroids	72	64	65	95	57	12
Pharmaceuticals	Oxycodone	0	0	27	137	236	74
	Hydrocodone	0	1	17	111	186	67
	Hydromorphone	29	35	28	28	11	3
	Benzodiazepines	30	44	27	23	26	6
	Methylphenidate	0	0	1	1	2	0

*Data for 2006 are preliminary and incomplete.
Source: United States Drug Enforcement Administration.

DEA bought its own cocaine. It sold cocaine to sellers in Colombia, who then smuggled it into the United States, where government agents bought it back.[73] Deposed Panamanian leader Manuel Noriega, who was indicted for drug trafficking, claims he received cocaine from the Central Intelligence Agency (CIA). Also implicated in the drug trade were the Haitian and Jamaican prime ministers.[74]

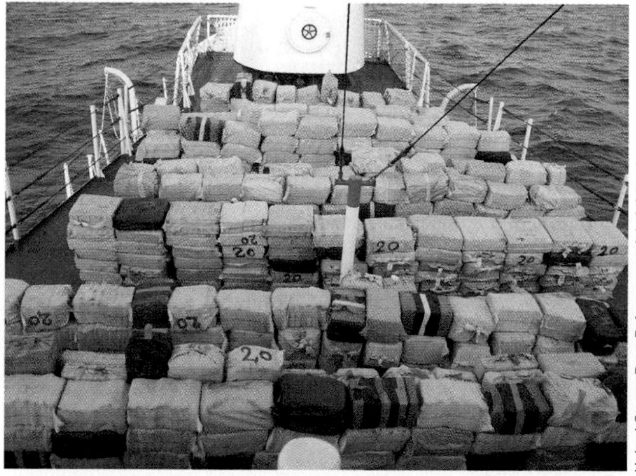
United States Drug Enforcement Administration

A record 42,845 pounds of cocaine—worth an estimated $300 million in drug revenues—bound for Mexican drug traffickers was seized by the U.S. Coast Guard from the Panamanian flagged motor vessel Gatun off the coast of Panama in 2007.

Interdiction is especially difficult because of numerous points of entry. Moreover, new trade agreements and the collapse of the Soviet Union have made it easier to ship drugs across borders.[75] It is virtually impossible to check every person, aircraft, vessel, and container crossing the border. Interdiction alone will not stop the flow of illegal drugs. Figure 4.3 shows the route by which cocaine is transported.

Nonetheless, progress has been made in curtailing the supply of drugs from other countries. Colombia has reduced cultivation by one-third since 2001.[76] Cultivation of the opium poppy was reduced by two-thirds between 2001 and 2005.[77] Moreover, heroin in the United States today is less pure than it was in the 1990s.[78] Opium comes primarily from four distinct geographical areas: South America (Colombia), Southeast Asia (primarily Burma, now known officially as Myanmar), Mexico, and Southwest Asia (primarily Afghanistan).[79] In 2005, over 1,700 kilograms (3,740 pounds) of heroin was seized in the United States.[80] The Bush administration shifted priorities in its attempt to prevent Colombia from processing more cocaine. Rather than continue with military aid to Colombia, economic assistance was aimed at promoting judicial reform and crop substitution is the focus.[81] Nonetheless, Buenaventura, a port city in Colombia, had 408 homicides in 2006, many of which stemmed from the drug trade. Buenaventura has the highest homicide rate in Colombia.[82] Table 4.5 shows

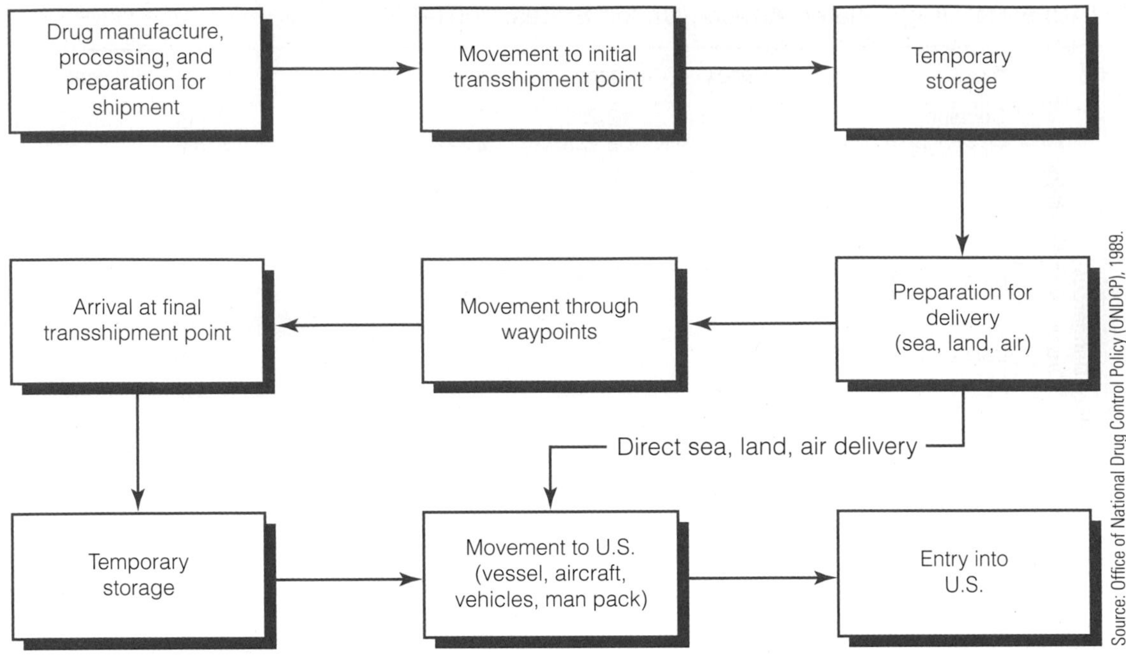

Figure 4.3 Cocaine Transportation

the amount of heroin, cocaine, marijuana, hashish, and methamphetamine seized from 2000 through 2007. Since 2000, cocaine shipments from Colombia to Europe, especially Spain and the Netherlands, have increased at a much greater rate than those to the United States.[83]

Opium production has escalated in many provinces formerly of the Soviet Union. In January 1992, the prime minister of Kazakhstan legalized cultivation of the opium poppy.[84] Opium poppy cultivation has also been reported in 17 of China's 30 provinces. Previously, the two primary regions supplying heroin to the United States were Southeast Asia and southwestern Asia, but in recent years Colombia and Mexico have increased production significantly.[85] In July 2000, Afghanistan's ruling Taliban almost totally eliminated the poppy crop in that country. However, opium production in Afghanistan subsequently soared, and opium now represents one-third of Afghanistan's gross national product.[86]

A major source of marijuana shipped to the United States is Colombia. Mexico and Canada are increasing their export of marijuana to the United States.[87] Other countries including Lebanon, Morocco, Pakistan, and Thailand are becoming more prominent in growing marijuana.

Prevention

Harm reduction is gaining favor as an approach to preventing drug abuse. Harm reduction, which started during the 1980s in European cities including Amsterdam, Rotterdam, and Liverpool, focuses on reducing the personal and social adverse effects

TABLE 4.5 DEA Drug Seizures, 2000–2007

Calendar Year	Cocaine (kg)	Heroin (kg)	Marijuana (kg)	Methamphetamine (kg)
2007	96,713	625	356,472	1,086
2006	69,826	805	322,438	1,711
2005	118,311	640	283,344	2,161
2004	117,854	672	265,813	1,659
2003	73,725	795	254,196	1,678
2002	63,640	710	238,024	1,353
2001	59,430	753	271,849	1,634
2000	58,674	546	331,964	1,771

Source: U.S. Department of Justice, 2008.

emanating from drug use.[88] It does not address reducing the supply of drugs or punishing the drug user. The goals of harm reduction are to reduce violence associated with the drug trade, lower death rates directly attributable to drugs, and curtail infectious diseases caused by drug use.[89] The concept of harm reduction is being applied to reducing nicotine dependency also. The assumption is that the more knowledge one has about tobacco smoking, the less likely it is that one will smoke.[90]

Efforts of harm-reduction advocates include providing sterile syringes to people who inject drugs to curtail the spread of HIV infection, as well as educational campaigns and increased treatment.[91] Advocates of harm reduction propose that physicians be allowed to prescribe methadone, heroin, and other drugs to addicts only to prevent addicts from buying drugs on the black market. Some addicts go to "shooting galleries" to inject themselves with drugs. Shooting galleries are unsafe due to the violence associated with them and because the environment is unsterile. Thus, some people advocate for a safe place for addicts to inject themselves. Another proposal is to establish drug analysis laboratories to test the purity and potency of drugs and thereby prevent drug users from taking contaminated drugs.

Although harm-reduction proponents do not believe that this policy will eliminate drug-related problems, they do believe that many of the problems will diminish. They think that drug abuse should be treated as a public health problem, not a criminal problem.[92] Opponents of the harm-reduction approach, on the other hand, believe that young people might get the wrong impression, that drug use is okay if it is done safely. Also, harm-reduction detractors believe that this approach ultimately could make it easier to legalize drugs.[93]

harm reduction A series of practical interventions that respond to the needs of drug users and the community where they live in an effort to reduce the harm caused by illicit drug use

normalization A term used by the Dutch for the practice of not prosecuting users of soft drugs such as marijuana

A number of countries have adopted a harm-reduction approach. In the United Kingdom, drug education emphasizes harm minimization.[94] In 1982, the Dutch government implemented a policy called **normalization**. Under this policy, using some drugs is not illegal, but it is illegal to traffic in drugs.[95] Small amounts of hashish can be purchased in youth centers and coffee shops, although it remains illegal to buy and use heroin or cocaine.[96] The Dutch believe their policy is pragmatic. The minister of justice contends that the policy removes the sale of hashish from the realm of hard crime and that the illegality of some drugs causes more harm than good.[97]

The risks of infectious diseases, violence, and social ostracism are compounded, say the Dutch, when drugs are illegal. The Dutch government does not forsake people who encounter drug problems. Treatment is provided to assist the physical and social well-being of addicts rather than to try to stop their addiction. An increasing number of addicts have entered treatment to achieve drug-free lifestyles.

What effect has the Dutch model had on drug use? The Netherlands has less drug use than the United States and other European countries.[98] The use of hard drugs such as cocaine and heroin has

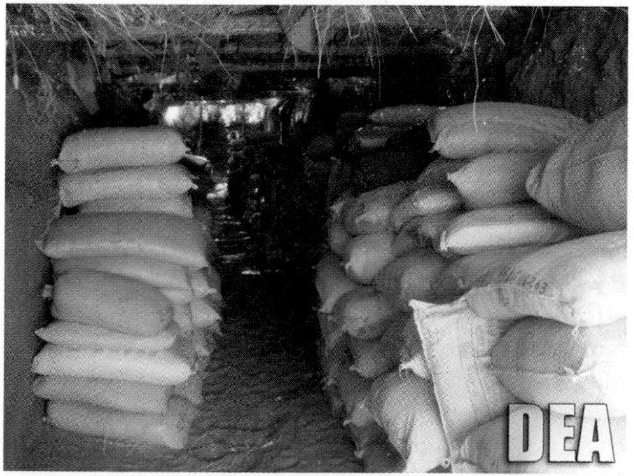

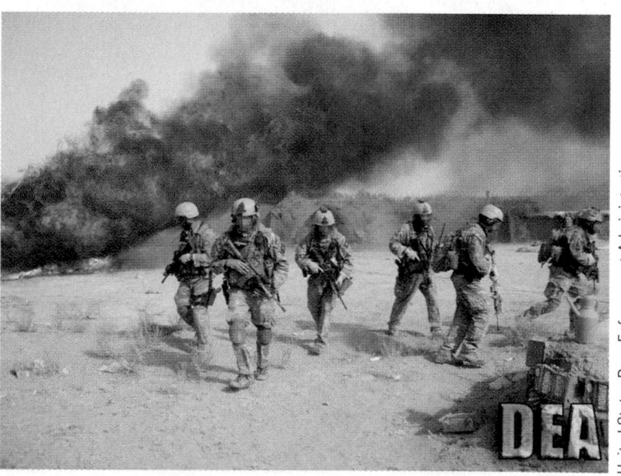

United States Drug Enforcement Administration

In June 2008, 262 tons of hashish were seized from narcotics laboratories and underground bunkers (shown on left) within Taliban-controlled areas of the Kandahar Province in Afghanistan, and the hashish bunkers were destroyed. This joint effort of the Afghan government and the DEA's Foreign-Deployed Advisory and Support Teams represented the largest known drug seizure to date.

declined, and long-term marijuana use has leveled off.[99] In addition to the Netherlands, other European countries have decriminalized marijuana.[100]

Starting in spring 2004, the Canadian government provided heroin to addicts to reduce heroin-related problems. The Swiss already have a heroin maintenance program. They feel that heroin distribution is one way to reduce the harm associated with heroin.[101] In the Netherlands it was found that prescribing heroin to addicts was less costly to society in terms of expense and reducing criminal behavior than prescribing methadone.[102] As these strategies illustrate, those individuals who support harm reduction do not support drug use, but they advocate for reducing the dangers associated with drug use.

Racism and Drug Enforcement

The War on Drugs is marred by some racial overtones. In enforcing drug laws in inner-city communities, police officers in Boston and Chicago, among other cities, have obtained questionable search warrants, ignoring the Fourth Amendment protection of people from unreasonable searches and seizures. Also, people of color tend to be stopped and searched more often than others in airports, bus depots, and train stations and on state highways, on the basis of "drug courier" profiles.[103]

Blacks comprise less than 15% of the population and use drugs in the same proportion as Whites. However, Blacks make up 32% of those arrested for drugs.[104] According to statistics from the Office of National Drug Control Policy, Whites use more than 70% of all illegal drugs, yet Blacks are seven times more likely to be sentenced to prison.[105] It is easier, says one writer, to arrest Black street-level drug sellers than White bankers laundering vast sums of drug money.[106] In Maryland, 90% of people jailed for drug convictions are Black, even though they make up 30% of the population.[107] The FBI estimates that one-third of Black male babies born in the United States in 2004 will to go to prison during their lifetime.[108] It is also possible that racism may lead to drug abuse. One study found that 12-year-old African Americans who experienced racism were twice as likely to use drugs by the time they became teens.[109]

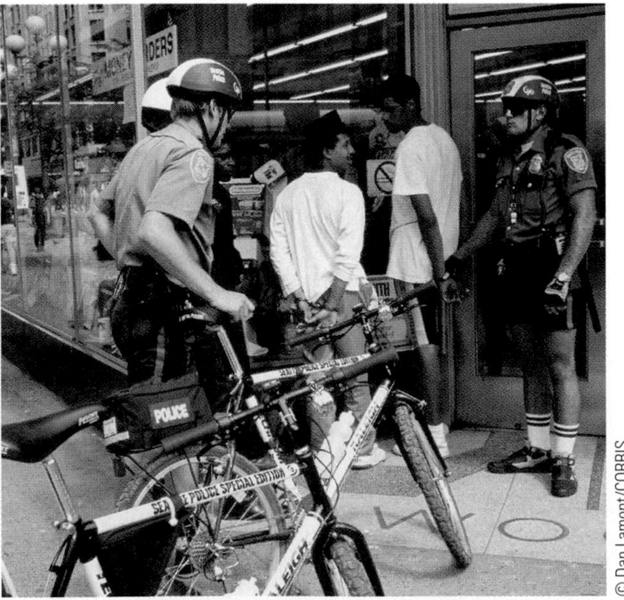

© Dan Lamont/CORBIS.

People of color tend to be stopped and searched more often than others in airports, bus depots, and train stations and on state highways, on the basis of "drug courier" profiles.

The disparity in drug sentencing becomes particularly apparent when crack cocaine and powder cocaine are discussed. Crack cocaine is more likely to be used by poor people, usually people of color, and powder cocaine is more likely to be used by middle-class people.[110] Among individuals convicted of crack cocaine offenses, 88% are Black and 6% are White.[111] Federal law mandates that a person possessing 5 grams of crack cocaine receive the same sentence as someone with 500 grams of powder cocaine. Many people think this 100-to-1 disparity is unjust. However, a number of judges have ruled that the more severe penalties for crack cocaine are justified and not discriminatory because crack is more addicting and less expensive than powder cocaine.[112] In 1995, the U.S. Sentencing Commission recommended lower penalties for crack cocaine, comparable to the penalties for powder cocaine. President Bill Clinton and the Congress rejected the commission's recommendation. Meanwhile, because of the severe penalty associated with crack, some dealers are recruiting more youths to sell the drug for them.[113]

Minority women who use drugs during pregnancy are subjected to more punishment and stigmatization than nonminority women.[114] One study found that Black women and their newborns were 1.5 times more likely to be tested for illegal drugs than non-Black women.[115] Drug use occurs more or less equally across racial and ethnic groups. A woman from a racial or ethnic minority who uses drugs while pregnant, however, is 10 times more likely to be reported to child protective services than a White woman.[116] Powder cocaine and crack cocaine produce harmful effects to the fetus, too, but crack cocaine has been portrayed in the media as especially deleterious. Nonminority women are more likely to use powder cocaine, and minority women more frequently use crack cocaine. Middle-class women who use cocaine tend to be treated, whereas poor women who use crack tend to be imprisoned. Crack-using pregnant women are subject to criminal prosecution on the grounds that they are engaging in child abuse. Even though alcohol is the drug that accounts for the majority of birth defects, women who use alcohol during pregnancy are not prosecuted.

Mandatory Minimum Drug Sentencing

One proposal for reducing drug-related problems is to mandate minimum drug sentences. Starting in 1984, the U.S. Congress has enacted an array of mandatory minimum penalties specifically focusing on drugs and violent crimes. Politicians from both political parties favor a mandatory minimum sentence for drug offenses because it demonstrates a "get-tough" approach to drug abuse. For example, federal law requires that an individual convicted of possessing one-half kilogram or more of cocaine be sentenced to a prison term of at least 5 years.

Are mandatory minimum drug sentences cost-effective for taxpayers, and do they curtail drug abuse and related consequences? It has been shown that mandatory minimum drug sentences have not acted as deterrents to further crime.[117] One individual who has argued against mandatory minimum drug sentencing is U.S. Supreme Court Justice Anthony Kennedy.[118]

Opponents of mandatory minimum drug sentences argue that they give no latitude to judges to determine appropriate punishments. A defendant's history and circumstances are not taken into account. Moreover, mandatory minimums may violate American standards for justice and equity. The benefit of removing one drug dealer is at best temporary, because there is no shortage of individuals willing to take that person's place, regardless of the possible consequences.

A comprehensive study found that mandatory minimum drug sentences for lower-level dealers were not cost-effective.[119] Less use of cocaine and a reduction of crime are achieved by better enforcement and by providing treatment rather than implementing mandatory minimum drug sentences. One study found that treatment is 15 times more effective for reducing serious crime than mandatory minimum sentencing.[120] Also, the longer low-level, nonviolent drug offenders spend in prison, the greater the likelihood that they will return to prison.[121] With the imposition of mandatory sentences, drug dealers incur more risk and, consequently, increase the cost of cocaine. The authors of the study speculated that mandatory sentences for higher-level dealers might be more cost-effective. Ironically, higher-level dealers are less likely than lower-level dealers to be caught with substantial amounts of cocaine in their possession.

Summary

During the American Colonial period, the first drug to be regulated was alcohol. The concern was over drunkenness, not moderate use. The temperance movement took shape in the late 1700s. To raise revenues, Congress imposed a tax on alcohol in 1791. Farmers in southwestern Pennsylvania objected, and President George Washington responded by sending in the militia, resulting in the Whiskey Rebellion.

The early 1800s witnessed a movement to restrict opium. Laws against opium did not arise from concern over its effects. Rather, they probably were attributable to anti-Chinese sentiment. One of the first nationwide drug laws was the Pure Food and Drug Act of 1906, which regulated over-the-counter or proprietary drugs. Although over-the-counter (OTC) drugs included opiates, cocaine, alcohol, and other drugs, the law did not limit these substances, but just stipulated that they had to be listed among the ingredients.

The next important law was the Harrison Act of 1914, which restricted the use of narcotics. Legal narcotic use was placed on a prescription basis.

Congress passed the Marijuana Tax Act in 1937 because of the efforts of Henry Anslinger, who believed that marijuana caused sexual promiscuity, mental illness, and violence. Despite testimony to the contrary by the American Medical Association, Congress passed the law to tax marijuana with little debate. The law imposed a tax on people prescribing, selling, and growing marijuana. In effect, the law prohibited recreational and medicinal use of marijuana.

Before 1938, the marketing of nonnarcotic drugs was largely uncontrolled. To ensure that drugs were safe and properly labeled, Congress enacted the Food, Drug, and Cosmetic Act in 1938. The law did not stipulate that drugs had to be effective, though. It did establish a system in which drugs were placed on a prescription basis. The manufacturers could determine whether a drug was listed as an OTC drug or as a prescription drug. This law was altered in 1951 with the passage of the Humphrey-Durham Amendment. More stringent guidelines for marketing drugs were adopted in the early 1960s.

The Comprehensive Drug Abuse Prevention and Control Act, more commonly known as the Controlled Substances Act, was enacted in 1970. This law repealed, replaced, or updated previous federal drug laws. Though the law addressed rehabilitation, research, and education, its main emphasis was on drug enforcement. The primary target was the drug dealer, not the user. The law established a drug schedule system in which drugs were placed in one of five schedules based on potential for abuse and medical utility. Penalties for possession, trafficking, distribution, and manufacturing are determined by the schedule.

To discourage individuals from using drugs, the Anti-Drug Abuse Act was passed in 1988. This law was directed at the drug user, and penalties included the loss of college loans and grants; forfeiture of one's car, boat, or airplane if drugs are seized on these vehicles; and removal from public housing. College students convicted of a drug-related offense may jeopardize their chance to receive federal financial assistance.

Many legal issues have evolved concerning drugs. Should drug paraphernalia be banned? Should drug use be decriminalized? Thousands of babies are born to drug-addicted women, and emergency room incidents continue to escalate. The cost of enforcement is enormous, prisons are overcrowded with people arrested on drug-related offenses, and crime and violence are perpetrated by drug dealers and their victims.

One country that decriminalized drugs with some success is the Netherlands. To the Dutch, decriminalization of drugs is pragmatic. They prefer to treat rather than prosecute drug users. Dutch officials contend that drug use not only has stabilized but also has decreased in some cities. The Swiss had the opposite experience.

Because there are many points of entry into the United States, stopping drugs from crossing the borders is not easy. The State Department is trying to stop drugs at their source while acreage allocated to growing drugs is increasing in many of the originating countries. Officials from other countries say that the problem is the insatiable appetite of Americans for drugs. Most of the cocaine coming into the United States arrives from South America, much heroin is sent from Asia, and Colombia is the largest exporter of marijuana.

Thinking Critically

1. One of the richest men at the inception of the United States was George Washington, who made his fortune from tobacco crops. If Congress had raised revenue by taxing tobacco instead of alcohol, what would have been the implications for society today?
2. Do you view narcotic addiction as a disease or as a crime? If addiction were a medical condition, would you view the addict differently than if addiction were a crime? Should the addict be a patient or an inmate? Why?
3. The case of thalidomide points to the necessity for regulating drugs. Drug regulations, however, can delay beneficial drugs from reaching the marketplace. Should testing procedures be relaxed when certain illnesses, such as AIDS, have a high mortality rate?
4. Students convicted of drug charges are not eligible to receive federal financial assistance. People who commit crimes such as robbery and murder are not denied student aid. Should students who have used drugs be held to a higher standard than others?
5. Legal and physical problems can arise from drug use. Harm may come from the effects of drugs or from their illegal status. If you were asked to reduce the adverse consequences of drugs, would you approach the drug issue as a legal problem or as a public health problem? What is your rationale?

Web Resources

DanceSafe
http://www.dancesafe.org
This organization engages in a harm-reduction strategy, attempting to reduce the harm of the drug Ecstasy by testing pills to determine whether the contents are Ecstasy or some type of adulterant.

U.S. Drug Enforcement Administration (DEA)
http://www.usdoj.gov/dea/index.htm
The DEA provides current data on drug seizures, drug arrests, and drugs coming into the United States as well as a wealth of other data.

NORML (National Organization for the Reform of Marijuana Laws)
http://www.norml.org/
As the title suggests, NORML strives to reduce the penalties associated with marijuana use.

Drug Policy Alliance Network
http://www.drugpolicy.org
The Drug Policy Alliance provides a library of information about various drugs. It also advocates for a sensible approach for regulating drugs.

Notes

1. D. W. Conroy, "Puritans in Taverns: Law and Popular Culture in Colonial Massachusetts, 1630–1720," in *Drinking Behavior and Belief in Modern History,* edited by S. Barrows and R. Room (Berkeley: University of California Press, 1991).
2. B. S. Katcher, "Benjamin Rush's Educational Campaign Against Hard Drinking," *American Journal of Public Health,* 83 (1993): 273–281.
3. D. F. Musto, *Drugs in America: A Documentary History* (New York: New York University Press, 2002).
4. M. L. Keire, "Dope Fiends and Degenerates: The Gendering of Addiction in the Early Twentieth Century," in *The American Drug Scene,* edited by J. A. Inciardi

and K. McElrath (Los Angeles: Roxbury Publishing Co., 2004).
5. E. Nadelmann, "Yes (Re: Drug Legalization)," *American Heritage* (February/March 1993): 421.
6. H. Kleber and J.A. Califano, "Legalization: Panacea or Pandora's Box," *World and I* (January 2006).
7. A. Goldstein and H. Kalant, "Drug Policy: Striking the Right Balance," *Science* (September 28, 1990): 1513–1521.
8. W. L. White, *Slaying the Dragon: The History of Addiction Treatment in America* (Bloomington, IL: Chestnut Health Systems/Lighthouse Institute, 1998).
9. Nadelmann, supra note 5.
10. Musto, supra note 3.
11. D. F. Musto, *The American Disease: Origins of Narcotic Control* (New Haven, CT: Yale University Press, 1973).
12. Musto, supra note 3.
13. J. F. Kauffman and G. E. Woody, *Matching Treatment to Patient Needs in Opioid Substitution Therapy* (Treatment Improvement Protocol, TIP Series 20) (Rockville, MD: U. S. Department of Health and Human Services, 1995).
14. D. F. Musto, "America's First Cocaine Epidemic," in *The American Drug Scene,* edited by J. A. Inciardi and K. McElrath (Los Angeles: Roxbury Publishing Company, 2004).
15. Center for Drug Abuse Treatment, *Alcohol, Tobacco, and Other Drug Abuse: Challenges and Responses for Faith Leaders* (Washington, DC: Substance Abuse and Mental Health Services Administration, 1995).
16. New York Medical Journal, 1915.
17. *Outlook* (1919), cited in Chapter 8 of E. M. Brecher, *Licit and Illicit Drugs* (Boston: Little, Brown, 1972).
18. Ibid.
19. Nadelmann, supra note 5.
20. "Cannabits," *Forbes* (November 10, 2003): 146.
21. J. F. Kauffman and G. E. Woody, *Matching Treatment to Patient Needs in Opioid Substitution Therapy* (Treatment Improvement Protocol, TIP Series 20) (Rockville, MD: U. S. Department of Health and Human Services, 1995).
22. J. Sullum, "Sex, Drugs and Techno Music," *Reason,* 33 (January 2002): 75–85.
23. Musto, supra note 3.
24. U.S. House of Representatives, Committee on Ways and Means, *Taxation on Marijuana: Hearings on H. R. 6385,* 75th Congress, 1st Session (1937).
25. M. Meadows, "Drug Research and Children," *FDA Consumer,* (January/February 2003): 36–40.
26. G. J. Annas and S. Elias, "Thalidomide and the Titanic: Reconstructing the Technology Tragedies of the Twentieth Century," *American Journal of Public Health,* 89 (1999): 98–101.
27. H. Burkholz, "Giving Thalidomide a Second Chance," *FDA Consumer,* 31 (1997): 12.
28. R. Goldberg, *Taking Sides: Clashing Views on Controversial Issues in Drugs and Society,* 5th ed. (Guilford, CT: McGraw-Hill/Doshkin, 2004).
29. P. Guthrie, "US Senate Passes FDA Reauthorization Act," *CMAJ: Canadian Medical Association Journal,* 177 (July 3, 2007): 23.
30. B. L. Muldrew, "Drug Enforcement: Controlled Substances Act Inapplicable to Medicinal Marijuana," *Journal of Law, Medicine and Ethics,* 32 (Summer 2004): 371–372.
31. D. M. Grilly, *Drugs and Human Behavior,* 4th ed. (Boston: Allyn & Bacon, 2001).
32. S. Wisotsky, "Beyond the War on Drugs," in *The Drug Legalization Debate,* edited by J. A. Inciardi (Newbury Park, CA: Sage Publications, 1991).
33. T. Green, "DPF's Policy Priorities," *Drug Policy Letter,* 38, no. 1 (1999): 8–12.
34. C. Dervarics, "Question Regarding Student Drug Use Returns in FAFSA Debate," *Diverse: Issues in Higher Education,* 24 (September 20, 2007): 12.
35. E. Goode, *Drugs in American Society,* 5th ed. (New York: Alfred A. Knopf, 1998).
36. J.P. Caulkins and P. Reuter, "Reorienting U.S. Drug Policy," *Issues in Science and Technology, 23,* no. 1 (Fall 2006): 79–85.
37. Q. Hardy, "That's Not Funny, Man," *Forbes Global,* 6 (November 10, 2003): 68.
38. J. Katz, "White House Tries to Ban the Bong," *Rolling Stone* (July 24, 2003): 54–55.
39. E. Nadelmann, "Commonsense Drug Policy," *Foreign Affairs,* 77 (1998): 111–126.
40. *National Drug Control Strategy* (Washington, DC: Government Printing Office, 2007).
41. P. Gorman, "Veteran Cops Against the War," *The World and I* (January 2006).
42. E. A. Nadelmann, "An Unwinnable War on Drugs," *New York Times,* April 26, 2001.
43. "Drug War Pushes U.S. Inmate Population Over 2 Million," *Drug Policy Alliance* (April 10, 2003): 2.
44. H. D. Kleber, "Our Current Approach to Drug Abuse—Progress, Problems, Proposals," *New England Journal of Medicine,* 330 (1994): 361–365.
45. D. T. Courtwright, "No (Re: Drug Legalization)," *American Heritage* (February/March, 1993): 431.
46. J. Q. Wilson, "Against the Legalization of Drugs," in *The American Drug Scene,* edited by J. A. Inciardi and K. McElrath (Los Angeles, Roxbury Publishing Company, 2004).
47. J. Q. Wilson, "A New Strategy for the War on Drugs," *Wall Street Journal,* April 13, 2000.
48. J. A. Inciardi and C. A. Saum, "Legalization Madness," *Public Interest,* 123 (1996): 72–82.
49. P. J. Goldstein, "Drugs, Violence, and Federal Funding: A Research Odyssey," *Substance Use and Misuse,* 33 (1998): 1915–1936.
50. J. Gray, "How to Win the War on Drugs," *Liberty,* 40 (May 2003): 33–34.
51. J. Tierney, "Lighting Up in Amsterdam," *New York Times,* August 26, 2006.
52. "Epidemiology of HIV/AIDS—United States, 1981–2005," *MMWR Weekly,* 55 (June 2, 2006): 589–592.
53. J. S. Wenner, "Drug War: A New Vietnam?" *New York Times,* June 23, 1990.
54. Nadelmann, supra note 5.
55. J. A. Inciardi and K. McElrath, *The American Drug Scene* (Los Angeles: Roxbury Publishing Company, 2004).
56. W. Block, "Drug Prohibition: A Legal and Economic Analysis," in *Drugs, Morality, and the Law,* edited by S. Luper-Foy and C. Brown (New York: Garland Publishing, 1994).
57. R. E. Barrett, "Curing the Drug-Law Addiction: The Harmful Side Effects of Legal Prohibition," in *Dealing with Drugs: Consequences of Government Control,* edited by R. Hamowy (Lexington, MA: D. C. Heath, 1987).
58. Inciardi and McElrath, supra note 55.
59. J. A. Inciardi, D. Lockwood, and A. E. Pottieger, *Women and Crack-Cocaine* (New York: Macmillan, 1993).
60. P. J. Goldstein, "The Drugs/Violence Nexus: A Tripartite Conceptual Framework," in *The American Drug Scene,* edited by J. A. Inciardi and K. McElrath (Los Angeles: Roxbury Publishing Company, 2004).
61. National Drug Control Strategy, supra note 40.
62. M. S. Scott and K. Dedel, *Clandestine Methamphetamine Labs* (Washington, DC: U.S. Department of Justice, Office of Community Oriented Policing Services, 2006).
63. *Pushing Back Against Meth: A Progress Report on the Fight Against Methamphetamine in the United States* (Washington, D.C.: Office of National Drug Control Policy, 2006).

64. *National Drug Threat Assessment* (Washington, D.C.: Drug Enforcement Agency, 2006).
65. National Drug Threat Assessment, supra note 64.
66. *National Drug Control Strategy—FY 2008 Budget Summary* (Washington, D.C.: Office of National Drug Control Policy, 2007).
67. ONDCP Drug Policy Information Clearinghouse, *Cocaine* (Rockville, MD: Office of National Drug Control Policy, 2007).
68. National Forensic Laboratory Information System (Arlington, VA: Office of Diversion Control, Drug Enforcement Administration, 2006).
69. Weil, "Letter from the Andes: The New Politics of Coca," *New Yorker,* 71 (1995): 70–80.
70. Ibid.
71. G.L. Fisher, *Rethinking Our War on Drugs: Candid Talk about Controversial Issues* (Westport, CT: Praeger, 2006).
72. Ibid.
73. T. G. Carpenter, "Washington's Unsavory Antidrug Partners," *USA Today Magazine* (November 2002): 20–22.
74. Ibid.
75. S. Flynn, "Worldwide Drug Scourge: The Expanding Trade in Illicit Drugs," *Brookings Review* (Winter 1993): 6–11.
76. National Drug Control Strategy, supra note 40.
77. Ibid.
78. Ibid.
79. ONDCP Drug Policy Information Clearinghouse, *Heroin* (Rockville, MD: Office of National Drug Control Policy, 2006).
80. National Drug Threat Assessment, supra note 64.
81. Carpenter, supra note 73.
82. S. Romero, "Cocaine Wars Turn Port Into Colombia's Deadliest City," *New York Times,* May 22, 2007.
83. J. Feroro, "Europe Expands as Market for Colombian Cocaine," *New York Times,* May 29, 2001.
84. Flynn, supra note 75.
85. Carpenter, supra note 73.
86. A. Mulrine and K. Whitelaw, "The Drug Trade's Collateral Damage," *U.S. News and World Report,* 143 (July 2, 2007): 33.
87. *Drug Trafficking in the United States* (Washington, D.C.: U.S. Drug Enforcement Agency, 2004).
88. R. J. MacCoun, "Toward a Psychology of Harm Reduction," *American Psychologist,* 53 (1998): 1199–1208.
89. Goldberg, supra note 28.
90. B. Rodu, "The Reduced Harm in Being Honest," *World Tobacco,* 218 (2007): 20–22.
91. MacCoun, supra note 88.
92. S. Bayes, "Making the Case for Harm Reduction," *Behavioral Healthcare,* 27 (July 2007): 43–44.
93. MacCoun, supra note 88.
94. "UK Votes to Decriminalize Marijuana," *Drug Policy Alliance Newsletter,* November 13, 2003.
95. S. Staley, *Drug Policy and the Decline of American Cities* (New Brunswick, NJ: Transaction Publishers, 1992).
96. E. Currie, "Toward a Policy on Drugs," *Dissent* (Winter 1993): 65–71.
97. B. Bollag, "Notes from Academe: The Netherlands," *Chronicle of Higher Education,* 13 (March 13, 1998): B2.
98. Staley, supra note 95.
99. "The Dutch Experiment," *New Scientist* (February 21, 1998): 30–31.
100. E. A. Nadelmann, "Common-Sense Drug Policy," in *The American Drug Scene,* edited by J. A. Inciardi and K. McElrath (Los Angeles: Roxbury Publishing Company, 2004).
101. "Canadian Heroin Study Seeks to Save Lives, Money," *Drug Policy Alliance Newsletter,* October 30, 2003.
102. G.W. Dijkgraaf, B. P. van der Zanden, C. A. J. M. de Borgie, P. Blanken, J. M. van Ree, and W. van den Brink, "Cost Utility Analysis of Coprescribed Heroin Compared with Methadone Maintenance Treatment in Heroin Addicts in Two Randomised Trials," *British Medical Journal,* 330 (June 4, 2005): 1294–1297.
103. I. Glasser and L. Siegel, "When Constitutional Rights Seem Too Extravagant to Endure: The Crack Scare's Impact on Civil Rights and Liberties," in *Crack in America: Demon Drugs and Social Justice,* edited by C. Reinarman and H. G. Levine (Berkeley: University of California Press, 1997).
104. "FBI Releases Crime Data Showing 40% Increase in Drug Arrests Over 10 Years," *Drug Policy Alliance Newsletter,* October 30, 2003.
105. Gorman, supra note 41.
106. T. Duster, "Pattern, Purpose, and Race in the Drug War: The Crisis of Credibility in Criminal Justice," in *Crack in America: Demon Drugs and Social Justice,* edited by C. Reinarman and H. G. Levine (Berkeley: University of California Press, 1997).
107. "Study: Racial Disparities in Maryland Drug Incarceration," *Drug Policy Alliance Newsletter,* October 14, 2003.
108. Gorman, supra note 41.
109. R. Gibbons, "Racism's Hidden Threat," *Diverse Issues in Higher Education,* 24 (May 17, 2007): 5.
110. C. Reinarman and H. G. Levine, *Crack in America: Demon Drugs and Social Justice,* edited by C. Reinarman and H. G. Levine (Berkeley: University of California Press, 1997).
111. E. Goode, "Drug Arrests at the Millennium," *Society* (July/August 2002): 41–45.
112. J. Elden, "Drug Sentencing Frenzy," *Progressive* (April 1995): 25.
113. Division of Epidemiology and Prevention Research, Community Epidemiology Work Group, "Epidemiologic Trends in Drug Abuse: December 1997" (Rockville, MD: National Institute on Drug Abuse, 1998).
114. C. S. Carter, "Perinatal Care for Women Who Are Addicted," *Health and Social Work,* 27 (August 2002): 166–174.
115. H.V. Kunins, E. Bellin, C. Chazotte, E. Du, and J. H. Arnsten, "The Effect of Race on Provider Decisions to Test for Illicit Drug Use in the Peripartum Setting," *Journal of Women's Health,* 16 (March 2007): 245–255.
116. S. R. Kendall, "Treatment Options for Drug-Exposed Infants," in *Medications Development for the Treatment of Pregnant Addicts and Their Infants,* edited by C. N. Chiang and L. P. Finnegan (NIDA Research Monograph 149) (Washington, DC: Government Printing Office, 1995).
117. M. Mauer, Congressional Testimony, June 26, 2007.
118. "Supreme Court Justice Kennedy Calls for Repeal of Mandatory Minimum," *Drug Policy Alliance Newsletter* (August 14, 2003).
119. P. Caulkins, C. P. Rydell, W. L. Schwabe, and J. Chiesa, *Mandatory Minimum Drug Sentences* (Santa Monica, CA: Rand, 1997).
120. M. E. Fitzgerald, "Women and Children: Casualties of War," *Drug Policy Letter,* 46 (May/June 2000): 10–12.
121. P. Ninemire, "Treatment, Not Prison," *America,* 196 (May 28, 2007): 13–15.

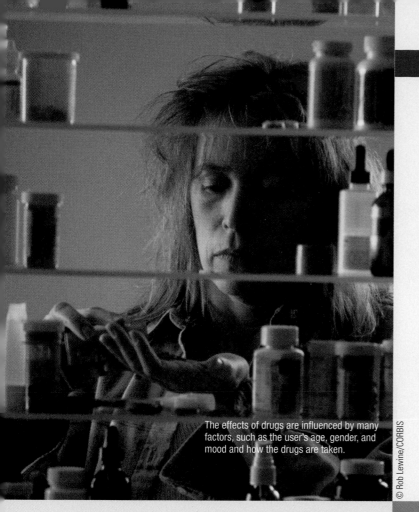

The effects of drugs are influenced by many factors, such as the user's age, gender, and mood and how the drugs are taken.

FACT OR FICTION?

1. Marijuana's effects are more profound when it is ingested than when it is smoked.
2. At one time LSD was given to patients in order to study mental illness.
3. People who engage in strenuous exercise actually emit a neurotransmitter that contributes to a "high" feeling.
4. The day of the week on which most heart attacks occur is Monday.
5. The most common cause of death for cigarette smokers is lung cancer.
6. Older men are more affected by a drug's effects than are older women.
7. Heroin today is purer than it was 20 years ago.
8. Mixing medications with wine causes more potential health problems than mixing medications with beer.
9. One's mood while taking psychoactive drugs will affect the experience derived from the drug.
10. The rate of injecting drugs, especially heroin, has decreased among users age 29 and younger.

Turn the page to check your answers

5

The Pharmacology and Physiology of Drug Use

Chapter Objectives

After completing this chapter, the reader should be able to describe:

- How neurons work
- The difference between a dendrite and an axon
- The effects of various neurotransmitters
- Functions of the reticular activating system, hypothalamus, cerebral cortex, limbic system, basal ganglia, and brain stem
- Factors that alter the effects of drugs
- How drugs interact with different systems of the body
- Differences between the sympathetic and parasympathetic branches of the autonomic nervous system
- The additive, antagonistic, and synergistic effects of drugs
- Differences among pharmacological tolerance, behavioral tolerance, cross-tolerance, and reverse tolerance
- How effects of drugs vary according to the way they are administered

FACT OR FICTION?

1. **Fiction:** The fact is—marijuana's effects are stronger when it is smoked, because the drug reaches the brain more quickly when smoked.
2. **Fact:** In the 1950s it was believed that schizophrenia could be studied by giving LSD to patients.
3. **Fact:** During strenuous exercise the human body produces endorphins, which give the individual a euphoric feeling.
4. **Fact:** It is believed that heart attacks occur most frequently on Monday, possibly from a weekend of heavy alcohol use.
5. **Fiction:** The fact is—despite popular perception, smokers are more likely to die from cardiovascular disease than from lung cancer.
6. **Fiction:** The fact is—because they have a higher percentage of fat, which increases the accumulation of drugs, women tend to be more affected by drugs than men.
7. **Fact:** The purity of heroin is much higher now than it was two decades previously.
8. **Fiction:** The fact is—the important factor is how much alcohol is consumed when using medications, not the type of alcohol that is consumed.
9. **Fact:** One's state of mind can influence whether a drug's effects are euphoric or dysphoric.
10. **Fiction:** The fact is—since 1995 the percentage of heroin users under age 29 who inject heroin has increased considerably.

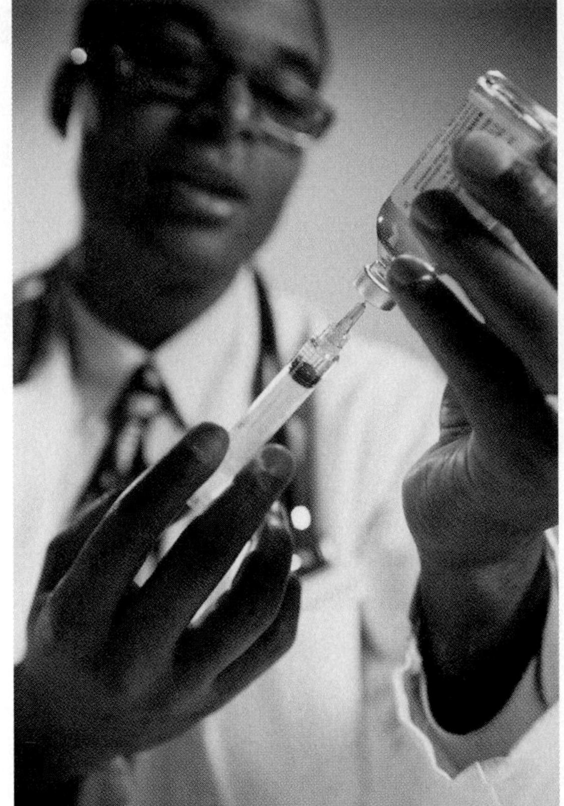
© Photodisc/PictureQuest.

Injected drugs reach the brain more quickly than drugs administered by other methods.

Different drugs produce different effects within the **psyche** and **soma**, and these effects also differ from one person to another. This chapter addresses the chemical or pharmacological effects associated with drugs. It explores factors that influence how drugs affect people and how people allow drugs to affect them.

Pharmacology

Ancient records show that humans have been using drugs to alter their mood and behavior for a long time.[1] The relationship or interaction between drugs and living organisms is called **pharmacology**. The pharmacology of drugs relates to the way in which they are administered, absorbed, distributed, metabolized, and excreted from the body. Ingesting drugs, for example, produces different effects than inhaling drugs. Smoking marijuana has a more profound effect than ingesting it. Chewed tobacco is absorbed differently from smoked tobacco. The effects of injected narcotics are more intense than the effects of narcotics taken in other ways.

Furthermore, drugs that act quickly and produce profound and intense effects are more likely to be abused than are drugs that act slowly. Injected drugs are absorbed quickly, reaching the brain in seconds. Not all drugs lend themselves to injection, though. Marijuana cannot be injected because its resin does not dissolve in water. Therefore, it is less likely to be abused than cocaine or narcotics that can be injected. Similarly, cocaine is more apt to be abused than caffeine because the effects of cocaine are much more powerful. Besides having a different chemical structure from caffeine, cocaine takes effect more quickly because of the way in which it is administered. Injected cocaine produces more powerful effects than snorted cocaine. Up through the early 1980s the most common route of administration was snorting or inhaling cocaine. With the introduction of crack cocaine at that time, smoking became the most popular route of administration.[2]

Alcohol is metabolized in the liver, and its primary site of absorption is the small intestine. It is removed through exhaling, urinating, and sweating at a rate of three-fourths ounce per hour. If cocaine is snorted, the mucous membranes in the nose absorb the drug quickly, and the effects are felt within minutes. Amphetamines taken orally produce peak effects in 2 to 3 hours and are eliminated in 2 to 3 days, whereas the peak effects from injected amphetamines are felt in less than 5 minutes.

The effects of caffeine are felt in 15 to 45 minutes. It is metabolized by the liver and eliminated primarily by the kidneys. Similarly, nicotine is metabolized by the liver and removed via the kidneys. When marijuana is smoked, about half of its psychoactive substance, tetrahydrocannabinol (THC), is absorbed through the lungs before entering the bloodstream. The organ that initially detoxifies the THC is the liver, and THC is removed primarily through the feces.

psyche Refers to the mind

soma From the Greek; literally means "body"

pharmacology The professional discipline that studies the relationships and interactions between living organisms and substances within them

central nervous system (CNS) The brain and spinal cord

neurons Messengers in the brain that transmit information via chemical and electrical processes

dendrites Parts of the neuron that allow nerve impulses to be transmitted to the nerve's cell body

axons Parts of the neuron that send nerve impulses away from the nerve's cell body

action potential The procedure by which the nerve impulse is sent down the axon

synapse The space between an axon and a dendrite

vesicles Saclike structure at the end of the axon

neurotransmitter A chemical substance manufactured in vesicles of the brain

Drug Actions

Drugs affect various organs within the body, including the nervous system. The nervous system consists of the **central nervous system (CNS)**, the autonomic nervous system (ANS), and the peripheral nervous system (PNS). The CNS, consisting of the brain and spinal cord, is composed of nerve cells called **neurons**. Neurons function as messengers in which information is communicated via synapse functions (Figure 5.1). Transmitting information *between* neurons is accomplished chemically and relaying information *within* the neuron occurs electrically through the exchange of ions. Chemical transmission is much more common than electrical transmission.

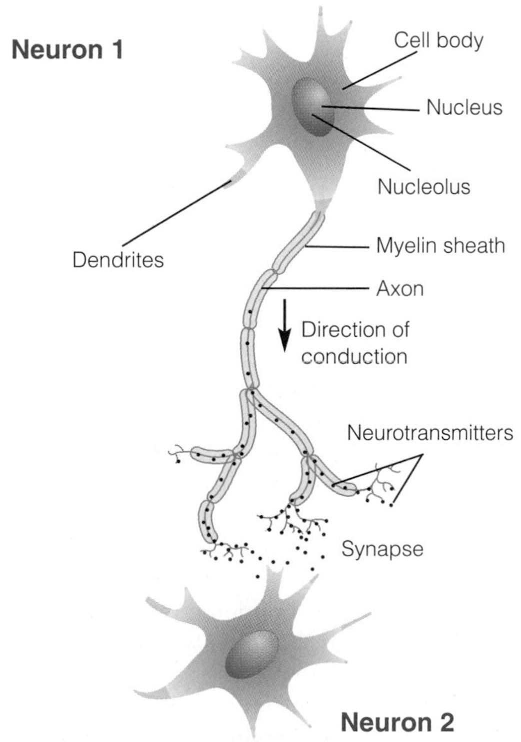

Figure 5.1 Neurons in the Brain

The Neuron

A neuron contains two types of nerve fibers: dendrites and axons. **Dendrites** allow nerve impulses to be transmitted to the nerve's cell body (soma), whereas **axons** send impulses away from the cell body. Each neuron has several dendrites but only one axon. Electrical impulses originate in the dendrite and pass through the cell body via the axon. This process is called the **action potential**.

For an electrical message to be sent from the axon of one neuron to the dendrite of another neuron, it must traverse the space, called a **synapse**, between them (Figure 5.2). The message sent through a neuron is electrical, but the process by which an impulse is transmitted from one neuron to another—from the axon of one neuron to the dendrite of another neuron—is chemical. Drugs are most likely to have their major effect at the synapse. Prolonged or repeated exposure to alcohol, for example, can cause changes in neurons that may lead to the development of alcoholism in susceptible people.[3] Anesthetic drugs obstruct pain impulses from being transmitted to the brain.

At the end of the axons are saclike structures known as **vesicles**. Manufactured within these vesicles are chemical substances called **neurotransmitters**, which cross the synapse to receptor sites. Chemicals in the receptor sites generate electrical

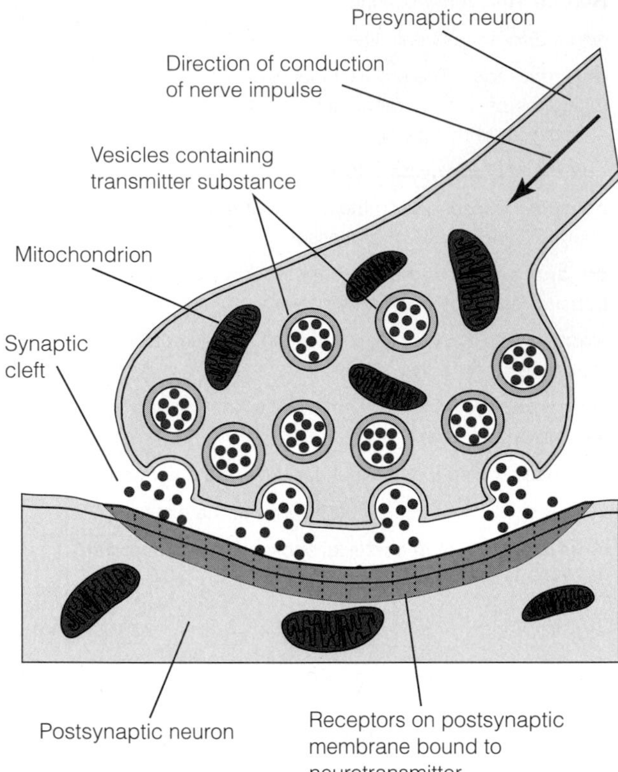

Figure 5.2 Synaptic Transmission

impulses. The neuron responsible for causing the neurotransmitter to be released at the synapse is called the presynaptic neuron. The neuron receiving the neurotransmitter is the postsynaptic neuron.

Drugs influencing the release, storage, and synthesis of neurotransmitters are classified as presynaptic, and drugs affecting neurotransmitters after they cross the synapse are classified as postsynaptic. Neurotransmitters linked to addiction include dopamine, norepinephrine, gamma-aminobutyric acid (GABA), and serotonin.[4]

Some drugs cause the nerve cell to become more sensitive. As sensitivity increases, activity and excitation of certain neurotransmitters increase. This action is exemplified by caffeine. The opposite effect, in which nerve cells become less sensitive, occurs with sedative-hypnotic drugs. Lessened sensitivity inhibits neurotransmitter release. This process is not as straightforward as it may seem. For example, antidepressants and cocaine produce the same biochemical effect, but their physiological effects differ.

In addition, many nerve cells contain **autoreceptors**, which may be situated on any part of the cell. Autoreceptors act when the nerve cell releases neurotransmitters and alter their synthesis, usually by reducing production of neurotransmitters. This is demonstrated with a drug such as LSD, which activates serotonin autoreceptors. The production of serotonin at the synapse decreases.

To summarize: Part of the nerve cell or neuron receives a stimulus, which is converted into an electrical nerve impulse. The nerve impulse is forwarded to the axon, which proceeds to send impulses to terminals, causing chemicals called neurotransmitters to be released. Neurotransmitters traverse the synapse to receptor sites on the next neuron. Some drugs speed up transmission of electrical impulses, and others slow them down. Two drugs that create opposite effects are minor tranquilizers and amphetamines. Minor tranquilizers produce a calming effect. Norepinephrine results in increased excitation.

Neurotransmitters

Most drugs affect brain activity by increasing or decreasing the activity of various neurotransmitters. Neurotransmitters enable the brain to receive, process, and respond to information by carrying impulses from one neuron to the next. Precisely how they do this is not well understood. Neurotransmitters affect cognition, our movement, and our emotions.[5] Also, it is believed that they are implicated with drug abuse and with some forms of mental illness, especially depression.[6] Some scientists are once again using LSD and other hallucinogens to determine whether certain types of mental disorders are improved by these drugs.[7] Some drugs mimic the action of neurotransmitters, and others block their action. The functions of selected neurotransmitters are described on the following pages.

Acetylcholine

Acetylcholine (ACH) is synthesized from a molecule of choline (derived from one's diet and naturally manufactured in the body) and acetyl CoA. Neurons containing acetylcholine are termed cholinergic and are linked to specific behaviors. Drugs that block the action of ACH receptors are called anticholinergic.

ACH acts as an excitatory transmitter in the skeletal muscles but functions as an inhibitory transmitter in the heart muscle. Reduced numbers of ACH receptors in the brain have been associated with Alzheimer's disease, a progressive condition resulting in memory loss. Also, ACH has been tied to aggression and depression.

A number of hallucinogenic drugs are found in plants and fungi including the *Datura* and the *Amanita muscaria* mushrooms. This is significant because substances in these plants and fungi interfere with the action of ACH and can produce hallucinations. These plants are called **anticholinergic hallucinogens**.

Before ACH can be inactivated, the enzyme **cholinesterase** must be present. This enzyme, located in the synapse, is nullified by cholinesterase inhibitors such as nerve gas. The continuous release of ACH resulting from a cholinesterase inhibitor arouses the postsynaptic membrane and can lead to seizures, respiratory depression, and death. Cholinesterase inhibitors are found in the insecticides used on plants, for example. Insecticides contain another highly toxic agent, nicotine, which mimics the action of ACH at the neuromuscular junction.

autoreceptors Units that alter the synthesis of neurotransmitters after they are released by the nerve cells

acetylcholine (ACH) A neurotransmitter synthesized from a molecule of choline and from acetyl CoA

anticholinergic hallucinogens Substances found in datura and Amanita muscaria mushrooms; interfere with the action of acetylcholine to produce hallucinations

cholinesterase An enzyme necessary for the metabolism of acetylcholine

serotonin An inhibitory neurotransmitter located in the upper brain stem; plays a role in regulating sensory perception, eating, pain, sleep, and body temperature

tryptophan An amino acid that affects serotonin levels, allowing one to fall asleep more easily

Serotonin

Serotonin is an inhibitory neurotransmitter situated in the upper brain stem (Figure 5.3). Serotonin plays a role in regulating pain, sensory perception, eating, sleep, and body temperature. At one time, serotonin was believed to be effective for studying the effects of LSD and other hallucinogens because it resembles the chemical structure of these drugs. Depression can result from excessive reabsorption of serotonin. Also, serotonin has been related to hallucinations, psychosis, and obsessive-compulsive disorder, and has been implicated with aggression or violence. Serotonin poisoning, often resulting from its use with other drugs, was responsible for 118 deaths in 2005.[8] Despite the potential problems with antidepressant drugs such as selective serotonin reuptake inhibitors (SSRIs), they are the type of antidepressant that is most often prescribed.[9]

Serotonergic neurons, or tryptaminergic neurons, might prevent overreaction to various stimuli associated with mood, sexual behavior, and motor activity. When functioning improperly, tryptaminergic hormones have been linked to mental illness. Because tryptaminergic neurons affect the release of hormones in the hypothalamus, they monitor the release of hormones from the anterior pituitary gland. These hormones include leuteinizing hormone (LH) and follicle-stimulating hormone (FSH) as well as prolactin, which is responsible for milk production in the nursing mother.

To synthesize serotonin in tryptaminergic neurons, the amino acid tryptophan is needed. High levels of **tryptophan** are found in milk and other protein-rich

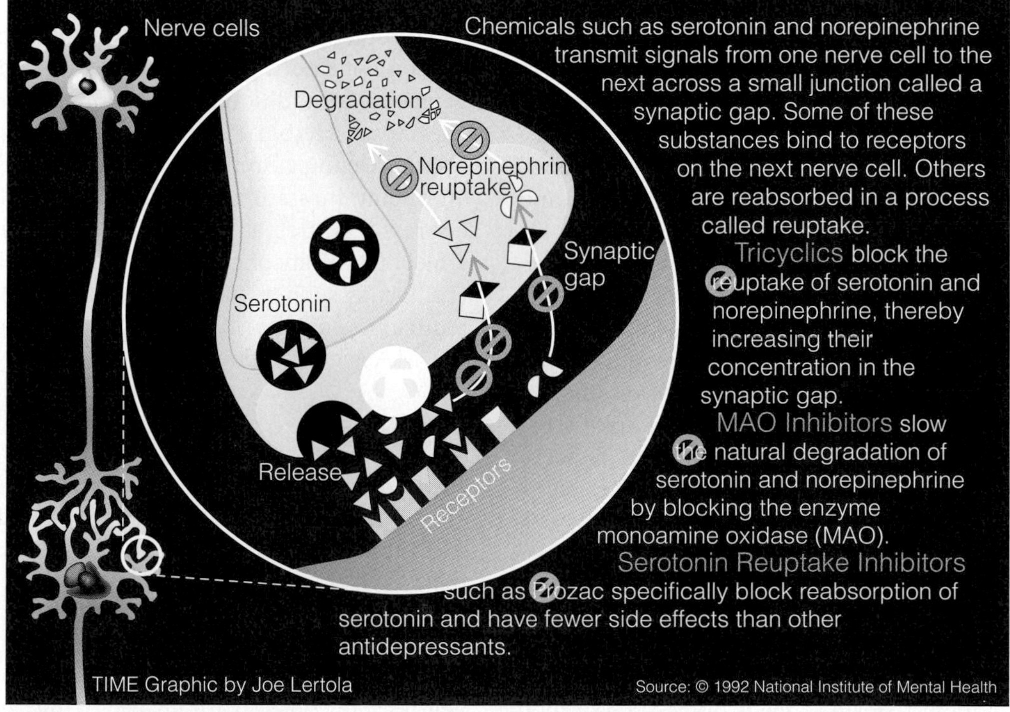

Figure 5.3 How the Drugs Work

foods. Drinking warm milk helps a person fall asleep because tryptophan enhances the brain's production of serotonin—which promotes relaxation.

Gamma-aminobutyric Acid

A second type of neurotransmitter that inhibits nerve impulses from being sent from one neuron to another is **gamma-aminobutyric acid (GABA)**. Drugs such as alcohol stimulate GABA, producing relaxation and feelings of decreased inhibition. Other drugs that increase the action of GABA are barbiturates and minor tranquilizers. The neurological disorder Huntington's chorea has been linked to GABA.

Catecholamines

Another group of neurotransmitters is **catecholamines**. Examples of catecholamine neurotransmitters are epinephrine, dopamine, and norepinephrine. Catecholamines function repeatedly because they are reabsorbed by the neuron that discharges them—a process known as **reuptake**. Catecholamines affect emotional states. An increase in catecholamines results in stimulation, whereas a decrease in catecholamines leads to depression. Drugs such as amphetamines and cocaine increase catecholamines initially, but this is followed by a depletion of the neurotransmitters. This explains the mood swings that individuals experience while using these drugs.

Dopamine plays a significant role in emotional, mental, and motor functions. It is speculated that dopamine can produce hyperactivity and tic and movement disorders such as Tourette's syndrome, affective disorders, and disorders of sexual activity and sexual drive. Dopamine levels are influenced by marijuana, affecting one's perception of pain, movement, and balance. Other drugs that alter dopamine levels include nicotine, heroin, and amphetamines.[10] Excessive dopamine has been related to schizophrenic symptoms, whereas Parkinson's disease can arise if neurons containing dopamine are destroyed. A drug that boosts dopamine levels is caffeine.[11] One study of 8,000 men showed that those men who drank two or more cups of coffee daily had a lower risk of developing Parkinson's disease.[12] Cocaine, on the other hand, is thought to deplete dopamine levels. In a study with laboratory animals, their desire for cocaine was lessened by dopamine agonists.[13]

In times of acute stress, **epinephrine**, or **adrenaline**, is released into the bloodstream. Epinephrine is integral to the **fight-flight-fright syndrome**. The release of epinephrine speeds up coronary blood flow and heart rate, among other effects. Because epinephrine causes the bronchi to dilate (expand), it is used to treat asthma. Figure 5.4 diagrams the fight-flight-fright mechanism, also called the stress response.

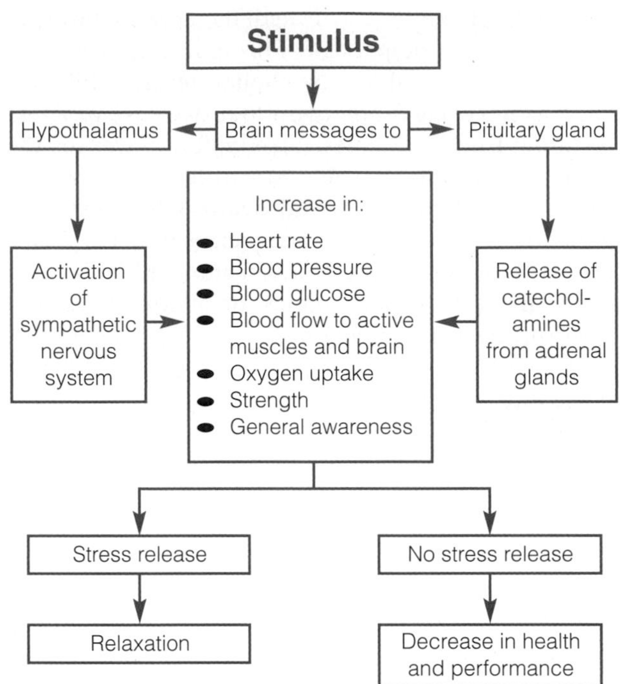

Figure 5.4 Fight-Flight-Fright Mechanism

Closely related to epinephrine is norepinephrine, also called noradrenaline. Norepinephrine inhibits its target neurons. Depending on the activity level of norepinephrine, a person can be aroused, depressed, or manic. In addition, norepinephrine increases motor activity. Heroin withdrawal symptoms are blocked by decreasing norepinephrine levels. Tobacco and amphetamines stimulate norepinephrine, and antidepressants such as Elavil and Triavil inhibit it. The effect of norepinephrine on mood is not always apparent. Drugs such as mescaline and MDMA (Ecstasy) reduce norepinephrine levels. At low doses, however, MDMA acts as a stimulant.

Peptides

Peptides are substances in which sequences of amino acids are linked. Whether peptides are truly transmitters is questionable because they modulate the activity of transmitters. One peptide group consists of **endorphins**, naturally occurring chemicals with opiate-like properties, which are found throughout the body. The term *endorphin* is derived from the words *endo*genous (naturally occurring) and m*orphin*e. Endorphins in the brain are called **enkaphalins**. The word *enkaphalins* comes from the Greek and means "in the head."

Endorphins and enkaphalins, whose actions are similar to those of morphine and heroin, are instrumental in moderating one's perception of pain. High levels of enkaphalins in the brain could be a causative factor in morphine dependency, and the absence of enkaphalins could account for the appearance of withdrawal symptoms. Chronic alcohol use impairs production of these neurotransmitters. Some postulate that alcohol withdrawal may arise from too little enkaphalin and endorphin stimulation.[14] Others say research supporting the role of endorphins in alcoholism or narcotic addiction is lacking.[15]

The brain emits endorphins when the person feels stress or pain. Also, endorphins are believed to be released during strenuous exercise, resulting in the "runner's high." Thus, an addiction to running or other forms of strenuous exercise could have a neurochemical basis. Endorphins have been linked to everything from obesity to sexual activity. They ameliorate the emotional response to pain. Opiates release endorphins, and acupuncture and electrical stimulation may cause them to be discharged as well. Table 5.1 provides a synopsis of selected neurotransmitters.

TABLE 5.1 Effects of Selected Neurotransmitters

Neurotransmitter	Effects
Acetylcholine (ACH)	An excitatory transmitter in the skeletal muscles but an inhibitory transmitter in the heart muscle; affects memory; linked to aggression and depression
Serotonin	An inhibitory neurotransmitter that plays a role in regulating sensory perception, eating, pain, sleep, and body temperature; a factor in hallucinations
Gamma-aminobutyric acid (GABA)	A type of neurotransmitter that produces relaxation and sleepiness
Catecholamines	A group of neurotransmitters that affects emotional states; an increase leads to stimulation and a decrease leads to depression; implicated in mood swings
Peptides	Substances linking amino acids; one type is endorphins, naturally occurring chemicals with opiate-like properties; they moderate perception of pain

gamma-aminobutyric acid (GABA) A type of neurotransmitter that produces relaxation and sleepiness

catecholamines A group of neurotransmitters that includes epinephrine, dopamine, and norepinephrine

reuptake A process by which a chemical is reabsorbed into the cell from which it was discharged

dopamine A neurotransmitter that affects emotional, mental, and motor functions

epinephrine A natural chemical, also called adrenaline, involved in the fight-flight-fright syndrome

adrenaline A hormone secreted by the adrenal gland in the fight-flight-fright response; another name for epinephrine

fight-flight-fright syndrome Psychological response of the body to stress, which prepares the individual to take action by stimulating the body's defense system

peptides Substances linking amino acids; include endorphins, which are naturally occurring chemicals with opiate-like properties

endorphins Naturally occurring chemicals with opiate-like properties

enkaphalins Endorphins found within the brain

reticular activating system (RAS) Part of the central nervous system; affects sleep, attention, and arousal

The Central Nervous System (CNS)

The CNS consists of the brain and spinal cord. Messages are transmitted from the brain to the muscles and organs and back to the brain through the spinal cord. The type of message depends on which part of the brain is sending it. The different parts of the brain and their functions are described next and are illustrated in Figure 5.5.

Reticular Activating System

Because the **reticular activating system (RAS)** has an extensive network of multiple synaptic neurons throughout the brain (like a telephone switchboard), its susceptibility to drugs is high. Many drugs, including barbiturates, LSD, alcohol, and amphetamines, affect the RAS extensively. Not surprisingly, the RAS plays a significant role in sleep, attention, and arousal.

For an individual to be aroused, the cortex has to be stimulated. The RAS alerts the cerebral cortex of important stimuli. If the stimuli generate alertness beyond conventional limits, hallucinations occur. Conversely, the RAS shuts down as one sleeps. Stimuli are forwarded to the brain constantly, but the cortex is aroused only if the message is consequential, such

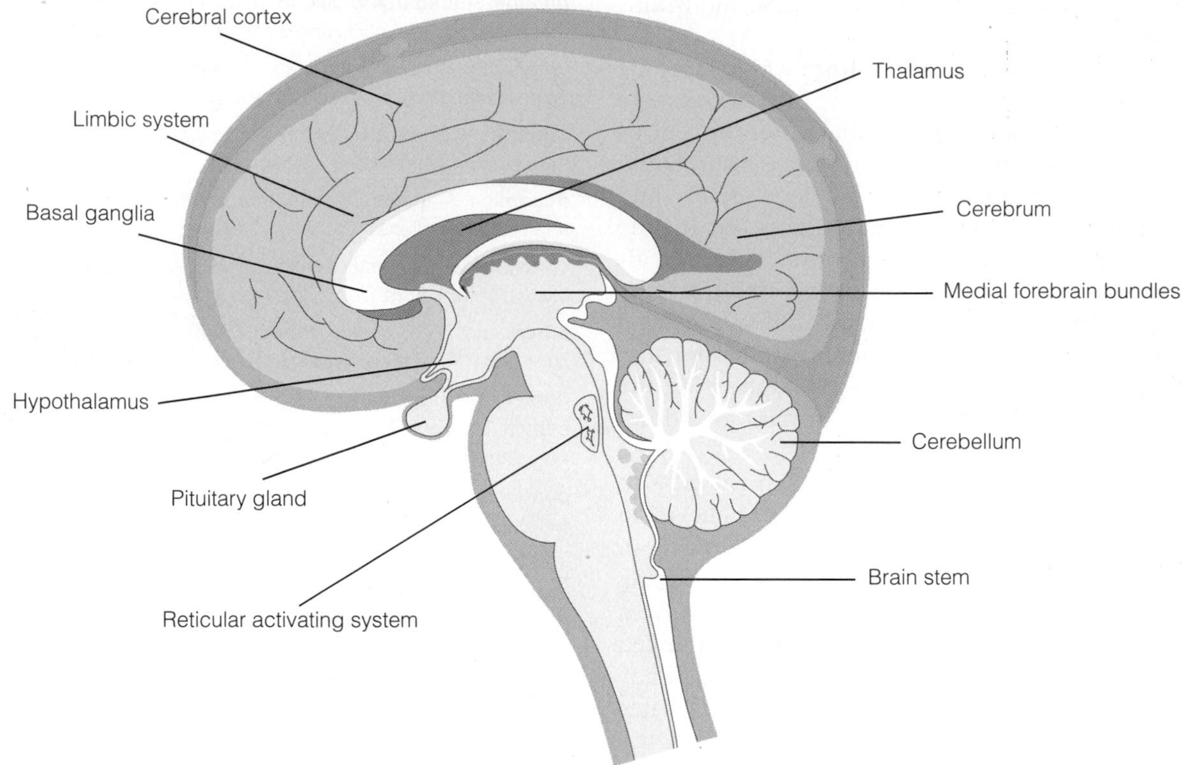

Figure 5.5 Cross Section of the Human Brain

as a baby crying. Sleeping through a thunderstorm but waking up to a baby's cry is a function of a properly functioning RAS.

The RAS is involved in helping to focus attention. Hyperactive children are thought to have an underactive RAS, suggesting that they are easily distracted. Stimulants activate the RAS, which filters out extraneous stimuli, enabling the hyperactive child to concentrate on a specific task.

Hypothalamus

Located near the base of the brain, the **hypothalamus** is comparable to a central computer from which many smaller computers receive their directions. The connection between the hypothalamus and the **pituitary gland** makes it possible. The pituitary gland regulates hormones that affect many behaviors, and many life-supporting functions originate from the hypothalamus. This helps to keep the body's biological systems in balance, called **homeostasis**. The hypothalamus has an effect on stress, heart rate, hunger, aggressiveness, body temperature, blood pressure, thirst, consciousness, and sexual behavior. It also has been linked to behavioral and chemical dependencies from alcohol to gambling to obesity.

Cerebral Cortex

The part of the brain that distinguishes humans from other mammals is the **cerebral cortex**, located in the **cerebrum**. The cortex is essential for most of our thought processes and for understanding information. This encompasses speech, motor movement, sensory perception, hearing, vision, and higher cognitive functions such as fine sensory discriminations, memory, language, abstract thought, and reasoning. The cortex influences personality and how we interpret emotions. The cortex is affected by almost all psychoactive drugs. For example, feelings of euphoria are activated by marijuana.

Limbic System

The **limbic system** combines many diverse structures in the cerebral hemispheres, where circuits relating to varied functions come together. The limbic system serves as the emotional center of the brain. For instance, if a person smells a perfume that his or her mother uses, that person might be reminded of his or her mother. This is largely a result of the ability of the limbic system to store and sort this information and then connect the memory with the emotion. Emotions regulated by the limbic system include sorrow, fear, pleasure, and anger.

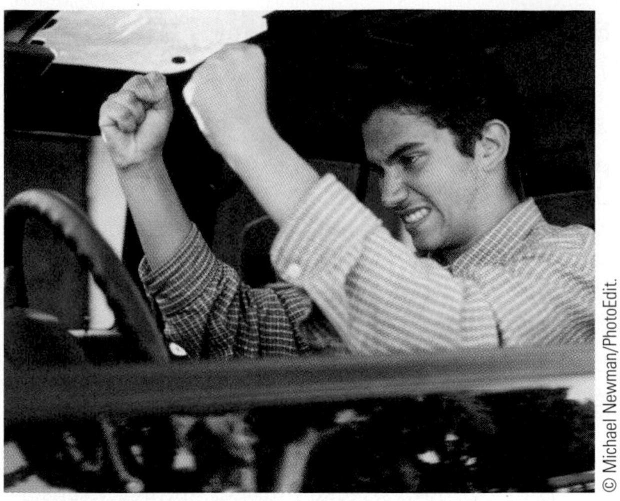

© Michael Newman/PhotoEdit.

The limbic system regulates emotions including anger and hostile behaviors.

hypothalamus Gland situated near the base of the brain; maintains homeostasis; affects stress, aggressiveness, heart rate, hunger, thirst, consciousness, body temperature, blood pressure, and sexual behavior

pituitary gland The "master gland"; responsible for controlling many bodily functions by secretion of hormones

homeostasis A condition in which the body's systems are in balance

cerebral cortex Part of the brain involved in intellectual functioning; affects speech, motor movement, sensory perception, hearing, vision, sensory discrimination, memory, language, reasoning, abstract reasoning, and personality

cerebrum Part of the brain that contains the cerebral cortex

limbic system Part of the central nervous system that plays a key role in memory and emotion

medial forebrain bundle (MFB) Serves as a communication route between the limbic system and the brain stem; affects pleasure and reward

basal ganglia Part of the central nervous system

periventricular system Part of the central nervous system implicated with punishment or avoidance behavior

Cocaine affects neurotransmitters in the limbic system, creating intense feelings of excitement and joy. Childress and colleagues found that the craving for cocaine can be induced by cocaine-related cues that cause activity in the limbic regions of the brain.[16] When cocaine is withdrawn, the outcome is severe withdrawal marked by depression, paranoia, irritability, and craving. However, when certain parts of the limbic system have lesions or are electrically stimulated, emotional disturbances, depersonalization, catatonia (immobility), and hallucinations can occur.

Depressants reduce electrical activity in the limbic system. This produces feelings of tranquility and relaxation rather than depression.

Medial Forebrain Bundle

Along each side of the hypothalamus is a **medial forebrain bundle (MFB)**, which serves as a communication route between the limbic system and the brain stem. By acting on this part of the brain, a part of the limbic system, amphetamines and cocaine produce intense euphoria. This is one reason that people repeat use of these drugs.

The MFB is significant in sexual response because the sensation of orgasm originates here. Laboratory rats, given the freedom to self-stimulate the MFB by pressing a lever in which electrodes were attached to the MFB, did so until they were completely exhausted. Animals have self-stimulated in preference to sex, food, or water, even though they had to endure electrical shocks to their feet. Humans whose MFB was stimulated while they were being operated on for brain tumors or other brain disorders have exhibited the pleasure response. Also, MFB stimulation alleviates feelings of depression.

Basal Ganglia

On both sides of the brain and below the cerebral cortex are the **basal ganglia**, which maintain involuntary motor control. The abilities to stand, walk, run, carry, throw, and lift are attributable largely to proper functioning of the basal ganglia. Excessive activity of, or damage to, the basal ganglia, however, can produce rigidity of facial, arm, and leg muscles, as well as spasms and trembling. An example of a condition that destroys the basal ganglia is Parkinson's disease. Drugs prescribed for schizophrenia can precipitate Parkinson's-like behavior. Also, the designer drug China white (fentanyl) has been linked to brain damage similar to that found in patients who have Parkinson's disease, and only small amounts of fentanyl can prove fatal.

Periventricular System

The **periventricular system**, composed of nerve cells above and to either side of the hypothalamus, is associated with punishment or avoidance behavior. People experience a distinct sense of discomfort or displeasure when the periventricular system is stimulated. When this system is aroused in animals, their behavior slows down or stops. The MFB and the periventricular system are coupled in that stimulation of one inhibits the other.

Brain Stem

The brain stem is located at the point where the brain and spinal cord join. It consists of the **medulla oblongata**, the **pons**, and the **midbrain**. The brain stem is responsible for regulating vital functions such as breathing, heartbeat, dilation of the pupil of the eye, blood pressure, and the vomiting reflex (the body's way of ridding the stomach of toxic substances).

In concert with the cerebellum, the brain stem governs muscle tone; with the hypothalamus, it controls the cardiovascular system; and, combined with the reticular activating system, it exerts some influence on arousal.

Drugs affecting the brain stem include alcohol and opiates. These drugs are capable of stopping breathing by depressing the respiratory system. Conversely, stimulants activate the medulla, causing vomiting and nausea.

Table 5.2 summarizes the actions of the parts of the brain discussed here.

TABLE 5.2 Actions of Various Parts of the Brain

Part of Brain	Actions
Reticular activating system (RAS)	Affects sleep, attention, and arousal
Hypothalamus	Maintains homeostasis; affects heart rate, hunger, thirst, consciousness, body temperature, blood pressure, and sexual behavior
Cerebral cortex	Affects speech, motor movement, sensory perception, hearing, vision, sensory discrimination, memory, language, reasoning, abstract thought, and personality
Limbic system	Plays a key role in memory and emotion
Medial forebrain bundle (MFB)	Serves as communication route between limbic system and brain stem; mediates pleasure and reward
Basal ganglia	Affects ability to stand, walk, run, carry, throw, and lift; can produce muscular rigidity of facial, arm, and leg muscles
Periventricular system	Implicated in punishment or avoidance behavior
Brain stem	Regulates vital functions such as breathing, heartbeat, dilation of pupils, and blood pressure, as well as vomiting reflex

The Peripheral Nervous System

Another component of the nervous system, the **peripheral nervous system (PNS)**, encompasses the somatic and autonomic nervous systems. The nerves associated with the PNS lie outside the skull and the spinal cord and serve as transmitting agents that link the brain and spinal cord to the body's extremities.

Somatic Nervous System

The **somatic nervous system** is a collection of nerves that control skeletal muscles and relay sensory information to the CNS and motor information back out. The cranial nerves are involved with our ability to taste, smell, chew, hear, and see, as well as movements of the face and tongue.

Autonomic Nervous System

The **autonomic nervous system (ANS)** regulates blood pressure, gastrointestinal and urinary functioning, body temperature, sweating, and other involuntary bodily functions. It is divided into two branches called the **sympathetic nervous system** and the **parasympathetic nervous system**, which frequently work in opposition to each other. The sympathetic branch relaxes bronchi in the lungs, inhibits intestinal and stomach glands, constricts blood vessels in the skin, increases heart rate, and dilates pupils of the eyes. The parasympathetic branch constricts bronchi, dilates blood vessels of the skin, increases action of the intestinal and stomach glands, decreases the heart rate, and constricts pupils of the eye.

The sympathetic nervous system enables the body to react to situations that require either fighting or fleeing (the fight-flight-fright syndrome) by increasing blood supply to the brain and muscles through the release of adrenaline. During acute stress and excitation, this system is especially active.

The parasympathetic system, in contrast, comes into play during calm situations. It allows the body to achieve a resting state following an emergency. Table 5.3 contrasts the effects of stimulating the sympathetic and parasympathetic systems.

Drugs that mimic actions of the sympathetic system are called **sympathomimetics**. Examples are amphetamines, cocaine, and caffeine. Drugs that mimic actions of the parasympathetic system are called **parasympathomimetics**. Examples are nicotine and the hallucinogen *Amanita muscaria*.

TABLE 5.3 Comparison of Sympathetic and Parasympathetic Systems

Sympathetic Effects	Parasympathetic Effects
Increases heart rate	Decreases heart rate
Constricts blood vessels	Dilates blood vessels
Slows down intestinal action	Increases intestinal action
Dilates pupils	Constricts pupils
Relaxes gall bladder	Constricts gall bladder

Drugs and Major Body Systems

The impact of drugs is not limited to the nervous system. Drugs affect the endocrine, cardiovascular, respiratory, and gastrointestinal systems as well.

Endocrine System

Many structures make up the endocrine system. Because these structures release hormones directly into the bloodstream rather than through ducts, the glands of the endocrine system are called ductless glands. Hormones released by the endocrine system have many effects ranging from stimulating the growth of new tissues to storing nutrients, maintaining homeostasis, and affecting metabolism and sexual behavior. The hypothalamus controls the endocrine system and the pituitary gland, the latter of which has been called the "master gland."

The pituitary gland consists of the anterior pituitary and the posterior pituitary. In females the anterior pituitary secretes FSH and LH, which cause women's ovaries to produce the sex hormones estrogen and progesterone. Besides regulating the menstrual cycle, estrogen is responsible for development of secondary sex characteristics. In males, FSH and interstitial cell-stimulating hormone (ICSH) produce androgen in the testicles. The primary androgenic hormone, testosterone, is produced in the testes and is necessary for sperm production and development of secondary sex characteristics.

Two hormones released by the posterior pituitary are oxytocin and vasopressin (also known as the antidiuretic hormone or ADH). Oxytocin causes uterine contractions during pregnancy and is administered sometimes to induce contractions during a difficult or slow labor. Vasopressin causes an increase in blood pressure and prevents urine from building up in the kidneys.

The adrenal glands, another part of the endocrine system, are located at the top of each kidney and secrete adrenaline and cortisol. Adrenaline prepares the body to fight or flee. Cortisol is administered primarily to treat inflammation and to diminish arthritic deterioration of the joints. Unfortunately, cortisol produces a number of undesirable side effects, so synthetic drugs similar to cortisol now are being used.

medulla oblongata One of two structures constituting the brain stem; helps control respiration, blood pressure, heart rate, and other vital functions

pons One of two structures constituting the brain stem, connecting the medulla with the brain stem

midbrain Part of the brain stem that connects the larger structures of the brain to the spinal cord

peripheral nervous system (PNS) Consists of the autonomic and somatic nervous systems

somatic nervous system Part of the nervous system that controls movement of the skeletal muscles

autonomic nervous system (ANS) Part of the peripheral nervous system that is automatic and involuntary

sympathetic nervous system A branch of the autonomic nervous system that releases adrenaline

parasympathetic nervous system Branch of the autonomic nervous system that includes acetylcholine and alters heart rate and intestinal activity

sympathomimetics Drugs that mimic actions of the sympathetic nervous system, which is involved with fight-flight-fright activity

parasympathomimetics Drugs that mimic actions of the parasympathetic system, which allows the body to rest during states of emergency

Cardiovascular System

The heart and blood vessels constitute the cardiovascular system. One arguably could state that the heart is the body's most important organ because people die within minutes when it stops functioning. The heart is responsible for pumping blood throughout the body, delivering nutrients and oxygen through the blood. Drugs that interfere with the heart's ability to contract present a danger. For example, alcohol can cause the heart muscle to degenerate, induce cardiac arrhythmia (irregular heartbeat), and increase blood pressure, which can bring about a heart attack. Heavy, short-term alcohol abuse over several days can cause "holiday heart syndrome," a condition marked by cardiac arrhythmia and symptoms similar to a heart attack.

A drug often implicated in cardiovascular disease is caffeine. Despite popular belief, there is insufficient proof that moderate caffeine use raises the risk of heart disease. A more in-depth look at the research on caffeine and heart disease is included in Chapter 11.

Cocaine has been found to be detrimental to the cardiovascular system. It produces a significant rise in heart rate and blood pressure, thereby increasing the risk for heart attack. Cocaine also is a vasoconstrictor, depriving the heart of needed blood. A particular concern is that cocaine use can produce cardiovascular damage in young people who appear healthy and have no history of heart disease. Further, cardiovascular problems can arise from only small to moderate amounts of cocaine.

Smoked drugs pose a special risk to the cardiovascular system because smoke interferes with the ability of the blood to distribute oxygen. There is much justified concern about the relationship between tobacco and lung cancer. Yet, smokers are far more likely to die from cardiovascular disease than from cancer. A smoker is twice as likely to have a heart attack as a nonsmoker. Nicotine in cigarettes raises the blood pressure, and carbon monoxide makes the heart work harder because the amount of oxygen delivered throughout the body is reduced. A positive note is that people who quit smoking have no greater risk of heart disease than nonsmokers after several years.

Marijuana, too, produces increased heart rate, called tachycardia. The heart rate is temporarily increased by as much as 50% after marijuana use. Patients with angina pectoris (chest pain related to diminished blood supply to the heart) are more susceptible to angina after smoking marijuana.

Respiratory System

Many drugs interfere with the functioning of the respiratory system. In particular, depressant drugs such as barbiturates, minor tranquilizers, alcohol, and narcotics can have tragic effects because they slow down respiration. Any depressant can cause breathing to stop. Combining depressants with other drugs can have a **synergistic effect**. For example, using alcohol and barbiturates together can be a deadly mix.

Stimulants such as amphetamines and cocaine increase the respiratory rate. Some stimulants can be beneficial. Tea, containing the stimulant theophylline, has been recommended for people with breathing difficulties because it causes the air passages to open.

Smoked tobacco is especially harmful to the respiratory system. Cigarette smoke impedes the cilia from removing mucus and other foreign matter from the lungs. Breathing becomes labored. Close to 70% of the particles in tobacco smoke stay in the lungs. Not only do smokers have more respiratory infections than nonsmokers, but their infections tend to be more severe. Marijuana, too, impairs the ability of the lungs to function properly. Because marijuana is inhaled more deeply and for longer periods than regular tobacco, more particles probably are retained from marijuana. Chronic marijuana smoking results in air passages becoming smaller. In addition, marijuana has as much tar and half again as many carcinogens as conventional tobacco.[17]

Gastrointestinal System

The gastrointestinal system, consisting of the esophagus, stomach, and intestines, enables the body to absorb nutrients and water and remove waste. Gastrointestinal disorders affect millions of people. Upset stomach, ulcers, constipation, and diarrhea are common maladies of modern society. To neutralize stomach acid, antacids containing sodium bicarbonate, calcium carbonate, aluminum hydroxide, or magnesium salts are ingested. Laxatives are used to relieve constipation.

Many drugs contribute to gastrointestinal disorders. Alcohol causes diarrhea, as well as irritation and inflammation of the stomach, small intestine, esophagus, and pancreas. Moreover, it eventually results in malnutrition by interfering with the absorption of nutrients. A combination that is especially harmful to the stomach is alcohol and aspirin, because it can cause excessive internal bleeding. Peyote can produce nausea and vomiting. Although narcotics cause constipation, they can be beneficial, even life-saving, to people suffering from diarrhea—a common cause of death in many underdeveloped countries.

Factors Influencing the Effects of Drugs

The effects of drugs are a function of their pharmacological or chemical makeup. A drug's pharmacology or chemistry, however, does not tell the whole story. Individual and cultural factors play a significant role, too.

Age

Infants and the elderly are more sensitive to the effects of drugs than people between those life stages. Drug actions are prolonged in infants and the elderly because they are less able to metabolize and excrete drugs.

In the United States, in 2006, more than 45,000 people ages 55 and older went to emergency rooms because of adverse drug reactions.[18] An estimated one in four elderly Americans living outside of an institution receive one or more prescription drugs that are unneeded or potentially harmful.[19] For example, people ages 50 or older who use selective serotonin reuptake inhibitors (SSRIs) are two times more likely to suffer from fragility fractures.[20] Two percent of adults age 55 or older are admitted for treatment from abusing prescription narcotic medications.[21] The American Medical Association calls substance abuse among the elderly a hidden epidemic.[22] An estimated 1.7 million Americans over age 50 are addicted to drugs.[23] Elderly women are more likely than men to be at risk for drug-related problems because they receive more prescriptions. This is partly because women see physicians more often than men do.

Tolerance for alcohol lessens as people age.[24] Blood alcohol concentrations are higher in the elderly when they drink, because they have less body fluid. Moreover, older people who drink alcohol are more likely to have problems sleeping.[25] One encouraging study, however, reported that older men and women drank less alcohol as they aged.[26] As people age, their percentage of body fat increases. Some drugs accumulate in adipose tissue, increasing the sensitivity to those drugs and the possibility of a toxic reaction. Antidepressant drugs serve as a good example. Although they are effective with 70% to 90% of the elderly who take them, they can precipitate glaucoma, impair the prostate gland, and cause delirium and confusion.

It is estimated that in the United States, 5.5% of women used an illegal drug while pregnant, 18% consumed alcohol, and 20% smoked cigarettes.[27] Intrauterine cocaine exposure has resulted in fetal growth retardation and preterm deliveries.

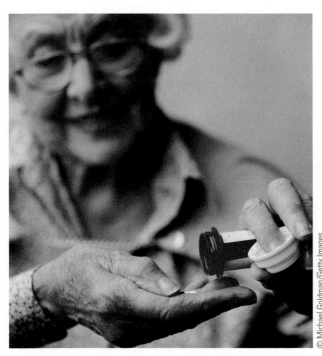

The rate of prescription drug use is higher among the elderly than any other age group.

synergistic effect An enhanced, unpredictable effect caused by combining two or more substances

teratogenic Refers to substances that cause harm to the fetus

threshold dose The smallest amount of a drug required to produce an effect

There is also some research showing that elementary-age children respond differently to drugs. The over-the-counter antihistamine diphenhydramine, commonly sold under the trade name Benadryl, has a strong sedating effect on adults. However, researchers in Denver found that this drug did not have a sleep-like effect on children. Moreover, these children scored as well on cognitive tests as children receiving placebos.[28]

Gender

Females and males respond to drugs differently. Differences in how drugs affect men and women are related to fat and water content, not gender per se. Women who weigh the same as men have a higher percentage of body fat and a lower percentage of water, making women more sensitive to the actions of drugs because fat stores drugs and water dilutes the amount of a drug in the bloodstream.

Hormones also make a difference. During the premenstrual phase of the menstrual cycle, women absorb ethyl alcohol more quickly. Females are especially affected by drugs during pregnancy. Many drugs traverse the placental barrier. Because the fetus lacks enzymes and its excretory system is not fully developed, drugs have a greater impact on the fetus than on the pregnant woman. Drugs causing damage to the fetus are called **teratogenic**. Finally, the use of tobacco, coffee, and alcohol during pregnancy increases the risk of miscarriages.

Dosage

The amount of a drug consumed—the dosage—plays a significant role in the effect of drugs. Before it produces an effect, the drug must be present in a certain amount. The smallest amount of a drug required to produce an effect is called the **threshold dose**. Typically, as the dosage increases, the effects become more pronounced. Because the effects of drugs are not always proportional, though, they do not affect everyone in the same way. If twice the amount of a drug is administered, it will not necessarily be twice as effective or potent. Some drugs work on an all-or-none basis in that they act either maximally or not at all.

On Campus

College students who have Friday classes before 10:00 AM drink less alcohol than students who have Friday classes after that time.

Source: P.K. Wood, K.J. Sher, and P.C. Rutledge, "College Student Alcohol Consumption, Day of the Week, and Class Schedule," *Alcoholism: Clinical and Experimental Research*, 31 (2007): 1195–1207.

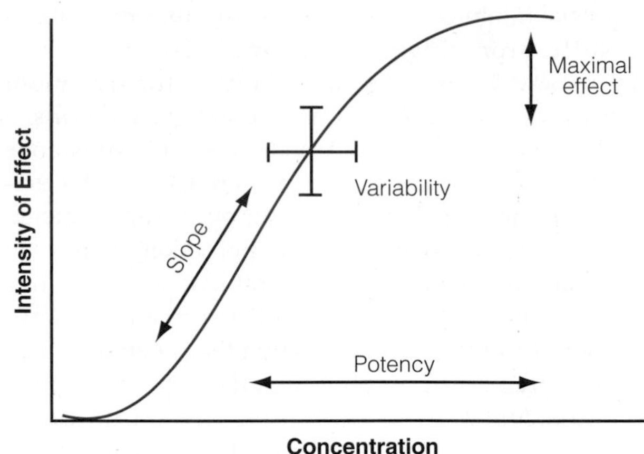

Figure 5.6 Dose-Response Curve

The amount necessary to achieve a specific response is called the **effective dose (ED)**. If a drug is identified as ED 50, it produces an effect in 50% of the population tested. The quantity required to cause death is the **lethal dose (LD)**. The safety of a drug is determined by the difference between its ED and LD. The greater the margin between the ED and LD, the safer the drug. When discussing the effects of drugs at different dosage levels, pharmacologists refer to the **dose-response curve** (Figure 5.6), which plots the specific effects that occur at specific doses. More pronounced effects take place as the dosage level goes up, although age, gender, size, and overall health also matter. Not surprisingly, there is less variability *within* a species than among species.

Purity and Potency

Many health-related problems that drug users experience arise from impurities rather than from the drugs themselves. The quality or **purity** of drugs, which varies greatly among illegal drugs, is a significant factor in the drug's effect. The Drug Enforcement Administration (DEA) found that the purity of heroin purchased in the mid-1970s was about 6%. In the early 1980s, purity was less than 4%, and it was more than 20% in the early 1990s. By 2001, the purity of heroin ranged from 51% to 69%. The purity of cocaine was as low as 53% and as high as 69%.[29]

Potency refers to a drug's ability to produce an effect relative to other drugs. The smaller the quantity required to elicit an effect, the more powerful the drug. Comparing heroin, morphine, and aspirin as pain relievers, heroin is the most potent, followed by morphine, then aspirin. Thus, a smaller amount of heroin than morphine or aspirin is needed to reduce pain to the same degree. Some drugs vary naturally in potency. For example, the percentage of THC, the psychoactive substance in marijuana, ranges from 4% to 9%.

Table 5.4 shows the average purity of cocaine, heroin, MDMA, and methamphetamines from 2001 to 2004.

Drug Interactions

The interaction of drugs with other drugs or certain foods can be hazardous. An estimated 25% of admissions to emergency rooms result from interactions between alcohol and medications.[30] The effects of drugs and food can be additive, antagonistic, or synergistic. Additive effects refer to the sum or cumulative effects of two or more substances mixed together. Combining

TABLE 5.4 Average Purity of Drug Samples Tested, by Percentage, 2001–2004

Drug	Type	2001	2002	2003	2004
Cocaine		78.0	77.0	82.0	84.0*
Heroin	South America	78.0	72.0	70.0	64.0
	Southwest Asia	69.0	64.0	62.0	67.0
	Southeast Asia	68.0	73.0	63.0	63.0
	Mexico	30.0	33.0	37.0	39.0
MDMA		53.6	50.6	55.6	53.9
Methamphetamine		39.1	43.6	57.2	60.6

*Representative of January through July 2004.
Source: Drug Enforcement Administration.

aspirin and alcohol, for example, increases the risk of intestinal and prolonged bleeding.

Antagonistic drugs negate the effects of other drugs. One commonly prescribed drug that is antagonistic is the antibiotic tetracycline. Mixing it with penicillin, milk, or antacids negates its actions, and penicillin is ineffective when used with milk or antacids. Using barbiturates with diphenhydramine (Benadryl) or dimenhydrinate (Dramamine) negates the effectiveness of both. Minor tranquilizers such as Valium, Miltown, and Librium reduce the effectiveness of oral contraceptives. It has been found that more than 150 prescription and over-the-counter medications interact negatively with alcohol.[31] Therefore, when obtaining a prescription, one should ask a pharmacist or physician about possible drug interactions.

The combination of some drugs has a synergistic effect. The combined effect of taking both drugs is greater than if the drugs' effects are simply added together. One way to illustrate this concept is to consider muscular strength. If a person has enough muscle mass in the bicep to lift 25 pounds of weight and enough muscle mass in the forearm to lift 25 pounds of weight, the person theoretically can lift 50 pounds. Because the muscles in the bicep and forearm work in concert, however, the person may be able to lift 100 pounds instead of 50.

Some drugs have this same type of synergism: Their effects when combined are much greater than the sum of their effects when administered individually. An example of such a synergistic combination of drugs is barbiturates and alcohol. Every year several thousand people die from combining these two drugs, either accidentally or intentionally. Table 5.5 shows some possible risks of mixing alcohol with other drugs.

Taking certain antidepressants with certain foods can result in hemorrhaging and stroke. People who eat foods containing tyramine—such as red wine, beer, chocolate, raisins, and aged cheeses—while taking an antidepressant monoamine oxidase (MAO) inhibitor can experience an increase in blood pressure to perilously high levels. Another dangerous mixture is oral contraceptives and tobacco. Women who smoke and take oral contraceptives have a greater chance of developing a heart attack, stroke, or blood clots. Also, the risk of a heart attack and stroke increases for smokers who are taking medication to relieve hypertension.

Tolerance

Tolerance has been defined as "a state of progressively decreasing responsiveness to a drug."[32] In developing tolerance, increasing amounts of a drug are required. Tolerance depends on dosage, the type of drug, and frequency of use. Even though a person may require a greater amount of a drug to achieve the desired results, the amount required to cause a fatal overdose does not necessarily increase. The types of tolerance are pharmacological, behavioral, cross, and reverse tolerance.

effective dose (ED) The amount of drug required to produce a specific response

lethal dose (LD) The amount of a drug required to result in death

dose-response curve Graphic representation of the effects of drugs at various levels

purity Quality of a substance; state of noncontamination of a drug

potency A drug's ability to produce an effect relative to other drugs; the less that is needed to produce a response, the more potent the drug

pharmacological tolerance Adjustment or compensation of the body to the presence of a given drug

behavioral tolerance Adjustment or behaviors learned by an individual to compensate for the presence of drugs

Pharmacological Tolerance

Pharmacological tolerance means that the body adjusts to or compensates for the presence of a particular drug. This could arise from the rapid deactivation or excretion of drugs resulting from repeated use. Therefore, to achieve the effect desired, the person has to increase either the amount or the frequency of use.

Depressant drugs provide an example. If the same dosage of a depressant is maintained over a long enough period, that dosage no longer has the desired effect. Similarly, an individual develops tolerance to alcohol, although not everyone has the same tolerance level. Some people are born with naturally higher tolerance levels, suggesting that they can drink more alcohol than others without feeling the effects of alcohol. Likewise, the capacity to reach a state of euphoria from amphetamines declines with regular use, although continued use can produce psychotic-like effects.

Behavioral Tolerance

Behavioral tolerance means that an individual *learns* to adjust to the presence of drugs. After repeated exposure to a drug, experienced drug users are more able to moderate their behavior than people who are less experienced with drugs. Individuals are capable of developing behavioral tolerance more quickly if they are offered an incentive.[33] In a sense, they are conditioned to the effects of the

TABLE 5.5 Drug Interactions with Alcohol

Symptom/Disorders	Medication (Brand Name)	Medication (Generic Name)	Some Possible Reactions with Alcohol
Allergies/Colds/Flu	Allegra®, Allegra-D®	Fexofenadin	Drowsiness, dizziness; increased risk for overdose
	Benadryl®	Diphenhydramine	
	Claritin®, Claritin-D®	Loratadine	
	Dimetapp® Cold & Allergy	Brompheniramine	
	Sudafed® Sinus & Allergy	Chlorpheniramine	
	Triaminic® Cold & Allergy	Chlorpheniramine	
	Tylenol® Allergy Sinus	Chlorpheniramine	
	Tylenol® Cold & Flu	Chlorpheniramine	
	Zyrtec®	Cetirizine	
Angina (chest pain), coronary heart disease	Isordil®	Isosorbide	Rapid heartbeat, sudden changes in blood pressure, dizziness, fainting
		Nitroglycerin	
Anxiety and epilepsy	Ativan®	Lorazepam	Drowsiness, dizziness; increased risk for overdose; slowed or difficulty breathing; impaired motor control; unusual behavior; and memory problems
	Librium®	Chlordiazepoxide	
	Paxil®	Paroxetine	
	Valium®	Diazepam	
	Xanax®	Alprazolam	
	Herbal preparations (kava kava)		Liver damage, drowsiness
Arthritis	Celebrex®	Celecoxib	Ulcers, stomach bleeding, liver problems
	Naprosyn®	Naproxen	
Blood clots	Coumadin®	Warfarin	Occasional drinking may lead to internal bleeding; heavier drinking also may cause bleeding or may have the opposite effect, resulting in possible blood clots, strokes, or heart attacks
Cough	Delsym®, Robitussin Cough®	Dextromethorpan	Drowsiness, dizziness; increased risk for overdose
	Robitussin A–C®	Guaifenesin + codeine	
Depression	Anafranil®	Clomipramine	Drowsiness, dizziness; increased risk for overdose; increased feelings of depression or hopelessness in adolescents (suicide)
	Effexor®	Venlafaxine	
	Elavil®	Amitriptyline	
	Lexapro®	Escitalopram	
	Luvox®	Fluvoxamine	
	Prozac®	Fluoxetine	
	Wellbutrin®	Bupropion	
	Zoloft®	Sertraline	
	Herbal preparations (St. John's wort)		
Diabetes	Glucophage®	Metformin	Abnormally low blood sugar levels, flushing reaction (nausea, vomiting, headache, rapid heartbeat, sudden changes in blood pressure)
	Micronase®	Glyburide	
	Orinase®	Tolbutamide	
Heartburn, indigestion, sour stomach	Tagamet®	Cimetidine	Rapid heartbeat, sudden changes in blood pressure (metoclopramide); increased alcohol effect
	Zantac®	Ranitidine	
High blood pressure	Accupril®	Quinapril	Dizziness, fainting, drowsiness; heart problems such as changes in the heart's regular heartbeat (arrhythmia)
	Hytrin®	Terazosin	
	Lopressor® HCT	Hydrochlorothiazide	
	Lotensin®	Benzapril	
	Minipress®	Prazosin	
	Vaseretic®	Enalapril	

drug. A person who frequently drinks alcohol often can function better under the influence of alcohol than someone who doesn't drink or one who drinks infrequently.

cross-tolerance Transference of tolerance to a drug to chemically similar drugs

reverse tolerance A drug user's experiencing of the desired effects from lesser amounts of the same drug

Cross-Tolerance

Cross-tolerance means that people who develop tolerance to a drug will develop tolerance to chemically similar drugs. If a person becomes tolerant to LSD, for example, he or she will develop tolerance to other hallucinogens, such as mescaline and peyote. Likewise, chronic alcohol users become tolerant not only to alcohol but to other depressants such as barbiturates and minor tranquilizers as well.

Reverse Tolerance

Reverse tolerance means that a drug user will feel the desired effects from lesser amounts of the drug. Hallucinogens and marijuana have been used as examples, though one possible explanation for reverse tolerance in marijuana is that it is stored in fatty tissue and later released as fat breaks down. Also, experienced marijuana users anticipate the drug's effects, and the learning process may play an important role. Reverse tolerance to alcohol seems to occur in the late stages of alcoholism because of progressive liver dysfunction in which the liver enzymes are inadequate to metabolize alcohol.

TABLE 5.5 Drug Interactions with Alcohol (*continued*)

Symptom/Disorders	Medication (Brand Name)	Medication (Generic Name)	Some Possible Reactions with Alcohol
High cholesterol	Crestor® Lipitor® Pravachol® Vytorin™ Zocor®	Rosuvastatin Atorvastatin Pravastatin Ezetimibe + simvastatin Simvastatin	Liver damage (all medications); increased flushing and itching (niacin), increased stomach bleeding (pravastatin + aspirin)
Muscle pain	Flexeril® Soma®	Cyclobenzaprine Carisoprodol	Drowsiness, dizziness; increased risk of seizures; increased risk for overdose; slowed or difficulty breathing; impaired motor control; unusual behavior; memory problems
Nausea, motion sickness	Dramamine®	Dimenhydrinate	Drowsiness, dizziness; increased risk for overdose
Pain (such as headache, muscle ache, minor arthritis pain), fever, inflammation	Advil® Aleve® Excedrin® Motrin® Tylenol®	Ibuprofen Naproxen Aspirin, acetaminophen Ibuprofen Acetaminophen	Stomach upset, bleeding and ulcers; liver damage (acetaminophen); rapid heartbeat
Seizures	Dilantin® Klonopin®	Phenytoin Clonazepam Phenobarbital	Drowsiness, dizziness; increased risk of seizures
Severe pain from injury, postsurgical care, oral surgery, migraines	Darvocet-N® Demerol® Percocet® Vicodin®	Propoxyphene Merepidine Oxycodone Hydrocodone	Drowsiness, dizziness; increased risk for overdose; slowed or difficulty breathing; impaired motor control; unusual behavior; memory problems
Sleep problems	Ambien® Lunesta™ Sominex® Unisom®	Zolpidem Eszopiclone Diphenhydramine Doxylamine	Drowsiness, sleepiness, dizziness; slowed or difficulty breathing; impaired motor control; unusual behavior; memory problems
	Herbal preparations (chamomile, valerian, lavender)		Increased drowsiness

Source: *Harmful Interactions: Mixing Alcohol with Medicines* (Rockville, MD: National Institute on Alcohol Abuse and Alcoholism, 2007).

Set and Setting

Two vital, interlocking components of the drug experience are set and setting. **Set** refers to the drug user's psychological makeup, personality, mood, and expectations when using drugs. **Setting** alludes to the social and physical environment in which drugs are taken. Set, then, deals with internal environment, and setting relates to the external environment. The effects of drugs on behavior depend greatly on one's attitudes toward drugs, emotional state, and previous experiences with drugs. If a person is depressed or anxious or previously had an unpleasant experience while taking drugs, the effects will be different than if one is in a happy mood or is looking forward to the drug's effects.

Placebos are inert substances capable of producing psychological and physiological reactions. A large percentage of prescriptions given to patients are placebos. They are effective because of expectations for the drug. Placebos may provide relief for 30% to 40% of patients for whom they are prescribed.[34]

The notion of a drug being euphoric or dysphoric depends a great deal on set. For example, people using cocaine who are under stress in their lives may be more susceptible to dysphoria from the drug. Someone in a hospital who is given morphine for analgesic purposes during surgery probably would not describe the effects of morphine in euphoric terms, whereas a person using morphine bought illegally may well describe the effects very differently.

On many college campuses heavy drinking is associated with football game days. For example, on football game days fans drink more alcohol and are more affected than nonfans. One study found that males drink more than females but that females experienced more adverse consequences. The age group that drank more alcohol was the 21 to 26 age group, as opposed to younger or older age groups.[35]

The portrayal of a drug's effects also is different if drugs are consumed alone or with friends at a party. To a large extent, setting determines set. Taking legal drugs among friends is likely to be viewed as drug *use*. Taking illegal drugs by oneself is likely to be seen as drug *abuse*.

Methods of Administration

How a drug enters the body has a significant bearing on its effects. The route of administration determines how quickly a drug takes effect, the amount of time it is active, its intensity, and how localized its actions are. Drugs enter the body via oral ingestion, injection, topical application to the skin, inhalation, suppositories, and implantation.

Oral Ingestion

Drugs can be consumed in the form of pills, liquids, tablets, or capsules. Though oral ingestion is one of the most convenient, safest, and most common ways to consume drugs, several factors make it difficult to control the dosage level. Once a drug enters the stomach, its effectiveness is reduced because it mixes with food, acid, and digestive enzymes in the gastrointestinal tract. Any food present slows the rate of absorption of the drug into the bloodstream. Drugs in the form of capsules and tablets must dissolve before they enter the bloodstream.

Disadvantages of taking drugs orally include the following[36]:

- Oral administration is not appropriate in emergencies because drugs are absorbed slowly.
- The slow absorption rate may reduce the amount of the drug to an insufficient level.
- People could fatally choke on a drug if they are not conscious.
- Some ingested drugs cause nausea and vomiting.
- Because conditions in the gastrointestinal tract are changing constantly, drug absorption is variable.

Injection

Parenteral drug use refers to injecting drugs. Injected drugs reach the brain quickly but carry many risks. Drugs such as heroin may not be lethal when they are smoked but may be lethal when they are injected. Injecting drugs with unsterile hypodermic needles poses a risk for infectious diseases including AIDS and hepatitis. Thousands of AIDS infections in women can be attributed to injection drug use. Needle-exchange programs report fewer addicts sharing needles even though the federal government prohibits its drug treatment funds to be used for such programs. Figure 5.7 shows the number of U.S. adult who contracted HIV/AIDS in recent years, and the source of the infection.

Drugs can be injected intravenously, intramuscularly, or subcutaneously.

Intravenous Injection

In intravenous injection, or mainlining, drugs are administered directly into the bloodstream. Within a minute after injection, the drug is distributed to all parts of the body in high concentration. Consequently, the effects of drugs are experienced quickly and fully when they are taken intravenously.

Further, drugs can be measured precisely when they are administered intravenously. Unlike drugs taken orally, drugs given intravenously do not mix with stomach contents. Thus, intravenous drugs do

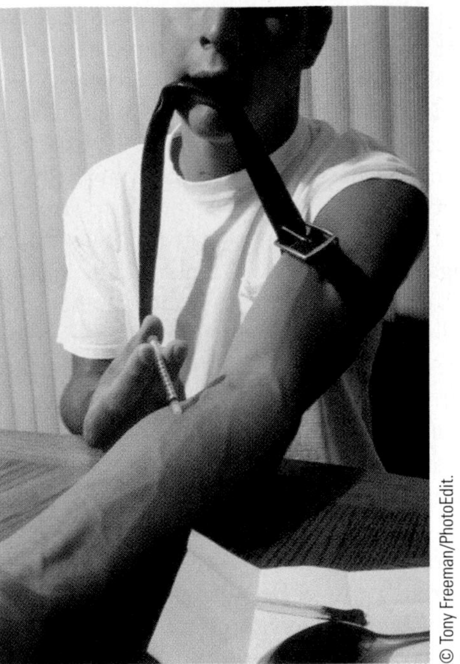

Health risks are associated with injected drug use.

not have to be absorbed first. Although these factors are seen as advantages, repeated intravenous injections increase the risk of clot formation as well as vessel irritation and collapse.

set The psychological state, personality, and expectations of an individual while using drugs

setting The physical and social environment in which drugs are used

parenteral drug use Drug administration by injection

Intramuscular Injection

In intramuscular injection, drugs are injected into muscle tissue. Because muscle tissue serves as a filter, drugs delivered intramuscularly are absorbed more slowly than drugs delivered intravenously. For example, the onset of euphoria after injecting heroin intravenously is 7 to 8 seconds. When it is injected intramuscularly, the onset of euphoria is 5 to 8 minutes.[37] The rate of absorption depends on the muscle receiving the drug. The more blood vessels the muscle has, the more quickly the drug is absorbed. Drugs injected into the deltoid muscle are absorbed more rapidly than the same drugs injected into the buttocks.

Subcutaneous Injection

Injecting drugs just below the layers of the skin is called subcutaneous injection. With this method, also known as skin-popping, drugs are absorbed less evenly. Although subcutaneous injection is safer than intravenous injection, skin irritation and abscesses can occur.

Figure 5.7 Proportion of AIDS Cases Among Adults and Adolescents, by Transmission Category and Year of Diagnosis, 1985–2006—United States and Dependent Areas

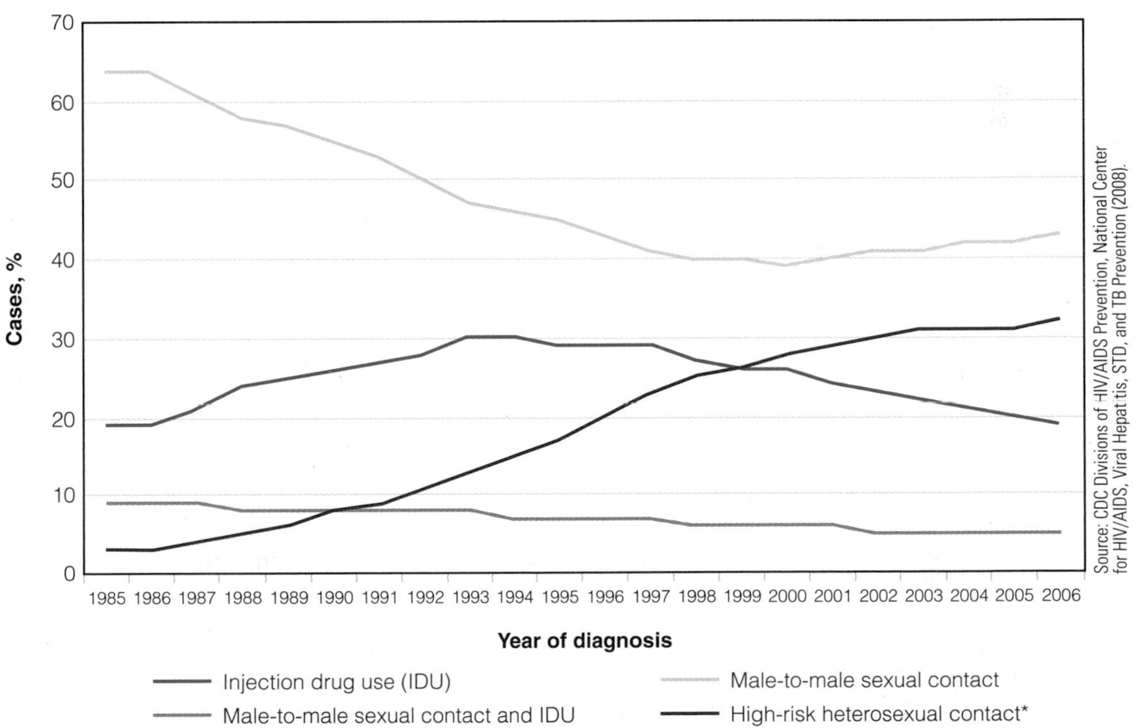

Note. Data have been adjusted for reporting delays and cases without risk factor information were proportionally redistributed.

* Heterosexual contact with a person known to have, or to be at high risk for, HIV infection.

Topical Application

Drugs can be applied to the skin and absorbed into the bloodstream by placing small disks or patches behind the ear or on the arm or chest. Called the **transdermal method**, it has limited popularity because of the uneven way in which drugs are absorbed. Also, drugs are introduced into the body slowly when applied topically. An advantage to transdermal application is that drugs are absorbed directly into the bloodstream at programmed rates. Transdermal patches have been used to relieve motion sickness, angina pectoris, and nicotine dependency.

Inhalation

Drugs can be absorbed into the bloodstream via the lungs through inhalation. The speed and efficiency of drugs entering the bloodstream are quite high because of the accessibility of the capillary walls of the lung. The actual amount of an inhaled drug that reaches the brain is variable, though. Nevertheless, inhaled drugs reach the brain in 5 to 8 seconds, though the effects usually are brief. Inhaled drugs irritate the lungs.

Inhaled drugs include volatile anesthetics such as glue, paint thinner, and gasoline, in addition to cigarettes, marijuana, and crack cocaine. Since 2002, inhalant use by male adolescents has remained stable while use among female adolescents has increased slightly.[38]

Summary

Drugs alter behavior by the way they affect the central nervous system (CNS). Consisting of the brain and spinal cord, the CNS has nerve cells, or neurons, that act as messengers. Within the neuron are dendrites and axons. Dendrites carry impulses to the neuron, and the axon carries impulses away from the neuron. The impulses that pass through the neuron are electrical, and those from the axon to the dendrite are chemical. To send electrical messages from the axon of one neuron to the dendrite of another neuron, the messages or impulses must cross a space called the synapse.

At the end of each axon are saclike structures or vesicles containing neurotransmitters. Neurotransmitters are chemicals discharged by one neuron that change electrical activity in another neuron. These chemicals have many effects on the mind and body. Acetylcholine (ACH) excites skeletal muscles but inhibits heart muscles. Serotonin helps regulate body temperature, sensory perception, eating, pain, and sleep. Gamma-aminobutyric acid (GABA) is linked to relaxation and sleepiness. Catecholamines affect emotional states such as arousal or depression, depending on whether their production is increased or decreased. Peptides, substances linking sequences of amino acids, consist of numerous chemicals including endorphins. Endorphins are believed to contribute to a natural high and modify one's perception of pain.

Various parts of the brain have their own functions. The reticular activating system (RAS) affects arousal, attention, and sleep. The hypothalamus helps to maintain homeostasis and one's response to stress, and the cerebral cortex enables one to process information and engage in higher-level thinking. The limbic system plays a key role in making a connection between memory and emotion. The medial forebrain bundle (MFB) is the center for pleasure and pain, and the basal ganglia help govern involuntary muscle control. The brain stem is involved in vital functions, including breathing, heartbeat, dilation of the pupils, and blood pressure.

Many factors besides pharmacology account for the way drugs affect people. Age is a factor; the very young and elderly have more difficulty metabolizing and excreting drugs. Because drugs collect in adipose tissue and women tend to have more adipose tissue than men, drugs have a greater effect on women.

The dosage has a bearing on the effects of drugs. The amount necessary to produce a desired effect is called effective dose, or ED, and the amount required to be fatal is the lethal dose, or LD. The difference between ED and LD is called the drug's margin of safety. The dose-response curve refers to specific behavioral effects at various levels.

The effects of drugs also depend on their purity and potency. Purity refers to quality and potency refers to strength, both of which vary greatly with illegal drugs. During the last 20 years the purity of illegal drugs has increased while their costs have decreased.

How drugs interact with other drugs and food may alter their effect. Some drugs cancel out the effects of other drugs, and other drugs act more powerfully when they are combined. Synergism refers to the added strength of drugs in combination.

Another concept relating to the effects of drugs is tolerance. The four types of tolerance are the following:

- Pharmacological tolerance: A drug has less effect because the body adjusts to the drug based on previous experiences with it.
- Behavioral tolerance: The person has learned to adapt to the effects of a drug.
- Cross-tolerance: A person adjusts to drugs that are chemically similar.
- Reverse tolerance: The person achieves the desired effects of a drug at decreasing levels.

Set and setting also affect how drugs affect people. Set is one's psychological state of mind when taking a drug. Setting is the environment in which one takes drugs.

Drugs can enter the body through various means. One of the most common and simplest ways is ingestion.

Because ingested drugs mix with the contents in the stomach, their rate of absorption is difficult to control. Drugs injected intravenously are distributed quickly and at high concentrations. Drugs injected intramuscularly are absorbed less quickly, and drugs injected subcutaneously are the least efficiently absorbed. In the last several years the number of people becoming HIV-infected as a result of injecting drugs has decreased. Inhaled drugs take effect quickly but are effective for a shorter time.

transdermal method Administration of drugs by applying them on the surface of the skin

Thinking Critically

1. An argument for legalizing drugs relates to purity and potency. If drugs were legal, proponents say, there would be more assurance regarding the quality and strength of drugs. What are the arguments against this line of reasoning?
2. Think back to the first time you consumed alcohol. Try to recall whom you were with, where you were, the effects of the alcohol, and how you felt while drinking the alcohol. Were you euphoric or dysphoric?

Web Resources

Drug Policy Alliance
http://drugpolicy.org
This site is a good source for information dealing with legal issues as they relate to drug laws.

University of Utah
http://learn.genetics.utah.edu/content/addiction/drugs/mouse.html
This Web site depicts the effects of drugs on the brain through the use of animated mice.

CASA–The National Center on Addiction and Substance Abuse at Columbia University
http://www.casacolumbia.org
This organization's Web site contains highlights of various studies it conducts and drug-related topics.

Notes

1. D. M. Grilly, *Drugs and Human Behavior,* 5th ed. (Boston: Allyn & Bacon, 2005).
2. Substance Abuse Mental Health Services Administration, Office of Applied Studies, *The Dasis Report: Cocaine Route of Administration Trends: 1995–2005* (Rockville, MD: September 13, 2007).
3. "From Genes to Geography: The Cutting Edge of Alcohol Research," *Alcohol Alert* (Rockville, MD: U. S. Department of Health and Human Services, 2000).
4. M. D. Lemonick and A. Park, "The Science of Addiction," *Time,* 170 (July 16, 2007): 42–48.
5. M. Wehrenberg and S. Prinz, *The Anxious Brain: The Neurological Basis of Anxiety Disorders and How to Effectively Treat Them* (New York: W.W. Norton and Company, 2007).
6. A. K. Ashton, D. A. D'Mello, B. D. Hefner, F. G. Leon, G. A. Matson, C. B. Montano, J. F. Pradko, N. Sussman, and B. Winsberg, "Applying Neuropharmacology When Treating Patients with Depression," *Journal of Family Practice,* 52 (December 2003): 34–42.
7. Blakeslee, "Scientists Test Hallucinogens for Mental Ills," *New York Times,* March 13, 2001.
8. J. E. Brody, "A Mix of Medicines That Can Be Lethal," *The New York Times,* February 27, 2007.
9. T. Blake, "Tracking the Ups and Downs of Antidepressants," *Nursing,* 37 (April 2007): 49–51.
10. *How Communities Can Strengthen Their Strategies to Fight Drug Abuse Using Research from the National Institute on Drug Abuse (NIDA)* (Boston: Join Together, 2000).
11. N. Boyce, "Storm in a Cup," *New Scientist* (January 29, 2000): 28–31.
12. B. Liebman, "Caffeine and Parkinson's Disease," *Nutrition Action Newsletter,* 27 (September 2000): 11.
13. P. E. M. Phillips, G. D. Stuber, M. L. Heien, R. M. Wrightman, and R. M. Carelli, "Subsecond Dopamine Release Promotes Cocaine Seeking," *Nature,* 422 (2003):614–618.
14. M. Oscar-Berman and K. Marinkovic, "Alcoholism and the Brain: An Overview," *Alcohol Research and Health,* 27 (2003): 125–133.
15. S. Peele, A. Brodsky, and M. Arnold, *The Truth About Addiction and Recovery* (New York: Simon and Schuster, 1991).
16. A. R. Childress, P. D. Mozley, W. McElgin, J. Fitzgerald, M. Reivich, and C. P. O'Brien, "Limbic Activation During Cue-Induced Cocaine Craving," *American Journal of Psychiatry,* 156 (1999): 11–18.
17. P. Zickler, "Marijuana Smoking Is Associated with a Spectrum of Respiratory Disorders," *NIDA Notes,* 21 (October 2006): 12–14.
18. Substance Abuse Mental Health Services Administration, *Drug Abuse Warning Network, 2006: National Estimates of Drug-Related Emergency Department Visits* (Rockville, MD: U.S. Department of Health and Human Services, 2008).
19. S. M. Willcox, D. U. Himmelstein, and S. Woolhandler, "Inappropriate Drug Prescribing for the Community-Dwelling Elderly," *Journal of the American Medical Association,* 272 (1994): 292–296.
20. G. Isaacson, "A Bone to Pick with Prozac," *Psychology Today,* 40 (October 2007): 23.
21. "Older Adults: Prescription Drugs and Alcohol Don't Mix," *SAMHSA News,* 12 (July/August 2004): 5.
22. "A Hidden Epidemic: Substance Abuse Among Older Americans Is Often Overlooked," *Prevention Pipeline,* 13 (March/April 2000): 3–6.
23. J. Kluger and J. Ressner, "Balding, Wrinkled and Stoned," *Time* (January 23, 2006): 54–56.
24. "Alcohol and Aging," *Alcohol Alert* (Rockville, MD: U.S. Department of Health and Human Services, April 1998).

25. K. J. Brower and J. M. Hall, "Effects of Age and Alcoholism on Sleep: A Controlled Study," *Journal of Studies of Alcohol,* 62 (2001): 3–6.
26. R. H. Moos, K. Schutte, P. Brennan, and B. S. Moos, "Ten-Year Patterns of Alcohol Consumption and Drinking Problems Among Older Women and Men," *Addiction,* 99 (2004): 829–838.
27. C. S. Carter, "Perinatal Care for Women Who Are Addicted: Implications for Empowerment," *Health and Social Work,* 27 (2002): 161–174.
28. "Study Highlights Need to Study Drug Effects Specifically on Children," *Medical Letter on the CDC & FDA* (June 10, 2001).
29. *Illegal Drug Price and Purity Report* (Washington, DC: U.S. Drug Enforcement Administration, 2002).
30. "Alcohol-Medication Interactions," *Alcohol Alert* (Rockville, MD: U.S. Department of Health and Human Services, 1994).
31. "Alcohol—An Important Women's Health Issue," *Alcohol Alert,* 62 (July 2004): 4.
32. R. M. Julien, *A Primer of Drug Action,* 11th ed. (New York, Worth Publishers, 2008).
33. "Developing Effective Addiction Treatments," *NIDA Notes,* 19 (April 2004): S8–S10.
34. W. A. Brown, "The Placebo Effect," *Scientific American,* 278 (1998): 90–95.
35. J. Haun, T. Glassman, V.J. Dodd, and G. Young, "Game-Day Survey Results: Looking at Football Fan Alcohol-Related Behaviors," *American Journal of Health Education,* 18 (March/April 2007): 91–98.
36. Grilly, supra note 1.
37. National Institute on Drug Abuse Research Report, *Heroin: Abuse and Addiction* (Rockville, MD: National Institute on Drug Abuse, 2000).
38. "Patterns and Trends in Inhalant Use by Adolescent Males and Females: 2002–2005," *The NSDUH Report.* (Rockville, MD: U.S. Department of Health and Human Services, March 15, 2007).

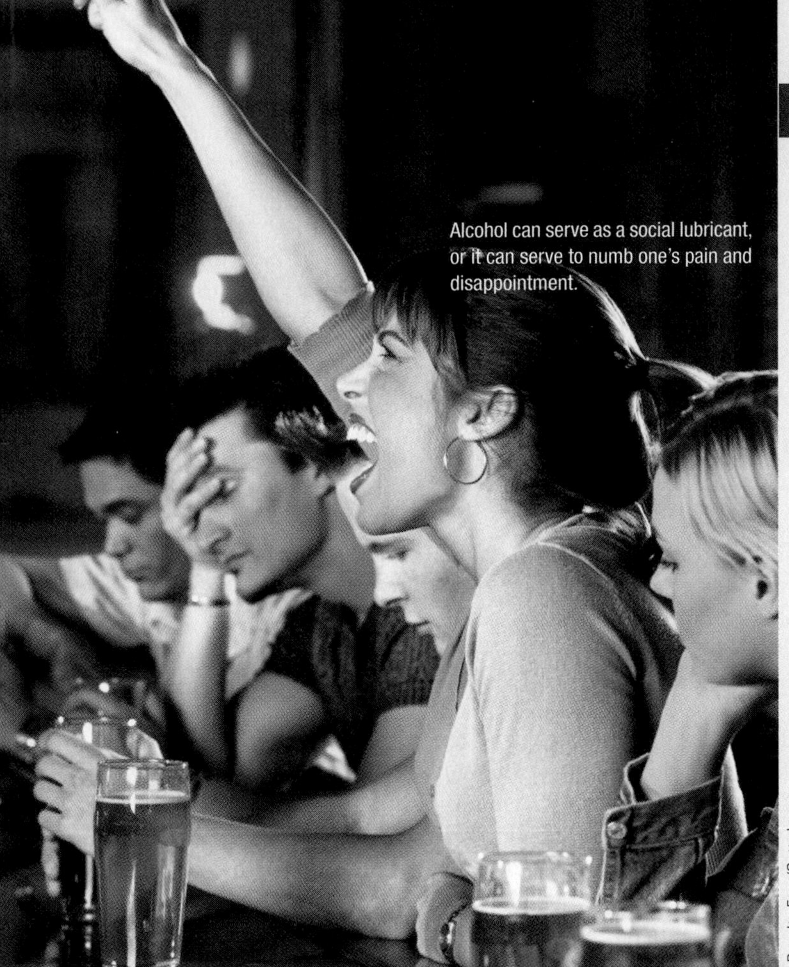

Alcohol can serve as a social lubricant, or it can serve to numb one's pain and disappointment.

FACT OR FICTION?

1. Nearly 10% of Americans indicated that they have been under the influence of alcohol while at work at least one time during the past year.
2. During Prohibition, alcohol-related deaths increased.
3. Some over-the-counter medicines, such as cough syrups, can contain as much as 10% alcohol.
4. Most college students reduce their binge drinking after graduating from college.
5. Overall, more Blacks drink alcohol than Whites, but Whites are more likely to drink heavily.
6. The younger one is when drinking alcohol for the first time, the more likely one will become a problem drinker.
7. Moderate alcohol drinkers have lower rates of cardiovascular disease than abstainers.
8. The only medical condition that is more prevalent in newborns than fetal alcohol syndrome is cerebral palsy.
9. At least one-fourth of people who drive under the influence of alcohol will be arrested.
10. Only two states have a drinking age below age 21 years.

Turn the page to check your answers

6 Alcohol

Chapter Objectives

After completing this chapter, the reader should be able to describe:

- Factors accounting for society minimizing its view of alcohol as a serious drug
- Roles of the Women's Christian Temperance Union, Anti-Saloon League, and National Prohibition Party in alcohol reform
- Events leading up to Prohibition as well as its repeal
- Differences among ethnic groups regarding patterns of alcohol consumption
- Factors affecting the rate of alcohol absorption
- The effects of alcohol on different systems in the body
- The effects of alcohol on the fetus
- Environmental and genetic factors that may be related to alcoholism
- The influence of culture on drinking patterns
- The effects of alcoholism on adult children of alcoholics

FACT OR FICTION?

1. **Fiction:** The fact is—fewer than 2% of Americans indicated that they were under the influence of alcohol while at work at least one time during the past 12 months.
2. **Fiction:** The fact is—when Prohibition first went into effect, alcohol-related deaths and illness related to alcohol use declined.
3. **Fact:** Some medications include as much as 10% alcohol.
4. **Fact:** Binge drinking peaks at age 21 and declines after that age.
5. **Fiction:** The fact is—more Whites drink alcohol than Blacks, but more Blacks will drink heavily.
6. **Fact:** Several studies link alcohol-related problems with the early onset of drinking.
7. **Fact:** People who drink no more than one to three drinks per day have less risk of cardiovascular disease than nondrinkers. People who drink more than three drinks per day have a higher risk of cardiovascular disease.
8. **Fiction:** The fact is—fetal alcohol spectrum syndrome affects more newborns than cerebral palsy, Down's syndrome, and spina bifida combined.
9. **Fiction:** The fact is—of the estimated 82 million drinking and driving trips in a given year when the driver has a blood alcohol concentration of .08 or higher, about 1.5 million drivers are arrested—less than 2%.
10. **Fiction:** The fact is—no state allows alcohol consumption before age 21.

No drug in history has had as much impact on the United States or the world as alcohol. Alcohol affects everyone, either by their own or someone else's use. Attitudes toward alcohol have run the gamut from reverence to dismay. It is believed to be the oldest drug known to humans. Primitive societies used alcohol ritually or socially to deal with anxiety created by an unstable environment.[1] Yet, alcohol is not always acknowledged as a drug, because of the following:

1. Alcohol is legal. This could lead one to believe that its effects are not negative or severe. If alcohol were bad for a person, the government would do more to limit its availability.
2. Parents and other role models consume alcohol as part of their lifestyle.

People drink alcohol for many reasons. They consume it to relax, to reduce their inhibitions, and for pleasure. They use it at family dinners, on festive occasions, at weddings, and to celebrate national holidays. Alcohol is part of the social fabric. It is difficult to think of a drug that serves as many cultural purposes as alcohol—or has caused as much havoc.

In this chapter we will explore the history of alcohol use in the United States, the role of alcohol in society, the extent of its usage, its effects on the individual, and its impact on the family. Treatment for alcoholism is discussed in Chapter 15.

History of Alcohol Use in the United States

We can trace the history of alcohol beginning with Colonial times, to the temperance movement, to Prohibition, to contemporary use.

Colonial Times

Alcohol use in the United States began when the Puritans disembarked from the Mayflower at Plymouth, Massachusetts. In one speculation, they anchored at Plymouth because their supply of beer and spirits was becoming depleted.[2] Alcohol was an integral component of Colonial life, and attitudes of early settlers toward alcohol were positive. Not only were beers and wines a part of daily living and used during festive situations, but alcohol was also considered a "good creature from God." Although drinking in moderation was acceptable, a person could be whipped, fined, and confined to the stocks for drunkenness in Massachusetts and Virginia.[3]

Two factors contributed to the importance of alcohol during Colonial times: sanitation and nutrition. Sanitary practices were lacking. Human and animal waste contaminated drinking wells, and tuberculosis probably was transmitted through cow's milk. Alcohol is a preservative.

Moreover, alcoholic beverages at that time contained important nutrients including vitamins, minerals, and yeast. Early settlers made wine from potatoes, apples, carrots, lettuce, wheat, cranberries, dandelions, squash, and so forth. Beer and wine were necessary drinks instead of recreational beverages. It was not uncommon for children as well as adults to drink alcohol on a daily basis.[4]

In 1640, the Dutch opened the first distillery on Staten Island.[5] One popular form of alcohol in the New World was rum. The rum trade became New England's largest and most profitable business. Yankee traders would ship "demon rum" to Africa's west coast to be traded for slaves. The slaves were transported to the West Indies, where they were used as barter for molasses, which then was taken back to New England and converted into rum. This practice finally ended

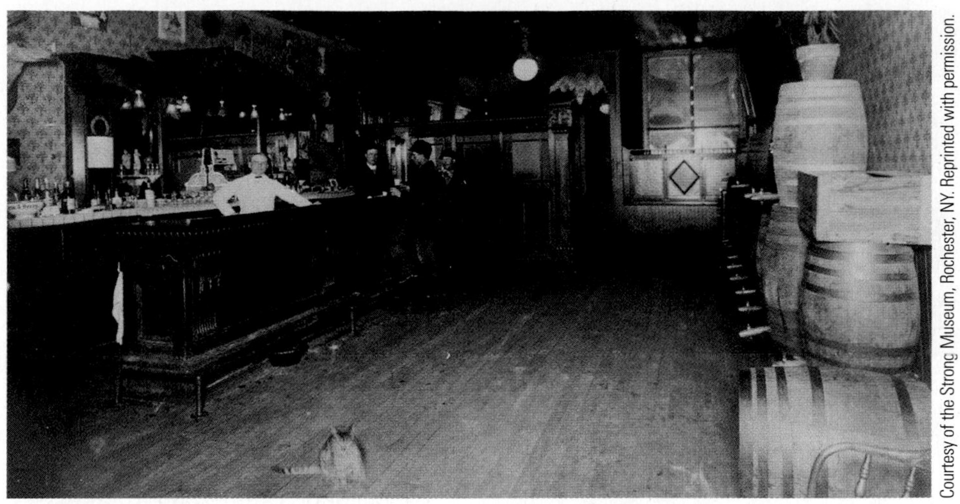
Courtesy of the Strong Museum, Rochester, NY. Reprinted with permission.

This photograph, circa 1905, depicts a typical saloon interior. The absence of tables allowed more floor space to accommodate customers.

when Congress passed legislation prohibiting slaves from being imported and when domestic whiskey became cheaper to produce.

Alcohol consumption peaked in the United States during Thomas Jefferson's presidency. Farmers took alcohol into the fields, employers gave it to employees on the job, and aspiring politicians gave alcohol to voters at polling places. Troops of the Continental Army received daily rations of rum or whiskey. Consumption of whiskey was extremely high by the end of the Civil War.[6] Figure 6.1 shows the rate of alcohol consumption from 1935 to 2004.

Dr. Benjamin Rush, a signer of the Declaration of Independence, was one of the first people to identify alcoholism as a disease.[7] In his 1784 publication, *An Inquiry into the Effects of Ardent Spirits upon the Human Body and Mind*, Rush described the harmful effects of alcohol.[8] The temperance movement followed shortly thereafter.

Temperance Movement

In the early 1800s, a movement to curb the escalating rate of alcohol use and abuse swept through the United States, though few people made the connection between excessive alcohol consumption and social problems. An alcohol-related problem was believed to be the individual's problem alone.[9] Increasingly, though, people recognized the larger problems emanating from uncontrolled alcohol use. Alcohol was seen as a major cause of crime and violence; for example, men who drank too much would steal and beat their wives. These observations led to the temperance movement, the initial purpose of which was to modify alcohol use, not to eliminate it. In essence, alcohol consumption in moderation was acceptable but habitual drunkenness was viewed as sinful.[10]

Rush did not condemn alcohol, but he was critical of uncontrolled drinking. He argued that alcohol,

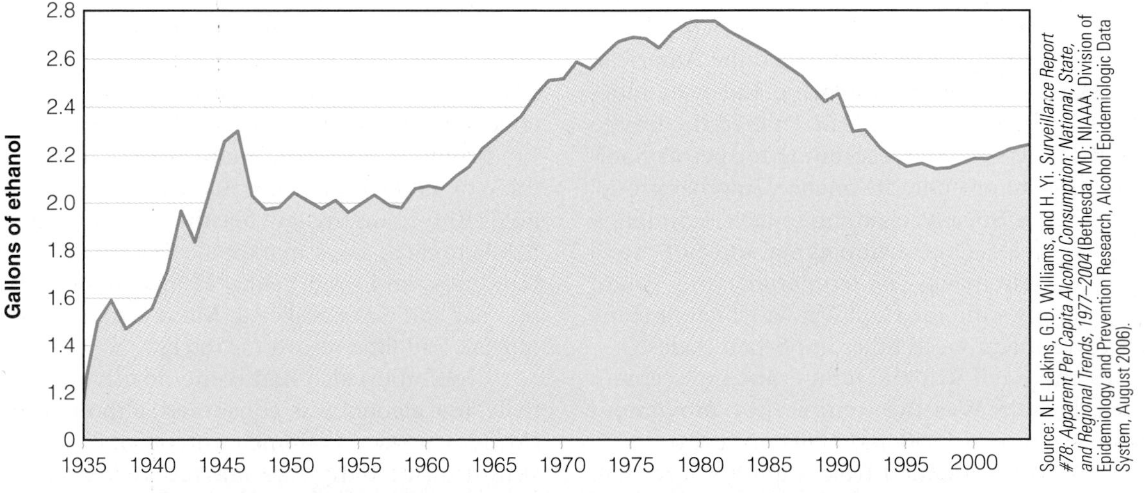

Source: N.E. Lakins, G.D. Williams, and H. Yi. *Surveillance Report #78: Apparent Per Capita Alcohol Consumption: National, State, and Regional Trends, 1977–2004* (Bethesda, MD: NIAAA, Division of Epidemiology and Prevention Research, Alcohol Epidemiologic Data System, August 2006).

Figure 6.1 Total Per Capita Ethanol Consumption, United States, 1935–2004

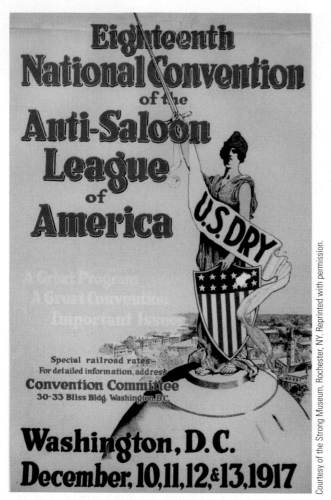

A poster printed for the Ohio Dry Convention in 1917 announced the Anti-Saloon League.

especially hard alcohol, interfered with the ability to earn a living and with family life. He believed that alcoholism was both a progressive disease culminating in addiction and a gradual form of suicide.[11]

Beginning in 1808, many independent organizations formed their own temperance groups. Not until 1826, however, did the American Society for the Promotion of Temperance, later called the American Temperance Society, come into being. Later the Independent Order of Good Templars entered the fray to combat the evils of liquor, recruiting former alcoholics in an effort to promote abstinence. Another group, the Temperance Society, claiming to have 1.5 million members, was a zealous campaigner and put much pressure on politicians. The temperance movement remained strong until the Civil War, at which time the federal government faced other important issues.

After the Civil War the temperance movement reasserted itself. Was the temperance movement successful? Between 1830 and 1840, annual per capita use of alcohol declined from slightly more than 7 gallons per adult to slightly more than 3 gallons.[12] Today, the average American adult drinks about 2 gallons of alcohol annually.

Three influential groups in alcohol reform were the Women's Christian Temperance Union (WCTU), the Anti-Saloon League, and the National Prohibition Party. The WCTU favored social reform, prayer, education, prevention, and legislation forbidding alcohol.[13] The WCTU published journals critical of alcohol, held programs for children, depicting alcohol as a substance to fear and loathe, and was responsible for laws mandating alcohol education.

The Anti-Saloon League grew into a powerful political force, campaigning for candidates who supported controls on alcohol. The National Prohibition Party was a major impetus in getting many states to ban alcohol. From 1880 to 1889, seven states passed prohibition laws, and 34 states passed similar legislation between 1907 and 1919, the year national prohibition was signed into law. In the meantime, two states repealed their laws banning alcohol.

Prohibition

Efforts to impose a national ban gathered strength in the early 1900s. Not only did states enact their own legislation, but it was illegal to ship alcoholic beverages to places where the sale and manufacture of liquor was forbidden and to use the postal service to advertise liquor. Sentiment for the federal government to exert control over alcohol was strong.

The United States had been at war since April 1917, and the hysteria that gripped the nation in its crusade against the Kaiser extended the firm belief that liquor sapped the nation's strength and willpower, and even depleted the cereal grains that could be used in bread for the troops and starving Europeans.[14]

The amendment to forbid alcohol, authored by Andrew Volstead, was adopted by the U.S. Senate in 1917 and the House of Representatives the next year. To become law, 36 states had to ratify the amendment. The only two states not ratifying the amendment were Rhode Island and Connecticut.[15] The Eighteenth Amendment, the Volstead Act, went into effect on January 16, 1920.

Prohibition spurred many problems. The illegal trade of alcohol was vigorous. Organized crime took hold. Enforcing the law became a serious dilemma. Adulterants in black market alcohol caused paralysis, blindness, and even death. Home brewing became popular and was not illegal. Many citizens and police officials had little regard for the law.[16]

Prohibition also had some positive effects. Initially, less alcohol was consumed, although the rates slowly increased.[17] Some contend that alcohol consumption actually had started to decline before 1920. In the early years of Prohibition, deaths from

distilled spirits Beverages such as whiskey, rum, gin, and vodka that are produced by boiling various solutions

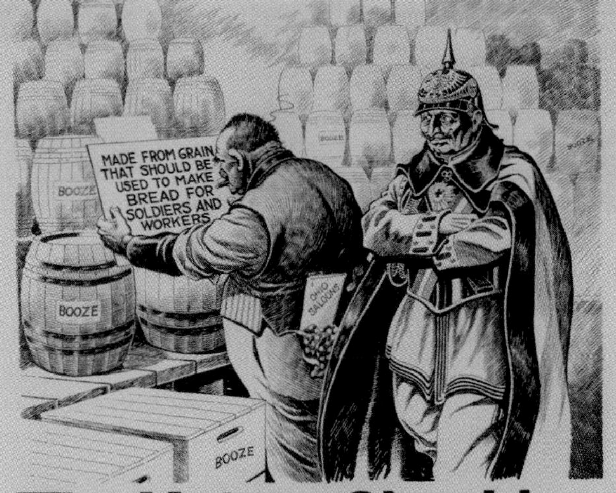

MADE FROM GRAIN THAT SHOULD BE USED TO MAKE BREAD FOR SOLDIERS AND WORKERS
BOOZE
BOOZE
BOOZE
OHIO SALOONS
The Kaiser Chuckles
Every Bushel of Grain that is diverted from supplying American Soldiers with Bread; from supplying American Workmen with Bread, is helping the Kaiser's game.
If the Kaiser could he would reach out his bloody hand and pat the man on the back who is boosting his game here in Ohio by voting wet.
Ohio has no grain to waste on beer or booze—now or ever—Ohio needs every ounce of grain for her soldiers and workers and for a hungry and starving world.
Vote Yes on Prohibition Nov. 5th.

A poster printed for the Ohio Dry Convention in 1917.

cirrhosis of the liver, alcohol-related deaths, automobile accidents, and hospital admissions for alcoholism declined.[18] Deaths from alcohol increased by the mid-1920s, but not at the same rate as before Prohibition.

Because of disregard for Prohibition and the need for jobs and tax revenue, the law was repealed in 1933[19] when Congress and the states approved the Twenty-first Amendment, repealing the Eighteenth Amendment. In terms of health, Prohibition seemed to be effective. In view of how it helped spur organized crime and social disruption, however, it was a failure. By the end of Prohibition, many rituals and social sanctions regulating drinking were no longer in place.

It should also be noted that several women's groups opposed Prohibition. One group, the Molly Pitcher Club, named after the Revolutionary War heroine, sought to have Prohibition overturned because the group found that Prohibition led to an increase in violence and lawlessness.[20] In 1929, Pauline Sabin, the first woman to serve on the Republican National Committee, and other influential women formed the Women's Organization for National Prohibition Reform (WONPR). Sabin and WONPR realized that Prohibition caused more problems than it cured. Through its political savvy and the argument that repealing Prohibition would serve to protect the home rather than destroy it, WONPR was instrumental in getting the Eighteenth Amendment overturned.

Current Alcohol Use

Most people who drink today are *social drinkers*. Their drinking patterns do not lead to long-term health or social problems, although they may experience immediate risks such as accidents. Social drinkers are able to abstain from alcohol at will.

By contrast, people who cannot abstain and develop medical and social difficulties are called *problem drinkers* or *alcoholics*. Whether one is labeled a problem drinker or an alcoholic depends on the criteria used. A person can abuse alcohol and not be an alcoholic. Problem drinkers do not necessarily drink daily or even frequently. Thus, drinkers are not easily categorized. Factors such as whether a person drinks at home alone or with friends or whether a person drives a car or takes a taxi after drinking have to be taken into account.

One factor affecting the extent of alcohol consumption is cost. As costs increase, consumption levels decrease. The alcohol use, however, declines among social drinkers, not heavy drinkers.[21] Although there are some concerns with the research, an increase in taxes on alcohol appears to reduce consumption.[22] U.S. politicians are cracking down on acceptable levels of alcohol in the blood to be classified as driving while intoxicated. At the same time, many states allow drive-through alcohol sales. The decline in alcohol drinking since the early 1980s has been reflected largely in less use of **distilled spirits** such as whiskey, vodka, gin, and rum.

Alcohol consumption rates vary greatly by state, from 1.28 gallons per capita in Utah to 4.07 gallons per capita in New Hampshire.[23] Abstinence, overall, is increasing for men and women. Rates of abstention for both sexes increase as people age; but as education and family income go up, abstinence rates go down.[24] Rates of abstinence *and* heavy drinking are greater in rural areas.[25] In essence, there are lower rates of moderate alcohol use in rural areas.

Other factors that might have played a role in increased abstinence over the past 25 years are the more politically conservative climate of the 1980s, the trend toward healthier lifestyles, and public awareness of alcohol-related risks. At the same time, however, the proportion of heavy drinkers in their 20s has increased slightly, along with problems related to alcohol dependency. Heavy drinking is more likely to occur if one drinks at an early age, has less education, and is friendly with others who also drink heavily. An encouraging point is that heavy drinking tends to decline over time.[26]

A number of variables correlate with drinking patterns:

- College students who are fraternity and sorority members have significantly higher alcohol consumption rates than students who are not affiliated with fraternities and sororities.[27] One study found that 86% of fraternity members are binge drinkers and 64% are frequent binge drinkers.[28]
- Gay, lesbian, and bisexual college students drink more alcohol than heterosexual students.[29]
- Full-time college students ages 18 to 21 have higher rates of binge drinking than nonstudents.[30]
- Alcohol-related problems are greater where there is more access to places to drink or buy alcohol.[31]
- Per capita alcohol consumption is highest in the Northeast and lowest in the West.[32]
- The rate of binge drinking increases steadily from ages 12 to 21 and then steadily decreases.[33]

Because more women are seeking treatment, one could surmise that drinking problems among women are increasing. This may be misleading because the stigma of women having drinking problems is diminishing and, therefore, many women who previously shunned treatment out of fear of being stigmatized are now getting help.

In regard to women's drinking patterns, the demographic subgroups that stand out include women who are unemployed, looking for work, or employed part-time outside the home. Drinking problems are more prevalent among women who are divorced, separated, or not married but living with a partner. Women in their 20s to early 30s, as well as women with husbands or partners who drink heavily, are at greater risk for becoming problem drinkers. For many women heavy drinking started after a health problem such as depression or reproductive difficulties.[34] Although females do not drink as often or as heavily as males, the gap is decreasing. Fifty-seven percent of males ages 12 or older have consumed alcohol within the past 30 days. Forty-five percent of females ages 12 or older drank alcohol within the past 30 days.[35]

The number of arrests on college campuses for alcohol and other drugs has increased dramatically in the last few years. This increase may reflect stricter enforcement policies by college administrators.[36] Table 6.1 shows the arrest and referral rates for alcohol and other drugs at colleges with the highest rates.

Drinking patterns vary with age. In one study, more than 43% of high school seniors had tried

TABLE 6.1 Four-Year Campuses with the Most Arrests in 2002

Campus	Arrests
Liquor arrests	
University of Wisconsin at Madison	837
Indiana University at Bloomington	804
Western Michigan University	732
Pennsylvania State University at University Park	707
Michigan State University	686
University of Maryland at College Park	610
University of Michigan at Ann Arbor	485
Colorado State University	455
Louisiana State University at Baton Rouge	443
University of Wisconsin at Oshkosh	395
Drug arrests	
Indiana University at Bloomington	313
University of Wisconsin at Oshkosh	170
Arizona State University main campus	168
Western Michigan University	146
University of Connecticut	139
Michigan State University	138
Pennsylvania State University at University Park	135
University of Maryland at College Park	123
University of Iowa	109
George Mason University	108
Weapons arrests	
University of Colorado Health Sciences Center	29
Michigan State University	25
University of Kansas Medical Center	17
University of California at Berkeley	16
State University of New York Upstate Medical University	15
University of Connecticut	13
University of North Carolina at Charlotte	13
Virginia Commonwealth University	12
Grambling State University	11
University of California at Irvine	10
Southwest Texas State University	10

Source: *Chronicle of Higher Education,* May 28, 2004.

alcohol within the previous 30 days, 25% consumed five or more drinks at one sitting, and 28% indicated that they had been drunk within the past month.[37] Another study revealed that two in five college students binge drink and 47% reported being drunk within the past 30 days.[38] Also, college students have been found to consume more alcohol on days of football games.[39]

Despite the reputation among young people for heavy drinking, 46% of individuals ages 18 to 24 abstain from alcohol. This percentage is greater than for people ages 25 to 34 (36%) and 35 to 44 (37%).[40] Heavy drinking among men and women was most prevalent in the 18 to 24 age group and declined in successive age groups. Married individuals have lower rates of heavy drinking than those who have never married or who are divorced.[41]

Even though Americans ages 60 and older have lower levels of alcohol use and abuse, alcoholism is increasing among the elderly.[42] Alcohol abuse among the elderly is not limited to the United States: one report cites alcohol abuse in Britain as becoming epidemic among the elderly.[43] Loneliness and isolation make the elderly more vulnerable to alcoholism. While some older people reduce alcohol use because of different stressors in their lives, for others, those same stressors may result in an increase in alcohol abuse.[44] Also, over one-third of male and female problem drinkers use alcohol to manage pain. Fifteen percent of male nonproblem drinkers and 13% of female nonproblem drinkers use alcohol to manage pain.[45]

Among those ages 60 and older, the prevalence of alcoholism, alcohol abuse, and problem drinking is estimated to be between 2% and 10%.[46] Older men are twice as likely as older women to have alcohol-related problems or late-life onset of alcoholism.[47] Older drinkers are more likely to experience hangovers from alcohol use.[48] Despite the increase in alcoholism among the elderly, the percentage of abstainers also increases in older age groups.[49] The greater proportion of abstainers among older age groups might be attributed to heavy drinkers' dying before they reach old age. More people ages 55 or older seek treatment for alcohol abuse than do people who are younger than age 55.[50]

Binge Drinking

Binge drinking typically starts at an early age and increases during adolescence. About eight percent of eighth-grade students report that they have had 5 or more drinks at one time.[51] Adolescents who binge drink are more likely to perform poorly in school as well as engage in other health risk behaviors such as having unprotected sex, smoking cigarettes, and committing suicide.[52] In a study of adolescents, nearly 14% met the criteria for heavy drinking but only 16% of that group acknowledged having a substance-abuse problem.[53] Students who stated that parties were "very" or "somewhat" important were far more likely to binge drink. Also, college athletes were more likely than nonathletes to engage in binge drinking.[54]

binge drinking Consuming five or more drinks (men) or four (women) in a short period of time

In a study of Canadian adolescents, 24% of students abstained from alcohol and another 22% had tasted alcohol but were not current drinkers.[55] The two reasons most commonly cited for not drinking were "bad for health" and "upbringing." Another Canadian study of college students found that drinking behavior was influenced by the perception of others' use of alcohol. Students who thought that other students drank heavily also engaged in heavy drinking.[56] Among persons ages 12 to 20, the ethnic group with the highest rate of binge drinking is American Indian/Alaska Native, followed by Whites, Hispanics, Blacks, and Asians.[57]

Drinking and Ethnicity

In regard to abstaining from alcohol use, 61% of Blacks abstained whereas 38% of Whites and 59% of Hispanics abstained. In contrast to White adolescents, Black adolescents drink less often, are older when they start, and are less likely to engage in heavy drinking.[58] Alcohol-related mortality is greater for Black and Hispanic men than for White and Asian American men.[59] Black men possibly have more alcohol-related problems than White men because of their higher unemployment rate, discrimination, poor living conditions, and inadequate health care, rather than alcohol use

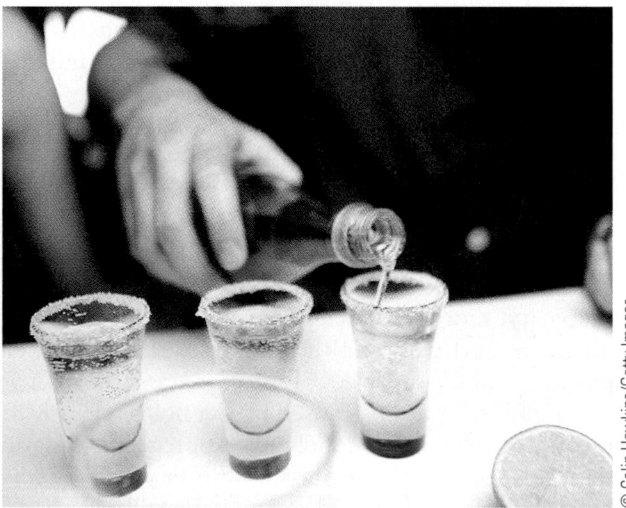

Binge drinking is prevalent on college campuses.

per se. Among individuals seeking alcohol treatment, the group most likely to seek help is American Indian or Native Alaskan.[60]

Any discussion of drinking patterns among Hispanics is complicated by their cultural diversity. Among the numerous Hispanic groups are Mexicans, Puerto Ricans, and Cubans. In contrast to men and women of Puerto Rican or Cuban origin, Mexican American men and women were more likely to either abstain from alcohol or to drink heavily. Also, Mexican American men and women had more alcohol-related problems than the other two groups. Drinking patterns seem to be affected by **acculturation**. The more acculturated a person becomes, the more he or she follows the drinking patterns of the adopted population.[61]

One study of Caucasian and Asian students found that Asian students were better able to resist social pressure to drink alcohol than Caucasian students.[62] Many Asians have a mutant gene that causes the alcohol-flush reaction when they drink alcohol. Because of this genetic mutation, the liver is less able to metabolize alcohol. Symptoms of the alcohol-flush reaction include facial flushing, heart palpitations, dizziness, and nausea.[63] Consequently, alcohol use and problems are less prevalent among Asian Americans than among all other major racial and ethnic groups in the United States. Significant differences are found, however, among Asian American subgroups.[64] Also, Asian Americans born in the United States have significantly higher alcohol usage than Asians who immigrated to the United States.[65]

In one California study, nearly half of Korean men abstained from alcohol, whereas one-third of Japanese, Chinese, and Filipino men did not use alcohol at all.[66] Korean and Filipino women had higher rates of abstinence than Chinese women, who in turn had higher rates than Japanese women. Chinese and Korean women showed no evidence of heavy drinking. Because heavy drinking is done with friends and on special occasions, drinking behavior has social controls. Problems related to alcohol are more likely when a person drinks for personal reasons, not social reasons.

Similarly, generalizing about drinking patterns of American Indians is unwise because of tribal diversity. Some tribes have a high incidence of alcohol abuse, and others are primarily abstinent. Despite the disparity, more American Indian adolescents overall drink and get drunk than adolescents of other ethnic groups.[67]

Examining deaths caused by alcohol is one way to assess the extent of alcohol-related problems among American Indians and Alaska Natives. Rates of suicides, accidents, homicides, and especially cirrhosis of the liver—conditions influenced by alcohol—are higher among American Indians and Alaska Natives than the general population.[68] Native Americans have the highest rates of alcohol-related deaths of all ethnicities in the United States.[69] The high incidence of accidents and homicides is attributed to binge drinking, which is characteristic of some tribes.

It is speculated that American Indians experience a flushing response similar to the flushing reaction in Asians but that it is milder and less unpleasant than the Asian flushing response.[70] This flushing reaction has little effect on drinking frequency or amount.

Alcoholic Beverages

Alcohol is a central nervous system depressant. Beverage alcohol, or **ethyl alcohol**, should not be confused with **methyl alcohol**, or wood alcohol. Methyl alcohol is extremely toxic and may lead to blindness and death. By using certain yeasts, the carbon, hydrogen, and oxygen of sugar and water are transformed into ethyl alcohol and carbon dioxide. This process, called **fermentation**, yields beverages that are about 14% alcohol.

The percentage of alcohol in a beverage can be increased by **distillation**, a procedure in which a solution containing alcohol is boiled.[71] Alcohol has a lower boiling temperature than other liquids. Therefore, during the heating process alcohol separates from the solution in the form of steam. The steam is captured in a cooling tube and turns back into a liquid. This distilled liquid contains a higher alcohol content.

To brew beer, sprouted barley is added to cereal grains such as corn, wheat, or rye to change the carbohydrates in the grains into sugar, while yeast changes the sugar into alcohol. The alcohol content of beer is about 5%, and beer advertised as having fewer calories also has less alcohol.

Fruit juices, particularly those with high sugar content, are used to make wine. The alcohol content of wine ranges from 8% to 14% generally. Wine coolers, a mixture of wine with various carbonated beverages, first introduced in the early 1980s, are about 4% alcohol by volume. Adding alcohol to slightly sweetened wines produces **fortified wines** such as sherry and port. These have a higher alcohol content. In the United States, labels on bottles of distilled alcohol, such as rum, gin, and whiskey, indicate the **proof** of the contents. The amount of alcohol is determined by dividing the proof in half. Thus, a bottle that is 80 proof is 40% alcohol. Figure 6.2 shows the equivalent content of alcohol for beer, wine, and hard liquor.

In a 2006 survey of high school students, it was found that 70% of 12th graders and 35% of eighth graders drank flavored alcoholic beverages called

STANDARD DRINK CONVERSION

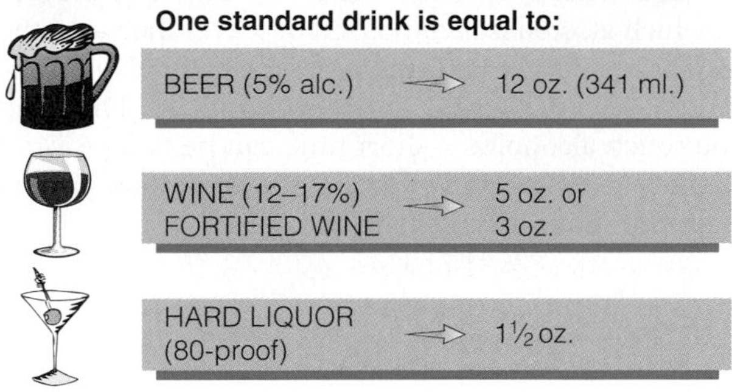

One standard drink is equal to:
BEER (5% alc.) 12 oz. (341 ml.)
WINE (12–17%) FORTIFIED WINE 5 oz. or 3 oz.
HARD LIQUOR (80-proof) 1½ oz.

One standard drink represents 13.6 grams of absolute alcohol

WINE: 1 bottle		
25 oz./750 ml.	5	5 standard drinks
40 oz./1.14 L.	5	8 standard drinks
25 oz. fortified	5	8 standard drinks

HARD LIQUOR: 1 bottle		
12 oz. (mickey)	5	8 standard drinks
25 oz./750 ml.	5	17 standard drinks
40 oz./1.14 L.	5	27 standard drinks

For light beer or light wine, standard drinks are calculated in terms of a ratio. For example, 12 oz. of a 2.5% light beer =0.5 SDs, while 12 oz. of a 4% light beer =0.8.

Figure 6.2 Standard Drink Conversion

alcopops.[72] These beverages, which were first marketed around 1995, are frequently shown in music videos. The appearance of alcopops in music videos is linked to their increased use.[73] The majority of American youths perceive alcopops to be less harmful than other alcoholic beverages.[74]

On Campus

A North Carolina study found that nearly one-fourth of college students drank high-energy alcoholic beverages. These beverages increase the likelihood of alcohol-related consequences.

Source: M. C. O'Brien, T. P. McCoy, S. D. Rhodes, A. Wagoner, and M. Wolfson, "Caffeinated cocktails: energy drink consumption, high-risk drinking, and alcohol-related consequences among college students," *Academic Emergency Medicine*, 15:453–460.

acculturation The adaptation and acceptance of cultural and social norms of a new environment

ethyl alcohol The form of alcohol that people consume

methyl alcohol Wood alcohol; not fit for human consumption

fermentation The process of transforming certain yeasts, carbon, hydrogen, and oxygen of sugar and water into ethyl alcohol and carbon dioxide

distillation A heating process that increases alcohol content

fortified wines Beverages produced by adding alcohol to slightly sweetened wines

proof Amount of alcohol in a beverage expressed as twice the percentage of the alcohol content

alcopops Malt, distilled alcohol-containing, or wine-containing beverages which have been flavored with fruit juices or other added ingredients; an example is Mike's Hard Lemonade

acetaldehyde Product of metabolism of alcohol by the liver; also found in tobacco smoke

Pharmacology of Alcohol

Alcohol is transformed in the liver into **acetaldehyde** and then to acetate, water, and carbon dioxide. It is eliminated from the body through urine, exhalation, and sweat. Alcohol leaves the body at a rate of approximately three-fourths ounce per hour. An ounce of distilled spirits, a bottle of beer, and a glass of wine all have about the same amount of alcohol. Thus, beer and wine are capable of producing the same intoxicating effect as hard liquor.

The primary site of absorption is the small intestine. Several factors affect the rate of absorption. If food is in the stomach, alcohol is absorbed more slowly. Wine and beer are absorbed less quickly than distilled spirits. Champagne is an exception. It contains carbon dioxide, which hastens absorption. Distilled spirits mixed with carbonated beverages are absorbed more quickly also. The speed at which food travels from the stomach to the small intestine is affected by strong emotions. Emotions such as anger and fear cause food, including alcohol, to be absorbed more quickly.

Males and females absorb alcohol at different rates. Because the average male body is larger and contains more water than the average female, males are less likely to feel the effects from the same amount of alcohol.[75] Another difference is that men have more gastric alcohol dehydrogenase activity, enabling them to metabolize alcohol more quickly than women. Hence, there is a greater buildup of alcohol in women, as alcohol leaves their bodies more slowly.

A woman herself does not always absorb alcohol at the same rate. In the premenstrual phase of her cycle, a woman absorbs alcohol more quickly than at

TABLE 6.2 Approximate Blood Alcohol Concentrations

Drinks (per hour)	Body Weight (pounds) 100	120	140	160	180	200	220	240
1	.04	.03	.03	.02	.02	.02	.02	.02
2	.08	.06	.05	.05	.04	.04	.03	.03
3	.11	.09	.08	.07	.06	.06	.05	.05
4	.15	.12	.11	.09	.08	.08	.07	.06
5	.19	.16	.13	.12	.11	.09	.09	.08
6	.23	.19	.16	.14	.13	.11	.10	.09
7	.26	.22	.19	.16	.15	.13	.12	.11
8	.30	.25	.21	.19	.17	.15	.14	.13
9	.34	.28	.24	.21	.19	.17	.15	.14
10	.38	.31	.27	.23	.21	.19	.17	.16

Source: Distilled Spirits Council of the United States.

TABLE 6.3 Effects of Alcohol at Varying Blood Alcohol Concentrations

BAC	Effects
0.05%	Less alert; less inhibited; slightly impaired judgment; slight euphoria
0.10%	Slower reaction time; impaired muscle control; reduced visual and auditory acuity; legal intoxication in most states
0.15%	Distorted perception and judgment; impaired mental and physical functions; less responsible behavior
0.20%	Markedly affected psychomotor ability; difficulty staying awake
0.25%	Inability to stand without help; grossly affected ability to comprehend
0.30%	Stuporous state; inability to respond to stimuli; not likely to remember events the next day
0.35%	Completely anesthetized; 1% will die at this BAC
0.40%	State of unconsciousness or coma; half will fatally overdose without medical intervention
0.50%	Deep coma or complete unconsciousness if not already dead

other times. Thus, she will feel the effects of alcohol faster. Also, women who take birth control pills absorb alcohol more quickly than women who do not.

The concentration of alcohol in the blood is referred to as **blood alcohol concentration (BAC)** or **blood alcohol level (BAL)**. The effect of alcohol on a person correlates with the percentage of alcohol in the person's bloodstream. Table 6.2 shows the percentage of alcohol in the body, or blood alcohol concentration, based on amount of alcohol consumed and body weight.

If alcohol is consumed at a rate exceeding the rate at which alcohol is metabolized or leaves the body, the BAC rises. As the BAC increases, behavioral and subjective effects become more pronounced. Drinking too much alcohol in a short time can be fatal. A brief summary of alcohol's effects at varying blood alcohol concentrations is shown in Table 6.3.

Effects of Alcohol

Alcohol accounts for 10% of all deaths in the United States each year, and the life expectancy of an alcoholic is reduced by 15 years. It affects every organ in the body. Two important factors that determine how alcohol affects the body are frequency of use and quantity consumed. The type of alcohol consumed does not matter. In a study of male and female adolescents, beer, wine, and distilled spirits produced equally damaging physical impairment.[76] In this section we will examine the acute and chronic effects of alcohol on the brain, liver, gastrointestinal tract, cardiovascular system, and immune system, as well as the relationship between alcohol and cancer. Figure 6.3 illustrates the effects of alcohol on various body systems.

The definition of moderate drinking for men is no more than two alcoholic drinks per day, and for women it is no more than one alcoholic drink per day. Light drinking would be less than this amount. There is no standard definition of heavy drinking, although a commonly accepted number for binge drinking is consumption of five or more drinks at one sitting for men and four or more drinks for women at one sitting.

Alcohol and the Brain

The brain is highly sensitive to the effects of alcohol. Five to six drinks daily will adversely effect cognitive functioning. The extent of impairment increases with higher levels of consumption. An estimated 15% to 30% of all nursing home patients are admitted because of permanent alcohol-induced brain damage.[77] Alcohol acts on the cerebrum, affecting judgment, reasoning, and inhibitions. It stimulates the release of serotonin, which could account for the disinhibiting effect of alcohol.

Alcohol acting on the cerebral cortex affects motor activity, and moods change quickly. Alcohol stimulates the release of dopamine, accounting for feelings of pleasure or euphoria. The senses are impaired when alcohol affects the cerebellum.

blood alcohol concentration (BAC)/blood alcohol level (BAL) Percentage of alcohol in the bloodstream

Many alcoholics experience memory loss and difficulty with problem-solving and decision-making.[78] At some level of consumption of alcohol, the medulla is sedated to the point that respiration could stop. A report released from the National Institute on Drug Abuse states that autopsy studies show chronic alcohol use shrinks the brain, especially in women.[79]

Although drinking small amounts of alcohol daily does not affect memory adversely, occasional large amounts could harm memory. A study of teenagers in the United Kingdom found that those who used excessive amounts of alcohol suffered from memory problems.[80] Alcohol-induced amnesia usually lasts a short time. Some people appear conscious and even function when they drink, but later they have no memory of what transpired. This condition, referred to as an alcohol-induced blackout, may be an early indication of alcoholism. Finally, prenatal exposure of the fetus to alcohol possibly affects attention and memory for the long term even with no more than one drink per day.[81]

One condition resulting from chronic alcohol abuse is Wernicke-Korsakoff syndrome, which occurs in about 20% of chronic alcohol users. This syndrome develops because alcohol impedes the body's ability to utilize thiamine, one of the B vitamins.[82] The person with this disorder is able to remember events or facts learned early in life but unable to recall recent events or facts. Other characteristics of this disease are disorientation, nerve damage, poor coordination, and rapid horizontal eye movement.

Chronic alcohol use is associated with neurotic and psychotic symptoms ranging from depressive reactions to generalized anxiety disorders and panic attacks. One study reported that about 20% of people diagnosed with a mood or anxiety disorder were alcoholic.[83] Among college students, those who have higher levels of social anxiety are more likely to consume alcohol.[84] People with mood disorders who self-medicate with alcohol and other drugs are more likely to exacerbate their problems and may be a greater risk for suicide.[85] Clinical depression is common. Depressed adolescents are more likely to drink alcohol and use other drugs than nondepressed adolescents.[86] It is unclear if alcohol abuse leads to depression or if depression leads to alcohol abuse. Nonetheless, one-third to one-half of alcoholics exhibit symptoms of depression at some time. Treating depression could help prevent relapse in recovering alcoholics.

Alcohol and the Liver

Chronic alcohol consumption increases the risk for cancer in many organs, including the liver.[87] Because the liver is the main site of metabolism of alcohol, heavy alcohol use can have devastating effects on

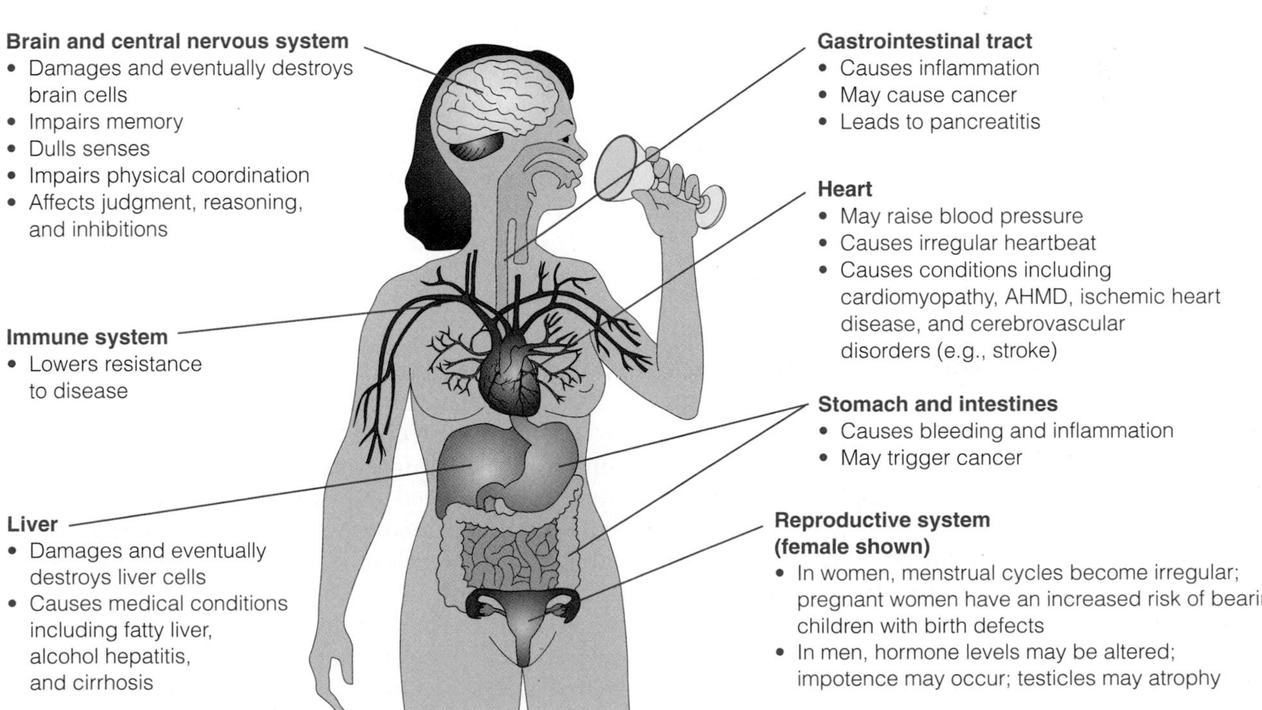

Brain and central nervous system
• Damages and eventually destroys brain cells
• Impairs memory
• Dulls senses
• Impairs physical coordination
• Affects judgment, reasoning, and inhibitions
Immune system
• Lowers resistance to disease
Liver
• Damages and eventually destroys liver cells
• Causes medical conditions including fatty liver, alcohol hepatitis, and cirrhosis
Gastrointestinal tract
• Causes inflammation
• May cause cancer
• Leads to pancreatitis
Heart
• May raise blood pressure
• Causes irregular heartbeat
• Causes conditions including cardiomyopathy, AHMD, ischemic heart disease, and cerebrovascular disorders (e.g., stroke)
Stomach and intestines
• Causes bleeding and inflammation
• May trigger cancer
Reproductive system (female shown)
• In women, menstrual cycles become irregular; pregnant women have an increased risk of bearing children with birth defects
• In men, hormone levels may be altered; impotence may occur; testicles may atrophy

Figure 6.3 Effects of Alcohol Use on Body Systems Over Time

Source: B. Q. Hafen and W. W. K. Hoeger, *Wellness: Guidelines for a Healthy Lifestyle*, (Englewood, CO: Morton Publishing, 1998), 341.

that organ. The three main conditions associated with overuse of alcohol are fatty liver, alcohol hepatitis, and cirrhosis. If one already has hepatitis C, then alcohol will exacerbate the condition, resulting in a shorter lifespan. The mean age of death for women with hepatitis C who drink heavily is reduced from 61.0 years to 49.1 years. The comparable reduction for males is 55.1 years to 50.0 years.[88] Cirrhosis is irreversible, even if alcohol use stops. Some signs of fatty liver are evident in 90% to 100% of heavy drinkers, whereas 10% to 35% develop alcohol hepatitis, and 10% to 20% develop cirrhosis.[89] Fatty liver can develop within a few days of heavy drinking. Symptoms of alcohol hepatitis include jaundice (a yellowish skin color), fatigue, low-grade fever, reduced appetite, dark urine, and occasional vomiting and nausea.

Cirrhosis of the liver, a deadly condition in which liver cells are destroyed, occurs in about 10% of long-term heavy drinkers.[90] A positive note is that since 1970, the rates of cirrhosis have declined in many countries, including the United States. The death rate from cirrhosis of the liver declined from 17.8 deaths per 100,000 people in 1970 to 9.7 deaths per 100,000 people in 2000.[91] The decline in rates of cirrhosis possibly can be attributed to earlier diagnosis and treatment, prevention programs, health promotion efforts, and misdiagnosis rather than to lower levels of consumption.[92]

Women are more susceptible than men to alcohol-related liver damage despite their lower levels of consumption. Also, women show symptoms of liver disease after shorter time spans of alcohol use. The elderly have seen an increase in alcohol-related liver diseases. Moreover, their prognosis is especially poor.[93] Generally, White males and females have lower rates of cirrhosis than non-White males and females. However, White males and females ages 65 and older have higher cirrhosis mortality rates than non-Whites.

Alcohol and the Gastrointestinal Tract

In moderate amounts, alcohol aids digestion by increasing the secretion of gastric juices in the stomach. Yet, alcohol can irritate the stomach, leading to internal bleeding. When alcohol is consumed on a regular basis, the esophagus and existing peptic ulcers are subject to inflammation.[94] Irritation of the esophagus is marked by chest pain and pain while swallowing. Alcohol abusers have higher rates of esophageal cancer and gastric carcinomas. Because a high proportion of abusers also smoke, it is difficult to delineate how much damage is attributable to alcohol use and how much is due to smoking. When alcohol is taken with aspirin, the inner lining of the stomach is especially prone to damage. Internal bleeding is especially common when alcohol and aspirin are taken together.

Heavy alcohol use is implicated in acute pancreatitis, a potentially fatal condition marked by severe abdominal pain, nausea, occasional diarrhea, tachycardia, vomiting, and fever. The pancreas secretes insulin and regulates blood sugar levels. More than three-fourths of chronic pancreatitis cases are related to heavy alcohol consumption. It is believed that alcohol abuse is the major cause of chronic pancreatitis.[95] Development of alcoholic pancreatitis occurs, typically, after 10 to 15 years of heavy drinking.

Alcoholics often incur malnutrition because alcohol interferes with the body's ability to utilize nutrients and also causes diarrhea, which leaches nutrients out of the body. Alcohol alters how the body metabolizes proteins, carbohydrates, lipids (fats), and minerals. Also, alcoholics tend to have poor eating habits and, as a result, often become anemic. Nutritional inadequacies are linked to liver disease, certain forms of cancer, pancreatic disease, and fetal alcohol syndrome in newborns. In young and middle-aged men, chronic alcohol use has been associated with the bone disorder osteoporosis.

Alcohol and the Cardiovascular System

Depending on the level of consumption, alcohol consumption can be both protective and harmful to the heart.[96] Degeneration of the heart muscle, known as alcoholic heart muscle disease (AHMD) or cardiomyopathy, occurs in about 2% of alcoholics, and less severe forms of this condition are found in most alcoholics. Other conditions include high blood pressure, cardiac arrhythmias, ischemic heart disease (deficient circulation of the blood to the heart), and cerebrovascular disorders such as strokes. Abnormal cardiac rhythms can result from years of heavy drinking, as well as from binge drinking. This "holiday heart syndrome" is more likely to occur around holidays and on Mondays after a weekend of binging. Symptoms of the holiday heart syndrome include irregular palpitations, dizziness, or chest pain.[97] It has been found that light drinkers who engage in binge drinking occasionally have higher death rates from coronary disease.[98]

Moderate alcohol consumption (no more than one drink per day for women or two drinks per day for men) has not been shown to cause high blood pressure, although blood pressure rises moderately during drinking. Nonetheless, it has been reported that men with hypertension who drink moderately have a decreased risk of a heart attack.[99] Stroke-like episodes sometimes appear within 24 hours after a drinking binge. Excessive alcohol use is believed to predispose people to stroke and sudden death.[100]

Many studies point to a positive relationship between moderate alcohol use and reduced coronary heart disease, particularly for people at risk for heart disease. In fact, regular, moderate alcohol use has been said to reduce the risk of heart disease by 40%. Guidelines published in May 2000 by the U.S. Department of Agriculture indicate that moderate alcohol use can benefit men older than age 45 and women older than age 55 (although the cardiovascular benefits of alcohol were not shown to benefit younger people).[101] The National Institute on Alcohol Abuse and Alcoholism (NIAAA) supports the idea that moderate alcohol use is beneficial cardiovascularly.[102] Although most studies focus on men, moderate alcohol use by women has been shown to reduce their cardiovascular risk as well.[103] In a 22-year study in Sweden, Theobold and associates found that moderate consumption of wine, but not of distilled spirits or beer, significantly reduced the risk of heart disease.[104] In France and Italy, where per capita wine consumption is more than six times greater than in the United States, mortality from heart disease is less than half that in the United States. The French, however, have higher rates of mortality from other causes.[105]

Red wine has been noted to be especially beneficial, although other forms of wine and beer possibly yield the same benefits to the heart. Moderate drinkers live longer and get fewer colds, and they are more likely to exercise and not smoke. Moderate use also might benefit the cardiovascular system by increasing high-density lipoproteins (HDLs).[106] Higher HDL levels are associated with reduced coronary artery disease. When discussing the benefits of moderate alcohol use, a potential problem is that some individuals cannot restrain themselves to drink moderately. In addition, moderate drinkers who occasionally binge drink are at greater risk for heart disease.[107]

Alcohol and the Immune System

Many studies show that moderate alcohol use reduces immunity.[108] Heavy drinkers are more prone to infections such as pneumonia and peritonitis. Alcohol interferes with the movement of white blood cells, which is important in fighting infections. A type of white blood cells, **T lymphocytes**, which help to resist infections, are notably deficient in alcoholics with severe liver disease.

T lymphocytes Type of white blood cells that help in fighting infections

In a study of alcoholic patients who use multiple drugs, many patients traded sex for money or drugs, and their rates of HIV infection and sexually transmitted diseases were high.[109] Among heterosexual alcoholics, the risk of contracting HIV was 10 times greater than for the general population.[110] Although the subjects in that study used other drugs, the researchers believed that alcohol was the primary factor because of its disinhibiting effect. A study of American and Australian homeless youth found that they were more prone to developing HIV because they were more likely to engage in high-risk behaviors, especially the Australian youths.[111] Another study of older African American drug users who abused alcohol noted that their level of risk for HIV/AIDS is similar to that of younger alcohol abusers.[112] Individuals who are chronic drinkers are more susceptible to HIV.[113]

Alcohol and Cancer

The relationship between alcohol and cancer is complex because the effects vary by quantity and cancer site. Considerable research links alcohol abuse and certain forms of cancer, especially cancers of the nasopharynx, esophagus, larnyx, and liver. A European study of more than 500,000 people found that the risk of colon cancer was 26% higher for those people who had more than two alcoholic drinks per day.[114] In another study that included 750,000 people, on the other hand, those who drank four to seven glasses of red wine per week were only 52% as likely to be diagnosed with prostate cancer.[115] Similarly, individuals who drank two or more glasses of wine per week had a 40% reduction in developing kidney cancer.[116]

There is a relationship between alcohol consumption and breast cancer. One study found that women who consume two or more alcoholic beverages daily had an 80% greater risk of breast cancer.[117] It is estimated that 4% of newly diagnosed cases of breast cancer among women in the United States can be attributed to chronic alcohol use.[118] A European study of more than 17,000 nurses reported that nurses who had 22 to 27 drinks per week had twice the risk of developing breast cancer as moderate drinkers.[119] In the Framingham study, in which about 5,000 women were tracked over 20 years, women who were light drinkers of any type of alcoholic beverage had no greater risk of breast cancer.[120] Female drinkers who take folate reduce their risk of breast cancer.[121]

Esophageal cancer is 10 times greater for people who consume 21 drinks per week than people who drink fewer than 7 drinks per week.[122] People who smoke and drink excessively have a 38 times greater risk of developing cancers of the mouth, throat, and esophagus.[123] Although alcohol abuse can cause high rates of esophageal cancer even among nonsmokers, alcohol and smoking combined produce a much higher rate, suggesting a synergistic effect.

Beer consumption is related to cancers of the lower gastrointestinal tract. This could be attributable to **congeners**—the nonalcoholic ingredients such as flavoring agents or other residual substances—rather than alcohol itself.

Alcohol and Women

Although female use of alcohol does not equal that of males, the gap is shrinking. Five percent of males ages 50 or older are alcohol dependent or abusive. Among women in the same age group, only 1.6% are alcohol dependent or abusive. However, in the 12 to 17 age group, more females abuse alcohol or are dependent than males. The percentages of females and males who are heavy alcohol users are nearly identical.[124] Female alcoholics are more likely than male alcoholics to have liver damage, hypertension, anemia, and malnutrition, despite having shorter histories of heavy drinking. Chronic heavy drinking also has been linked to menstrual disorders, which can cause fertility problems. Even five or fewer drinks per week reduce the chance for conception.[125] Because women are more affected by alcohol, they tend to have more accidents and bone fractures, especially older women.

Estimates indicate that women account for one-third of all people dependent on alcohol.[126] Women have different treatment needs than men, but few treatment facilities are geared to meet the specific needs of women. Of women in alcohol treatment, one study found that 70% reported some form of childhood sexual abuse.[127] Another study indicated that women who were victims of childhood sexual abuse initiated drinking alcohol around ages 12 and 13.[128] A study of female college students noted a relationship between drinking habits and the expectation of being sexually victimized.[129]

Fetal Alcohol Spectrum Disorders

Fetal alcohol spectrum disorders is a general term describing various effects that occur as a result of women who drink alcohol while pregnant. These effects can be behavioral, physical, and/or mental. In addition, they can produce learning disabilities.[130] The leading known cause of mental retardation is fetal alcohol spectrum disorders (FASD).[131] Unfortunately, diagnosing FASD is difficult because the physical markers for in-utero alcohol use are not apparent.[132]

Alcohol traverses the placenta and interferes with fetal development. The fetus is especially vulnerable during the first trimester of pregnancy. Unfortunately, many women drink alcohol before realizing they are pregnant. Yet, a study of more than 188,000 women in the United States found that 2% engaged in binge drinking while pregnant.[133]

The National Institute on Alcohol Abuse and Alcoholism's Four Criteria for Defining Fetal Alcohol Syndrome:

- Maternal drinking during pregnancy
- A characteristic pattern of facial deformities
- Growth retardation
- Brain damage, which often is manifested by intellectual difficulties or behavioral problems

Source: National Institute on Alcohol Abuse and Alcoholism, *Alcohol Alert* No. 50, December 2000.

In addition to a smaller brain at birth, children with FASD are marked by head and facial anomalies such as a small head, flat cheeks, and thin lips, as well as retarded growth, central nervous system problems, and malformations of many major organs in the body. As these children get older, they exhibit behavioral problems including hyperactivity, short attention span, poor impulse control, and poor coordination. An Australian study found that women who drank more than one drink per day or who engaged in binge drinking had children with learning, attention, and intellectual problems.[134] Children of mothers who used alcohol while pregnant were studied over a period of 25 years. After 25 years, there was a higher likelihood of attention, arithmetic, spatial-visual memory, and IQ deficits as well as increased alcohol problems and psychiatric disorders.[135]

Children with FASD also suffer from eye-related problems, although they are not the only people who have eye-related problems from alcohol. Chronic alcoholism is associated with a significantly increased risk of cataracts, color vision deficiencies, and problems with the cornea.[136] Also, there may be a link between prenatal alcohol exposure and iron-deficiency anemia in infancy. The prenatal effects of alcohol may be exacerbated by iron deficiency.[137] FASD is irreversible but preventable.

Since 1989, the U.S. Surgeon General's office has required that all alcoholic beverages bear a label warning pregnant women of the hazards of drinking. Unlike labels on cigarette packages, these labels are not uniform and are difficult to see. Nevertheless, after the labels were introduced, drinking by pregnant women decreased, although most women who reduced their alcohol consumption were low-risk drinkers.[138] One study reported that women who are most likely to drink during pregnancy tend to be younger, less educated, single, and unemployed.[139] Research showed that, of pregnant women exposed to various health messages, 80% reduced their alcohol use and 61% completely abstained.[140]

The British Medical Association issued a report advising women who are pregnant or who plan on becoming pregnant to stop all alcohol consumption.[141] The inference is that even moderate alcohol use is not advisable. A study by the Alan Guttmacher Institute found that half of the doctors it surveyed believe that occasional alcohol use during pregnancy will not increase the risk of adverse outcomes, despite the fact that since the early 1980s the federal government has advised women to refrain from consuming alcohol during pregnancy.[142]

What is the incidence of FASD? In the United States it is estimated that 40,000 babies are born each year with FASD, costing the country up to $6 billion.[143] FASD is estimated to occur in 10 per live 10,000 births,[144] though FASD possibly is underdiagnosed.[145] In the United States, FASD rates are highest among American Indians and lowest among Asians. To quantify exactly how much alcohol the mother has to drink to cause FASD would be difficult. Some women consume two drinks daily and produce children with FASD, whereas other mothers can drink the same amount and not have babies with FASD. Some neurobehavioral problems have appeared with as few as seven drinks per week.[146] A woman who consumes four to six drinks per day has a one-third chance of bearing a child with FASD. One thing is clear, though: The more a pregnant woman drinks, the more likely it is that FASD will develop.

Many women who drink heavily in early pregnancy have higher rates of miscarriages, suggesting that FASD rates may be underreported. A perplexing point is that not all women who drink excessively deliver offspring with FASD. Therefore, maternal or genetic factors may account for some women bearing children with characteristics of FASD.

congeners The nonalcoholic ingredients in some forms of alcohol, such as flavoring agents or other residual substances

Alcohol-Related Issues

Alcohol has been implicated in violent behavior, suicide, criminal activity, automobile accidents, premature death and disability, and loss of productivity in industry. Next we will explore underage drinking, the distinction between an alcoholic and a problem drinker, and symptoms associated with alcohol withdrawal.

Underage Drinking

The social cost of underage drinking, in terms of violence, suicide, and educational failure, is estimated to be $53 billion annually.[147] An estimated 1.5% of 12- to 13-year-olds engage in binge drinking. For 14- and 15-year-olds, the percentage is 8.9%, and for 16- to 17-year-olds it is 20%.[148] High school students who engaged in binge drinking ten or more times were 6 times more likely to drink and drive.[149] There is no difference in binge drinking rates between high school males and females.[150] The vast majority of college students drink alcohol. One study reported that 19.3% injured themselves, 6.6% got into a fight, and 2.0% were coerced into sex at some point in the previous 12 months.[151] One group that has received little attention is community college students, although their drinking rates are believed to be lower because these students on average are older.[152] The alcoholic beverage of choice is beer, especially among male adolescents. The health and social costs associated with underage drinking are expected to rise because the number of underage youth will increase during the next decade. Problems associated with underage drinking include injuries and deaths caused by automobile crashes and alcohol-induced violence, unplanned and unprotected sex, poor academic performance and dropping out of school, illegal behavior, and delinquency. A less obvious consequence is economic in that money spent on alcohol is not spent on more constructive pursuits.

In the early 1970s many states lowered the legal age for purchasing alcohol from 21 to 18. Subsequently, the number of alcohol-related fatalities among people in that age group increased. To address this disturbing trend, in 1984 the federal government attempted to standardize the drinking age at 21. States that did not raise the drinking age to 21 risked losing federal highway funds. By 1988, all states were in compliance with the age 21 limit. Addressing drinking by students, especially younger students, is important because it has been demonstrated that the younger one is when drinking is initiated, the more likely one will develop an alcohol dependency.[153]

On Campus

A current study in the Midwest found that 83% of college students drank alcohol to celebrate their 21st birthday. Of these, 34% of men and 24% of women drank 21 or more drinks. It is estimated that 1,400 people die each year from accidental alcohol poisoning.

P. C. Rutledge, A. Park and K. J. Sher, "21st Birthday Drinking: Extremely Extreme," *Journal of Consulting and Clinical Psychology*, 2008 (76): 511–516.

Problem Drinking

The terms *alcoholic* and *problem drinker* are not synonymous. An individual who is an alcoholic is a problem drinker, but a problem drinker is not necessarily an alcoholic. The concept of "alcoholic" focuses on one's inability to control drinking. Alcoholics are dependent on alcohol. The problem drinker encounters interpersonal, financial, or social problems from his or her drinking. The problem drinker may drink infrequently—once a month, once a year, or even less—but has problems when consuming alcohol at those times. A problem drinker may drink considerably less alcohol than a social drinker. Therefore, by focusing on the amount of alcohol consumed, one may assume incorrectly that a social drinker has more alcohol-related problems than an occasional drinker. Depending on how one defines alcohol abuse, it is estimated that the number of alcohol abusers in the United States ranges from 10 to 20 million. A common symptom of problem drinking is **blackouts**, characterized by temporary memory loss, which may result from the capacity of alcohol to disrupt protein synthesis in the neuron. Blackouts appear to be more common then previously believed. Also, the number of older people experiencing blackouts from alcohol has increased over the past few decades.[154]

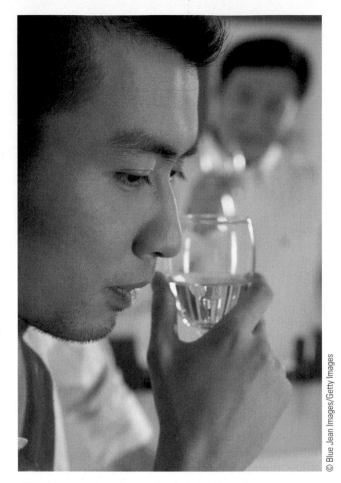
© Blue Jean Images/Getty Images

Alcoholism affects 1 out of every 10 Americans.

Alcoholism

Alcoholism has many definitions, none of which is universally accepted. Some consider it to be a disease. The disease concept gained popularity with the decline of the temperance movement and the failure of the movement to prohibit alcohol. The notion that alcoholism is a disease identifies the individual as having some kind of personal defect rather than placing the blame on failed social policies. The idea that alcoholism is a progressive disease that follows a series of stages was promoted by E. M. Jellinek. His ideas have been dismissed because most alcoholics do not follow consistent patterns.

The 1994 revision of the *Diagnostic and Statistical Manual of Mental Disorders* (*DSM-IV*) discarded the term *alcoholism* in favor of **alcohol abuse** and **alcohol dependence**. Alcohol abuse refers to continued drinking despite recurring social, interpersonal, and legal problems. Alcohol dependence is predicated on the presence or absence of tolerance and withdrawal. According to the U.S. Department of Health and Human Services, alcohol dependence is "a disease that is characterized by abnormal alcohol-seeking behavior that leads to impaired control over drinking."[155]

Increasingly, mental health experts are viewing alcohol abuse on a continuum with a range of treatments. Whether alcoholism is considered a disease is important. As a society, we are not likely to hold people at fault for having a disease. Thus, if alcoholism is a disease, drunkenness can be used as a legal defense. Also, if alcoholics run afoul of the law, they receive treatment rather than punishment.

Two common threads that run through the various definitions of alcoholism are the following:

1. Alcoholics are unable to control their drinking.
2. Some physical, social, or psychological consequence will result from their drinking.

Some research suggests that alcoholics or problem drinkers can benefit from a controlled drinking program.[156] Even though only a minority of people drink excessively, we all have to face alcohol abuse when we encounter drunk drivers, family members who drink too much, and people who become violent after drinking.

Definitions of Alcoholism/Alcoholic

American Medical Association: Significant impairment that is directly associated with persistent and excessive use of alcohol. Impairment may involve physiological, psychological, or social dysfunction.

American Psychiatric Association: Patients whose alcohol intake is great enough to damage their physical health, or their personal or social functioning, or when it has become a prerequisite to normal functioning.

National Council on Alcoholism and Drug Dependency: A disease in which there is impaired control over drinking, preoccupation with alcohol, continued use of alcohol in the face of adverse consequences, and distorted thinking.

American Society of Addiction Medicine: A primary, chronic disease with genetic, psychological, and environmental factors influencing its development and manifestations. The disease is often progressive and fatal. It is characterized by continuous or periodic impaired control over drinking, preoccupation with alcohol, use of alcohol despite adverse consequences, and distortions in thinking, most notably denial.

Withdrawal

Like other depressants, alcohol can create dependency. Thus, an alcohol-dependent person who stops drinking undergoes withdrawal symptoms. The first 5 days of withdrawal are the most severe, although withdrawal symptoms can last for weeks. The craving for alcohol is one obvious symptom of withdrawal. Other characteristics of alcohol withdrawal are the following:

1. *Delirium tremens (DTs):* A potentially fatal withdrawal symptom marked by delusions, confusion, and disorientation. The person might feel bugs crawling on the skin. The initial phase of DTs lasts from 1 day to 1 week. DTs cannot be cured, and medical supervision is necessary. During withdrawal, a sedative sometimes is administered to ease the discomfort.
2. *Extreme arousal:* Characterized by anxiety, irritability, absence of hunger, and inability to get to sleep. This state of arousal is actually a rebound effect, as an alcoholic is typically depressed.
3. *Auditory and visual hallucinations:* Visions and imaginary perceptions occur in about one-fourth of alcoholics during withdrawal.
4. *Physiological symptoms:* Include elevated temperature and blood pressure, fast pulse, dilation of pupils, and increased perspiration (may last for 2 or 3 days), increased sensitivity to sounds and touch, and grand mal seizures.
5. *Cognitive symptoms:* Impaired concentration, memory, and judgment.

blackouts A common symptom of problem drinking; characterized by temporary memory loss

alcoholism Condition in which an individual loses control over intake of alcohol

alcohol abuse A state characterized by physical, social, intellectual, emotional, or financial problems resulting from the use of alcohol

alcohol dependence Condition in which one's body requires alcohol or else withdrawal symptoms will occur; also marked by tolerance

Causes of Alcoholism

In the 1800s, a common view of alcoholism was that it was a matter of personal choice. Today, theories explaining the causes of alcoholism range from heredity to sociocultural reasons to differences in biochemistry to personality differences to interpersonal factors. No single theory provides a definitive explanation.[157] A family history of alcoholism is strongly linked to children's alcoholism. According to the *Ninth Special Report to the U.S. Congress on Alcohol and Health* in 1997, "a positive family history for alcoholism is one of the most consistent and powerful predictors of a person's risk for developing the disease." Regardless of the cause for alcoholism, it has been shown that drinking at an early age is associated with later alcoholism. One study found that among alcoholics, 47% had problems with alcohol by age 21.[158] In the following pages we will examine various theories that seek to explain factors contributing to alcoholism.

Genetics

One way to determine whether alcoholism is genetic is by studying identical twins. Four decades ago a researcher found that if one identical twin was alcoholic, the chance of the other twin being alcoholic was 71%.[159] The odds of fraternal twins both being alcoholic was 32%. More recent twin studies found that the heritability of alcoholism for males was 50%. The heritability for female twins was nil.[160] However, women tend to become addicted to alcohol more quickly than men.[161]

These studies suggest that genetics could well be a predisposing factor. Twins, however, are socially closer than nontwin siblings and, therefore, their relationship might lead to imitative behavior. However, Danish twins born to an alcoholic parent but adopted by the age of 6 weeks to nonalcoholic parents had a higher rate of alcoholism than adopted children born to nonalcoholic parents.[162] Other studies corroborate that children born to alcoholic parents but adopted during infancy and reared by others were at greater risk for alcoholism.[163] Using adoption studies to determine the possible presence of a genetic link to alcoholism has been criticized on the grounds that adoption agencies are biased in how they decide where to place children, and that there is no standard definition of alcoholism.

According to the National Institute on Alcohol Abuse and Alcoholism, between 50% and 60% of alcoholism vulnerability has a genetic basis.[164] Recent studies suggest that many genes may play a role in the development of alcoholism,[165] but one of the difficulties is identifying these specific genes. It is speculated that some neurotransmitters such as serotonin or gamma-aminobutyric acid may be linked to alcoholism.[166] The genetic predisposition to alcoholism may involve a lack of physiological sensitivity to the effects of alcohol, which can lead to heavy drinking. One study reported that there is a relationship between eating disorders and alcohol abuse.[167]

Finally, even if genetics is a factor, environmental conditions such as marriage have an ameliorating effect. And, even though the rate of alcoholism among children of alcoholics is higher, most children of alcoholics do not become alcoholics. Practically speaking, children of alcoholics should be mindful of the greater risk but understand that they are not consigned to a life of alcoholism if one or both parents are alcoholics.

Psychosocial Factors

The psychological and social bases for alcoholism include how individuals start using alcohol, the reinforcing qualities of alcohol, and individual traits of people who become alcoholics. Those who believe that alcoholism is a personality disorder view alcoholics as immature and fixated in their development. Most people use alcohol socially and do not progress further. Progression from social drinking to dependence is influenced by psychological state and expectations regarding alcohol's effects, the setting in which alcohol is used, and its pharmacological properties. Drinking alone or with others makes a difference in terms of alcohol consumption. For example, individuals are more likely to drink heavily when they are in a group than when they are alone.

A current study found that 20% of alcoholics have a concurrent mood or anxiety disorder. Also, 20% of people with a mood or anxiety disorder had a concurrent substance abuse disorder.[168] Personality variables such as history of antisocial behavior, high levels of depression, and low self-esteem have been linked to alcohol abuse.[169] There is research demonstrating that people who lack impulse control have higher rates of alcoholism.[170] For many women, alcohol problems stem from family conflict, difficulties with their offspring, and depression.[171]

Alcohol problems during adolescence and adulthood have been linked to antisocial behavior in childhood. The relationship between alcohol and depression occurs among adolescents also.[172] Because alcohol produces mild euphoria and reduces anxiety, its use is reinforcing. Whether alcohol abuse is the reason for certain personality characteristics or certain personality traits contribute to one becoming an alcoholic is unclear. Interestingly, there is little relationship between one's personality as an alcoholic and one's prealcoholic personality.[173] Also, many people displaying antisocial behaviors early in life do not become alcohol abusers, and many abusers did not behave antisocially early in life.

People's expectations about alcohol have been shown to be predictors of alcohol dependence. Alcohol abusers anticipate the effects of alcohol to be positive. Likewise, if using alcohol is viewed as helpful in coping with negative moods, the potential for abuse is higher. The adolescents at greatest risk for developing alcohol-related problems think alcohol is socially enhancing.

College students who expect positive outcomes from drinking alcohol likewise are heavier drinkers. Abuse is more common among people who believe that alcohol enhances their social and physical enjoyment, potency, aggression, sexual performance and responsiveness, and social competence. However, individuals who expected alcohol to increase their sexual risk-taking behavior did engage in more sexual risk-taking behaviors.[174]

Alcohol is linked to sexual behavior. One study of college students found that 32% drank alcohol prior to having unprotected vaginal sex.[175] One-third of high school students report they are sexually active and one-fourth of these students used alcohol or another drug before their last sexual intercourse.[176] Another study of 18- to 25-year-olds noted that alcohol dependence is associated with a greater number of sexual partners—ten or more partners.[177] Many adolescents expect alcohol to have a disinhibiting effect and, consequently, engage in risk-taking sexual behavior.

In one study, two groups of college students were given alcohol. Subjects in one group were told that the alcohol would interfere with their ability to perform a task, and subjects in the other group were told that alcohol would not affect their performance. Based on their expectations regarding alcohol, members of the group that were told they would be adversely affected did more poorly on the assigned task.[178] A similar experiment also found that students did more poorly on a cognitive test after drinking because of the expectation that they would perform more poorly.[179]

Culture

An important variable related to drinking patterns is the attitude of a given culture, subculture, or group that implicitly or explicitly establishes its own rules for behavior. Alcohol abuse is low in any group in which most group members agree on drinking customs, values, and sanctions. Moreover, groups that accept moderate drinking, but not heavy drinking, abuse alcohol less. Among Canadian college students, the degree of alcohol use is dictated by their perceptions of how much other students drink. If they perceive that other students drink a lot, then those students will drink comparably. Likewise, students will limit their drinking if they perceive that other students drink very little.[180] In an international survey of college students in 21 developed and developing countries, the highest rates of drinking were in Belgium, Colombia, Ireland, Poland (men), and England (women).[181]

Religious groups such as the Muslims and the Mormons advocate abstinence. The greater one's religious commitment, the less likely one is to drink heavily and the more likely one will abstain.[182] When alcohol is used ritualistically (in religious ceremonies or for special occasions) or is consumed for social reasons, heavy drinking is minimal. Alcoholism rates are higher if alcohol is used for personal reasons such as relaxing or coping with problems.

Alcohol policies vary greatly across cultures. In Japan, where alcohol is readily available and there are few restrictions on alcohol advertising, overall rates of consumption have declined, although Japanese women have increased their alcohol use.[183] In England, 34% of men and 20% of women drank more than the recommended amount of alcohol.[184] To curb underage drinking, Switzerland increased taxes on alcohol. France launched a campaign against drinking and driving, resulting in a 20% reduction in road deaths. The European Union (EU) is monitoring binge drinking among teenagers because it increased from 47% to 57% in Ireland and from 37% to 50% in Norway during the last decade.[185] Because alcohol consumption in Ireland rose 49% from 1989 to 2001, and because there has been a significant increase in alcohol-related admissions to treatment programs, the Irish government is restricting alcohol advertising.[186] In Russia premature death rates are very high. It is believed that excessive drinking is an important factor in the high mortality rate.[187]

The mere fact that alcohol is available or restricted is not a factor in rates of alcoholism. Forbidding children from drinking small amounts of alcohol does not affect whether they ultimately become alcoholics. Attitudes toward alcohol, reasons for its use, and demonstrating how it can be consumed responsibly are more important in whether children drink abusively.

Alcohol and Society

Alcohol can devastate friends, families, neighbors, and others with whom the drinker is involved. The media regularly report family violence, criminal activity, suicides, accidents, and automobile fatalities attributed to alcohol. Heavy drinkers are often victims of violence-related injuries.[188] Various surveys reveal that 6% to 11% of elderly patients admitted to hospitals, 20% of elderly people in psychiatric wards, and 14% of elderly people in emergency rooms show symptoms of alcoholism.[189] Among individuals visiting emergency rooms, 13.1% of women and 32.8% of men were classified as at-risk drinkers.[190] In a separate study of emergency room patients, it was found that drinking doubles the risk of injury.[191] Alcoholism is a factor in 25% of all hospital admissions. Nonetheless, the revenue from taxes on alcoholic beverages exceeds the money spent on health care costs resulting from alcoholism.

In the United States, it is estimated that 8% to 9% of the population suffer from post-traumatic stress disorder. A strong relationship has been found between trauma, post-traumatic stress disorder, and alcohol abuse.[192]

Automobile Accidents

The leading cause of death among youth ages 15 to 20 is motor vehicle crashes. Yet, almost 30% of high school seniors have indicated that they drove a car while impaired or rode with someone else who was impaired.[193] The age group with the highest rate of drunk-driving fatal crashes is 21 to 34. This age group accounts for 43% of all drunk-driving fatal crashes (see Figure 6.4).[194] Although laws against drinking and driving appear to affect light and moderate drinkers, heavy drinkers continue to drive.[195]

In 2006, over 17,000 people died as a result of alcohol-related motor vehicle accidents in the United States. Alcohol was a factor in nearly 40% of all traffic deaths.[196] The rate of alcohol-related traffic deaths declined from the early 1980s to the mid-1990s and has since leveled off.[197] Most fatalities occur between 6:00 P.M. and 6:00 A.M. and on Saturdays.[198] Drivers in reported crashes with suspended, revoked, or no licenses were five times more likely to be drinking than were drivers with valid licenses. However, it has been found that revoking a driver's license immediately has more impact than waiting until there is a conviction.[199] One study looked at the impact of Mothers Against Drunk Driving (MADD) Victim Impact Panels on individuals who attended a school for people convicted of driving while intoxicated. The study found that the Victim Impact Panel was no more effective than the information approach used with the DWI school.[200]

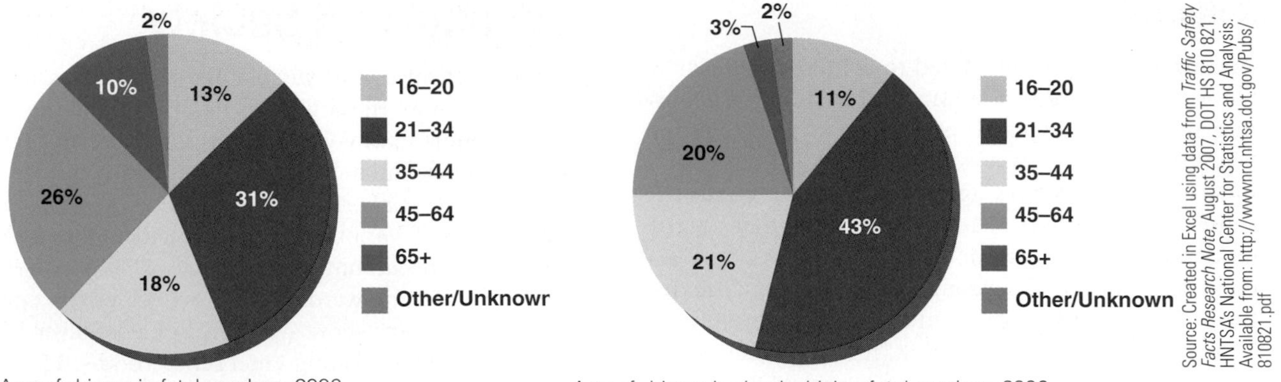

Age of drivers in fatal crashes, 2006

Age of drivers in drunk-driving fatal crashes, 2006

Source: Created in Excel using data from *Traffic Safety Facts Research Note*, August 2007, DOT HS 810 821, HNTSA's National Center for Statistics and Analysis. Available from: http://wwwnrd.nhtsa.dot.gov/Pubs/810821.pdf

Figure 6.4 The Rate of Drunk-Driving Fatal Crashes by Age

Recognizing that having patrons who get into automobile accidents is bad for business, some bar owners have agreed to give out vouchers for taxis to their patrons. Patrons are more likely to use taxi vouchers if the workers at the bar promote them.[201] The message against drinking and driving has reached many 16- to 20-year-old drivers. It is estimated that raising the drinking age to 21 has reduced fatalities involving 18- to 20-year-old drivers by 13% and has saved an estimated 19,121 lives since 1975.[202] Gender is an important variable. Seventy-three percent of drivers in alcohol-related crashes are males.[203]

Statistics from the National Highway Traffic Safety Administration (NHTSA) reveal that in 2006 about 13% of the drunk-driving traffic fatalities involved 16- to 20-year-olds.[204] The NHTSA recommends that for drivers younger than age 21, the maximum BAC should be .02, and exceeding that limit should result in suspension of the driver's license immediately. It is estimated that 1,651 pedestrians were under the influence of alcohol when they were killed by an automobile.[205]

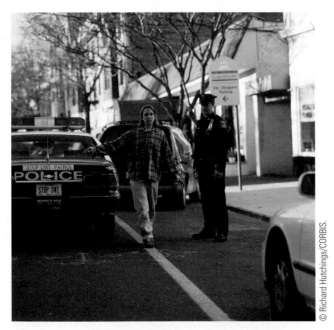

© Richard Hutchings/CORBIS.

The rate of "driving while intoxicated" convictions in the United States has increased since the late 1990s.

Alcohol affects the driver in the following ways:[206]

1. A driver who is under the influence of alcohol processes information more slowly than one who is not.
2. Alcohol-impaired drivers are more likely to look to the center of their visual field and not use their peripheral vision.
3. Alcohol-impaired drivers are less able to attend to multiple sources of information.
4. People who drink moderately (.05 BAC) underestimate hazards when they drive.[207]

In 1998, the U.S. Senate debated whether there should be a national .08 BAC standard for drunk driving. Senator Paul Wellstone of Minnesota argued in favor of a .08 standard, citing that it would reduce alcohol-related fatalities by 5% to 8%.[208] Senator Jack Reed of Rhode Island concurred, noting that states with a .08 standard had 16% fewer fatal automobile deaths.[209] Senator Frank Lautenberg of New Jersey supported the .08 standard, claiming that countries such as Canada, Ireland, Great Britain, and Germany have successfully implemented such restrictions.[210] Rick Berman of the American Beverage Institute maintained that the evidence suggesting that a BAC of .08 lowers the fatal automobile rate is inconclusive.[211]

Not all U.S. senators believe that a national .08 standard is appropriate. In 1998, Senators Trent Lott of Mississippi,[212] Don Nickles of Oklahoma,[213] and Craig Thomas of Wyoming[214] agreed that the issue of drunk driving has to be addressed, but that the federal government should not intervene in the states' right to decide. They asserted that the federal government should not usurp the responsibilities of individual states.

Accidents

Not only is alcohol use implicated with fatal falls, but alcohol in the body also impedes recovery from traumas.[215] A person with a blood alcohol level of .10 is three times more likely than a nondrinker to have a fall.[216] A German study noted that 53% of fatal falls down stairs were attributable to alcohol.[217] A review of several studies found that between 33% and 61% of persons who died as a result of burns had been drinking before being burned.[218]

The U.S. Coast Guard reported that 697 boaters died in 2005 and that alcohol was implicated in one-fourth of those fatalities.[219] In Australia it was found that alcohol contributed to 30% of all drowning fatalities associated with recreational aquatic activity and 35% of drownings associated with boating.[220] Skiing accidents are more likely to occur if skiers drink within 12 hours before skiing.[221] The accidents may result from the residual effects of a hangover or from fatigue. It is believed that many workplace accidents result from heavy alcohol use from the previous day.[222] One study found that over 9% of workers were hung over while at work.[223] The professions with the highest rate of heavy alcohol users are food service workers (17.4%) followed by construction workers (15.1%).[224]

Suicide

It is estimated that about 7% of alcoholics commit suicide. However, nearly 16% of men and 10% of women entering alcohol treatment have contemplated suicide.[225] One study reported that alcohol is more likely to result in women committing or attempting suicide.[226] Alcohol is linked to about two-thirds of suicide attempts. It seems to be connected more with people who commit suicide impulsively than with those who premeditate suicide. Alcohol consumption immediately before the suicide attempt is a more significant risk factor than habitual alcohol use.[227] The suicide rate is especially high for alcoholics who have depression.[228] Suicide rates increase dramatically as the use of distilled spirits goes up but are not related to increased use of beer and wine.[229]

Among adolescents, alcohol has been implicated with attempting and committing suicide.[230] As the BAL increases, the likelihood of using firearms for purposes of suicide also goes up.

Family Violence

Many studies show a relationship between alcohol abuse and domestic violence.[231] Alcohol is more likely to be involved in partner violence than in nonpartner violence.[232] Many studies indicate a relationship between alcohol dependence and physical abuse.[233] As the amount and frequency of alcohol use escalate, so does the probability of violence. Conversely, a reduction in intoxication reduces victimization.[234] High doses of alcohol significantly increase aggression.[235] Various studies report that 30% to 90% of violent crimes occurred when the offender was under the influence of alcohol.[236] In one study, 37% of crime victims had consumed alcohol before being victimized.[237] In two-thirds of all homicides, the victim, assailant, or both had been drinking.[238] Moreover, women who are victims of violence or other traumatic events have higher rates of alcohol dependence.[239]

Alcohol also is related to child abuse, though studies linking the two do not account for variables such as socioeconomic status. Nevertheless, children who are abused are more likely to become alcohol dependent as adults.[240] Also, a connection has been identified between women who physically abuse children and alcohol abuse or dependency. Yet, cross-cultural studies show that alcohol does not have to lead to aggressive behavior.[241] One could speculate that alcohol is used as an excuse for this behavior. In other words, the relationship between aggression and alcohol use may depend on the culture where alcohol is consumed.

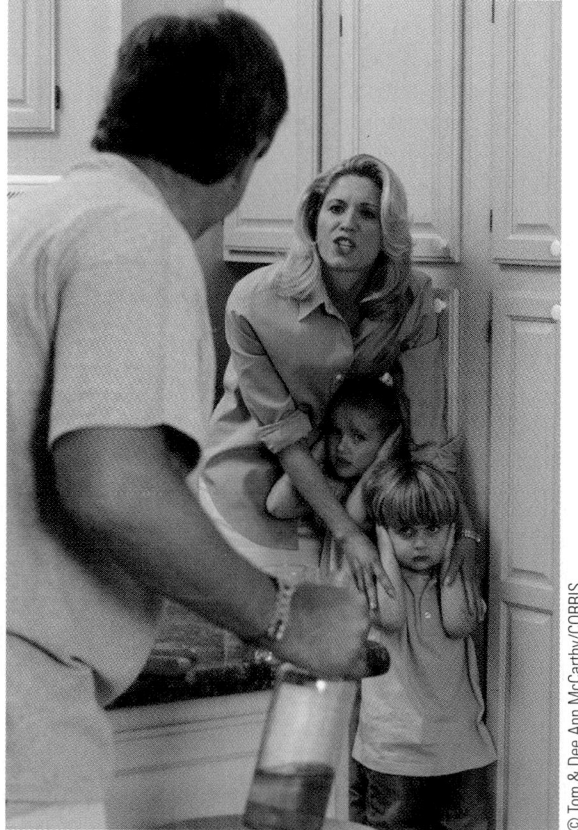

There is a strong relationship between heavy alcohol use and spousal abuse, as well as child abuse.

Children of Alcoholics

Children reared by an alcoholic parent carry a burden. Because of the shame and unpredictability of having an alcoholic parent, many children do not bring friends to their homes or have few friends. These children often experience sleep difficulties, depression, loneliness, and stomach problems. They are more likely to be delinquent and commit suicide. Some children of alcoholics are cognitively impaired in their verbal skills, planning goals, responding to stimuli, memory, and abstract thinking.[242] Attention deficit hyperactivity disorder (ADHD) is 2.5 to 3 times more likely to occur in children whose mothers have an alcohol use disorder.[243] It is not unusual for children of alcoholics to lie, suppress feelings, and withdraw from close relationships. Moreover, they may demonstrate anger toward the nondrinking for not providing support and protection.[244]

The harmful effects of parental alcohol abuse do not end with childhood. Adult children of alcoholics (ACOAs) find it hard to receive and give love. They devalue themselves, are easily depressed, develop inordinate feelings of responsibility, fear abandonment, handle authority poorly, and feel guilt when asserting themselves.[245] To avoid feelings of failure and self-deprecation, they have a great need to be in control.[246] Children often go to great lengths to hide a parent's drinking problem. Secrecy and denial are key elements of a family with an alcohol problem. Many ACOAs, however, are not significantly different from adults with nonalcoholic parents in terms of psychological well-being, personality characteristics, and adult development.[247] ACOAs should recognize the following four points:

1. The family affected by alcoholism is not a normal family.
2. Responsibility and blame for an alcoholic family do not rest with them.
3. Growing up in an alcoholic household, although extremely painful, can be a learning experience.
4. ACOAs have to acquire skills to form healthy relationships.

Individuals can find support from the group Adult Children of Alcoholics, which operates similarly to Alcoholics Anonymous. Despite the difficulties, growing up in an alcoholic household does not doom a child to an unhappy, unfulfilling adulthood. Many children are resilient and transcend the frightful situations in which they find themselves.

Although the ACOA movement is beneficial to many people, it does have its detractors. One criticism is that, although ACOA meetings foster support and fellowship, they also may foster feelings of being a victim. This allows some adult children to blame their alcoholic parents for many of the problems they have. Healthy children in healthy families also grow up with conflict and disappointment, and conflict and disappointment during the formative years do not necessarily lead to problems during adulthood. Some studies have found that ACOAs have no more psychological problems than those who are not raised in an alcoholic household.[248] It has been noted that adult children of alcoholics do not have higher rates of substance abuse, defensiveness, or codependency.[249] One study found that adolescent sons of alcoholic fathers had strong senses of identity. This may be due to these adolescents maturing at a faster rate than peers.[250]

■ Summary

No drug is used more extensively or serves as many functions as alcohol. It played an integral role in the early history of the United States, when it was viewed positively because it contained nutrients and because other beverages were often unsanitary. The rum trade was instrumental to the economic prosperity of the United States. Concern over immoderate drinking and alcohol's role in the breakdown of the family eventually led to the temperance movement and to politically active groups such as the Women's Christian Temperance Union (WCTU), the Anti-Saloon League, and the National Prohibition Party.

National prohibition of alcohol, the Eighteenth Amendment, went into effect in 1920. At first it reduced alcohol-related illnesses and deaths. But the law was difficult to enforce, illegal alcohol posed hazards, and there was widespread contempt for the law. In 1933, Prohibition was repealed by the Twenty-first Amendment.

Most people who drink alcohol are social drinkers. Drinking behavior varies according to geography, sex, race, and age. Generally, men drink more alcohol than women; some ethnic groups, such as Asian Americans, drink less than other groups, and older people consume less alcohol than younger people. Among college students, about 40% engage in binge drinking on a regular basis.

Ethyl alcohol is a central nervous system depressant consisting of carbon, hydrogen, and oxygen. Beer is about 5% alcohol, and table wine is around 10% to 12% alcohol. Distilled spirits contain approximately 40% to 50% alcohol. Alcohol is absorbed primarily in the small intestine. Food in the stomach, carbon dioxide in the beverage, emotional state, and body size affect the rate of absorption. The liver is responsible for metabolizing alcohol. The body metabolizes alcohol at a rate of three-fourths ounce per hour.

Alcohol affects every organ in the body. It affects the brain by altering inhibitions, judgment, coordination, and memory. Alcohol acts on the liver by causing fatty liver, alcohol hepatitis, and cirrhosis of the liver. The esophagus and existing peptic ulcers become inflamed from alcohol consumption. Alcohol adversely affects the heart muscle, contributing to poor circulation, raises blood pressure, and increases the risk of stroke. Alcoholics are more prone to infections. Alcohol is associated with cancer of the pharynx, esophagus, larynx, and liver. Women who drink while pregnant can deliver children with fetal alcohol spectrum disorder (FASD), a condition characterized by mental retardation and other physical anomalies.

Alcoholics use alcohol chronically and are unable to control their drinking. They differ from problem drinkers, who consume alcohol infrequently or occasionally but encounter emotional, social, financial, or interpersonal problems when they drink. Alcoholism has been shown to run in families. Studies dealing with twins and alcoholism indicate a possible relationship. Another theory suggests that alcoholism arises from the reinforcement of euphoria or reduction of tension produced by alcohol. Drinking patterns are affected greatly by cultural practices. Cultures that accept drunkenness, allow alcohol to be used for personal reasons, and find intoxication amusing have higher rates of alcoholism.

Everybody in society pays for the problems associated with alcohol. On college campuses, arrests for alcohol offenses increased greatly in the late 1990s. Much money goes toward treating people with alcohol-related illnesses. Half of all fatalities from automobile accidents are linked to alcohol. Alcohol use is high among those who die from accidents and suicides, and it is connected to family violence. Many children growing up in households in which one or both parents are alcoholics are left with emotional scars. Many women receiving alcohol treatment were abused as children.

Most people who drink do so without harm to themselves or others. Yet, too many people have suffered from their own use of alcohol or from the drinking of someone else.

Thinking Critically

1. Drinking behavior is often regulated by social norms. Friends, for example, exert an influence on alcohol use. How would you characterize the norms of your friends regarding alcohol use? Do they accept moderate use? Excessive use? Abstinence? Have your norms changed in response to your friends' norms?
2. Wine coolers are popular with young people. They are sweet and are packaged similarly to soft drinks (in 12-ounce to 2-liter bottles), and advertisements are directed toward young people. What restrictions would you put on advertising and packaging of these alcoholic beverages, if any?
3. Although a person can develop cirrhosis without drinking alcohol, most cases are alcohol-induced. Because many cases of cirrhosis would not occur if people did not drink excessively, should insurance companies and tax dollars pay to treat people whose condition was brought on by their own behavior?
4. Some research shows that moderate consumption of alcohol is healthful. Other guidelines advocate no alcohol intake. Do you think moderate alcohol drinking is healthy or unhealthy, and what is your rationale?
5. Warning labels pointing out the dangers of alcohol on the developing fetus are found on alcohol containers and in places where alcohol is served. Do you think these labels have any value? Would they alter your decision to drink alcohol if you were pregnant?
6. If alcoholism is accepted as a disease to which a person is genetically predisposed, should an alcoholic be held responsible for developing this disease? If a person has cancer or diabetes, is the person responsible for these conditions? What are the implications of calling alcoholism a disease?

Web Resources

National Institute on Alcohol Abuse and Alcoholism
http://www.niaaa.nih.gov
This site provides research on the causes, consequences, treatment, and prevention of alcoholism and alcohol-related problems.

National Council on Alcoholism and Drug Dependence
http://www.ncadd.org
This site contains objective information and referral for individuals, families, and others seeking intervention and treatment.

Alcohol: Problems and Solutions
http://www2.potsdam.edu/hansondj/index.html
This site deals with many controversial issues such as underage drinking policies regarding alcohol advertising.

Notes

1. J. D. Levin, *Introduction to Alcoholism Counseling: A Biosocial Approach* (Washington, DC: Taylor and Francis, 1995).
2. J. Kinney, *Loosening the Grip: A Handbook of Alcohol Information*, 9th ed. (New York: McGraw-Hill, 2008).
3. D. W. Conroy, "Puritans in Taverns: Law and Popular Culture in Colonial Massachusetts, 1630–1720," in *Drinking Behavior and Belief in Modern History*, edited by S. Barrows and R. Room (Berkeley: University of California Press, 1991).
4. J. McMullen, "Underage Drinking: Does Current Policy Make Sense?" *Lewis and Clark Law Review*, 10 (Summer 2006): 333–365.
5. Kinney, supra note 2.
6. M. Rudin, "Beer and America: It Came Over with the Mayflower and Stayed on to Be the Unchallenged Drink of Democracy," *American Heritage* (June/July 2002): 28–38.
7. Levin, supra note 1.
8. D. F. Musto, "Alcohol in American History," *Scientific American*, 274 (1996): 78–83.
9. Rudin, supra note 6.
10. V. B. Stolberg, "A Review of Perspectives on Alcohol and Alcoholism in the History of American Health and Medicine," *Journal of Ethnicity in Substance Abuse*, 5 (April 2006): 39–106.
11. W. L. White, *Slaying the Dragon: The History of Addiction Treatment in America* (Bloomington, IL: Chestnut Health Systems/Lighthouse Institute, 1998).
12. Musto, supra note 8.
13. Kinney, supra note 2.
14. D. F. Musto, *The American Disease: Origins of Narcotic Control* (New Haven, CT: Yale University Press, 1973), 89–90.
15. Center for Substance Abuse Treatment, Alcohol, Tobacco, and Other Drug Abuse: *Challenges and Responses for Faith Leaders* (Washington, DC: Substance Abuse and Mental Health Services Administration, 1995).
16. D. J. Hanson, *Preventing Alcohol Abuse* (Westport, CT: Praeger, 1995).
17. S. Staley, *Drug Policy and the Decline of American Cities* (New Brunswick, NJ: Transaction Publishers, 1992).
18. H. A. Siegel and J. A. Inciardi, "A Brief History of Alcohol," in *The American Drug Scene*, edited by J. A. Inciardi and K. McElrath (Los Angeles: Roxbury Publishing Company, 2004).
19. J. S. Blocker, "Did Prohibition Really Work? Alcohol Prohibition as a Public Health Innovation," *American Journal of Public Health*, 96, (February 2006): 233–244.
20. S. Ehlers, "How American Women Repealed Prohibition," *Drug Policy Letter* (Winter 1998): 23–24.
21. Alcohol and Health, *Tenth Special Report to the U.S. Congress* (Rockville, MD: U.S. Department of Health and Human Services, 2000).
22. D. J. Young and A. Bielinska-Kwapisz, "Alcohol Consumption, Beverage Prices and Measurement Error," *Journal of Studies on Alcohol*, 64 (2003).
23. N. E. Lakins, G. D. Williams, and H. Yi, *Surveillance Report #78: Apparent Per Capita Alcohol Consumption: National, State, and Regional Trends, 1970–2004.* (Bethesda, MD: National Institute on Alcohol Abuse and Alcoholism, Division of Epidemiology and Prevention Research, August 2006).
24. Alcohol and Health, Tenth Special Report, supranote 21.
25. T. F. Borders and B. M. Booth, "Rural, Suburban, and Urban Variations in Alcohol Consumption in the United States: Findings from the National Epidemiologic Survey on Alcohol and Related Conditions," *Journal of Rural Health*, 23 (Fall 2007): 314–322.
26. K. L. Delucchi, H. Metzger, and C. Weisner, "Alcohol in Emerging Adulthood: 7-Year Study of Problem and Dependent Drinkers," *Addictive Behaviors*, 33 (January 2008): 134–142.
27. H. Wechsler, J. Lee, M. Kuo, and H. Lee, "College Binge Drinking in the 1990s," in *The American Drug Scene*, edited by J. A. Inciardi and K. McElrath (Los Angeles: Roxbury Publishing Company, 2004).
28. B. D. Caudill, S. B. Crosse, B. Campbell, J. Howard, B. Luckey, and H. T. Blane, "High-risk Drinking Among College Fraternity Members: A National Perspective," *Journal of American College Health*, 55 (2006): 141–155.
29. K. DeBord, P. Wood, K. Sher, and G. Good, "Gay, Lesbian and Bisexual Students More Alcohol-Involved," *Journal of College Student Development*, 39 (1998): 157–168.
30. "Alcohol Use and Risks Among Young Adults by College Enrollment Status," *The NSDUH Report* (October 31, 2003): 1.
31. E. R. Weitzman, A. Folkman, R. L. Folkman, and H. Wechsler, "The Relationship of Alcohol Outlet Density to Heavy and Frequent Drinking and Drinking-Related Problems Among College Students at Eight Universities," *Health and Place*, 9 (2003): 1–6.
32. T. M. Nephew, G. D. Williams, H. Yi, A. K. Hoy, F. S. Stinson, and M. C. Dufour, *Surveillance Report #62: Apparent Per Capita Alcohol Consumption: National, State, and Regional Trends, 1977–2000* (Rockville, MD: National Institute on Alcohol Abuse and Alcoholism, 2003).
33. Results from the 2006 National Survey on Drug Use and Health: *National Findings* (Rockville, MD: U.S. Department of Health and Human Services, 2007).
34. "The Marital Status and Substance Use Among Women," *The NSDUH Report* (May 28, 2004): 1–6.
35. "Gender Differences in Alcohol Use and Alcohol Dependence or Abuse: 2004 and 2005," *The NSDUH Report* (August 2, 2007): 1–4.
36. E. Hoover, "Most College Officials Wring Their Hands over Alcohol Abuse, But How They Treat the Problem Differs Widely," *The Chronicle of Higher Education* (March 26, 2004): A35.
37. L. D. Johnston, P. M. O'Malley, J. G. Bachman, and J. E. Schulenberg, *Monitoring the Future: National Results on Drug Use, 2008*, (Bethesda, MD: National Institute on Drug Abuse, 2008).
38. L. D. Johnston, P. M. O'Malley, J. G. Bachman, and J. E. Schulenberg, *Monitoring the Future: National Results on Drug Use, 1975–2007, Volume II, College Students and Adults Ages 19–45* (Bethesda, MD: National Institute on Drug Abuse, 2008).
39. J. Haun, T. Glassman, V. J. Dodd, and G. C. Young, "Game-Day Survey Results: Looking at Football Fans Alcohol-Related Behaviors," *American Journal of Health Education*, 38 (March/April 2007): 91–96.
40. National Center for Health Statistics, *National Health Interview Survey*, 1997–2005. (Atlanta, GA: Centers for Disease Control and Prevention, 2006).
41. Ibid.
42. W. L. Adams and N. S. Cox, "Epidemiology of Problem Drinking Among Elderly People,"

in *Older Adults' Misuse of Alcohol, Medicines, and Other Drugs*, edited by A. M. Gurnack (New York: Springer, 1997).
43. J. Johnson, "Binge Drinking Among Pensioners Is Soaring," *Sunday Express* (December 24, 2006).
44. S. A. Wood, "Developmental Issues in Older Drinkers' Decisions: To Drink or Not to Drink," *Alcoholism Treatment Quarterly*, 24 (2006): 99–118.
45. P. L. Brennan, K. K. Schutte, and R. H. Moos, "Pain and Use of Alcohol to Manage Pain: Prevalence and 3-Year Outcomes Among Older Problem and Non-Problem Drinkers," *Addiction*, 100 (2005): 777–786.
46. Council on Scientific Affairs, "Alcoholism in the Elderly," *Journal of the American Medical Association*, 275 (1996): 797–800.
47. S. S. DeHart and N. G. Hoffmann, "Screening and Diagnosis: Alcohol Use Disorders in Older Adults," in *Older Adults' Misuse of Alcohol, Medicines, and Other Drugs*, edited by A. M. Gurnack (New York: Springer, 1997).
48. F. MacRae, "Hangovers Hit Older People Harder," *Daily Mail* (November 6, 2006).
49. Adams and Cox, supra note 42.
50. "Numbers Increasing in Substance Abuse Treatment," *SAMHSA News*, 12 (July/August 2004): 6.
51. Johnston et al., supra note 37.
52. J. W. Miller, T. S. Naimi, R. D. Brewer, and S. E. Jones, "Binge Drinking and Associated Health Risk Behaviors Among High School Students," *Pediatrics*, 119 (January 2007): 76–86.
53. A. T. McLellan, T. A. Hagan, and J. Durell, "Supplemental Social Services Improve Outlook in Public Addiction Treatment," *Addiction*, 93 (1998): 1489.
54. J. A. Ford, "Alcohol Use Among College Students: A Comparison of Athletes and Nonathletes," *Substance Use and Misuse*, 42 (2007): 1367–1377.
55. L. Feldman, B. Harvey, P. Holowaty, and L. Shortt, "Alcohol Use Beliefs and Behaviors Among High School Students," *Journal of Adolescent Health*, 24 (1999): 48–58.
56. H. W. Perkins, "Misperceptions of Peer Drinking Norms in Canada: Another Look at the 'Reign of Error' and Its Consequences Among College Students," *Addictive Behaviors*, 32 (November 2007): 2645–2656.
57. Results from the 2006 National Survey on Drug Use and Health: *National Findings* (Rockville, MD: U.S. Department of Health and Human Services, 2007).
58. National Center for Health Statistics, supra note 40.
59. "Alcohol and Minorities," *Alcohol Alert* (Rockville, MD: U.S. Department of Health and Human Services, January 1998).
60. C.S. Lieber, "Hepatic and Other Medical Disorders of Alcoholism: From Pathogenesis to Treatment," *Journal of Studies on Alcohol*, 59 (1998): 9–25.
61. K. Bloomfield, T. Stockwell, G. Gmel, and N. Rehn, "International Comparisons of Alcohol Consumption," *Alcohol Research and Health*, 27 (2003): 95–109.
62. T. P. Oei and C. L. Jardim, "Alcohol Expectancies, Drinking Refusal Self-Efficacy and Drinking Behavior in Asian and Australian Students," *Drug & Alcohol Dependence*, 87 (March 2007): 281–287.
63. T. Wall, K. Schoedel, H. Z. Ring, S. E. Luczak, D. M. Katsuyoshi, and R. F. Tyndale, "Differences in Pharmacogenetics of Nicotine and Alcohol Metabolism: Review and Recommendation for Future Research," *Nicotine and Tobacco Research*, 9 (September 2007): 459–474.
64. D. Sue, "Use and Abuse of Alcohol by Asian Americans," *Journal of Psychoactive Drugs*, 19 (1987): 57–66.
65. F. Y. Wong, Z. J. Huang, E. E. Thompson, J. M. DeLeon, M. S. Shah, R. J. Park, and T. D. Do, "Substance Use Among a Sample of Foreign- and U.S.-Born Southeast Asians in an Urban Setting," *Journal of Ethnicity in Substance Abuse*, 6 (2007): 45–66.
66. H. H. Kitano and I. Chi, "Asian-Americans and Alcohol Use," *Alcohol Health and Research World*, 11 (1986–1987): 42–47.
67. Johnston et al., supra note 37.
68. Kinney, supra note 2.
69. C. L. Ehlers, "Variations in ADH and ALDH in Southwest California Indians," *Alcohol Health and Research World*, 30 (2007): 14–17.
70. K. Gill, M. E. Elk, Y. Liu, and R. A. Deitrich, "An Examination of ALDH2 Genotypes, Alcohol Metabolism and the Flushing Response in Native Americans," *Journal of Studies in Alcohol*, 60 (1999): 149–158.
71. A. Goldstein, *Addiction: From Biology to Drug Policy* (New York: W. H. Freeman, 2001).
72. Johnston et al., supra note 37.
73. J. Van den Bulck, K. Buellens, and J. Mulder, "Television and Music Video Exposure and Adolescent Alcopop Use," *International Journal of Adolescent Medicine and Health*, 18 (January–March 2006): 107–114.
74. "Surveys: California Youths Discuss Appeal of Alcopops," *Alcoholism and Drug Abuse Weekly*, 18 (March 20, 2006): 6–7.
75. *Effects of Alcohol on Women* (Rockville, MD: Substance Abuse and Mental Health Services Administration, 2007).
76. S. Hansell, H. R. White, and F. M. Vali, "Specific Alcoholic Beverages and Physical and Mental Health Among Adolescents," *Journal of Studies on Alcohol*, 60 (1999): 209–218.
77. M. A. Schuckit, "Alcoholic Patients with Secondary Depression," *American Journal of Psychiatry*, 140 (1983): 711–714.
78. J. Ling, T. M. Heffeman, T. Buchanan, J. Rodgers, A. B. Scholey, and A. C. Parrott, "Effects of Alcohol on Subjective Ratings of Prospective and Everyday Memory Deficits," *Alcoholism: Clinical and Experimental Research*, 27 (2003): 970–974.
79. "Imaging and Alcoholism: A Window on the Brain," *Alcohol Alert* (Rockville, MD: U.S. Department of Health and Human Services, 2000).
80. T. M. Heffernan and J. Bartholomew, "Does Excessive Alcohol Use in Teenagers Affect Their Everyday Prospective Memory," *Journal of Adolescent Health*, 39 (2006): 138–140.
81. M. Testa, B. M. Quigley, and R. D. Eiden, "The Effects of Prenatal Alcohol Exposure on Infant Mental Development: A Meta-analytical Review," *Alcohol and Alcoholism*, 38 (2003).
82. G. Sechi and A. Serra, "Wernicke's Encephalopathy: New Clinical Settings and Recent Advances in Diagnosis and Management," *Lancet Neurology*, 6 (May 2007): 442–455.
83. "Largest Ever Comorbidity Study Reports Prevalence and Co-occurrence of Alcohol, Drug, Mood, and Anxiety Disorders," *NIH News* (August 2, 2004): 1–2.
84. C. Neighbors, N. Fossos, B. A. Woods, P. Fabiano, M. Sledge, and D. Frost, "Social Anxiety as a Moderator of the Relationship Between Perceived Norms and Drinking," *Journal of Studies of Alcohol*, 68 (2007): 91–96.
85. J. Bolton, B. Cox, I. Clara, and J. Sareen, "Use of Alcohol and Drugs to Self-Medicate Anxiety Disorders in a Nationally Representative Sample," *The Journal of Nervous and Mental Disease*, 194 (November 2006): 818–825.
86. "Depression and the Initiation of Alcohol and Other Drug Use Among Youths Aged 12 to 17," *The NSDUH Report* (May 3, 2007).

87. H. K. Seitz and P. Becker, "Alcohol Metabolism and Cancer Risk," *Alcohol Research and Health*, 30 (2007): 38–47.
88. C. M. Moon, Y. Yoon, H. Yi, and D. L. Lucas, "Alcohol and Hepatitis C Mortality Among Males and Females in the United States: A Life Table Analysis," *Alcoholism: Clinical and Experimental Research*, 31 (February 2007): 285–292.
89. "Alcohol and the Liver: Research Update," *Alcohol Alert* (Rockville, MD: U.S. Dept. of Health and Human Services, 1998).
90. Lieber, supra note 57.
91. Y. H. Yoon, H. Yi, B. F. Grant, F. S. Stinson, and M. C. Dufour, *Surveillance Report #63: Liver Cirrhosis Mortality in the United States, 1970–2000* (Rockville, MD: National Institute on Alcohol Abuse and Alcoholism, 2003).
92. R. G. Smart and R. Mann, "Recent Liver Cirrhosis Declines: Estimates of the Impact of Alcohol Abuse Treatment and Alcoholics Anonymous," *Addiction*, 88 (1993): 193–198.
93. H. K. Seitz and F. Stickel, "Alcoholic Liver Disease in the Elderly," *Clinics in Geriatric Medicine*, 23 (November 2007): 905–921.
94. R. Fields, *Drugs in Perspective* (New York: McGraw-Hill, 2007).
95. A. Vonlaufen, J. S. Wilson, R. C. Pirola, and M. V. Apte, "Role of Alcohol Metabolism in Chronic Pancreatitis," *Alcohol Research and Health*, 30 (2007): 48–54.
96. W. C. Kerr and Y. Yu, "Population-Level Relationships Between Alcohol Consumption Measures and Ischemic Heart Disease Mortality in U.S. Time-Series," *Alcoholism: Clinical and Experimental Research*, 31 (November 2007): 1913–1919.
97. J. Dirks, "Supporting Your Patients Through Holiday Heart Syndrome," *Nursing*, 37 (February 2007): 64–66.
98. J. Rehm, G. Gmel, C. T. Sempos, and M. Trevisan, *Alcohol-Related Morbidity and Mortality* (Rockville, MD: National Institute on Alcohol Abuse and Alcoholism, 2003).
99. J. W. Beulens, E. B. Rimm, A. Ascherio, D. Spiegelman, H. J. Hendriks, and K. J. Mukamal, "Alcohol Consumption and Risk for Coronary Heart Disease Among Men with Hypertension," *Annals of Internal Medicine*, 146 (2007): 10–19.
100. K. Reynolds, B. Lewis, J. D. Nolen, G. L. Kinney, B. Sathya, and J. He, "Alcohol Consumption and Risk of Stroke: A Meta-Analysis," *Journal of the American Medical Association*, 289 (2003): 579–588.
101. "New Advice on Drinking," *Prevention Pipeline*, 13 (July/August 2000): 6–8.
102. *National Institute on Alcohol Abuse and Alcoholism Five Year Strategic Plan, FY 08–13* (Rockville, MD: NIAAA, 2007).
103. J. M. Dorn, K. Hovey, B. A. Willaims, J. L. Freudenheim, M. Russell, T. H. Nochajski, and M Trevisan, "Alcohol Drinking Pattern and Non-Fatal Myocardial Infarction in Women," *Addiction*, 102 (May 2007): 730–739.
104. H. Theobold, L. O. Bygren, J. Cartensen, and P. Engfeldt, "A Moderate Intake of Wine Is Associated with Reduced Total Mortality from Cardiovascular Disease," *Journal of Studies on Alcohol*, 62 (2001): 652–656.
105. Lieber, supra note 60.
106. E. Kronish, "Drink to Your Health," *Self*, 29 (November 2007): 95.
107. J. H. O'Keefe, K. A. Bybee, and C. J. Lavie, "Alcohol and Cardiovascular Health: The Razor-Sharp Double-Edged Sword," *Journal of the American College of Cardiology*, 50 (September 2007): 1009–1014.
108. Alcohol and Health, Tenth Special Report, supranote 21.
109. M. Windle, "The Trading of Sex for Money or Drugs, Sexually Transmitted Diseases (STDs), and HIV-Related Risk Behaviors Among Multisubstance-Using Alcoholic Inpatients," Drug and *Alcohol Dependence*, 49 (1997): 33–38.
110. A. L. Avins, W. J. Woods, C. P. Lindan, E. S. Hudes, W. Clark, and S. B. Hulley, "HIV Infection and Risk Behaviors Among Heterosexuals in Alcohol Treatment Programs," *Journal of the American Medical Association*, 271 (1994): 515–518.
111. N. G. Milburn, J. A. Stein, E. Rice, M. J. Rotheram-Borus, S. Mallet, D. Rosenthal, and M. Lightfoot, "AIDS Risk Behaviors Among American and Australian Homeless Youth," *Journal of Social Issues*, 63 (September 2007): 543–565.
112. S. D. Johnson, C. Striley, and L. B. Cotter, "Comorbid Substance Use and HIV Risk in Older African American Drug Users," *Journal of Aging & Health*, 19 (August 2007): 646–658.
113. A. K. Singh, Y. Jiang, and S. Gupta, "Effects of Chronic Alcohol Drinking on Receptor-Binding, Internalization, and Degradation of Human Immunodeficiency Virus 1 Envelope Protein gp 120 in Hepatocytes," *Alcohol*, 41 (December 2007): 591–607.
114. "Heavy Alcohol Consumption Increases Cancer Risk," *AORN Journal*, 86 (November 2007): 823.
115. "Some Alcohol Consumption May Lower Risk of RCC," *Urology Times*, 35 (August 2007): 30.
116. J. P. Greving, et al., "Alcoholic Beverages and Risk of Renal Cell Cancer," *British Journal of Cancer*, 97 (2007): 429–433.
117. C. I. Li, K. E. Malone, P. L. Porter, N. S. Weiss, M. T. Tang, and J. R. Daling, "The Relationship between Alcohol Use and Risk of Breast Cancer by Histology and Hormone Receptor Status among Women 65–79 Years of Age," *Cancer Epidemiology, Biomarkers & Prevention*, 12 (2003): 1061–1066.
118. H. K. Seitz and B. Maurer, "The Relationship Between Alcohol Metabolism, Estrogen Levels, and Breast Cancer," *Alcohol Research & Health*, 30 (2007): 42–43.
119. L. S. Morch, et al., "Alcohol Drinking, Consumption Patterns and Breast Cancer Among Danish Nurses: A Cohort Study," *The European Journal of Public Health* (2007).
120. L. Zhang, "The Influence of Parental Drinking and Closeness on Adolescent Drinking," *Journal of Studies on Alcohol*, 60 (1999): 245–251.
121. S. M. Zhang, W. C. Willett, J. Selhub, D. J. Hunter, E. L. Giovannucci, M. D. Holmes, G. A. Colditz, and S. E. Hankinson, "Plasma Folate, Vitamin B6, Vitamin B12, Homocysteine, and Risk of Breast Cancer," *Journal of the National Cancer Institute*, 95 (2003): 373–380.
122. Alcohol and Health, Tenth Special Report, supra note 21.
123. "Alcohol and Tobacco," *Alcohol Alert* (Rockville, MD: U.S. Department of Health and Human Services, 1998).
124. "Gender Differences in Alcohol Use and Alcohol Dependence or Abuse: 2004 and 2005," *The NDSUH Report* (August 2, 2007).
125. T. K. Jensen, N. H. I. Hjolland, T. B. Henriksen, et al., "Does Moderate Alcohol Consumption Affect Fertility? Follow-Up Study Among Couples Planning First Pregnancy," *British Medical Journal*, 317 (1998): 505–512.
126. C. S. North, "Alcoholism in Women," *Postgraduate Medicine*, 100 (1996): 221–224, 230–232.
127. J. Howard, *Substance Abuse Treatment for Persons with Child Abuse and Neglect*

Issues (Rockville, MD: Center for Substance Abuse Treatment, 2000).

128. C. E. Sartor, M. T. Lynskey, K. K. Bucholz, V. V. McCutcheon, E. C. Nelson, and A.C. Heath, "Childhood Sexual Abuse and the Course of Alcohol Dependence Development: Findings from a Female Twin Sample," *Drug & Alcohol Dependence*, 89 (July 10, 2007): 139–144.
129. B. Benson, C. Gohm, and A. Gross, "College Women and Sexual Assault: The Role of Sex-Related Alcohol Expectancies," *Journal of Family Violence*, 22 (August 2007): 341–351.
130. Substance Abuse and Mental Health Services Administration, *The Physical Effects of Fetal Alcohol Spectrum Disorders* (Rockville, MD: U.S. Department of Health and Human Services, 2007).
131. "Fetal Alcohol Exposure and the Brain," *Alcohol Alert* (Rockville, MD: U. S. Department of Health and Human Services, December 2000).
132. D. L. Caprara, K. Nash, R. Greenbaum, J. Rovet, and G. Koren, "Novel Approaches to the Diagnosis of Fetal Alcohol Spectrum Disorder," *Neuroscience & Biobehavioral Reviews*, 31 (February 2007): 254–260.
133. J. Tsai, R. L. Floyd, P.P. Green, and C. A. Boyle, "Patterns and Average Volume of Alcohol Use Among Women of Childbearing Age," *Maternal & Child Health Journal*, 11 (September 2007): 437–445.
134. F. V. O'Callaghan, M. O'Callaghan, J. M. Najman, G. M. Williams, and W. Bor. "Prenatal Exposure and Attention, Learning and Intellectual Ability at 14 Years," *Early Human Development*, 83 (2007): 115–123.
135. A. Streissguth, "Offspring Effects of Prenatal Alcohol Exposure from Birth to 25 Years: The Seattle Prospective Longitudinal Study," *Journal of Clinical Psychology in Medical Settings*, 14 (June 2007): 81–101.
136. Y. Hiratsuka and G. Li, "Alcohol and Eye Diseases: A Review of Epidemiologic Studies," *Journal of Studies on Alcohol*, 62 (2000): 397–402.
137. R. C. Carter, S. W. Jacobson, C. D. Molteno, and J. L. Jacobson, "Fetal Alcohol Exposure, Iron-Deficiency Anemia, and Infant Growth," *Pediatrics*, 120 (September 2000): 559–567.
138. S. B. Blum, "Preventing Fetal Alcohol Syndrome: Where Are We Now?" *Addiction*, 91 (1996): 473–475.
139. G. R. Leonardson and R. Loudenburg, "Risk Factors for Alcohol Use during Pregnancy in a Multistage Area," *Neurotoxicology and Teratology*, 25 (2003): 651–658.
140. L. A. Kaskutas, T. Greenfield, M. E. Lee, and J. Cote, "Reach and Effects of Health Messages on Drinking During Pregnancy," *Journal of Health Education*, 29 (1998): 11–19.
141. L. Hitchen, "Doctors Advise Women Not to Drink Alcohol During Pregnancy," *BMJ: British Medical Journal*, 334 (June 9, 2007): 1186.
142. D. Hollander, "Pregnancy and Alcohol: Many Obstetrician-Gynecologists Are Unsure About Risks or How to Assess Women's Use," *Family Planning Perspectives*, 32 (2000): 308–310.
143. Substance Abuse and Mental Health Services Administration, *The Effects of Alcohol on Women* (Rockville, MD: U.S. Department of Health and Human Services, 2007).
144. Substance Abuse and Mental Health Services Administration, supra note 130.
145. Alcohol and Health, Tenth Special Report, supra note 21.
146. Ibid.
147. F. Joyce, "Underage Alcohol Use Linked with Violence, Suicide: Social Cost of $53 Billion," *Pediatric News*, 37 (December 2003): 18.
148. Results from the 2006 National Survey on Drug Use and Health: *National Findings* (Rockville, MD: U.S. Department of Health and Human Services, 2007).
149. J. W. Miller, T. S. Naimi, R. D. Brewer, and S. E. Jones, "Binge Drinking and Associated Health Risk Behaviors Among High School Students," *Pediatrics*, 119 (2007): 76–85.
150. Ibid.
151. M. P. Haines, G. Barker, and R. M. Rice, "The Personal Protective Behaviors of College Student Drinkers: Evidence of Indigenous Protective Norms," *Journal of American College Health*, 55 (2006): 69–75.
152. W. DeJong, *Community College Presidents' Role in Alcohol and Other Drug Abuse Prevention* (Washington, D.C.: U. S. Department of Education, Higher Education Center for Alcohol and Other Drug Prevention, 2006).
153. R. W. Hingson, T. Heeren, and M. R. Winter, "Age at Drinking Onset and Alcohol Dependence," *Archives of Pediatrics and Adolescent Medicine*, 160 (2006): 739–746.
154. J. Brown, "Raising Nurses' Awareness in Older People," *Nursing Times*, 103 (February 6, 2007): 30.
155. Alcohol and Health, Tenth Special Report, supra note 21.
156. Goldberg, *Taking Sides: Clashing Views on Controversial Issues in Drugs and Society* (Guilford, CT: McGraw-Hill/ Dushkin, 2008).
157. *National Institute on Alcohol Abuse and Alcoholism Five Year Strategic Plan, FY 08–13* (Rockville, MD: NIAAA, 2007).
158. R. W. Hingson, et al., "Age at Drinking Onset and Alcohol Dependence. Age at Onset, Duration and Severity," *Archives of Pediatrics & Adolescent Medicine*, 160 (July 2006): 739–746.
159. L. Kaij, *Alcoholism in Towns: Studies on the Etiology and Sequelae of Abuse of Alcohol* (Stockholm: Alonquist and Winkell, 1960).
160. Alcohol and Health, Tenth Special Report to the U. S. Congress, supra note 21.
161. K. Springer and B. Kantrowitz, "Alcohol's Deadly Triple Threat," *Newsweek* (May 10, 2004): 89–92.
162. D. W. Goodwin, "Is Alcoholism Hereditary?" *Archives of General Psychiatry*, 25 (1971): 545–549.
163. C. R. Cloninger, "Inheritance of Alcohol Abuse," *Archives of General Psychiatry*, 38 (1981): 861–868.
164. "The Genetics of Alcoholism," *Alcohol Alert* (Rockville, MD: National Institute on Alcohol Abuse and Alcoholism, July 2003).
165. Ibid.
166. "The Genetics of Alcoholism," supra note 164.
167. A. B. Kampov-Polevoy, J. C. Garbutt, and E.Khalitov, "Family History of Alcoholism and Response to Sweets," *Alcoholism: Clinical and Experimental Research*, 27 (2003): 1743–1749.
168. B. F. Grant, F. S. Stinson, D. A. Dawson, S. P. Chou, M. C. Dufour, W. Compton, R. P. Pickering, and K. Kaplan, "Prevalence and Co-occurrence of Substance Abuse Disorders and Independent Mood and Anxiety Disorders: Results from the National Epidemiologic Survey on Alcohol and Related Conditions," *Archives of General Psychiatry*, 61 (2004): 807–816.
169. K. R. Merikangas, M. Stolar, D. E. Stevens, J. Gouilet, M. A. Preisig, B. Fenton, H. Zhang, S. S. O'Malley, and B. J. Rounsaville, "Familial Transmission of Substance Use Disorders," *Archives of General Psychiatry*, 55 (1998): 973–979.
170. B. Porjesz, H. Begleiter, and J. C. Garbutt, "Reduced Frontal Lobe Activity and Impulsivity May Be Linked to Alcoholism Risk," *Alcoholism: Clinical & Experimental Research*, 31 (January 2007): 156–165.

171. S. Nolen-Hoeksema, M. M. Wong, H. Fitzgerald, and R. A. Zucker, "Depressive Symptoms Over Time in Women Partners of Men with and without Alcohol Problems," *Journal of Abnormal Psychology*, 115 (2006): 601–609.
172. R. M. Crum, C. L. Storr, N. Ialongo, and J. C. Anthony, "Is Depressed Mood in Childhood Associated with an Increased Risk of Initiation of Alcohol Use During Early Adolescence?" *Addictive Behaviors*, 33 (January 2008): 24–40.
173. J. Kinney, supra note 2.
174. K. C. Davis, C. S. Hendershot, W. H. George, J. Norris, and J. R. Heiman, "Alcohol's Effects on Sexual Decision Making: An Integration of Alcohol Myopia and Individual Differences," *Journal of Studies on Alcohol & Drugs*, 68 (November 2007): 843–851.
175. J. L. Brown and P.A. Vanable, "Alcohol Use, Partner Type, and Risky Sexual Behavior Among College Students: Findings from an Event-Level Study," *Addictive Behaviors*, 32 (December 2007): 2940–2952.
176. "Behaviors Among High School Students—United States, 1991–2001," *Morbidity and Mortality Weekly Report*, 51 (2002): 856–859.
177. P. A. Cavazos, et al., "The Relationship Between Alcohol Problems and Dependence, Conduct Problems and Diagnosis, and Number of Sex Partners in a Sample of Young Adults," *Alcoholism: Clinical & Experimental Research*, 31 (December 2007): 2046–2052.
178. E. J. Sharkansky and P. R. Finn, "Effects of Outcome Expectancies and Disinhibition on Ad Lib Alcohol Consumption," *Journal of Studies on Alcohol*, 59 (1998) 198–206.
179. M. T. Fillmore, J. L. Carscadden, and M. Vogel-Sprott, "Alcohol, Cognitive Impairment and Expectancies," *Journal of Studies on Alcohol*, 59 (1998): 174–179.
180. H. W. Perkins, "Misperceptions of Peer Drinking Norms in Canada: Another Look at the Reign of 'Error' and Its Consequences Among College Students," *Addictive Behaviors*, 32 (November 2007): 2645–2656.
181. C. Dantzer, J. Wardle, R. Fuller, S. Z. Pampalone, and A. Steptoe, "International Study of Heavy Drinking: Attitudes and Sociodemographic Factors in University Students," *Journal of American College Health*, 55 (September/October, 2006): 83–89.
182. N. Chawla, C. Neighbors, M. A. Clayton, C. M. Lee, and M. E. Larimer, "Attitudes and Perceived Approval of Drinking as Mediators of the Relationship Between the Importance of Religion and Alcohol Use," *Journal of Studies on Alcohol & Drugs*, 68, (May 2007): 410–418.
183. "Japan: Alcohol Today," Addiction, 102 (December 2007): 1849–1862.
184. The Information Centre, *Statistics on Alcohol: England 2007*, National Health Service, 2007.
185. "News from Around the World," *AIM: Alcohol in Moderation Digest*, 13 (March/April 2004): 2.
186. "Ireland's Health Minister Announces Plans to Curb Alcohol Abuse," *AIM Research Highlights* (May 2003): 2–3.
187. N. Eberstadt, "Save the Russians," *Foreign Policy*, 160 (May/June 2007): 42–43.
188. C. J. Cherpitel, A. R. Meyers, and M. W. Perrine, "Alcohol Consumption, Sensation Seeking and Ski Injury: A Case-Control Study," *Journal of Studies on Alcohol*, 59 (1998): 216–221.
189. "Alcohol and Aging," *Alcohol Alert* (Rockville, MD: U.S. Department of Health and Human Services, 1998).
190. E. A. Fleming, et al., "At-Risk Drinking and Drug Use Among Patients Seeking Care in an Emergency Department," *Journal of Studies on Alcohol and Drugs*, 68 (2007): 28–35.
191. S. Bazargan-Hejazi, T. Gaines, D. Naihua, and C. J. Cherpitel, "Correlates of Injury Among ED Visits: Effects of Alcohol, Risk Perception, Impulsivity, and Sensation Seeking Behaviors," *American Journal of Drug & Alcohol Abuse*, 33 (January 2007): 101–108.
192. B. D. Grinage, "Diagnosis and Management of Post-traumatic Stress Disorder," *American Family Physician*, 68 (2003): 2401–2409.
193. P. M. O'Malley and L. D. Johnston, "Drugs and Driving by American High School Seniors, 2001–2006," *Journal of Studies on Alcohol and Drugs*, 68 (2007): 834–842.
194. National Highway Traffic Safety Administration (NHTSA), "2006 Traffic Safety Annual Assessment-Alcohol-Related Fatalities," *Traffic Safety Facts Research Note*, August 2007.
195. R. E. Mann, R. G. Smart, G. Stoduto, E. M. Adlaf, E. Vingilis, D. Beirness, R. Lamble, and M. Asbridge, "The Effects of Drinking-Driving Laws: A Test of the Differential Deterrence Hypothesis," *Addiction*, 98 (2003): 1531–1536.
196. National Highway Traffic Safety Administration (NHTSA), supra note 194.
197. R. Hingson and M. Winter, "Epidemiology and Consequences of Drinking and Driving," *Alcohol Research and Health*, 27 (2003): 63–78.
198. Ibid.
199. A. C. Wagenaar and M. M. Maldonado-Molina, "Effects of Drivers' License Suspension Policies on Alcohol-Related Crash Involvement: Long-Term Follow-Up in Forty-Six States," *Alcoholism: Clinical & Experimental Research*, 31 (August 2007): 1399–1406.
200. M. Polasek, E. M. Rogers, W. G. Woodall, H. Delaney, D. Wheller, and N. Rao, "MADD Victim Impact Panels and Stages-of-Change in Drunk-Driving Prevention," *Journal of Studies on Alcohol*, 62 (2001): 344–350.
201. B. G. Simon-Morton and A. S. Cummings, "Evaluation of a Local Designated Driver and Responsible Server Program to Prevent Drinking and Driving," *Journal of Drug Education*, 27 (1997): 321–333.
202. "Alcohol and Transportation Safety," *Alcohol Alert* (Rockville, MD: U. S. Department of Health and Human Services, April 2001).
203. National Highway Traffic Safety Administration (NHTSA), supra note 194.
204. Ibid.
205. Ibid.
206. Hingson and Winter, supra note 197.
207. H. A. Deery and A. W. Love, "The Effect of Moderate Dose of Alcohol on the Traffic Hazard Perception Profile of Young Drinking Drivers," *Addiction*, 91 (1996): 815–827.
208. P. Wellstone, "Should Congress Pass a .08 Blood Alcohol Concentration (BAC) Drunk Driving Standard?" *Congressional Digest*, 77 (1998): 178–180.
209. J. Reed, ibid., 180–182.
210. F. Lautenberg, ibid., 186–188.
211. R. Berman, ibid., 189–191.
212. T. Lott, ibid., 179.
213. D. Nickles, ibid., 181–183.
214. C. Thomas, ibid., 187–189.
215. Alcohol and Health, Tenth Special Report, supra note 21.
216. Kinney, supra note 2.
217. R. Bux, M. Parzeller, and H. Bratzke, "Causes and Circumstances of Fatal Falls Downstairs," *Forensic Science International*, 171 (September 2007): 122–126.
218. Alcohol and Health, Tenth Special Report, supra note 21.
219. M. Nace, "Tips for Your Boat," *Mobility Forum: The Journal of the Air Mobility Command's Magazine*, 16 (May/June 2007): 25–27.
220. S. Diplock and K. Jamrozik, "Legislative and Regulatory Measures

for Preventing Alcohol-Related Drownings and Near-Drownings," *Australian and New Zealand Journal of Public Health*, 30 (August 2006): 314–317.

221. C. J. Cherpitel, "Alcohol and Violence-Related Injuries: An Emergency Room Study," *Journal of Studies on Alcohol*, 59 (1998): 216–221.
222. J. Howland, A. Almeida, D. Rohsenow, S. Minsky, and J. Greece, "How Safe Are Federal Regulations on Occupational Alcohol Use?" *Journal of Public Health Policy*, 27 (2006): 389–404.
223. M. R. Frone, "Prevalence and Distribution of Alcohol Use and Impairment in the Workplace: A U.S. National Survey," *Journal of Studies on Alcohol*, 67 (2006): 147–156.
224. Substance Abuse and Mental Health Services Administration News Release, *Nationwide Survey Shows Most Illicit Drug Users and Heavy Alcohol Users Are in the Workplace and May Pose Special Problems* (Rockville, MD: U.S. Dept. of Health and Human Services, July 2007).
225. K. R. Conner, Y. Li, S. Meldrum, P. R. Duberstein, and Y. Conwell, "The Role of Drinking in Suicidal Ideation: Analyses of Project MATCH Data," *Journal of Studies on Alcohol*, 64 (2003): 402–408.
226. K. R. Conner, et al., "Transitions to, and Correlates of, Suicidal Ideation, Plans, and Unplanned and Planned Suicide Attempts Among 3,729 Men and Women with Alcohol Dependence," *Journal of Studies on Alcohol and Drugs*, 68 (September 2007): 654–662.
227. G. Borges and H. Rosovsky, "Suicide Attempts and Alcohol Consumption in an Emergency Room Sample," *Journal of Studies on Alcohol*, 57 (1996): 543–548.
228. J. R. Cornelius, A. M. Salloum, J. Mezzich, M. D. Cornelius, H. Fabrega, J. G. Ehler, R. F. Ulrich, M. E. Thase, and J. J. Mann, "Disproportionate Suicidality in Patients with Comorbid Major Depression and Alcoholism," *American Journal of Psychiatry*, 152 (1995): 358–364.
229. P. J. Gruenewald, W. R. Ponicki, and P. R. Mitchell, "Suicide Rates and Alcoholism Consumption in the United States, 1970–1989," *Addiction*, 90 (1995): 1063–1075.
230. "Youth Drinking: Risk Factors and Consequences," *Alcohol Alert* (Rockville, MD: U.S. Department of Health and Human Services, July 1997).
231. L. J. Roberts and B. S. McCrady, *Alcohol Problems in Intimate Relationships: Identification and Intervention* (Rockville, MD: National Institute on Alcohol Abuse and Alcoholism, 2003).
232. G. Gmel and J. Rehm, "Harmful Alcohol Use," *Alcohol Research and Health*, 27 (2003): 52–62.
233. D. A. Dawson, B. F. Grant, S. P. Chou, and F. S. Stinson, "The Impact of Partner Alcohol Problems on Women's Physical and Mental Health," *Journal of Studies on Alcohol and Drugs*, 68 (2007): 66–75.
234. J. P. Shepherd, I. Sutherland, and R.G. Newcombe, "Relations Between Alcohol, Violence and Victimization in Adolescence," *Journal of Adolescence*, (2006): 539–553.
235. S. T. Chermack and S. T. Taylor, "Alcohol and Human Physical Aggression: Pharmacological Versus Expectancy Effects," *Journal of Studies on Alcohol*, 56 (1995): 449–456.
236. Gmel and Rehm, supra note 232.
237. Ibid.
238. Kinney supra note 2.
239. D. G. Kilpatrick, "Victimization and Posttraumatic Stress Disorder," in *Drug Addiction Research and the Health of Women*, edited by C. L. Wetherington and A. B. Roman (Rockville, MD: National Institute on Drug Abuse, 1998).
240. B. Jancin, "Childhood Sexual Abuse Linked to Later Alcohol Problems," *Family Practice News*, 33 (April 1, 2003): 36.
241. Hanson, supra note 16.
242. *National Clearinghouse for Alcohol and Drug Information*, "Children of Alcoholics: Important Facts" (Rockville, MD: Substance Abuse and Mental Health Services Administration, 2000).
243. L. Knouse, "Genetic Association Between Maternal Alcohol Use and Child ADHD," *ADHD Report*, 15 (February 2007): 13.
244. *Children of Alcoholics: Getting Past the Games Addicted Parents Play* (Do It Now Foundation, 2007).
245. J. A. Stein, M. B. Leslie, and A. Nyamathi, "Relative Contributions of Parent Substance Use and Childhood Maltreatment to Chronic Homelessness, Depression, and Substance Abuse Problems among Homeless Women," *Child Abuse and Neglect*, 26 (2002): 1011–1020.
246. T. L. Cermak and A. A. Rosenfeld, "Therapeutic Considerations with Adult Children of Alcoholics," in *Children of Alcoholics*, edited by M. Bean-Bayog and B. Stimmel (New York: Haworth Press, 1987).
247. S. H. Tweed and C. D. Ryff, "Adult Children of Alcoholics: Profiles of Wellness Amidst Distress," *Journal of Studies of Alcohol*, 52 (1991): 133–141.
248. H. E. Doweiko, *Concepts of Chemical Dependency*, 7th ed. (Pacific Grove, CA: Brooks/Cole), 2007.
249. A. L. Jones, D. M. Perara-Diltz, K. M. Salyers, J. M. Laux, and W. S. Cochrane, "Testing Hypothesized Differences Between Adult Children of Alcoholics (ACOAs) and Non-ACOAs in a College Student Sample," *Journal of College Counseling*, 10 (Spring 2007): 19–26.
250. B. Gavriel-Fried and M. Teichman, "Ego Identity of Adolescent Children of Alcoholics," *Journal of Drug Education*, 37 (2007): 83–95.

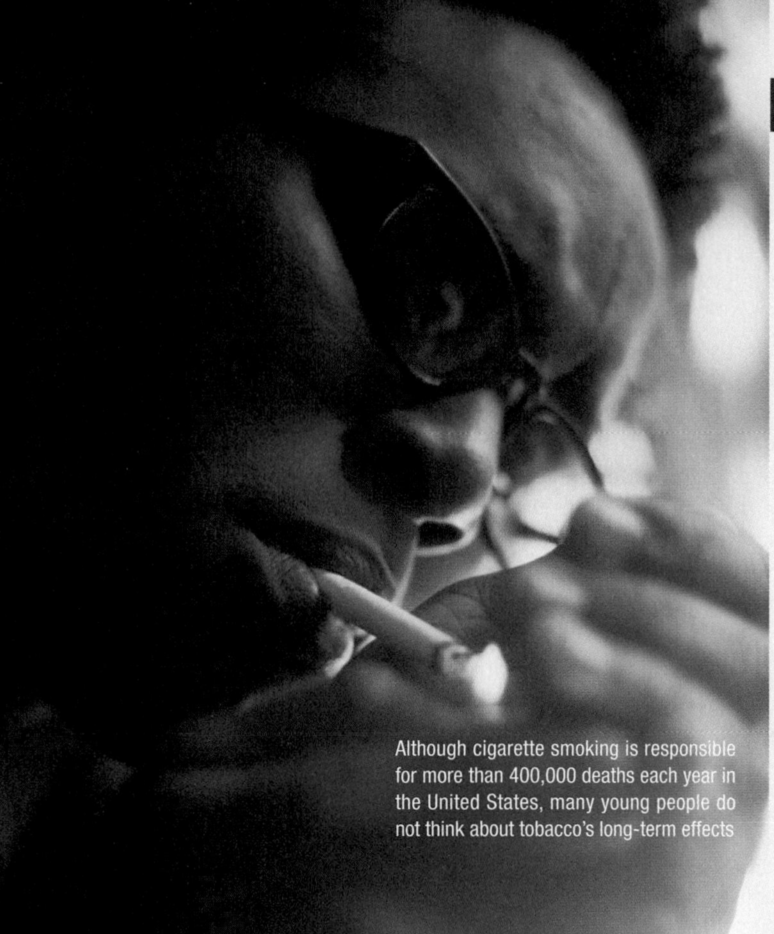

Although cigarette smoking is responsible for more than 400,000 deaths each year in the United States, many young people do not think about tobacco's long-term effects

FACT OR FICTION?

1. In a survey of more than 20,000 Americans, approximately one-half are in favor of totally banning smoking in restaurants.
2. The younger one is when smoking is initiated, the more likely one will become nicotine dependent.
3. The state with the highest percentage of adult smokers is Utah.
4. Less than half as many adults smoke today compared with 40 years ago.
5. The number of people dying from tobacco-related illnesses is about the same as people dying from alcohol-related illnesses.
6. Smokers are more likely to die from heart disease than from lung cancer.
7. Nicotine is absorbed more quickly from cigarettes than from chewing tobacco.
8. More nicotine and carbon monoxide come from the burning end of a cigarette than from what the smoker exhales.
9. To prevent youth smoking, most states in the United States have increased funding for tobacco prevention since 2000.
10. People who stop smoking by age 35 avoid 90% of the health risks attributed to tobacco.

Turn the page to check your answers

7 Tobacco

Chapter Objectives

After completing this chapter, the reader should be able to describe:

- The importance of tobacco to the U.S. colonies
- Factors that led to the popularization of cigarettes
- Medical costs linked to tobacco use
- Trends in tobacco use over the past century
- Difficulties in teaching young people about the adverse physical effects of tobacco
- Factors associated with tobacco dependence
- The connection between tobacco and heart disease, cancer, and respiratory conditions
- The effects of maternal smoking on fetal development
- The influence of advertising on tobacco use
- The success rate of various smoking cessation techniques

FACT OR FICTION?

1. **Fact:** Of people surveyed regarding the ban on restaurant smoking, 50.6% support a total ban.
2. **Fact:** There is a strong relationship between early use of cigarettes and tobacco dependence.
3. **Fiction:** The fact is—Utah has the lowest percentage of adult smokers with 10.4%. Kentucky has the highest percentage at 27.5%.
4. **Fact:** In the 1960s, about half of American male adults smoked cigarettes. Today, the rate is less than 25%. Smoking by American women has declined from 34% to 18%.
5. **Fiction:** The fact is—more than 400,000 Americans die from tobacco-related illnesses, compared with 100,000 dying from alcohol-related illnesses.
6. **Fact:** Heart disease is the leading cause of death associated with cigarettes.
7. **Fiction:** The fact is—chewing tobacco results in quicker absorption of nicotine compared with cigarette smoking.
8. **Fact:** Because the burning end of the cigarette is intensely hot, more nicotine and carbon monoxide come from it than from the smoker.
9. **Fiction:** The fact is—in the last several years, states have reduced funding for tobacco prevention programs.
10. **Fact:** At every age there are benefits associated with quitting smoking, although there are more benefits if one quits at a younger age.

One of the most pervasive and destructive drugs known to humankind is tobacco, and it is legal. It is entrenched in the culture, having played an integral role in the history of the United States, especially in financing the War of Independence. Efforts to regulate tobacco in the United States started in the latter part of the 1800s. Antitobacco legislation was characterized by two themes: (a) fire hazards created by smoking and (b) the morality of smoking.[1] By the beginning of the 1900s, these issues had become less important because of the economic benefits associated with the tobacco industry and states' viewing cigarette taxes as an important source of revenue. Today tobacco is a $45 billion industry and continues to be a significant source of revenue to state and federal governments.

In 1995, a Food and Drug Administration proposal to regulate nicotine as a drug was unsuccessful. The current emphasis is on controlling the sale and promotion of cigarettes and smokeless tobacco to minors and the effects of secondhand smoke. In the adult population the rate of smoking has declined and is about half of what it was 30 years ago. The public perception of tobacco use has become increasingly negative. What once was simply viewed as a "dirty practice" is seen now as a life-threatening addiction.

Nicotine is the addictive ingredient in tobacco. C. Everett Koop, former U.S. Surgeon General, was the first government official to warn people of the dangers of tobacco. He claimed that nicotine dependence is as powerful as heroin and cocaine dependence. One could argue that nicotine is more addictive because it is more available, but alcohol is as available as nicotine and most drinkers do not become alcoholics, whereas 90% of smokers become dependent.

In 1988, the American Psychiatric Association recognized nicotine dependency as a disorder. Depression is common among smokers, and antidepressants are prescribed for some people who are trying to stop smoking. In a study of more than 1,200 Finnish smokers who were psychiatric patients, the likelihood of a suicide attempt was 100% higher than among nonsmokers.[2] In addition, it has been shown that there is a link between adolescents who are depressed and smoking.[3]

Nicotine comes from the green tobacco plant, a member of the genus *Nicotiana*. Although this plant has 60 species, only the *Nicotiana rustica* and *Nicotiana tabacum* species are smoked. The tobacco from these plants is used in cigars, cigarettes, pipes, snuff, and chewing tobacco. This chapter focuses on the history of tobacco, the extent of tobacco use, the medical effects of smoking on oneself and others, and techniques for smoking cessation.

History of Tobacco Use

A stone carving in southern Mexico dating back to between A.D. 600 and 900 depicts smoke being blown through a pipe. Historians believe that people of that time used tobacco to ward off evil spirits and to communicate with a higher power. During his travels, Columbus received gifts of dried tobacco leaves. Upon returning to Europe, he passed along seeds from the tobacco plant, which the Europeans planted. Tobacco use became popular among Europeans.

At first only wealthy people used tobacco because it was expensive. In time, tobacco became affordable to most people, and thousands of tobacco shops were operating in London by the early 1600s.

Even though tobacco was well accepted, not everyone was enamored with it. In the 17th century, Pope Urban VIII and Pope Innocent X condemned its use. Sultan Murad IV of Constantinople hanged or beheaded soldiers who smoked, and the czar of Russia slit the nostrils of smokers. Despite these measures, tobacco use continued. When the Thirty Years' War

(1618–1648) was in progress, smoking was transported into Eastern Europe.

Tobacco was thought to have medical value.[4] During the plague of 1614, some people thought it warded off the illness. Further, tobacco was used to treat skin diseases; internal and external disorders; injuries; and diseases of the eyes, ears, mouth, and nose. Some people believed smoke could be used to breathe life into another person.

In 1828, when nicotine was isolated and identified as poisonous and addictive, tobacco's reputation as a medicinal agent declined. For the next 30 years, religious leaders, physicians, and educators in the United States and Europe questioned the medical value of tobacco. Moreover, it was attacked for causing mental illness, delirium tremens, impotence, and sexual perversions. Despite the warnings, tobacco continued to be used for pleasure.

Tobacco in the American Colonies

An early settlement in the New World was Jamestown, named after King James I of England. During the early 1600s, the brutal winters and food shortages took their toll on Jamestown residents. As a last resort before abandoning the settlement, Englishman John Rolfe convinced the settlers to plant tobacco. The tobacco crop flourished, and the Jamestown community began to prosper.[5]

Soon thereafter, tobacco farming spread to other communities. Tobacco was established as a valuable commodity and was used as a form of currency. Tobacco farming ultimately contributed to the wealth of many individuals. Ironically, tobacco production, financed by the French government, provided the funds for the Colonial settlers to fight the Revolutionary War against England.

Mechanization and Marketing

When the United States was in its infancy, tobacco was used in snuff, cigars, and pipes, not cigarettes. Chewing tobacco was popular, particularly during the expansion westward. While traveling on horses and in carriages, people found it easier to chew tobacco than handle it. Cigarettes were seen as cheap alternatives to other forms of tobacco.

Until the late 1800s, cigarettes were rolled by hand, and the best workers produced only four cigarettes per minute. This situation changed after the cigarette-rolling machine was patented in 1883. The Duke Company of North Carolina, under the leadership of James ("Buck") Buchanan Duke, bought the rights to the cigarette-rolling machine, which produced 120,000 cigarettes daily. This mass production enabled the Duke Company to cut cigarette prices in half. The cost of a box of 10 cigarettes was 5 cents. Other companies soon got into the business of mass-producing cigarettes.

Another influential and innovative person in the tobacco industry was Richard Joshua Reynolds. In 1891, Reynolds put saccharine in tobacco to sweeten it and to give it a longer shelf life. In 1907, he introduced Prince Albert, a new brand of tobacco used for pipes and cigarettes. The promotional literature stated that because the leaves of Prince Albert were sterilized in a licorice casing, it was "the most delightful and harmless tobacco for cigarettes and pipe smokers."

Reynolds introduced other brands, too, including Camel cigarettes. Camels were considered unique because they combined Turkish and domestic tobacco leaves. They were less expensive than other cigarettes, and their popularity skyrocketed. Other companies began to produce cigarettes similar to Camels. The American Tobacco Company came out with Lucky Strike, and Liggett and Myers produced Chesterfield.

The Duke Company extended its marketing campaign to entice women to smoke. Cigarettes were the first of the tobacco products marketed to women. Women who smoked, however, were subject to tarnished reputations. They were seen as promiscuous, and it was rumored that they would grow moustaches and become infertile.

Subsequently, cigarettes were marketed to young males. As an enticement, cigarette companies included colorful cards in their packages, and the cards were traded like baseball cards are traded today. In addition, cigarettes were less costly and milder than cigars, which increased their popularity with this segment of the population.

Opposition and Escalation

One of the first critics of tobacco was physician Benjamin Rush. In 1798, he condemned tobacco for its adverse health effects. Later, the Women's Christian Temperance Union (WCTU) and other groups supported controlling the use and sale of tobacco products. Several states banned the sale of tobacco to children. Wisconsin and Nebraska went further, making possession of cigarettes illegal for children and adults alike. In 1893, Charles Hubbard, the president of the New York Board of Education, was able to get 25,000 New York students to pledge not to smoke until age 21.

Despite efforts to depict cigarette smoking as an undesirable practice, smoking continued to grow in popularity. During World War I, the YMCA, the U.S. Army, and other groups distributed cigarettes to soldiers. After the war, cigarette sales escalated further.

The morality of smoking and concerns about its medical effects took a back seat to the public's desire.

Moreover, cigarette taxes contributed to the government's revenue. During World War II, cigarette manufacturers including the makers of Lucky Strike donated cigarettes to soldiers in combat—which was seen as a patriotic gesture.

Costs of Smoking

One factor that has been shown to reduce the demand for cigarettes is an increase in their cost. Many states are currently raising cigarette taxes, with proceeds going to various programs such as smoking prevention, hospital treatment for the uninsured, and school construction. The federal government also amasses substantial tax revenues from tobacco sales. One benefit of raising cigarette taxes is that people are discouraged from smoking. However, higher taxes encourage a black market for cigarettes.[6] For young people the Internet is an increasingly popular source for less-expensive cigarettes. In addition, proof of age is not required.[7]

Extent of Tobacco Use

In 2008, 20.4% of high school seniors had smoked within the previous 30 days, and less than 5.7% smoked at least one-half pack or more cigarettes daily. This represents a significant decline from 16 years earlier, when these figures were 28.3% and 10.7%, respectively.[8] Among ethnic groups, American Indians and Alaska Natives had the highest rate of smoking, followed by Whites, Blacks, and Asians.[9]

The rate of smoking increased until 1964, when the Public Health Service issued the publication *Smoking and Health: Report of the Advisory Committee to the Surgeon General.* This report unequivocally identified smoking as a serious health hazard. Since the time of that publication, more than 43 million people have quit smoking, and smoking rates among adults continue to decline steadily. These data seem confusing because the total *number* of smokers has increased; however, the *percentage* of people who smoke has decreased. Of those who do smoke, the number of cigarettes smoked per capita has not decreased; people who smoke tend to smoke heavily.

Today, filtered cigarettes are more popular than unfiltered cigarettes. The percentage of people smoking filtered cigarettes increased from 2% in 1952 to 60% in 1963, to 90% in the mid-1980s.[10] Although levels of **tar** and **nicotine** in cigarettes have been sharply reduced, this decrease has contributed to a rise in the number of cigarettes smoked, as smokers seek to take in the same amount of nicotine. People who smoke low-tar and low-nicotine cigarettes inhale more deeply, hold the smoke in their lungs longer, or smoke more of the cigarette.

Demographics of Smoking

More adult males smoke than adult females, although females are gaining on men. Since 1955, smoking rates for White and Black men and women have declined sharply. The drop has been greater for White men than for Black men. The smoking prevalence rates for White and Black women are nearly identical. The overall number of male and female smokers has declined, but the greatest declines have been for men.

Tobacco companies market their products to women by linking smoking to independence and equality. Also, many women fear that they will gain weight if they stop smoking. Middle-aged women who stop smoking gain on average more than 6 pounds over 2 years. The weight gain is reduced, however, by increasing their exercise.[11]

A study of college students found that 26% smoked cigarettes. Among young adults of the same age who were not in college, 44% smoked.[12] The increase applied to all ethnic groups, but Whites had higher smoking rates than Blacks or Asians. Also, freshmen, sophomores, and juniors had higher smoking rates than seniors and fifth-year students. Students attending public colleges showed a greater increase in smoking rates than students at private colleges. Eleven percent of students smoked their first cigarette at or after age 19, 28% became regular smokers at or after age 19, and 18% had made five or more attempts to quit in the year preceding the survey.

Teens who have older siblings who smoke are more likely to smoke than teens whose older siblings do not. Similarly, parents who smoke and are not as concerned about the health effects of smoking are more likely to have children who smoke.[13] Also, smoking rates are highly correlated with education and occupation. People with a high school education or less

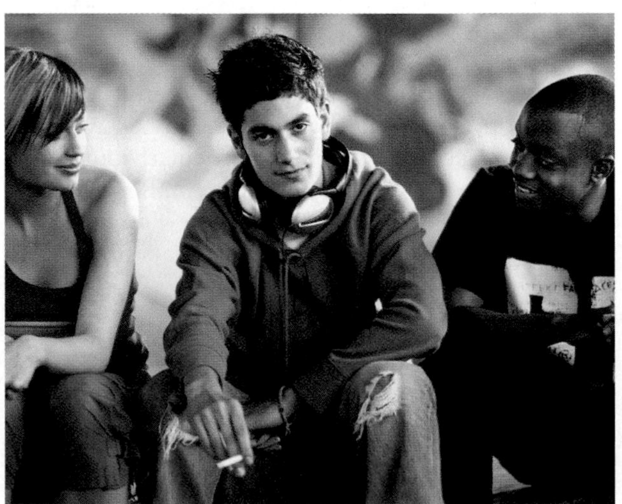

While cigarette smoking by adults has declined significantly, smoking by adolescents has declined only slightly.

are more likely to smoke than those who have gone to college, and a higher percentage of blue-collar workers smoke than white-collar workers. Individuals receiving psychiatric services or treatment for alcohol-related problems have higher prevalence rates.

tar A carcinogenic component of tobacco

nicotine Psychoactive component in tobacco responsible for stimulation and tobacco dependence

snuff A form of smokeless tobacco

Women and Smoking

The differences between men and women are diminishing. Currently, approximately 18.5% of women and 23.4% of men smoke cigarettes. In 1965, 52% of men and 34% of women smoked.[14]

Among women, as with the general population, one's level of education is correlated with smoking behavior. For example, less-educated women (those with an education through 11th grade) are three times more likely to smoke than women with 16 years or more of education.

Since 1980, about 3 million women in the United States have died prematurely from smoking-related diseases. Smoking is a major cause of coronary heart disease, although that risk declines substantially within 1 to 2 years after cessation. It is estimated that cigarette smoking reduces a woman's life span by 14 years. Lung cancer is the leading cause of cancer death among U.S. women, accounting for 25% of all cancer deaths among women. In addition, smoking is more dangerous for women than men because women cannot repair lung damage as readily as men.[15] Other types of cancer that are more common with women smokers include cancers of the pharynx, bladder, pancreas, kidney, and liver.

Women are subject to a number of other medical problems related to smoking. For example, peptic ulcers and cataracts are more common for smokers. Postmenopausal women have lower bone density than nonsmoking women. Also, women smokers are at greater risk for hip fractures. Women smokers have higher rates of depression, although it is not clear whether smoking precedes depression or depression precedes smoking.[16] Women smokers are more prone to rheumatoid arthritis, cataracts, and macular degeneration.[17]

Women's Health and Smoking

- Lung cancer is the leading cause of cancer deaths for women, surpassing breast cancer in 1987.
- Thirty-five-year-old and older female smokers are 12 times more likely to die prematurely from lung cancer than nonsmoking females.
- In 2007, about 70,880 women died from lung and bronchus cancer.
- Thirty-five-year-old and older female smokers are 10.5 times more likely to die from emphysema and chronic bronchitis, also known as chronic obstructive pulmonary disease (COPD), than nonsmoking females.
- The annual death rate for female smokers is 178,408.

Source: *Women and Smoking Fact Sheet,* American Lung Association, 2007.

Smokeless Tobacco

Use of smokeless tobacco—which consists of **snuff** and chewing tobacco—has nearly tripled in the last two decades. In 1986 the U.S. Congress banned television and radio advertisements for smokeless tobacco, but its use continues.

The nicotine in smokeless tobacco is absorbed quickly into the bloodstream through the mucous lining of the mouth, making it highly addicting. Thus, smokeless tobacco users reportedly have more difficulty stopping than cigarette users do. The nicotine level in one dip of snuff equals that in four cigarettes. Some people argue that smokeless tobacco is a desirable alternative to cigarettes. However, smokeless tobacco has a higher level of NNK, a known carcinogen, than regular tobacco.[18]

Based on the National Survey on Drug Use and Health, about 28.6% of Americans have used tobacco products in the previous month, although only 3.2% used smokeless tobacco in the past month.[19] The age group with the highest percentage of smokeless tobacco use is 18 to 20.[20] Of high school seniors, 2.7% use smokeless tobacco daily,[21] a lower percentage than in previous years. For example, in 1987, 5.1% of high school seniors used smokeless tobacco daily. Regionally, southerners have the highest rate of use. States with the highest prevalence of use are West Virginia, Mississippi, Wyoming, Arkansas, and Kentucky.

High school athletes are more likely than nonathletes to use smokeless tobacco. One reason is that students perceive smokeless tobacco as less physically damaging than other tobacco products. Most junior high school students and almost half of high school students who use smokeless tobacco believe they are either not at risk or at very little risk.

Smokeless tobacco cessation programs are effective. In a study of college athletes, 35% quit using smokeless tobacco after an intervention program, in contrast to 16% of college athletes in a control group.[22] Recent studies show that the nicotine patch is effective for getting smokeless tobacco users to abstain from use. Its long-term effectiveness, however, is not as promising.[23]

Although one could argue that smokeless tobacco is less harmful than cigarettes, smokeless tobacco produces many adverse health effects.[24] Besides cosmetic effects including discoloration of the teeth and bad breath, tobacco can cause gum recession, dental cavities, and leukoplakia, a precancerous condition marked by a white patch in the mouth that is reversible once one stops chewing. Chewing tobacco has been linked to cancers of the gum, mouth, larynx, pharynx, and esophagus. The risk of oral cancer is four times greater for smokeless tobacco users than for nonusers. Smokeless tobacco raises the blood pressure for up to 90 minutes after use, constricting blood vessels, and it can cause an irregular heartbeat, cardiovascular disease, and stroke. One study that looked at the mortality rates of male cigarette smokers who switched to smokeless tobacco found that those who changed to smokeless tobacco had a lower mortality rate but that their mortality rate was higher than former smokers who did not use smokeless tobacco.[25]

Tobacco Use in Other Countries

Smoking has increased greatly in parts of the world, possibly because of lax regulations and aggressive marketing. In Japan, almost two-thirds of the males smoke. China has an estimated 300 million smokers, 90% of which are men; 9 of 10 adult males there smoke. Tobacco use will kill an estimated 100 million of the 300 million smokers in China if the increase in smoking persists, and half of these deaths will occur during middle age.[26] One-third of all cigarettes are smoked in China.[27]

To capitalize on the high smoking rate in China, the R. J. Reynolds Company built its own cigarette factory there. China is the world's leading cigarette producer and the United States is second. It is estimated that cigarette smoking caused 4.8 million deaths on a worldwide basis in 2000.[28]

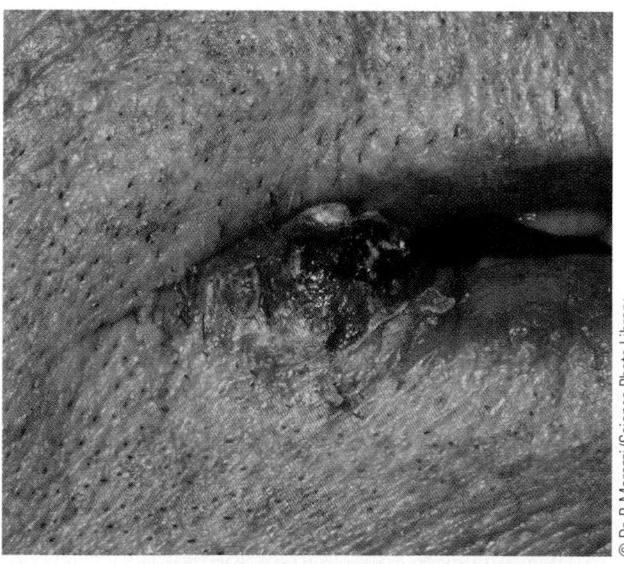

Smokeless tobacco was the cause of this squamous cell carcinoma in the oral cavity.

About three-fourths of Vietnamese men smoke. Philip Morris, the producer of Marlboro cigarettes, built a factory in Vietnam to augment its market share in that country. Interestingly, the cost of Marlboro and other Western cigarettes there is between 70 cents and $1, much less than in the United States. The cost of cigarettes is lower in developing countries than in industrialized countries, and their rates of smoking-related deaths are nearly the same as those in developed countries.[29]

Smoking rates in industrialized countries are decreasing, but in underdeveloped countries the trend is going in the opposite direction. Smoking has declined about 1% each year in industrialized countries, whereas rates in Africa increased 18% faster than the population. In Asia and Latin America, rates increased 7% faster than the population.[30] Smoking rates around the world vary from 40% in Cuba to 37% in Kuwait, Chile, Russia, Belarus, and Bangladesh. Other smoking rates are Nigeria at 6%, Salvador at 8%, Ghana at 8%, South America and Mexico at 15%, Argentina at 33%, Central Europe at 29%, and the European Union at 28%.[31] Table 7.1 shows the rate of smoking at various countries within the World Health Organization European Region.

The World Health Organization (WHO) is aggressively trying to curb smoking rates throughout the world. Meanwhile, U.S. tobacco companies export more than $2 billion worth of tobacco products. The U.S. government is pressuring Japan, South Korea, and Taiwan to eliminate restrictions on importation of foreign cigarettes. Unlike cigarette packages in the United States, the packages sent to Asian countries have no warning labels. Traditionally, Asian women have had low rates of cigarette use. Now, though, advertisements for cigarettes are targeting women and adolescents. In 1993, the French government banned all tobacco advertisements. Recently the European Union banned all tobacco advertisements, although some countries are disregarding the ban.[32]

Clove Cigarettes and Bidis

An alternative to traditional tobacco cigarettes is clove cigarettes. Manufactured in Indonesia, **clove cigarettes**, also known as kreteks, are made up of 60% tobacco and 40% ground cloves. They are aromatic and give smokers the impression they are safer because one of clove's components, **eugenol**, makes inhalation easier. It anesthetizes the back of the throat and thereby inhibits the coughing reflex that normally accompanies smoking of regular cigarettes.

Contrary to this expectation, some people who smoke clove cigarettes develop fluid in their lungs, bloody phlegm, and wheezing. Less serious effects are respiratory tract infections, shortness of breath, vomiting, and nausea. Clove cigarettes are not safe; in fact, numerous deaths have resulted from their use. They

clove cigarettes Cigarettes made from tobacco and cloves; contain more tar, nicotine, and carbon monoxide than commercial cigarettes

eugenol Ingredient in clove cigarettes that provides aroma and reduces coughing reflex

TABLE 7.1 Comparable Estimates of Adult Daily Smoking Prevalence in Selected Countries in the WHO European Region

Country	Male Prevalence (%) 2002	Male Prevalence (%) 2005	Female Prevalence (%) 2002	Female Prevalence (%) 2005
Austria	40.4	41.3	36.5	40.0
Azerbaijan	—	—	0.4	0.4
Belarus	57.7	57.7	16.8	16.8
Bosnia and Herzegovina	48.0	45.7	30.6	31.1
Bulgaria	41.3	41.3	23.4	23.4
Croatia	37.2	35.1	24.7	25.2
Czech Republic	30.1	30.0	21.5	20.7
Denmark	30.2	28.4	25.8	24.0
Finland	25.9	24.9	18.2	18.6
France	31.3	30.6	23.3	23.6
Germany	32.6	31.7	22.7	22.4
Hungary	39.3	39.0	29.1	29.7
Iceland	22.8	19.4	22.8	19.7
Israel	31.5	27.4	15.2	15.1
Italy	31.6	29.1	16.1	15.5
Kazakhstan	36.8	36.5	6.3	6.5
Lithuania	37.2	37.2	14.0	14.0
Luxembourg	34.4	33.8	27.7	28.0
Netherlands	32.4	31.7	27.1	27.6
Norway	27.4	26.1	24.7	23.7
Poland	40.2	37.6	23.5	23.3
Portugal	39.1	37.0	—	—
Romania	39.3	39.3	18.4	18.4
Russian Federation	64.4	64.9	20.4	21.6
Serbia and Montenegro (Serbia)	50.8	48.6	—	—
Slovakia	35.0	34.8	15.1	15.5
Spain	35.5	32.7	25.5	27.1
Sweden	16.3	14.4	19.4	18.1
Switzerland	25.3	23.6	18.8	17.7
Turkey	45.4	45.1	13.6	14.6
Ukraine	58.1	57.7	15.5	18.7
United Kingdom	28.8	28.8	27.9	27.9
Uzbekistan	19.3	19.1	0.6	0.6

Source: *The European Tobacco Control Report 2007.* Copenhagen, WHO Regional Office for Europe, 2007:143.

have higher levels of tar, nicotine, and carbon monoxide than commercial cigarettes.[33] Clove cigarettes also have higher levels of harmful particulates such as eugenol, anethole, and coumarin than conventional cigarettes.[34]

The Centers for Disease Control and Prevention (CDC) estimate that up to 3% of high school students and 2% of middle school students have smoked clove cigarettes. At the present time there is a bill in the United States Senate and House of Representatives regarding whether clove should be added to cigarettes. Like artificial or natural flavors such as strawberry, chocolate, and cocoa, clove is included in cigarettes to increase their appeal to children. Philip Morris, the largest cigarette manufacturer in the United States, introduced a clove-flavored version of Marlboro in Indonesia.[35] Clove cigarettes account for 90% of the cigarettes smoked in Indonesia.[36]

A recent fad, especially among teens, is **bidis**. These small cigarettes from India come in colorful packages and in different flavors. In India bidis are especially popular because they sell for one-fifth of what traditional cigarettes sell for.[37] Contrary to popular belief, bidis are not safe alternatives because they contain higher concentrations of nicotine. An estimated 2% of high school seniors smoked bidis in 2007.[38]

Light Cigarettes

In recent years many smokers have switched to "light" cigarettes, believing that they are a safer alternative to regular cigarettes. Light cigarettes, which are advertised as having less tar and nicotine, were introduced into the U.S. market in the late 1960s and account for nearly 85% of the cigarettes sold.[39] Although it is stated that light cigarettes deliver less tar and nicotine than regular cigarettes, they do not contain less tar and nicotine. Moreover, when people smoke light cigarettes, they receive about the same amount as those individuals who smoke regular cigarettes. Another problem with low-nicotine cigarettes is that smokers compensate for the lower levels of nicotine by changing smoking behaviors in order to get more of it.[40]

One study found that more than a third of smokers switched to light cigarettes to reduce their health risk. Also, many teen smokers believe that light cigarettes are less addictive.[41] Unfortunately, smoking a light cigarette does not reduce one's exposure to the carcinogens in tobacco. Nor is the risk to one's coronary system reduced: Blood pressure and heart rates are no different in light cigarette smokers as compared to regular cigarette smokers.[42]

Not only are light cigarettes marketed as a safer alternative to regular cigarettes, but many people believe that it is easier to quit use of light cigarettes than regular cigarettes. It has been reported, however, that light cigarette smokers actually have a lower rate of smoking cessation than those individuals who smoke regular cigarettes.[43] It is an illusion to think that light cigarettes are safer than regular cigarettes.

Cigars

One trend in the 1990s was the resurgence of cigar smoking. Indicative are magazines devoted to cigar smoking, cigar bars, and restaurants hosting cigar nights. From 1993 to 1999, the use of cigars and cigarillos (little cigars) increased 70%. In the United States in 2006, an estimated 5.3 billion cigars were smoked. This represents an increase of 9% from the previous year.[44] The promotion of little cigars is being addressed by attorneys general in 40 states. Little cigars, which some people consider to be cigarettes disguised in brown paper, are taxed at a lower rate than cigarettes and have fewer restrictions placed on their promotion.[45] It is believed that flavored little cigars are especially appealing to young people.[46]

Most cigar smokers are male, but an increasing number of women are taking up cigar smoking. The percentage of adolescents smoking cigars has risen also. Unlike cigarettes, cigars have no health warnings. Table 7.2 highlights cigar smoking by various age groups and by gender.

Although many people believe that cigars are a safe alternative to cigarettes, this is not necessarily true. People who switch from smoking cigarettes continue to inhale with cigars. Many health hazards are associated with cigar smoking. Nicotine levels are higher in cigars than in cigarettes.[47] Cigar smokers have a 34% higher cancer rate than nonsmokers; rates of cancers of the mouth, throat, and esophagus are higher among cigar smokers than cigarette smokers.

The lung cancer rate for cigar smokers is higher than that of nonsmokers, but it is lower than that of cigarette smokers. Individuals who smoke several cigars daily have a slightly increased risk for coronary heart disease and chronic obstructive pulmonary disease. The degree of danger is related to how many cigars one smokes and the depth of inhalation.[48]

TABLE 7.2 Lifetime, Past Year, and Past Month Use of Cigars, 2005

Age	Lifetime	Past Year	Past Month
12–17	14.1%	9.8%	4.2%
18–25	43.2	24.2	12.0
26 or older	38.1	8.9	4.7
Male	55.8	18.1	9.6
Female	18.0	4.5	1.8

Source: SAMHSA, Office of Applied Studies, *National Survey on Drug Use and Health,* 2005.

Characteristics of Smoking and Smokers

bidis Flavored cigarettes from India that have considerably higher concentrations of nicotine than regular cigarettes

Despite the harm that comes from tobacco products, many people continue to use them, and some people who smoke are unaware of the dangers. Tobacco use tends to have triggers, such as following a meal or while talking on the phone, drinking coffee, or being around other smokers. Unlike most other drugs, cigarettes do not interfere with *most* daily behaviors. A person can read a book, drive a car, and talk to a friend while smoking or chewing tobacco.

Some people use tobacco to be more alert, and others use it to relax. Although using tobacco for stimulation and for sedation seems paradoxical, the state of the smoker and the chemical properties of tobacco play a large role in their effects. Many smokers describe their first cigarette of the day as extremely pleasurable. Some claim that cigarettes curtail anxiety, sadness, and boredom. Tobacco contains acetaldehyde, a chemical with sedating properties similar to those of alcohol. Thus, depending on one's expectations or desires, tobacco can produce an arousing or a relaxing effect.

Nicotine and Performance

Nicotine improves cognitive performance slightly. The short-term memory and concentration of smokers are enhanced by nicotine for up to a half hour after smoking. Memory, attention, and reasoning ability decline 4 hours after the last cigarette. Because nicotine may improve memory, there is research into its possible benefits for patients with Alzheimer's disease.[49]

Tobacco Use by Young People

Most people begin smoking during childhood or adolescence. In fact, 89% of current adult smokers initiated their use by age 19.[50] Though it takes an average of 2 to 3 years after one begins smoking to become a regular smoker, the earlier in life one tries a cigarette, the more likely it is that one will become a regular smoker. One study involving Massachusetts sixth-grade students found that many students could become dependent within two days of when they initiated smoking.[51] It is estimated that over 4,000 young people ages 12 to 17 try cigarette smoking for the first time each day.[52] By eighth grade, 3.1% of students smoke on a daily basis. This is less than the 10.4% who were current smokers in 1996, a significant difference. Slightly more eighth-grade boys smoke than eighth-grade girls. In terms of ethnicity, Blacks have the lowest rate of smoking, followed by Hispanics, then Whites.[53]

On Campus

The rate of cigarette smoking among college students is less than one-third that of comparable-age individuals who do not attend college.

Source: *Monitoring the Future: National Survey Results on Drug Use,* 1975–2008 (2008).

One study found a strong relationship between smoking and early childhood misbehavior. Based on teacher ratings, children who misbehaved most were the most likely to be smokers as adults.[54] Curiosity is given as the most common reason for first trying cigarettes. One predictor of tobacco use among boys is aggressive/disruptive behavior, as early as the first grade. A behavioral intervention program to reduce aggressive behaviors had a positive effect on the initiation of smoking.[55] Another predictor is parents' and friends' smoking.[56]

Teenage smoking rates have gone up as expenditures for cigarette advertisements increased.[57] Of all smokers, 80% began as teenagers. An important factor in whether adolescents smoke is the neighborhood of residence. Prosocial activities within neighborhoods reduce the likelihood of smoking.[58] It is also beneficial when retailers refuse to sell cigarettes to minors. In random compliance checks, it was found that 10.9% of retailers sold cigarettes to minors. This figure is greatly reduced from the 40.1% that sold cigarettes to minors in 1997.[59]

Young people smoke to appear mature, to display independence, to cope with stress, or to bond with peers. Adolescent smoking has a high correlation with psychological distress.[60] Also, there is a strong relationship between depression and smoking.[61] Moreover, it has been demonstrated that there is a connection between nicotine dependence and low self-esteem.[62] A study spanning 25 years showed that adolescents who smoked 20 or more cigarettes daily were several times more likely than those who smoke 20 or fewer cigarettes a day to develop agoraphobia, generalized anxiety disorder, and panic disorder.[63] On the other hand, a study of late adolescent and young adult females who described themselves as having a personally meaningful spirituality found that they had lower rates of cigarette use.[64] Other studies confirm that regular religious attendance correlates with lower smoking rates.[65]

Peers seem to be more important than parents in determining whether young people smoke, although children of parents who stop smoking are not as likely to take up smoking and are more likely to quit smoking.[66] The most important factors in whether a teenager smokes are if the teenager's friends smoke, if the perceived benefits outweigh the risks, and if the teenager's household includes smokers.[67] One study found that the influence for smoking starts as early as sixth grade.[68] This is not to suggest that parental smoking is not a factor. Parents who smoked and were not especially concerned about the effects of smoking were more likely to have children who smoke.[69] Similarly, parents who strongly disapproved of smoking were less likely to have children who smoked.[70] Children of women who smoked during pregnancy had a higher rate of smoking than children whose mothers did not smoke.[71] Also, there may be a genetic connection between parental smoking and nicotine dependence in adolescents.[72]

Smoking is a form of experimentation for many young people, and whether they continue depends to some extent on whether they perceive the physiological effects of smoking as negative and whether they receive further social reinforcement for smoking.[73] It has been shown that very few youths are aware of the chemicals in cigarettes, even though most claim to be knowledgeable about this.[74]

Many studies demonstrate that most young people who use marijuana and other illegal drugs began with cigarettes, not alcohol.[75] Cigarette smoking in conjunction with alcohol use, however, is a strong predictor of illegal drug use. Also, smoking correlates highly with binge drinking.[76] Data from the CDC show a link between cigarette use and other behaviors.

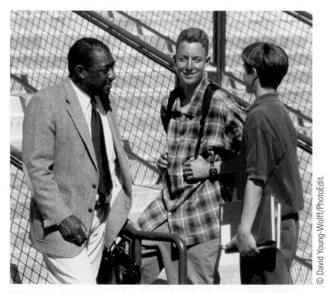
© David Young-Wolff/PhotoEdit.

Parents and respected adults influence teenagers' decision to smoke.

Cigarette Brands Most Preferred by Cigarette Smokers Ages 12 to 17

- Marlboro—48%
- Newport—23.2%
- Camel—10.1%
- Kool—2.7%
- Parliament—2.0%

Source: Substance Abuse and Mental Health Services Administration, *National Household Survey on Drug Abuse* (Department of Health and Human Services, 2002).

Compared with nonsmokers, smokers are less likely to wear seat belts, to use condoms, and to participate on a sports team and are more likely to get into fights, have sexual intercourse (and with more partners), and use steroids.

Teens are three times more responsive to cigarette advertisements than adults are.[77] To counter this, U.S. Food and Drug Administration (FDA) regulations banning tobacco advertisements on billboards within 1,000 feet of schools and playgrounds went into effect in 1997. Also, cigarettes cannot be sold in packs of fewer than 20 or given as samples. To get around the ban on the advertising of tobacco products, tobacco marketers place tobacco brand names in commercials for other products.[78]

As taxes on cigarettes have increased, the rate of use has decreased.[79] Federal taxes have been more effective than state taxes because people in low-tax states would smuggle cigarettes into high-tax states. In a study of smokers in Massachusetts, after a 25-cent increase went into effect, 3.5% of adult smokers quit smoking, 35% considered quitting, and 19% cut back their smoking or switched to lower-cost cigarettes.[80] One effective strategy for reducing teen smoking is better enforcement of laws for selling cigarettes to teens.[81] However, more teens are buying cigarettes through the Internet.[82] Of teenage smokers, 21% considered quitting and 26% cut back.

When teaching young people about the dangers of tobacco, one challenge is that harmful effects take years to appear, if they show up at all. Therefore, teenagers do not contemplate the risks of their behaviors. Although students know of the long-term negative health consequences of tobacco use, this knowledge does not dissuade them from smoking.[83] Emphasizing the short-term or cosmetic effects may have a greater impact. For instance, smoking causes premature wrinkles—a consequence that is of more concern to teens than the more serious long-term effects. Also, teens are more likely to respond to immediate effects such as smelly clothes and bad breath.

Only in the last few years have tobacco prevention programs been evaluated rigorously. Many programs operate on the assumption that if young people have knowledge about the hazards of tobacco, they will not begin to use tobacco or will cease using it. Most programs that are information based have been shown to be ineffective in reducing the onset of smoking. Programs geared to teaching young people about the social pressures to smoke and how to tactfully refuse cigarettes are more effective as deterrents. This is especially true if tobacco prevention programs are started before smoking is initiated.[84] Emphasizing an adolescent's psychological well-being may help because depression and anxiety symptoms play a role in the initiation of smoking.[85] Some smoking prevention programs strive to delay the onset of smoking. These programs have had mixed success.[86]

Social influence programs stress the role of peers, culture, and the media. Stressing social influences makes sense because most young people who use tobacco first do so in a social context. Some social influence programs have reduced smoking by adolescents. Moreover, the cost of drug prevention results in huge financial savings in terms of health care costs.[87] Another reason that smoking prevention programs are important is that young people who take up smoking, especially before age 15, are much more likely to use illegal drugs.[88]

Tobacco prevention programs, especially those that operate outside of schools, seem to be more effective with high-risk youths. Community organizations and groups have the potential to reach young people who do not respond to in-school programs. Preventive interventions might be improved by targeting parent, school, and community outcomes with an emphasis on social norms, peer influence, and acceptance of deviant behaviors.[89]

As suggested above, the younger one is when smoking is initiated, the more likely it is that one will become nicotine dependent.[90] Figure 7.1 highlights the rates of nicotine dependence for young smokers.

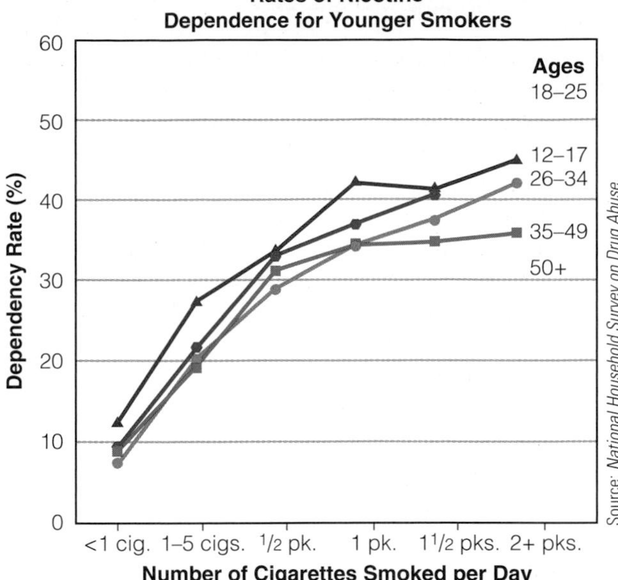

Figure 7.1 **Data from the National Household Survey on Drug Abuse show that the rate of nicotine dependence is higher among those younger than age 25 than in other age groups and that the dependence in these younger people develops with less exposure to nicotine.**

Nicotine Tolerance and Dependence

When people first attempt to smoke or chew, they may experience palpitations, dizziness and nausea, perspiration, and vomiting. Experienced smokers and chewers, however, build up tolerance quickly, some in a matter of weeks. Most people who use tobacco products continue to do so because nicotine is addictive. The term *addiction*, however, typically is associated with narcotics, not nicotine—which ignores the addictiveness of nicotine. Tobacco industry documents dating back to the 1960s describe the addictive properties of nicotine.[91] Nevertheless, the addictive quality of nicotine might be exaggerated in the United States.[92] Half of the people in the United States who have smoked no longer do so. Moreover, most people who quit are able to do so without the benefit of nicotine replacement.

Millions of people smoke 20 to 50 cigarettes daily. Few drugs are used as often. The compulsion for cigarette smoking was illustrated during World War II, when German prisoners of war traded food for cigarettes. Information about the harmful effects of smoking is well known. Most smokers would like to quit, and most are aware that smoking causes cancer.

Despite the desire to quit and the knowledge that cigarettes are detrimental, people continue to smoke. The effects of nicotine are highly reinforcing. Nicotine reaches the brain in a few seconds. To compensate for the reduction of nicotine in the blood, smokers simply light up another cigarette. Not everyone who uses tobacco products becomes addicted, though. The percentage of tobacco users who become addicted is not known. Nevertheless, nicotine addicts exhibit symptoms characteristic of other forms of addiction. They develop tolerance, have a strong desire for continued use, and undergo withdrawal. Rituals connected to smoking, such as lighting a cigarette after eating and when talking on the phone, become ingrained in one's behavior. A sense of comfort comes from rituals, and suddenly stopping these rituals is difficult.

Symptoms of Withdrawal

Although nicotine withdrawal is not fatal and varies from one person to another, the symptoms can be uncomfortable. The severity of withdrawal symptoms

Nicotine Withdrawal Symptoms

- Lower heart rate
- Tremors
- Aggressiveness
- Hunger
- Heart palpitations
- Headaches
- Anxiety
- Lower blood pressure
- Shorter attention span
- Increased circulation
- Insomnia
- Fatigue
- Drowsiness
- Craving for nicotine

is somewhat proportional to nicotine intake: The more one takes in, the greater the withdrawal symptoms. The symptoms are most acute 24 to 48 hours after tobacco use is ended, although the nicotine craving can remain for weeks or even years.

Symptoms of withdrawal include lower heart rate and blood pressure, difficulty maintaining attention, heightened aggressiveness, increased peripheral blood flow, insomnia, tremors, and hunger. Additional symptoms include heart palpitations, headaches, drowsiness, fatigue, and anxiety. The strongest symptom is a craving for nicotine. Numerous studies in England found that exercise, even as little as five minutes, ameliorates nicotine withdrawal symptoms.[93]

Pharmacology of Tobacco

Nicotine is one of about 4,000 chemical substances found in tobacco smoke. It has been used as an insecticide (60 mg can cause human death) and is carcinogenic. Nicotine is a stimulant with characteristics similar to those of amphetamines and cocaine. Nicotine injected intravenously is 5 to 10 times more reinforcing than cocaine injected intravenously. Nicotine releases the neurotransmitter **norepinephrine**, which is responsible for producing stimulation. As with other stimulants, depression follows arousal.

Even though nicotine speeds up blood flow to the skeletal muscles, smokers tend to have cold feet and hands because of the constriction of blood vessels. Nicotine also interferes with the ability to urinate and occasionally causes diarrhea.

Nicotine is absorbed almost immediately by the lungs and can reach the brain in as little as 10 seconds. One factor contributing to its addictiveness is the speed with which it works, since drugs that provide immediate relief are more likely to be repeated. Smokers feel the effects of nicotine every time they inhale. One way to reduce nicotine levels may be to smoke fewer cigarettes, but unfortunately, the amount of nicotine taken into the body is not reduced much because smokers will just smoke more of each cigarette.

After nicotine is absorbed in the body, it is distributed quickly throughout. Besides traversing the blood and brain, nicotine passes through the placenta of a pregnant woman to the fetus and has been found in breast milk. The liver metabolizes almost all of the nicotine before it is excreted by the kidneys. Nicotine stays in the body for 8 to 12 hours.

Physical Effects on the Individual

As early as the 1950s the tobacco industry was aware that tobacco use was linked to illness. Figure 7.2 depicts the health effects on the human body. It is believed that tobacco manufacturers have the technology to produce cigarettes containing fewer toxic chemicals,[94] but if tobacco companies produce and advertise a safer cigarette, this implies that cigarettes already on the market are unsafe, leaving them open to further litigation.

The World Health Organization (WHO) identified smoking as the single most important preventable cause of death in Europe.[95] Today, it is estimated that smoking is responsible for nearly 1 in 5 deaths in the United States.[96] Cigarette smoking is one of the leading *preventable* causes of disability and death in the United States. More Americans have died from smoking than from World War II and the Vietnam War combined. Cigarette smoking is the most prominent behavioral cause of lung cancer, other respiratory diseases, and cardiovascular diseases. Cigarette smoking is responsible for more than 440,000 deaths annually.[97]

The use of tobacco products represents one of the most serious public health problems today. If 440,000 people in the United States were to die from influenza, tuberculosis, smallpox, measles, or any other preventable disease, the situation would be deemed catastrophic. Health care professionals would mobilize forces. Yet according to the CDC, adult male smokers lose 13.2 years of life and female smokers lose on average 14.5 years.[98]

Either directly or indirectly, society bears the cost of tobacco-related problems, and smokers pay the price of impaired health. It is estimated that cigarette smoking is responsible for $167 billion in annual health-related economic losses in the United States—$75 billion in direct medical costs and $92 billion in lost productivity. In total, the economic cost of smoking is about $3,561 per adult smoker.[99] As shown in Table 7.3, a greater percentage of smokers compared to nonsmokers miss 5 or more days of work per month.[100] Moreover, family members of smokers make four more visits per year to health care facilities than families of nonsmokers. Nonsmokers pay for the health care costs of smokers through higher taxes and insurance premiums.

norepinephrine A neurotransmitter that may help regulate appetite and reduce fatigue

carbon monoxide Gas in cigarette smoke that interferes with oxygen-carrying capacity of blood

Heart Disease and Strokes

Although cigarette smoking is most often associated with lung cancer, smoking causes more cardiovascular deaths than cancer deaths. Each year, 170,000 premature deaths from coronary heart disease are attributed to smoking, and smoking is implicated in 30% of all deaths from coronary heart disease. In the United States, smoking is believed to be the most important modifiable risk factor related to heart disease. Of people younger than age 40 who undergo coronary bypass operations, the majority are smokers. Nonetheless, heart disease due to smoking has declined significantly. When New York City implemented its smoking ban in 2004, the number of people who went to hospitals due to heart attacks declined by 4,000.[101] The risk of a heart attack increases among women older than age 35 who smoke cigarettes and use oral contraceptives. Moreover, the likelihood of experiencing a stroke increases for women who smoke and use oral contraceptives.[102] Also, women smokers who are taking oral contraceptives are more likely to have brain hemorrhages.[103]

Autopsies performed on U.S. service personnel who died in the Korean and Vietnam Wars revealed that cardiovascular disease begins early in life. Also, smoking is linked to type 2 diabetes in women. Diabetes is a major risk factor for cardiovascular disease.

Cardiovascular damage is correlated with the frequency and length of time a person smokes. Nicotine raises the heart rate and blood pressure, forcing the heart to work harder. Cigarettes also produce **carbon monoxide**, which impedes the oxygen-carrying capacity of the blood.[104] Because carbon monoxide impairs circulation, cholesterol deposits increase. This can lead to arteriosclerosis, a condition more common in smokers than in nonsmokers.

Another condition related to tobacco is Buerger's disease, which can result in amputation of the extremities as a result of poor circulation. Buerger's disease affects mostly young male tobacco users. Tobacco cessation reduces the chances of limb amputation.[105] Smokers also are at greater risk of dying from strokes. Carbon monoxide and nicotine affect the adhesiveness

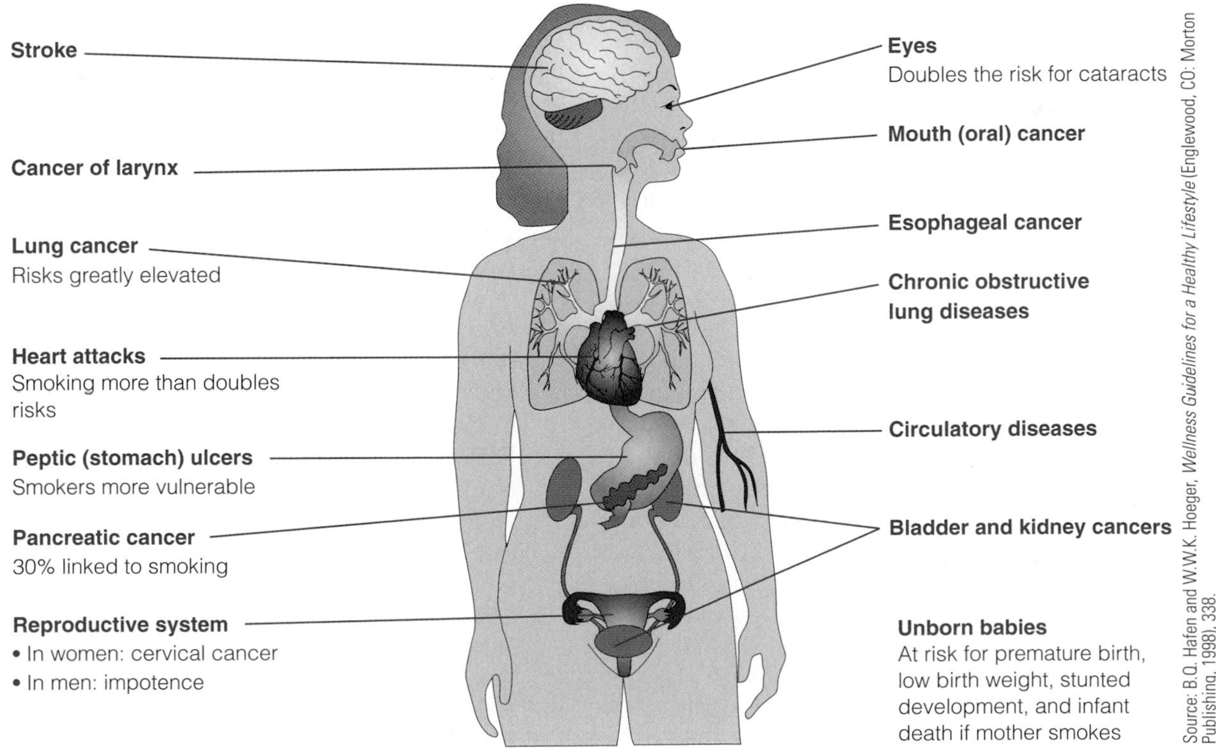

Source: B.Q. Hafen and W.W.K. Hoeger, *Wellness Guidelines for a Healthy Lifestyle* (Englewood, CO: Morton Publishing, 1998), 338.

Figure 7.2 Health Effects of Smoking

TABLE 7.3 Percentages of Full-Time Workers Ages 18 to 64 Who Missed 5 or More Days of Work in the Past Month Due to Illness or Injury

Age	Past Month Smokers	Past Month Nonsmokers
18–25	4.5%	3.5%
26–34	3.5%	3.3%
35–44	4.1%	2.6%
45–64	4.7%	3.0%

Source: *The NSDUH Report*, May 17, 2007. Office of Applied Studies, Substance Abuse and Mental Health Services Administration (SAMHSA). Available at http://oas.samhsa.gov/2k7/workMissed/workMissed.htm.

of platelets in the brain, hastening the formation of clots and the possibility of strokes. Finally, nicotine interferes with blood flow to the brain by constricting blood vessels, which also can result in strokes.

Respiratory Diseases

Two common respiratory conditions caused by smoking are chronic coughing (smoker's cough) and shortness of breath. More serious conditions are chronic bronchitis and emphysema, which appear almost exclusively in smokers and are referred to as chronic obstructive pulmonary disease (COPD). Bronchitis develops as a result of smoke irritating the bronchi, or air passages, which go from the windpipe to the lungs. Tar builds up on the cilia (hairlike structures that rid the body of foreign matter), and breathing becomes more labored. Because the cilia become less effective, smokers cough persistently and regurgitate phlegm. Not only does smoking reduce lung functioning during childhood and adolescence, but also the lung functioning of infants is reduced if mothers smoke during pregnancy.[106] An especially puzzling scenario is that of asthmatics who smoke. It was found that high school students with asthma used cigarettes, cigars, marijuana, and inhalants at rates equal to or greater than high school students without asthma.[107]

Emphysema is a disabling, incurable disease caused by the lungs' inability to retain normal elasticity and normal amounts of air. The lungs' inability to absorb oxygen as a result of smoking disables the lungs' tiny air sacs, causing shortness of breath. People with emphysema often die from cardiovascular problems. Women are especially vulnerable to respiratory problems. Current female smokers who are ages 35 or older are more than 10 times more likely to die from emphysema than nonsmoking females.[108]

Cancer

Besides carbon monoxide, other gases in tobacco smoke include ammonia, benzopyrene, hydrogen cyanide, nitrosamines, and vinyl chloride. These are just some of the nearly four dozen gases in tobacco smoke that are capable of producing cancer. Most of the cancer-causing substances are found in the tar of tobacco, though nicotine has been implicated in cancer as well. Cigarette packages are required to list levels of tar.

Cancer rates linked to tobacco use are increasing. Cigarette smoking is responsible for at least 30% of all cancers deaths and 87% of lung cancer deaths.[109] More women now die from lung cancer than from breast cancer. Lung cancer is the most common type of cancer in men also. Rates of lung cancer are higher in Black smokers than in White smokers, possibly because Blacks metabolize nicotine more rapidly than Whites, not because they smoke more. One study found that women are considerably more likely than men to develop lung cancer, even if their smoking rates are equivalent.[110]

Cigarette smoking is the leading risk factor for developing cancers of the larynx, mouth, esophagus, pancreas, and bladder. The chances of developing cancers of the oral cavity, pancreas, esophagus, kidney, larynx, trachea, and bladder are greater among smokers than among nonsmokers. Men who smoked $2\frac{1}{2}$ packs of cigarettes a day for 30 to 39 years had a significantly higher risk of developing non-Hodgkin's lymphoma.[111] Oral and pharyngeal cancers account for almost 8,000 deaths annually in the United States. The warning signs of oral cancer include the following:

- A sore in the mouth that does not heal (most common symptom)
- A white or red patch on the gums, tongue, tonsil, or lining of the mouth that will not go away
- A lump or thickening in the cheek
- A sore throat or a feeling that something is caught in the throat
- Difficulty chewing or swallowing
- Difficulty moving the jaw or tongue
- Numbness of the tongue or other area of the mouth
- Swelling of the jaw that causes dentures to fit poorly or become uncomfortable
- Loosening of the teeth or pain around the teeth or jaw
- Voice changes
- A lump or mass in the neck
- Weight loss

The Impact of Smoking during Pregnancy

The carbon monoxide in tobacco smoke interferes with the fetus. Babies born to women who smoke during pregnancy weigh less and are more likely to be delivered prematurely than babies born to women who do not smoke while pregnant. Pregnant smokers have a higher incidence of spontaneous abortions (miscarriage) than nonsmokers, as well as higher rates of stillbirths. One Swedish study involving more than 500,000 women found that smokers had a considerably higher rate of stillbirths than nonsmokers.[112] Smoking also significantly reduces fertility in women. A Danish study reported that smoking during pregnancy may reduce the likelihood of sons' future fertility by reducing sperm count.[113]

Sudden infant death syndrome (SIDS), in which infants suddenly stop breathing, occurs at a higher rate among babies of women who smoked during pregnancy. According to the Foundation for the Study of Infant Deaths (FSID), maternal smoking is the most important avoidable risk factor for SIDS.[114] Congenital malformations such as cleft lip and cleft palate are also more likely in children of smokers. There is evidence that children of mothers who smoke during pregnancy have higher rates of psychological problems such as attention problems and hyperactivity, although it is difficult to prove that maternal smoking causes these problems.[115]

While many women stop smoking once they become pregnant, various studies show that 15% to 37% of women smoke while pregnant.[116] Older women were less likely to quit smoking during pregnancy. An important factor in whether pregnant adolescent girls continued to smoke was having friends who smoke. It was reported that females who initiate smoking prior to age 15 are likely to continue to smoke during pregnancy.[117] A British study reported that women smokers had a 40% reduced chance of becoming pregnant.[118]

Tobacco and Physical Activity

Although smokers claim they are more alert and aroused after smoking, their ability to engage in physical activity is impaired demonstrably. The mucous membranes of the trachea and the bronchial tubes enlarge as a result of smoking, restricting the ability to get air in and out of the lungs. The alveoli in the lungs receive less oxygen, so respiratory demands, especially during exercise, are harder to meet. Conversely, the role of physical activity in one's lifestyle is important in whether one initiates smoking. A Finnish study found that physically inactive adolescents were more likely to smoke as adults.[119]

Smoking also impairs sexual activity. Carbon monoxide hampers production of the male sex hormone testosterone. Sexual excitement and erection in males diminish because nicotine constricts the blood vessels. The number of sperm in male smokers is reduced significantly, and sperm motility is sluggish.

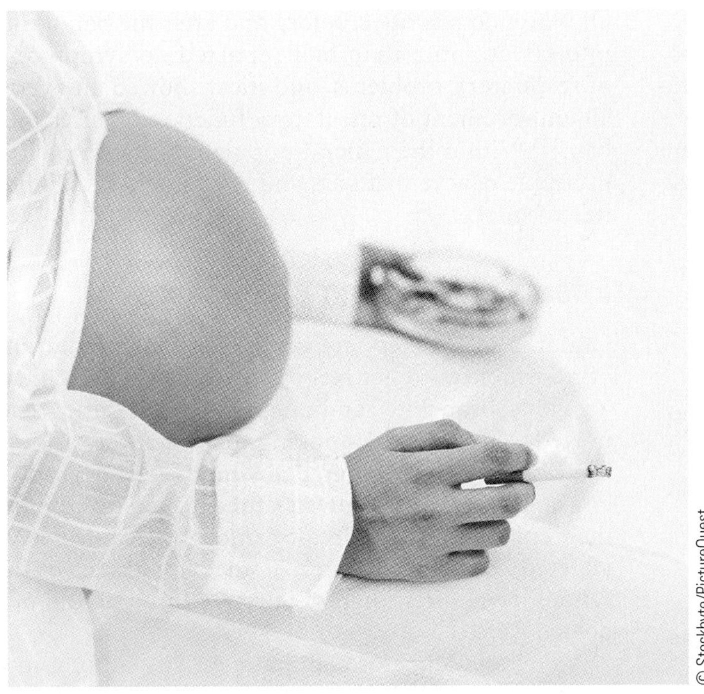

© Stockbyte/PictureQuest

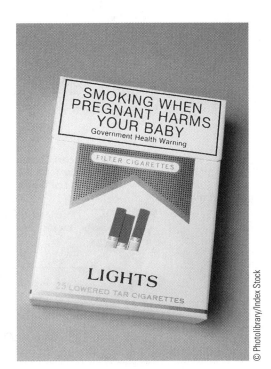

© Photolibrary/Index Stock

Pregnant women who smoke increase the risk of having preterm pregnancies and babies with low birth weights.

Numerous studies have noted that smoking causes erectile dysfunction in a significant number of men.[120]

Passive Smoke

The detrimental effects of tobacco are not limited to smokers. **Passive smoke**, also called involuntary or **environmental tobacco smoke (ETS)** and secondhand smoke, is a major source of indoor air pollution in the home and workplace. Passive smoke is blamed for 3,800 lung cancer deaths each year and accounts for 8,000 to 26,000 new asthma cases in children.[121] The extent of harm is related to the degree of exposure. Some critics claim that studies linking passive smoking to lung cancer are biased.[122] Nonetheless, the economic impact of environmental tobacco smoke is estimated at nearly $10 billion in terms of costs for medical care, mortality, and morbidity.[123]

Many nonsmokers report emotional discomfort from being around people who are smoking. Passive smoke is classified as mainstream or sidestream smoke. **Mainstream smoke** is the smoke that smokers exhale after inhaling. Figure 7.3 shows the composition of mainstream smoke. **Sidestream smoke** is the smoke that comes from the burning end of the cigarette, pipe, or cigar. Because sidestream smoke does not pass through a filter and burns at a hotter temperature, it contains more nicotine and carbon monoxide than mainstream smoke. Children of smokers have five times as much cotinine (a byproduct of nicotine) in their urine as children of nonsmokers.[124]

Laws against smoking in public places were precipitated by research pointing out the effects of sidestream smoke. Not only are there more restrictions on indoor smoking, but a number of communities are prohibiting smoking in public parks.[125] The following discussion examines the effects of tobacco smoke on nonsmokers and children of smokers.

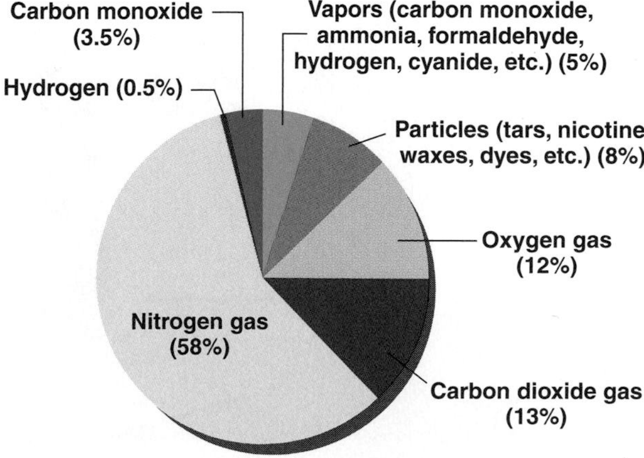

Figure 7.3 Chemical Composition of Mainstream Smoke

Effects on Nonsmokers

Besides irritating the nose and eyes, passive smoke causes many significant health problems. Environmental tobacco smoke has been linked to lung and urinary tract problems and to cancers of the liver and pancreas. Passive and active smoke increase the risk of breast cancer.[126] Lung cancer rates are higher for people who live with a smoker, and passive smoke at work increases the risk of lung cancer also.[127] For example, a Canadian study reported that people exposed to a lot of secondhand smoke, such as workers in bars and restaurants, have three times the risk of developing lung cancer.[128] Nonsmoking men and women who develop emphysema, chronic bronchitis, and asthma from exposure to passive smoke are more likely to develop lung cancer later.[129] According to a report from the U.S. Surgeon General, for nonsmokers who live with smokers, secondhand smoke increases the risk of heart disease by 25% to 30% and the risk of lung cancer 20% to 30%.[130] Nonsmokers married to smokers have three times the rate of heart attacks of people with nonsmoking spouses.[131] Also, there is some evidence that the risk of dementia increases due to secondhand smoke.[132]

The Environmental Protection Agency officially declared secondhand smoke a carcinogen in 1993.[133] Starting on January 1, 1998, tobacco smoking was prohibited from all bars and taverns in California. Of bartenders studied before and after the ban went into effect, more than half reported no symptoms of respiratory problems, and most showed an overall improvement of respiratory functioning after the ban.[134] Within the general population, the majority of people believe that bars and restaurants should be free of smoke.[135]

Effects on Children of Smokers

Children of smokers are more likely than children of nonsmokers to get respiratory infections including colds, bronchitis, and pneumonia. One study reported that maternal smoking increased the risk of bronchitis by 14%.[136] Yet, many mothers who smoke downplay the harmful effects of their smoking around their children.[137] Children of smokers are adversely affected academically because they are absent from school more often than children whose parents do not smoke.[138]

The incidence of asthma is greater among infants and young children who have been subjected to sidestream smoke. In fact, the general likelihood of ill health is more significant if both parents smoke.

Furthermore, some of the adverse effects from parental smoking are emotional; maternal smoking during pregnancy was associated with higher rates of depression, anxiety, and associated substance abuse in adolescents ages 16 to 18.[139] In addition, women who smoke while pregnant have toddlers who are more likely to exhibit more negative behaviors, such as physical aggression and hyperactivity-impulsivity.[140] It has also been shown that preadolescents were more likely to smoke if their mothers smoked during pregnancy.[141] One study found that passive smoke increased the risk of sickle cell anemia 1.9 times.[142] It has also been reported that passive smoke significantly increased the risk of dental cavities in children.[143]

passive smoke Tobacco smoke present in the air from someone else's smoking and inhaled by others

environmental tobacco smoke (ETS) Smoke in the air as a result of someone smoking

mainstream smoke Smoke exhaled by a smoker

sidestream smoke Smoke that comes from the burning end of a cigarette, pipe, or cigar

Rights of Smokers versus Nonsmokers

Balancing the rights of people who smoke against the rights of people who are opposed to smoking is difficult. Despite the detrimental effects of tobacco on health, should people be penalized for an addiction that is hard to overcome?

Antismoking Legislation

To discourage minors from smoking, federal legislation in 1997 established a minimum age of 18 to purchase tobacco products, and anyone under age 27 must show photo identification. The federal law represents a culmination of much state and local legislation. Numerous legislative efforts to limit smoking were initiated in the 1980s. By the end of 1995, about 1,006 local tobacco control ordinances against smoking had been initiated. The tobacco industry countered by getting state legislators to introduce statewide laws that would take precedence over local laws. In the 2008 presidential race, candidates were asked whether they would support a federal ban on public smoking. The candidates expressed their disapproval of smoking but felt that prohibiting public smoking was the responsibility of various states.[144]

Despite the efforts of tobacco companies, more than 75% of state legislators have supported measures to limit the purchase of tobacco products, especially by minors.[145] Even in Greensboro, North Carolina, home of several large tobacco companies, residents voted to restrict smoking. San Francisco voters approved legislation that forbade smoking not just in public areas but in the private workplace as well. A Massachusetts law stipulated that all new police officers and firefighters were forbidden from smoking—on and off the job. The U.S. Congress required cigarette packages and advertisements to include one of four health warnings, which are rotated every 3 months (see Figure 7.4).

Concerns regarding passive smoking prompted every federal agency to limit or prohibit smoking in public areas and workplaces. In 1994, the U.S. Department of Labor proposed a ban on workplace smoking, affecting about 6 million worksites. The Department of Defense implemented its own ban.

Questions Related to Rights of Smokers and Nonsmokers

- Does a person have the right to engage in self-destructive behavior?
- Does society have a moral obligation to help others overcome self-destructive behaviors?
- Should a person be penalized if he or she is addicted to nicotine?
- Does society have a responsibility to help a person who has an addiction?
- Does it matter if the substance to which a person is addicted is legal?
- Should a person be stigmatized for a behavior over which he or she has little control?
- Are smokers ultimately helped by being stigmatized?

SURGEON GENERAL'S WARNING:
Cigarette Smoke Contains Carbon Monoxide

SURGEON GENERAL'S WARNING:
Smoking Causes Lung Cancer, Heart Disease, Emphysema and May Complicate Pregnancy.

SURGEON GENERAL'S WARNING:
Smoking by Pregnant Women May Result in Fetal Injury, Premature Birth, and Low Birth Weight.

SURGEON GENERAL'S WARNING:
Quitting Smoking Now Greatly Reduces Serious Risks to Your Health.

Figure 7.4 Warnings from the Surgeon General Required for Tobacco Products

In New Zealand it was found that workers disapproved of smoking in the workplace.[146]

In New York City, tobacco advertisements are banned on all city-owned billboards and on private outdoor advertising media within 1,000 feet of a school.

Based on support prompted by a statewide initiative, the state of California spent $28 million on an advertising campaign to dissuade individuals from smoking. This initiative passed despite tobacco companies' spending $15 million to defeat it. To finance this antismoking effort, a cigarette tax of 25 cents per pack was implemented. In essence, smokers contributed to the campaign to persuade them to stop smoking. Cigarette sales declined, and lung cancer rates dropped.[147]

In 1990, airline passengers on all commercial flights within the continental United States, including Puerto Rico and the Virgin Islands, were forbidden from smoking. This ban extended to flights to Alaska and Hawaii that were shorter than 6 hours. Foreign airlines flying in the United States have cooperated in the effort to prohibit smoking. In 1990, Amtrak passenger trains banned smoking in first-class cars in the northeast corridor, but passengers are permitted to smoke in sleeping compartments and in smoking cars.

Exposure to workplace environmental tobacco smoke has been found to double the risk of lung cancer.[148] To reduce workplace smoking, many companies offer financial incentives (in some cases, disincentives) to workers. Some companies require workers who smoke to pay more than nonsmokers toward health insurance costs. Companies and individuals alike benefit from these incentives: The worker is less likely to become ill, health insurance expenses of the companies are lower, and absenteeism is reduced. Another reason that employers may want to prohibit workplace smoking is because of the significant legal risks posed by employees exposed to secondhand smoke. In a number of cases, employers have been sued by employees whose health was compromised by secondhand smoking.[149]

Although no law requires fast-food restaurants to ban smoking, many have implemented their own bans. An estimated 25% of customers and 40% of workers at fast-food restaurants are younger than age 18. Taco Bell restaurants and one-third of the members of the National Council of Chain Restaurants have not allowed smoking since March 1994.

One concern that restaurant owners express is that a smoking ban will result in a significant loss of business; however, a study of the first 13 U.S. cities to ban smoking found no loss in customers.[150] When New York City prohibited smoking in restaurants, concern likewise was raised that tourism and restaurant sales would decline. Instead, tourists spent more money.[151] Like New York, the revenues of restaurants in California increased after the ban on indoor smoking went into effect.[152]

One factor that affects both state revenues and the purchase of cigarettes is the sales tax on them. Table 7.4 shows the cigarette taxes in 2007 and how the states compare with each other.

The Master Settlement Agreement

If smokers become sick, who is responsible? Should the responsibility lie with tobacco companies or with the smoker? Legislation passed in November 1998 requires the tobacco industry to pay $206 billion among all 50 states. In exchange for this payment, 46 states agreed to end their litigation against the four largest tobacco companies.[153] The purpose of the fine is to compensate states for medical costs resulting from cigarette smoking and to create a $500 million fund to educate young people about the risks of smoking.[154] The Master Settlement Agreement states that tobacco companies are no longer liable for addiction or dependence claims, class action suits, and claims of punitive damages. The people who bear the brunt of this legislation are smokers, because the cost will be passed on to them.

Another aspect of the Master Settlement Agreement was that tobacco companies were totally banned from sponsoring football, basketball, baseball, soccer, and hockey. Each tobacco company was allowed to sponsor one other sport per year. The language has been interpreted broadly. Sponsorship of the Winston Cup racing series, for example, may entail sponsorship of the entire racing season. In addition, tobacco companies may sponsor a race car on which the name of the cigarette is shown repeatedly.[155]

In 2004, then New York Attorney General Eliot Spitzer sued Brown & Williamson Tobacco Corporation for violating the Master Settlement Agreement. Spitzer maintained that Brown & Williamson was promoting KOOL cigarettes through its hip-hop music sponsorship.[156]

Individuals have also sued tobacco companies. In a case in New Jersey, a man was awarded $400,000 for the death of his 58-year-old wife, who died after smoking for 42 years. That award later was overturned, with the court ruling that the woman was 80% at fault for her own death. Critical issues in the case were the absence of health warnings before 1966 and the fact that the woman was not informed properly of the risks.

In June 2001, a Los Angeles jury awarded a smoker with lung cancer $3 billion in punitive damages and $5.5 billion in general damages from the Philip Morris Companies. The jury stated that the

TABLE 7.4 State Cigarette Excise Tax Rates and Rankings

State	Tax	Rank	State	Tax	Rank
Alabama	$0.425	42nd	Nebraska	$0.64	35th
Alaska	$2.00	6th	Nevada	$0.80	32nd
Arizona	$2.00	6th	New Hampshire	$1.33	22nd
Arkansas	$0.59	38th	New Jersey	$2.58	2nd
California	$0.87	30th	New Mexico	$0.91	29th
Colorado	$0.84	31st	New York	$2.75	1st
Connecticut	$2.00	6th	North Carolina	$0.35	45th
Delaware	$1.15	25th	North Dakota	$0.44	41st
DC	$2.00	6th	Ohio	$1.25	23rd
Florida	$0.339	46th	Oklahoma	$1.03	26th
Georgia	$0.37	43rd	Oregon	$1.18	24th
Hawaii	$2.00	6th	Pennsylvania	$1.35	21st
Idaho	$0.57	39th	Rhode Island	$2.46	4th
Illinois	$0.98	28th	South Carolina	$0.07	51st
Indiana	$0.995	27th	South Dakota	$1.53	17th
Iowa	$1.36	20th	Tennessee	$0.62	36th
Kansas	$0.79	33rd	Texas	$1.41	19th
Kentucky	$0.30	47th	Utah	$0.695	34th
Louisiana	$0.36	44th	Vermont	$1.99	14th
Maine	$2.00	6th	Virginia	$0.30	47th
Maryland	$2.00	6th	Washington	$2.025	5th
Massachusetts	$2.51	3rd	West Virginia	$0.55	40th
Michigan	$2.00	6th	Wisconsin	$1.77	15th
Minnesota*	$1.504	18th	Wyoming	$0.60	37th
Mississippi	$0.18	49th	Puerto Rico	$1.23	NA
Missouri	$0.17	50th	Guam	$1.00	NA
Montana	$1.70	16th	Northern Marianas	$1.75	NA

* Tax stamp includes 75-cent health impact fee and 27.4-cent cigarette sales tax.

Source: Campaign for Tobacco-Free Kids. *State Cigarette Excise Tax Rates & Rankings*. October 15, 2008. Available from http://tobaccofreekids.org/research/factsheets/pdf/0097.pdf.

cigarette manufacturer was guilty of fraud, negligence, and making a defective product. Philip Morris is appealing the verdict.[157]

Some maintain that cigarette companies did their own research in the 1950s, which revealed a link between cigarettes and lung cancer, but that this information was not made public. On January 4, 1954, tobacco companies took out full-page advertisements in newspapers throughout the United States with a circulation of 50,000 or more pledging that they would cooperate closely with individuals interested in safeguarding the public's health. Yet tobacco companies continue to court politicians.

Legislative actions against tobacco companies are spreading to countries outside of the United States. Lawsuits against these companies are pending in Israel, Argentina, Guatemala, Venezuela, Bolivia, Nicaragua, Finland, France, Japan, Norway, Sri Lanka, Thailand, and Turkey.[158]

Cessation Techniques

Most smokers say they would like to stop. It usually takes several attempts. The first few months are critical. Forty-one percent of smokers who want to quit are successful for 1 day, but less than 5% were able to abstain during the next 3 to 12 months.[159] Also, how much people smoke affects how much difficulty they have with stopping. Heavy smokers may need comprehensive cessation programs to stop, and lighter smokers require less intervention.[160] Withdrawal symptoms can be intense, leading to anxiety and a depressed mood. Most people on average require five to seven attempts to quit before they are successful.[161]

The younger a person is when trying to quit smoking, the greater is the benefit. The pulmonary function of people who stopped smoking by age 40 was no worse than that of nonsmokers, but the same was not true for people who waited to quit until age 60.[162] Unfortunately, young people have an especially difficult time stopping smoking. Moreover, state funding for tobacco cessation programs has declined.[163] One study found that teenage smokers have a hard time coping with stress without cigarettes and that their friends who smoke often criticize them for trying to stop smoking.[164] Interestingly, less-educated young adult smokers (ages 18 to 24) have higher rates of smoking but they attempt to quit smoking at the same rate as more-educated young adult smokers.[165]

Stopping the use of smokeless tobacco is more difficult than quitting cigarettes. A number of smokeless tobacco users switch to cigarettes, although few cigarette users switch to smokeless tobacco.[166]

One reason that people have trouble overcoming tobacco dependency is that many activities trigger smoking. People are cued into smoking when waking up, having a cup of coffee, finishing a meal, talking on the phone, driving a car, or drinking alcohol. Smokers who are active alcoholics are less likely to stop smoking than smokers with no history of alcoholism, suggesting that discontinuing alcoholism may increase the potential for successful smoking cessation.[167]

Many smokers are concerned about gaining weight once they stop. Most weight gain occurs during the first year after quitting. The average weight gain is 8 to 13 pounds, although quitters who take up exercise experience less weight gain.[168]

Being paired up with a buddy doubles one's chances of stopping smoking, regardless of the type of treatment.[169] Confidence, not overconfidence, in one's ability to stop smoking is a crucial variable in how long one remains abstinent. Despite the array of smoking cessation programs available, 90% of smokers in the United States who quit do so without benefit of any formal treatment program. Generally, nicotine replacement therapy, such as nicotine gum, nicotine patches, and nicotine inhalers, helps many smokers to stop. On the other hand, drug therapy, aversive techniques, behavior modification, hypnosis, and acupuncture have not been proven conclusively to help.[170] Various cessation techniques are described in the following sections.

Nicotine Gum and Lozenges

If a person is addicted to nicotine, then it would seem logical to fulfill the need for nicotine through a safe source and gradually reduce the need for it. This is the premise of nicotine gum (such as Nicorette) and other nicotine replacement systems. Nicotine gum has been available through prescription since 1984, and beginning in 1996 it could be purchased without a prescription. Nicotine gum reduces withdrawal symptoms associated with cigarettes, but it does not provide the same satisfaction as cigarettes, because nicotine gum is absorbed more slowly. Nicotine is absorbed irregularly and unpredictably, limiting its success. In one study in which free nicotine patches or nicotine gum were offered, 53% of smokers indicated they would seriously consider quitting.[171] One interesting twist is that some people who have never smoked but who have used nicotine gum have become dependent on the gum.[172]

Nicotine gum was less effective with women than with men in another study.[173] Among college students, 24% indicated that nicotine gum was just as harmful as cigarettes.[174] Lozenges containing nicotine might aid smoking cessation. It has been shown that nicotine lozenges increase the likelihood of smoking cessation by 10% when compared to a placebo.[175] Side effects of nicotine lozenges include insomnia, nausea, hiccups, coughing, heartburn, headache, and gas.[176] When asked if they prefer a nicotine mouth spray to nicotine gum, most smokers preferred the nicotine spray even though the mouth spray was no more effective than the gum.[177]

Nicotine Patches

As of 1996, the nicotine patch, containing 30 mg of nicotine, became available as an over-the-counter drug. Nicotine patches consist of synthetic rubber in which nicotine is slowly dissolved.[178] The patch eases withdrawal symptoms that accompany tobacco cessation. Early studies with the nicotine patch demonstrated that it was effective for helping smokers quit. Various studies found that abstinence rates for those using nicotine patches ranged from 23% to 61% in the first six weeks but that success declined afterwards.[179] An English study involving young smokers found that nicotine patches were beneficial in smoking cessation.[180]

Some users report skin rashes. The biggest drawback, however, is that when people continue to smoke while wearing the patch, they receive dangerously high levels of nicotine. In an out-of-court settlement, the Ciba-Geigy Corporation, which sells the nicotine patch Habitrol, changed its advertisements because consumers believed that the patch is more effective than it actually is. Ciba-Geigy was required to include information that pregnant women, nursing mothers, and people with cardiovascular disease should check with their physicians before using the patch. One current study, however, found that nicotine patches do not increase the risk of coronary artery disease.[181]

rapid smoking Aversive smoking-cessation technique in which one smokes rapidly to exceed tolerance and becomes ill

Nicotine Inhalers

The FDA approved the nicotine inhaler in 1996. Similar to nasal inhalers, the nicotine nasal spray pumps small amounts of nicotine from small tubes into the nose. A common side effect is nasal and sinus irritation. Therefore, it is not recommended for people with nasal or sinus conditions, allergies, or asthma. Also, it is not recommended for use exceeding 6 months.

One study reported that nicotine inhalers were more effective if smokers were given the inhalers by a health care provider as opposed to buying the inhalers over the counter.[182] In a review of numerous studies, nicotine replacement therapy was found to double smoking cessation rates compared with a placebo.[183]

Drug Therapy

There are a number of drug therapies that have been developed to treat nicotine addiction. In 1997 the FDA approved the drug Zyban, also known as buproprion and originally prescribed as an antidepressant, for smoking cessation. How Zyban works is unclear, but it does seem to reduce the desire for nicotine. According to one study, Zyban helped 49% of smokers quit for one month.[184] Side effects associated with Zyban are dry mouth, difficulty sleeping, and skin rash. Convulsions and loss of consciousness occur in 1 of every 1,000 people who take the drug. It is contraindicated for people with epilepsy, eating disorders, and women who are pregnant or breastfeeding.

The most recent drug developed for nicotine addiction is varenicline (Chantix). One study involving both varenicline and buproprion found that only 14% of those who took varenicline stopped smoking after one year and only 6% who took buproprion had stopped smoking.[185] Buproprion is used for major depressive disorders and seasonal affective disorder also.[186] Unfortunately, one side effect of buproprion, especially when taken with Prozac, is delirium.[187] Varenicline has been shown to be three times more effective than a placebo.[188] The drug does not appear to be affected by food and it is well-tolerated by users.[189] As of 2007, the cost for a 3-month supply of varenicline was approximately $360.[190]

Antianxiety drugs have been given to smokers who are trying to quit, and these drugs reduce irritability in these individuals. In a pilot study, Prozac was found to help some individuals maintain their abstinence from cigarettes when it was combined with either group therapy or the nicotine patch.[191] Prozac reduces appetite, and this feature may appeal to people who are concerned about weight gain when they quit smoking. Currently, three vaccines are being developed to prevent nicotine addiction. The vaccinations will be tested to determine whether they are effective for smoking cessation.[192]

Aversive Techniques

One aversive technique is to have smokers engage in **rapid smoking** until they exceed their tolerance levels and become ill. The point is to make smoking an unpleasant experience. This technique is similar to negative reinforcement. An obvious drawback is that it may seriously endanger health, especially of a person with a cardiovascular problem. Another aversive technique is to give the drug taker—in this case, the smoker—an electric shock when he or she is engaging in drug use. This technique has been applied to alcohol treatment, and its benefits are short-term at best.

Behavior Modification

The premise of many programs is to change behaviors linked to smoking. Basically, the smoker learns new or alternative behaviors to use in place of smoking. For example, if a person typically smokes after dinner, he or she could take a walk instead. If someone is accustomed to smoking while talking on the telephone, he or she could keep paper and pencils next to the telephone to doodle in lieu of smoking. People can be taught to avoid or deal with situations in which the temptation to smoke might be a problem. Many behavior modification programs include support groups or a buddy system in which the buddy is called when the urge to smoke strikes. Behavioral therapy programs achieve a cessation rate of approximately 20%. These programs have higher success rates when they are augmented with other types of treatment.[193]

Hypnosis

Hypnosis is successful with some people. It seems to work best with people who want it to work; it is most effective with motivated individuals. By the same token, if a person is motivated, the specific program undertaken might not matter. Hypnosis might provide the excuse to motivate people to stop smoking, although hypnosis was not found to be particularly effective for getting pregnant women to stop smoking.[194] One study found that hypnosis as a smoking cessation technique is more effective with men than women.[195]

Acupuncture

The evidence supporting the effectiveness of acupuncture is minimal.[196] The mechanism by which acupuncture stops the desire to smoke is unclear. Nevertheless, advocates of acupuncture claim that it reduces the physical symptoms of withdrawal. They also state that acupuncture reduces the desire for smoking because the process causes endorphins to be released.[197] Acupuncture sessions typically are 30 minutes long, and smokers receive treatment for anywhere from 2 days to 3 months.

Summary

Tobacco played an integral role in the history of the United States because tobacco crops were vital to the survival of the colonial settlement Jamestown, enabling it to prosper. The French government helped finance tobacco farming in the New World, and these funds were used to help the colonies defeat the British during the Revolutionary War.

Initially, tobacco was used in pipes, snuff, and cigars. Cigarette sales increased when the cigarette-rolling machine was developed, because cigarettes became more plentiful and less costly. R. J. Reynolds added saccharine to cigarettes, giving them a sweeter taste and a longer shelf life. At first men used tobacco, then cigarettes were marketed for women, though women were criticized for smoking. Later, young people became the target of cigarette advertisements.

The health cost of tobacco translates to economic loss. Concern over the health effects of tobacco has led to a decline in the percentage of people who smoke. In 1964, when the Office of the U.S. Surgeon General issued its report describing tobacco's hazards, about 50% of adults smoked. Many people subsequently changed to filtered, low-tar, and low-nicotine cigarettes. Light cigarettes deliver the same amount of tar and nicotine as regular cigarettes. They have not been proven to be a safe alternative.

Smoking rates have gone down for men and women alike, though the rate for men has declined more drastically than that for women. Tobacco use correlates with education and occupation. Smoking rates have declined in industrialized countries but have increased in less-developed countries.

People smoke to be more alert, to relax, and to improve their short-term cognitive ability. Children growing up in homes in which parents smoke are more likely to smoke themselves because parents serve as role models. Peers are an important factor, particularly for adolescents. Teens often follow the behavior of peers with whom they associate. When compared with nonsmoking teens, teens who smoke have lower self-esteem, more anxiety, and lower perceptions of internal control. One difficulty in teaching young people about the dangers of tobacco is that the harmful effects take years to appear. Smoking rates have, however, begun to decline among adolescents.

Nicotine is an addictive and carcinogenic component of tobacco. Nicotine is a stimulant that is absorbed almost immediately by the lungs, reduces blood flow, and reaches the brain in seconds. During pregnancy, nicotine is passed to the fetus through the placenta.

Of the more than 400,000 Americans who die each year from smoking, most die from cardiovascular disease. Smoking is the most common factor responsible for sudden death in males. Women who smoke and use oral contraceptives are at greater jeopardy for heart attacks. Smoking increases the risk for strokes, bronchitis, and emphysema. Also, the tar in tobacco increases the risk of cancer. Most deaths from lung cancer are a result of cigarette smoking.

Women who smoke while pregnant deliver babies who weigh less than the typical newborn. Pregnant women also are more likely to have miscarriages and stillbirths, and their babies die more often than others from sudden infant death syndrome (SIDS).

Passive smoke is linked to health problems for nonsmokers. Mates of smokers are more likely to develop heart conditions, and children of smokers are more likely to have respiratory problems.

Federal agencies now forbid or limit smoking in public areas, and many state and local laws regulate public smoking. The 1998 tobacco agreement placed further restrictions on the promotion of tobacco products. Airlines have banned smoking on most flights. Some companies offer incentives to workers to quit smoking.

Smoking cessation is difficult. Because smoking is tied to many other behaviors, breaking the link is difficult. People who quit tend to believe that they were responsible for their success, rather than a program, and they have lower relapse rates.

Thinking Critically

1. In 1989, R. J. Reynolds test-marketed a new cigarette called Uptown, targeted specifically to African American men and women. Although this marketing campaign was dropped, can you find examples of tobacco products promoted more heavily to minorities, young people, or other groups?

2. Televised sporting events such as baseball often show players chewing tobacco. Yet, athletes are seen as role models. Should sport figures be encouraged to publicize the dangers of smokeless tobacco?
3. Nicotine use has been described as a habit and as an addiction. Former U.S. Surgeon General C. Everett Koop claimed tobacco to be as addictive as cocaine and heroin, yet millions of people have quit smoking. Do you believe tobacco use is addictive or is a habit? Why?
4. The cost of health insurance continues to climb. Should smokers be required to pay more for health insurance? How about people who do not exercise or consistently overeat?
5. Nicotine can pass through the placenta and enter the bloodstream of the fetus. What might be done to dissuade women from smoking during pregnancy?

Web Resources

CDC's Tobacco Information and Prevention Source
http://www.cdc.gov/tobacco
This site contains current information on smoking prevention programs.

American Lung Association
http://www.lungUSA.org
The American Lung Association's Web site includes statistics on teen smoking.

Notes

1. P. D. Jacobson and J. Wasserman, *Tobacco Control Laws: Implementation and Enforcement* (Santa Monica, CA: Rand, 1997).
2. A. Tanskanen, H. Viinamaki, J. Hintikka, H. Koivumaa-Honkanen, and J. Lehtonen, "Smoking and Suicidality Among Psychiatric Patients," *American Journal of Psychiatry,* 155 (1998): 129–130.
3. J. S. Vogel, D. P. Hurford, J. V. Smith, and A. Cole. "The Relationship Between Depression and Smoking in Adolescents," *Adolescence* 38 (Spring 2003): 57–75.
4. M. R. Digby, "Tobacco, Seduction and Puritanism," *Quadrant,* 51 (July/August 2007): 40–46.
5. C. Cottrell, "Journey to the New World: London and the New Colony," *History Today,* 57 (May 2007): 25.
6. K. E. Warner, "Tobacco," *Foreign Policy,* (May/June 2002): 20–28.
7. K. M. Ribisl, R. S. Williams, and A. E. Kim, *Internet Cigarette Sales* (Washington, D.C.: Briefing to the Congressional Task Force on Tobacco and Health, July 17, 2006).
8. L. D. Johnston, P. M. O'Malley, J. Bachman, and J. E. Schulenberg, *Monitoring the Future: National Survey Results on Drug Use, 1975–2008: Volume 1, Secondary School Students* (Bethesda, MD: National Institute on Drug Abuse, 2008).
9. *Results from the 2007 National Survey on Drug Use and Health: National Findings* (Rockville, MD: Substance Abuse and Mental Health Services Administration, 2008).
10. D. R. Shopland and C. Brown, "Changes in Cigarette Smoking Prevalence in the U.S.: 1955 to 1983," *Annals of Behavioral Medicine,* 7 (1985): 5–8.
11. I. Kawachi, R. J. Troisi, A. G. Rotnitzky, E. H. Coakley, and G. A. Colditz, "Can Physical Activity Minimize Weight Gain in Women After Smoking Cessation?" *American Journal of Public Health,* 86 (1996): 999–1004.
12. "College Students Less Likely Than Other High School Graduates to Use Illicit Drugs and Cigarettes; More Likely to Use Alcohol." *CESAR Fax,* 12 (March 10, 2003): 1.
13. B. Kalesan, J. Stine, and A. J. Alberg, "The Joint Influence of Parental Modeling and Positive Parental Concern on Cigarette Smoking in Middle and High School Students," *Journal of School Health,* 76 (October 26, 2006): 402–407.
14. American Lung Association, *Trends in Tobacco Use* (Epidemiology and Statistics Unit, 2006).
15. E. Crain, "Evil New Evidence on Smoking," *Cosmopolitan,* 243 (September 2007): 268.
16. *Women and Smoking: A Report of the Surgeon General* (Rockville, MD: U.S. Department of Health and Human Services, 2001.)
17. American Cancer Society, *Women and Smoking,* (Atlanta, GA: American Cancer Society, 2007).
18. S. S. Hecht, S. G. Carmella, S. E. Murphy, W. T. Riley, C. Le, X. Luo, M. Mooney, and D. K. Hatsukami, "Similar Exposure to a Tobacco-Specific Carcinogen in Smokeless Tobacco Users and Cigarette Smokers," *Cancer Epidemiology Biomarkers and Prevention,* 16 (2007): 1567–1572.
19. *Results from the 2007 National Survey on Drug Use and Health,* supra note 9.
20. Ibid.
21. Johnston et al., supra note 8.
22. M. M. Walsh, J. F. Hilton, C. M. Masouredis, L. Gee, M. A. Chesney, and V. L. Ernster, "Smokeless Tobacco Cessation Intervention for College Athletes: Results After 1 Year," *American Journal of Public Health,* 89 (1999): 228–234.
23. R. Mathias, "Nicotine Patch Helps Smokeless Tobacco Users Quit, but Maintaining Abstinence May Require Additional Treatment," *NIDA Notes,* March 2001.
24. D. A. Savitz, R. E. Meyer, J. M. Tanzer, S. Mirvish, and F. Lewin, "Public Health Implications of Smokeless Tobacco Use as a Harm Reduction Strategy," *American Journal of Public Health,* 96 (November 2006): 1934–1939.
25. S. J. Henley, C. J. Connell, P. Richter, C. Husten, T. Pechacek, E. E. Calle, and M. J. Thun, "Tobacco-Related Disease Mortality Among Men Who Switched from Cigarettes to Spit Tobacco," *Tobacco Control,* 16 (2007): 22–28.
26. B. Liu, R. Peto, Z. Chen, J. Bordham, P. Wu, J. Li, T. C. Campbell, and J. Chen, "Emerging Tobacco Hazards in China, Retrospective Proportional Mortality Study of One Million Deaths," *British Medical Journal,* 317 (1998): 1411–1422.

27. H. Restall, "All the Tobacco in China," *Opinion Journal* (October 26, 2007).
28. M. Ezzati and A. D. Lopez, "Estimates of Global Mortality Attributable to Smoking in 2000," *The Lancet*, 362 (2003): 847–852.
29. Ibid.
30. S. Chapman and J. Richardson, "Tobacco Excise and Declining Tobacco Consumption: The Case of Papua, New Guinea," *American Journal of Public Health*, 80 (1990): 537.
31. N. Naurath and J. M. Jones, "Smoking Rates Around the World—How Do Americans Compare," *Gallup Poll News Service* (August 17, 2007).
32. "EU Takes Action Against States Breaking the Tobacco Sponsorship Ban," *World Tobacco*, 216 (November, 2006): 10.
33. S. Farrer, "Alternative Cigarettes May Deliver More Nicotine Than Conventional Cigarettes," *NIDA Notes*, 18 (August 2003): 8–10.
34. G. M. Polzin, S. B. Stanfill, C. R. Brown, D. L. Ashley, and C. H. Watson, "Determination of Eugenol, Anethole, and Coumarin in the Mainstream Cigarette Smoke of Indonesian Clove Cigarettes," *Food and Chemical Toxicology*, 45 (October 2007): 1948–1953.
35. G. Harris, "Path to Tobacco Includes Compromise and Criticism," *The New York Times*, (July 17, 2007).
36. T. Wright, "Altria Seeks Indonesian Smokers," *Wall Street Journal—Eastern Edition* (July 2, 2007).
37. S. Dinakar, "Bye-Bye Bidis," *Forbes Asia*, 2 (February 13, 2006): 26–27.
38. Johnston et al., supra note 8.
39. H. A. Tindle, N. A. Rigotti, R. B. Davis, E. M. Barbeau, I. Kawachi, and S. Shiffman, "Cessation Among Smokers of 'Light' Cigarettes: Results from the 2000 National Household Interview Survey," *American Journal of Public Health*, 96 (August 2006): 1498–1504.
40. M. Siegel, "Unsafe at Any Level," *The New York Times* (January 28, 2007).
41. A. Fugh-Berman, "Light Cigarettes Carry Heavy Risks," *Women's Health Activist*, 31 (September–October, 2006): 11.
42. "Light Cigarettes Heavy on the Heart," *Family Practice News*, 37 (August 15, 2007): 11.
43. D. C. Arias, "Light Cigarettes May Hamper Quitting," *The Nation's Health*, 36 (September 2006): 14.
44. American Cancer Society, *Cigar Smoking* (Atlanta, GA: 2007).
45. "Attorneys General Take on Cigarette-like Little Cigars," *Tobacco Retailer*, 9 (June 2006): 10.
46. M. Bierne, "Anti-Smoking Proponents Not Sugarcoating Efforts," *Brandweek*, 47 (October 23, 2006): 18.
47. A. Hyland, K. M. Cummings, D. R. Shopland, and W. R. Lynn, "Prevalence of Cigar Use in 22 North American Communities: 1989 and 1993," *American Journal of Public Health*, 88 (1998): 1086–1098.
48. T. G. Shanks and D. M. Burns, "Disease Consequences of Cigar Smoking," in *Cigars: Health Effects and Trends* (Smoking and Tobacco Control Monograph 9) (Washington, DC: National Cancer Institute, 1998).
49. J. L. Lopez-Arrieta and F. J. Sanz, "Nicotine for Alzheimer's Disease," *Cochrane Database for Systematic Reviews* (2007).
50. P. M. Lantz, P. D. Jacobson, and K. E. Warner, "Youth Smoking Prevention: What Works?" *Prevention Researcher*, 8 (April 2001): 1–6.
51. K. Ash, "Adolescent Smoking," *Education Week*, 26 (August 15, 2007): 12.
52. Substance Abuse and Mental Health Services Administration, Office of Applied Studies, "A Day in the Life of American Adolescents: Substance Abuse Facts," *The OAS Report* (October 18, 2007).
53. Johnston et al., supra note 8.
54. C. L. Storr, B. A. Reboussin, and J. C. Anthony, "Early Childhood Misbehavior and the Estimated Risk of Becoming Tobacco-Dependent," *American Journal of Epidemiology*, 160 (2004): 126–130.
55. S. G. Kellam and J. C. Anthony, "Targeting Early Antecedents to Prevent Tobacco Smoking: Findings from an Epidemiologically Based Randomized Field Sample," *American Journal of Public Health*, 88 (1998): 1490–1495.
56. C. Jackson, L. Henriksen, D. Dickinson, L. Messer, and S. B. Robertson, "A Longitudinal Study Predicting Patterns of Cigarette Smoking in Late Childhood," *Health Education and Behavior*, 25 (1998): 436–447.
57. W. S. Choi, J. S. Ahluwalia, K. J. Harris, and K. Okuyemi, "Progression to Established Smoking: The Influence of Tobacco Marketing," *American Journal of Preventive Medicine*, 22 (2002): 228–233.
58. Y. Xue, M. A. Zimmerman, and C. H. Caldwell, "Neighborhood Residence and Cigarette Smoking Among Urban Youths: The Protective Role of Prosocial Activities," *American Journal of Public Health*, 97 (October 2007): 1865–1872.
59. Substance Abuse and Mental Health Services Administration, *FFY 2006 Annual Synar Reports: Youth Tobacco Sales* (2007).
60. S. Weinrich, "Psychological Correlates of Adolescent Smoking in Response to Stress," *American Journal of Health Behavior*, 20 (1996): 52–60.
61. Vogel et al., supra note 3.
62. M. S. Guillon, M. A. Crocq, and P. E. Bailey, "Nicotine Dependence and Self-Esteem in Adolescents with Mental Disorders," *Addictive Behaviors*, 32 (April 2007): 758–764.
63. J. G. Johnson, P. Cohen, D. S. Pine, D. F. Klein, S. Kasen, and J. S. Brook, "The Association between Cigarette Smoking and Anxiety Disorders during Adolescence," *Journal of the American Medical Association*, 284 (2000): 2348–2351.
64. J. D. Kass, "Can Cigarette Smoking in Young Women Be Prevented by Enhanced Spirituality?" in *Problems of Drug Dependence, 1996*, edited by L.S. Harris (Proceedings of the 58th Annual Scientific Meeting, NIDA Research Monograph 174) (Rockville, MD: National Institute on Drug Abuse, 1997).
65. F. A. Curlin, "Spirituality and Lifestyle: What Clinicians Need to Know," *Southern Medical Journal*, 99 (October 2006): 1170–1171.
66. A. J. Farkas, J. M. Distefan, W. S. Choi, E. A. Gilpin, and J. P. Pierce, "Does Parental Smoking Cessation Discourage Adolescent Smoking?" *Preventive Medicine*, 28 (1999): 213–218.
67. M. Q. Wang, E. C. Fitzhugh, and J. M. Eddy, "Social Influences on Adolescents' Smoking Progress," *Prevention Researcher*, 8 (April 2001): 6–7.
68. J. A. Hall and T. W. Valente, "Adolescent Smoking Networks: The Effects of Influence and Selection on Future Smoking," *Addictive Behaviors*, 32 (December 2007): 3054–3059.
69. B. Kalesan, J. Stine, and A. J. Alberg, "The Joint Influence of Parental Modeling and Positive Parental Concern on Cigarette Smoking in Middle and High School Students," *Journal of School Health*, 76 (October 2006): 402–407.
70. R. McGee, S. Williams, and A. Reeder, "Parental Tobacco Smoking Behaviour and Their Children's Smoking and Cessation in Adulthood," *Addiction*, 11 (2006): 1193–1201.
71. S. Perlstein, "Smoking Mothers, Smoking Children," *Pediatric News*, 38 (January 2004): 48.

72. D. B. Kandel, M. C. Hu, P. C. Griesler, and C. Schaffran, "On the Development of Nicotine Dependence in Adolescents," *Drug and Alcohol Dependence,* 91 (November 2007): 26–39.
73. Johnston et al., supra note 8.
74. Campaign for Tobacco-Free Kids, *Nationwide Survey of Teens and Adults* (March 2007).
75. G. B. Lindsay and J. Rainey, "Psychosocial and Pharmacologic Explanations of Nicotine's 'Gateway Drug' Function," *Journal of School Health,* 67 (1997): 123–126.
76. S. A. Everett, G. A. Giovino, C. W. Warren, L. Crossett, and L. Kann, "Other Substance Use among High School Students Who Use Tobacco," *Journal of Adolescent Health,* 23 (1998): 289–296.
77. R. W. Pollay, "Hacks, Flacks, and Counter-Attacks: Cigarette Advertising, Sponsored Research, and Controversies," *Journal of Social Issues,* 53 (1997): 53–74.
78. L. Zwarun, "Ten Years and 1 Master Settlement Agreement Later: The Nature and Frequency of Alcohol and Tobacco Promotion in Televised Sports, 2000 through 2002," *American Journal of Public Health,* 96 (August 2006): 1492–1497.
79. "America's Choice: Reducing Tobacco Addiction and Disease," *American Journal of Public Health,* 94 (2004): 174–176.
80. L. Biener, R. H. Aseltine, B. Cohen, and M. Anderka, "Reactions of Adult and Teenaged Smokers to the Massachusetts Tobacco Tax," *American Journal of Public Health,* 88 (1998): 1389–1391.
81. H. Ross and F. J. Chaloupka, "The Effect of Public Policies on Youth Smoking," *Southern Economic Journal,* 70 (2004): 796–815.
82. K. M. Ribisl, R. S. Williams, and A. E. Kim, "Internet Sales of Cigarettes to Minors," *The Journal of the American Medical Association,* 290 (2003): 1356–1359.
83. A. W. Waltenbaugh and M. J. Zagummy, "Optimistic Bias and Perceived Control among Cigarette Smokers," *Journal of Alcohol and Drug Education,* 47 (March 2004): 20–33.
84. S. Sussman, C. W. Dent, D. Burton, A. W. Stacy, and B. R. Flag, *Developing School-Based Tobacco Use Prevention and Cessation Programs* (Thousand Oaks, CA: Sage Publications, 1995).
85. G. C. Patton, J. B. Carlin, C. Coffey, R. Wolfe, M. Hibbert, and G. Bowes, "Depression, Anxiety, and Smoking Initiation: A Prospective Study over 3 Years," *American Journal of Public Health,* 88 (1998): 1518–1522.
86. L. Ranney, C. Melvin, L. Lux, E. McClain, L. Morgan, and K. Lohr, *Tobacco Use: Prevention, Cessation, and Control* (Rockville, MD: Agency for Healthcare Research and Quality, 2006).
87. J. P. Caulkins, R. L. Pacula, S. Paddock, and J. Chicsa, *School-Based Drug Prevention: What Kind of Drug Use Does It Prevent* (Santa Monica, CA: Rand Distribution Services, 2002).
88. S. Lai, H. Lai, J. B. Page, and C. B. McCoy, "The Association between Cigarette Smoking and Drug Abuse in the United States," *Journal of Addictive Diseases,* 19 (2000): 11–24.
89. B. Simons-Morton, A. D. Crump, D. L. Haynie, K. E. Saylor, P. Eitel, and K. Yu, "Psychosocial, School, and Parent Factors Associated with Recent Smoking Among Early-Adolescent Boys and Girls," *Preventive Medicine,* 12 (1999): 138–148.
90. D. B. Kandel and K. Chen, "Extent of Smoking and Nicotine Dependence in the United States: 1991–1993," *Nicotine and Tobacco Research,* 2 (2000): 263–274.
91. E. Bianco, "Tobacco Industry Marketing Strategies and Women," *Women's Health Journal,* July–December 2003: 64–67.
92. R. J. DeGrandpre, "What's the Hook? Smoking Is More Than a Chemical Bond," *Reason,* 28 (1997): 8.
93. "Exercise May Help Fight Cigarette Cravings," *CA—A Cancer Journal for Clinicians,* 57 (July/August 2007): 188–189.
94. M. Day, "Caring for the Customer," *New Scientist,* (March 6, 1999): 4–5.
95. Global Youth Tobacco Survey Collaborating Group, "Differences in Worldwide Tobacco Use by Gender," *Journal of School Health,* 73 (2003): 207–215.
96. American Cancer Society, *Cigarette Smoking* (Atlanta, GA: American Cancer Society, 2007).
97. "January 11, 2004 Marks the 40th Anniversary of the Inaugural Surgeon General's Report on Smoking and Health," *Tobacco Information and Prevention Source (TIPS),* June 2, 2004.
98. American Cancer Society, *Cigarette Smoking* (Atlanta, GA: American Cancer Society, October 2007).
99. The Centers for Disease Control, *Economic Facts about U.S. Tobacco Use and Production* (Atlanta, GA: Centers for Disease Control, July 2007).
100. The NSDUH Report, *Work Absences and Past Month Cigarette Use: 2004 and 2005* (Rockville, MD: Substance Abuse and Mental Health Services Administration, May 17, 2007).
101. A. Ramirez, "Report Says Smoking Ban Helps to Cut Heart Attacks," *The New York Times,* September 28, 2007.
102. "Combined Oral Contraceptives and Stroke," *WHO Drug Information,* 20 (2006): 131–132.
103. A. D. Walling, "Effects of Oral Contraceptive Use in Older Smokers," *American Family Physician,* 69 (2004): 1248.
104. *NIDA Info Facts, Cigarettes and Other Nicotine Products* (Bethesda, MD: National Institute on Drug Abuse, 2004).
105. K. Bone, "Phytotherapy for Buerger's Disease," *Townsend Letter: The Examiner of Alternative Medicine,* 288 (July 2007): 154–156.
106. *The Health Consequences of Smoking: A Report of the Surgeon General* (Atlanta: Centers for Disease Control and Prevention, 2004).
107. S. E. Jones, S. Maerkle, L. Wheeler, D. M. Mannino, and L. Crossett, "Tobacco and Other Drug Use among High School Students with Asthma," *Journal of Adolescent Health,* 39 (2006): 291–294.
108. American Lung Association, *Women and Smoking Fact Sheet* (June 2007).
109. American Cancer Society, supra note 98.
110. P. G. Norton, "Women Smokers More Likely to Develop Lung Cancer: Annual CT Detects Early," *Internal Medicine News,* 37 (February 1, 2004): 36.
111. D. S. Freedman, P. E. Tolbert, R. Coates, E. A. Brann, and C. R. Kjeldsberg, "Cigarette Smoking and Non-Hodgkin's Lymphoma," *American Journal of Epidemiology,* 148 (1998): 833–841.
112. C. Barclay, "Obstetrics and Gynaecology: Smoking Increases Risk of Stillbirth," *The Practitioner* (July 31, 2007):11.
113. "Women Who Smoke in Pregnancy May Affect Sons' Future Fertility," *Nursing Standard,* 21 (September 5, 2007): 16–17.
114. "Smoking Key SIDS Factor," *Royal College of Midwives Journal,* 10 (November/December 2007): 454.
115. T. M. Button, B. Maughan, and P. McGuffin, "The Relationship of Maternal Smoking to Psychological Problems in Offspring," *Early Human Development,* 83 (November 2007): 727–732.
116. W. Hofhuis, J. C. de-Jongste, and P. J. Merkus, "Adverse Health Effects of Prenatal and Postnatal Tobacco Smoke Exposure on Children,"

Archives of Disease in Childhood, 88 (2003): 1086–1090.

117. X. Chen, B. Stanton, S. Shankaran, and X. Li, "Age of Smoking Onset as Predictor of Smoking Cessation during Pregnancy," *American Journal of Health Behavior,* 30 (2006): 247–258.
118. Z. Kmietowicz, "Smoking Is Causing Impotence, Miscarriages, and Infertility," *British Medical Journal,* 328 (2004): 364.
119. U. M. Kujala, J. Kaprio, and R. J. Rose, "Physical Activity in Adolescence and Smoking in Young Adulthood: A Prospective Twin Cohort Study," *Addiction,* 102 (2007): 1151–1157.
120. S. A. Linnebur. "Tobacco Education: Emphasizing Impotence as a Consequence of Smoking," *American Journal of Health System Pharmacy,* 63 (December 15, 2006): 2509–2512.
121. *Reducing Tobacco Use: A Report of the Surgeon General* (Atlanta: Centers for Disease Control and Prevention, 2000).
122. J. B. Lopas and J. Q. Shi, "Reanalysis of Epidemiological Evidence on Lung Cancer and Passive Smoking," *British Medical Journal,* 320 (2000): 417–418.
123. D. F. Behan, M. O. Eriksen, and Y. Lin, *Economic Effects of Environmental Tobacco Smoke* (Society of Actuaries, 2005).
124. "Prescribing Notes: Smokers' Children Have Five Times Risk," *Pharmacy Today* (July 12, 2007): 18.
125. "More Parks Consider Smoking Bans," *Parks and Recreation,* 42 (June 2007): 21.
126. T. L. Lash and A. Aschengrau, "Active and Passive Cigarette Smoking and the Occurrence of Breast Cancer," *American Journal of Epidemiology,* 149 (1999): 5–12.
127. A. J. Wells, "Lung Cancer from Passive Smoking at Work," *American Journal of Public Health,* 88 (1998): 1025–1029.
128. A. Picard, "Secondhand Smoke Can Triple Risk of Lung Cancer," *Globe and Mail* (July 12, 2001).
129. S. T. Mayne, J. Buenconsejo, and D. T. Janerich, "Previous Lung Disease and Risk of Lung Cancer Among Men and Women Nonsmokers," *American Journal of Epidemiology,* 149 (1999): 13–20.
130. *The Health Consequences of Involuntary Exposure to Tobacco Smoke: A Report of the Surgeon General, 2006* (Rockville, MD: U.S. Department of Health and Human Services, 2006).
131. Mayne et al., supra note 129.
132. M. J. Friedrich, "Researchers Report New Clues to Dementia," *Journal of the American Medical Association,* 298 (July 11, 2007): 161–163.
133. *The Health Consequences of Smoking: A Report of the Surgeon General,* supra note 106.
134. M. D. Eisner, A. K. Smith, and P. D. Blanc, "Bartenders' Respiratory Health After Establishment of Smoke-Free Bars and Taverns," *Journal of the American Medical Association,* 280 (1998): 1909–1914.
135. W. Feigleman and J. A. Lee, "Are Americans Receptive to Smokefree Bars?" *Journal of Psychoactive Drugs,* 38 (June 2006): 133–141.
136. E. A. Simoes, "Maternal Smoking, Asthma, and Bronchiolitis: Clear-Cut Association or Equivocal Evidence," *Pediatrics,* 119 (June 2007): 1210–1212.
137. J. E. Robinson and A. J. Kirkcaldy, "You Think That I'm Smoking and They're Not: Why Mothers Still Smoke in the Home," *Social Sciences and Medicine,* 65 (August 2007): 641–652.
138. F. D. Gilliland, K. Berhane, T. Islam, M. Wenten, E. Rappaport, E. Avol, W. J. Gauderman, R. McConnell, and J. M. Peters, "Environmental Tobacco Smoke and Absenteeism Related to Respiratory Illness in Schoolchildren," *American Journal of Epidemiology,* 157 (2003): 861–869.
139. D. M. Ferguson, L. J. Woodward, and L. J.Horwood, "Maternal Smoking During Pregnancy and Psychiatric Adjustment in Late Adolescence," *Archives of General Psychiatry,* 55 (1998): 721–727.
140. S. C. Huijbregts, J. R. Seguin, M. Zoccolillo, M. Boivin, and R. E. Tremblay, "Associations of Maternal Prenatal Smoking with Early Childhood Physical Aggression, Hyperactivity-Impulsivity, and Their Co-Occurrence," *Journal of Abnormal Child Psychology,* 35 (April 2007): 203–215.
141. M. D. Cornelius, S. L. Leech, L. Goldschmidt, and N. L. Day, "Prenatal Tobacco Exposure: Is It a Risk for Early Tobacco Experimentation?" *Nicotine and Tobacco Research,* 2 (2000): 45–52.
142. M. G. Burke, "Linking Environmental Tobacco Smoke to Sickle Cell Crises," *Contemporary Pediatrics,* 21 (2004): 119–120.
143. "Passive Smoking and Children's Teeth," *Archives of Disease in Childhood,* 88 (2003): 783.
144. A. Simendinger, "Secondhand Politics," *National Journal,* 39 (September 8, 2007): 57–58.
145. A. O. Goldstein, J. E.Cohen, B. S. Flynn, N. H. Gottleib, L. J. Solomon, G. S. Dana, K. E.Bauman, and M. M. Munger, "State Legislators' Attitudes and Voting Intentions Toward Tobacco Control Legislation," *American Journal of Public Health,* 87 (1997): 1197–1200.
146. G. W. Thompson and N. Wilson, "Public Attitudes About Tobacco Smoke in Workplaces: The Importance of Workers' Rights in Survey Questions," *Tobacco Control,* 13 (2004): 206–207.
147. J. K. Ibrahim and S. A. Glantz, "The Rise and Fall of Tobacco Control Media Campaigns, 1967–2006," *American Journal of Public Health,* 97 (August 2007): 1383–1396.
148. L. Stayner, J. Bena, A. J. Sasco, R. Smith, K. Steenland, M. Kreuzer, and K. Straif, "Lung Cancer Risk and Workplace Exposure to Environmental Tobacco Smoke," *American Journal of Public Health,* 97 (March 2007): 545–552.
149. L. Zellers, M. A. Thomas, and M. Ashe, "Legal Risks to Employers Who Allow Smoking in the Workplace," *American Journal of Public Health,* 97 (August 2007): 1376–1382.
150. S. A. Glantz and L. R. Smith, "The Effect of Ordinances Requiring Smoke Free Restaurants on Restaurant Sales in the United States," *American Journal of Public Health,* 83 (1993): 1214–1221.
151. J. W. Cherner, "Smoke-free New York City—One Year Later," *Smokefree,* March 30, 2004.
152. L. Stolzenberg and S. J. D'Alessio, "Is Nonsmoking Dangerous to the Health of Restaurants?—The Effect of California's Indoor Smoking Ban on Restaurant Revenues," *Evaluation Review,* 31 (February 2007): 75–92.
153. R. Rajkumar, C. Gross, and H. P. Forman, "Is the Tobacco Settlement Constitutional?" *Journal of Law, Medicine and Ethics,* 34 (Winter 2006): 748–752.
154. M. Grossman and F. J. Chaloupka, "Cigarette Taxes: The Straw to Break the Camel's Back," *Public Health Reports,* 112 (1997): 291–297.
155. L. Zwarun, "Ten Years and 1 Master Settlement Agreement Later: The Nature and Frequency of Alcohol and Tobacco Promotion in Televised Sports, 2000 through 2002," *American Journal of Public Health,* 96 (August 2006): 1492–1497.
156. "Spitzer Sues Brown and Williamson for Targeting Youth," *Reuters,* June 17, 2004.
157. J. Sterngold, "A Jury Awards a Smoker with Lung Cancer $3 Billion from Philip Morris," *New York Times,* June 7, 2001.

158. R. A. Daynard, C. Bates, and N. Francey, "Tobacco Litigation Worldwide," *British Medical Journal,* 320 (January 8, 2000): 111–120.
159. "January 11, 2004 Marks the 40th Anniversary of the Inaugural Surgeon General's Report on Smoking and Health," supra note 97.
160. M. C. Willemsen, H. de Vries, G. Van Breukelsen, and R. Genders, "Long-Term Effectiveness of Two Dutch Work Site Smoking Cessation Programs," *Health Education and Behavior,* 25 (1998): 418–435.
161. A. Jain, "Treating Nicotine Addiction: Extracts from Best Treatments," *British Medical Journal,* 327 (2003): 1394–1395.
162. C. Frette, E. Barrett-Connor, and J. L. Clausen, "Effect of Active and Passive Smoking on Ventilatory Function in Elderly Men and Women," *American Journal of Epidemiology,* 143 (1996): 757–765.
163. T. C. Orleans, "Helping Young Adult Smokers Quit: The Time Is Now," *American Journal of Public Health,* 97 (August 2007): 1353.
164. G. Falkin, C. S. Fryer, and M. Mahadeo, "Smoking Cessation and Stress Among Teenagers," *Qualitative Health Research,* 17 (July 2007): 812–823.
165. L. I. Solberg, S. E. Asche, R. Boyle, M. C. McCarty, and M. J. Thoele, "Smoking and Cessation Behaviors Among Young Adults of Various Educational Backgrounds," *American Journal of Public Health,* 97 (August 2007): 1421–1426.
166. B. Chakravorty and S. Chakravorty, "Cessation Related Perceptions and Behavior of Former and Current Smokeless Tobacco Users," *Journal of American College Health,* 46 (1997): 133–138.
167. N. Breslau and E. L. Peterson, "Smoking Cessation in Young Adults: Age at Initiation of Cigarette Smoking and Other Suspected Influences," *American Journal of Public Health,* 86 (1996): 214–220.
168. A. Jain, supra note 161.
169. R. West, M. Edwards, and P. Hajek, "A Randomized Controlled Trial of a 'Buddy' System to Improve Success at Giving Up Smoking in General Practice," *Addiction,* 93 (1998): 1007–1011.
170. American Cancer Society, *Guide for Quitting Smoking* (Atlanta: American Cancer Society, November 13, 2003).
171. T. D. Gardina, A. Hyland, U. E. Bauer, and M. Cummings, "Which Population-Based Interventions Would Motivate Smokers to Think Seriously About Stopping Smoking?" *American Journal of Health Promotion,* 18 (2004): 405–408.
172. J. Etter, "Addiction to the Nicotine Gum in Never Smokers," *BMC Public Health,* 159 (July 17, 2007): 159.
173. D. K. Hatsukami, K. Perkins, S. E. Lukas, M. Rukstalis, K. T. Brady, and C. L. Wetherington, "Drugs of Abuse and Gender Differences," in *Problems of Drug Dependence,* 1996, edited by L. S. Harris (Proceedings of the 58th Annual Scientific Meeting, NIDA Research Monograph 174) (Rockville, MD: National Institute on Drug Abuse, 1997).
174. S. Y. Smith, B. Curbow, and F. A. Stillman, "Harm Perception of Nicotine Products in College Freshmen," *Nicotine and Tobacco Research,* 9 (September 2007): 977–982.
175. S. Shiffman, "Use of More Nicotine Lozenges Leads to Better Success in Quitting Smoking," *Addiction,* 102 (May 2007): 809.
176. American Cancer Society, supra note 170.
177. C. T. Bolliger, X. Van Biljon, and A. Axelsson, "A Nicotine Mouth Spray for Smoking Cessation: A Pilot Study of Preference, Safety and Efficacy," *Respiration,* 74 (2007): 196–201.
178. P. Thomas, "Nicorette Nicotine Patches," *Ecologist,* 37 (April 2007): 30–31.
179. I. Barker and R. Bushby, "Patches Help Pupils Quit," *Times Educational Supplement,* (January 12, 2007): 3.
180. "Nicotine Patch Demonstrated to Be Safe in Smokers with CAD," *Formulary,* 42 (May 2007): 321.
181. Thomas, supra note 178.
182. S. J. Leischow, J. Ranger-Moore, M. L. Muramoto, and E. Matthews, "Effectiveness of the Nicotine Inhaler for Smoking Cessation in an OTC Setting," *American Journal of Health Behavior,* 28 (2004): 291–301.
183. L. Smeeth and G. Fowler, "Nicotine Replacement Therapy for a Healthier Nation," *British Medical Journal,* 317 (1998): 1266–1267.
184. American Cancer Society, supra note 170.
185. "Varenicline Effect for Smoking Cessation," *Pulse,* 67 (January 18, 2007): 32.
186. "Buproprion Hydrochloride," *Brown University Geriatric Psychopharmacology Update,* 11 (August 2007): 8.
187. F. Y. Lam, "Delirium Associated with Buproprion and Fluoxetine," *Brown University Psychopharmacology Update,* 18 (March 2007): 2–3.
188. "Varenicline: A New Option to Help Smokers Quit," *Drugs & Therapy Perspectives,* 23 (April 2007): 1–4.
189. L. A. Potts and C. L. Garwood, "Varenicline: The Newest Agent for Smoking Cessation," *American Journal of Health-System Pharmacy,* 64 (July 1, 2007): 1381–1384.
190. B. L. Love and T. Merz, "Varenicline (Chantix) for Smoking Cessation," *American Family Physician,* 76 (July 15, 2007): 279–280.
191. K. K. Downey, L. M. Schuh, M. E. Tancer, J. A. Hopper, and C. R. Schuster, "Treatment of Nicotine Dependence with Fluoxetine, Nicotine Patch, and Group Therapy," in *Problems of Drug Dependence,* edited by L. S. Harris (Proceedings of the 59th Annual Scientific Meeting, NIDA Research Monograph 178) (Rockville, MD: National Institute on Drug Abuse, 1997).
192. C. L. Garwood and L. A. Potts, "Emerging Pharmacotherapies for Smoking Cessation," *American Journal of Health-System Pharmacy,* 64 (August 2007): 1693.
193. S. I. Rennard and D. M. Daughton, "Smoking Cessation," *Chest,* 117 (May 2000): 360–371.
194. A. Valbo and T. Eide, "Smoking Cessation in Pregnancy: The Effect of Hypnosis in a Randomized Study," *Addictive Behaviors,* 21 (1996): 29–35.
195. J. P. Green, S. J. Lynn, and G. H. Montgomery, "A Meta-Analysis of Gender Smoking Cessation, and Hypnosis: A Brief Communication," *International Journal of Clinical & Experimental Hypnosis,* 54 (April 2006): 224–233.
196. American Cancer Society, supra note 170.
197. M. T. Cabioglu, N. Ergene, and U. Tan, "Smoking Cessation After Acupuncture Treatment," *International Journal of Neuroscience,* 117 (May 2007): 571–578.

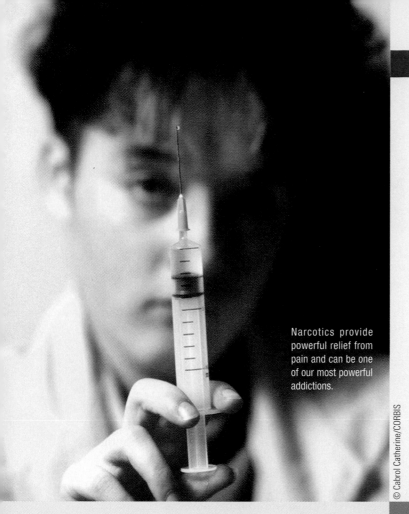

Narcotics provide powerful relief from pain and can be one of our most powerful addictions.

FACT OR FICTION?

1. At one time heroin was given to morphine addicts to help them break their addiction to morphine.
2. Mexican heroin, which is black, is more potent than heroin from other countries.
3. Over the past two decades, the purity of heroin has increased and the price has decreased.
4. Heroin users are likely to become violent while taking the drug.
5. Codeine, which can be found in cough syrup, is a mild narcotic.
6. Heroin is considered a performance-enhancing drug because it improves concentration.
7. Because NEPs have been shown to reduce the transmission of HIV infection, the federal government provides funding for NEPs in selected large cities.
8. Women are more likely to die from drug overdoses than men.
9. Although heroin has the reputation of being an extremely addictive drug, it is more difficult to withdraw from alcohol than from heroin.
10. Although methadone is given to patients to treat their heroin addiction, it is possible to become addicted to methadone.

Turn the page to check your answers

8

Narcotics

Chapter Objectives

After completing this chapter, the reader should be able to describe:

- Reasons that opium and morphine became prevalent in the United States in the 1800s
- The impact of the Harrison Act of 1914 on the type of person who used opiates
- The profile of the typical heroin user
- How political events affected the availability of narcotics
- Potential medical dangers related to using nonsterile hypodermic needles
- Needle-exchange programs and their effect on rates of HIV transmission
- Factors that influence the intensity of heroin withdrawal
- How narcotic antagonists work
- The medical uses of narcotics
- Advantages and disadvantages of methadone maintenance programs

FACT OR FICTION?

1. **Fact:** When heroin was first developed, it was viewed as a cure for morphine addiction even though it is more powerful than morphine.
2. **Fiction:** The fact is—black heroin is less potent than heroin from other countries, which is white.
3. **Fact:** Because world production of opium increased, the supply is more plentiful. This resulted in higher purity and lower cost.
4. **Fiction:** The fact is—heroin puts users in a stupefied state; thus, they are lethargic and nonviolent.
5. **Fact:** Although codeine is a regulated drug and a narcotic, it is a cough suppressant.
6. **Fiction:** The fact is—because heroin makes one sleepy and passive, it impedes performance instead of improving it.
7. **Fiction:** The fact is—the federal government acknowledges that needle-exchange programs reduce the transmission of HIV but refuses to provide any funding.
8. **Fiction:** The fact is—more men than women die from drug overdoses.
9. **Fact:** Withdrawing from alcohol is more life-threatening than withdrawing from heroin.
10. **Fact:** Methadone can be a highly addictive drug.

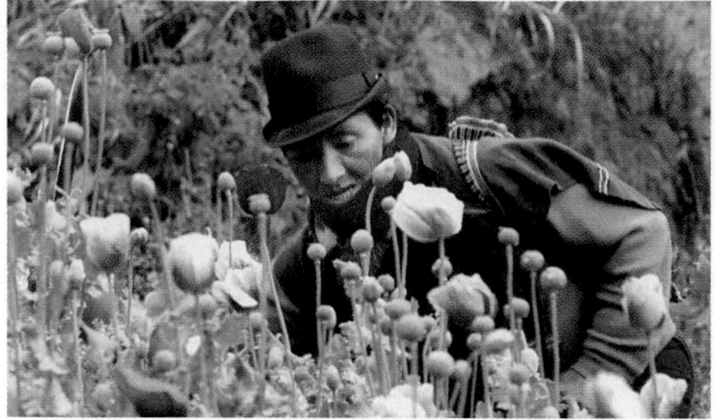

Throughout history, opium has figured prominently in the economic vitality of some countries.

The sedating, painkilling, sleep-inducing effects of opium have been noted for several thousand years. Painkilling drugs derived from opium include morphine and heroin. Law enforcement agencies often refer to opium-based drugs as narcotics. The term *narcotic* is derived from the Greek word meaning "stupor."

Throughout history, opium has figured prominently in wars between nations, in the economic vitality of some countries, in medicine, and in the work of lyricists and authors. In the 1800s, opium was plentiful in the United States. More than 70,000 Chinese workers came to the United States in the mid-1800s to build railroads and work in the mines in California. With them came their penchant for smoking opium and for opium dens. Before long, smoking opium was linked to the criminal underworld, and the Chinese were guilty by association.

Morphine use escalated during the 19th century. It was used to relieve pain, diarrhea, and dysentery—conditions that were prevalent during the Civil War.[1] Soldiers routinely injected themselves, and thousands became dependent. Morphine use and dependency were not limited to U.S. soldiers. The drug was used extensively during the Franco-Prussian and Prussian-Austrian wars. Morphine abuse was boosted by development of the hypodermic needle in the mid-1850s. The hypodermic needle hastened the effects of morphine. Also, injected morphine was believed to be nonaddicting.

In the 19th century no restrictions were placed on what could go into medicines. By 1906, opium and its derivatives were found in more than 50,000 medicines. Drugs containing opiates were used for treating mental illness, headaches, toothaches, coughs, tuberculosis, and pneumonia. Morphine and heroin could be bought in any local store, and prescriptions were not required. People who did not have easy access to stores where drugs were sold could easily get a hypodermic syringe kit and **laudanum**—another form of opium—through a Sears, Roebuck and Company mail-order catalog.

The typical patent medicine user was a middle- or upper-class, 30- to 50-year-old, White woman who was genteel and took opiates regularly for medicinal reasons.[2] Patent medicines containing opium and morphine were also used nonmedically, especially by women who frowned on alcohol use during this period of alcohol temperance. Many members of the Women's Christian Temperance Union (WCTU) worked for alcohol reform during the day and took "women's tonics" (containing laudanum) in the evening.[3] Many people continued using these medicines, because they feared the withdrawal symptoms. Ironically, the drug promoted to help people overcome morphine dependency was heroin. Factors contributing to morphine addiction during the latter part of the 19th century included the following:

- Importation of Chinese workers
- The Civil War
- Development of the hypodermic needle
- Inclusion in patent medicines

By the late 1800s, an estimated 4.59 per 1,000 people were dependent on opiates.[4] This figure is

laudanum A drug derived from opium

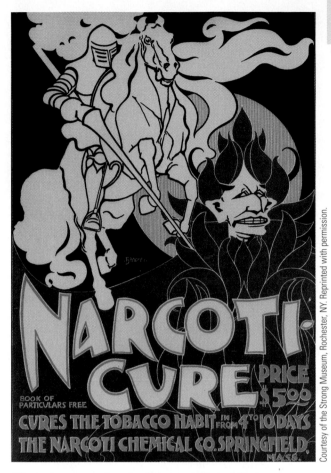

Courtesy of the Strong Museum, Rochester, NY. Reprinted with permission.

Narcotics were advertised as a cure for addiction to tobacco.

much higher proportionately than today's rate of addiction. The United States was known as the "dope fiend's paradise."

National concern regarding narcotics culminated in passage of the Harrison Act of 1914 (see Chapter 4). Because this law made narcotic use without a prescription illegal, the typical opiate addict shifted from a middle-class woman to a young, lower-class man. In a dramatic change, opiates, which once were viewed as good medicine, now were considered evil.[5] Likewise, perceptions of the opiate addict went from that of an unfortunate victim to one of a deviant criminal who was a threat to society.

Extent of Narcotic Use

According to government estimates, in 2006, 338,000 Americans had used heroin in the previous month.[6] Afghanistan is the largest producer of illicit opium, with Myanmar, formerly Burma, second.[7] Other prominent producers include Pakistan, Vietnam, Iran, Laos, China, Thailand, and Mexico. Distribution of heroin from Mexico, called black tar heroin, is limited to the southwestern border of the United States.[8] Though known mostly for its cocaine trade, Colombia is now producing opium. Worldwide production levels are shown in Table 8.1.

Increasing quantities of opium are coming from Central Asian republics that once were under the domain of the Soviet Union.[9] Although Mexico is responsible for 2% of the world's illicit opium, its entire crop is converted to heroin and shipped to the United States.[10] Not only are enormous amounts of

TABLE 8.1 Worldwide Potential Illicit Opium Production 2002–2007 (all figures in Metric Tons)

Country	2007	2006	2005	2004	2003	2002
Afghanistan	8000	5644	4475	4950	2865	1278
Myanmar (Burma)	270	230	380	330	484	630
Colombia*	in process	37		30	63	68
Guatemala			4	12		
Laos	5.5	8.5	28	50	200	180
Mexico	in process	108	71	73	101	58
Pakistan**		36	32		44	4.3
Thailand						9
Vietnam						10
Total Opium	8275.5	6063.5	4990	5445	3757	2237.3

* In 2007, the survey areas were reduced. The 2005 survey could not be conducted due to cloud cover. The reported number is a weighted average of previous years' cultivation.
** The 2005 and 2006 surveys included only the Bara River Valley growing area.
Source: *International Narcotics Control Strategy Report 2008* (Washington, DC: U.S. Department of State, 2008).

opium being produced, but it is relatively pure. In 2006, the purity of heroin from South America was 36.1% while Mexican heroin was 30% pure.[11]

Use in the United States

During the 1930s, morphine abuse exceeded heroin abuse in the United States. By the following decade, heroin addiction was greater. After World War II, heroin use gradually expanded to ghetto areas in many large cities. Heroin was relatively cheap: A person could get high by buying as little as a dollar's worth. Eventually heroin use spread from poor urban neighborhoods to middle-class suburban areas. Heroin use increased greatly beginning in the late 1960s and early 1970s.

Heroin use has become fashionable in some parts of the country. As a result, heroin-related visits to the emergency room and deaths in recent years have increased. According to the most recent data from the Drug Abuse Warning Network (DAWN), 189,780 people went to emergency rooms as a result of using heroin. Whites comprised the majority of those episodes.[12]

In the United States, there are more than 800,000 people addicted to heroin and other narcotics.[13] The National Survey on Drug Use and Health reports that 91,000 people ages 12 and older tried heroin for the first time in the previous 12 months.[14] Most heroin users are older, chronic users who inject the drug. Nevertheless, the number of younger users, who are more likely to snort or smoke heroin, is increasing.[15] Table 8.2 shows the percentage of students using heroin in 2007.

Not everyone who uses heroin or other narcotics becomes dependent on them. Some heroin users take the drug occasionally or on weekends. Precise figures on the number of people who fit this description are not available. These users, called **chippers**, take narcotics in a controlled way. Occasional heroin use contradicts the commonly held notion that a person is either an abstainer or an addict. In an older study comparing compulsive narcotic users to controlled users, controlled users fit the following pattern:

- Seldom used the drug more than once a day
- Could keep opiates around without using them
- Avoided opiates when known addicts were present
- Did not use opiates to alleviate depression
- Seldom, if ever, binged on opiates
- Knew the opiate source or dealer
- Took opiates for recreation or relaxation
- Did not take opiates to escape from life's daily hassles[16]

TABLE 8.2 Percentage of Students Reporting Heroin Use, 2008

Student Heroin Use	Eighth Grade (%)	Tenth Grade (%)	Twelfth Grade (%)
Past month	0.4	0.4	0.4
Past year	0.9	0.8	0.7
Lifetime	1.4	1.2	1.3

Source: *Monitoring the Future*, 2008.

Generalizing about the extent of heroin addiction is difficult, because patterns of drug abuse deviate sharply. An estimated 68% of heroin addicts admitted into treatment are male, 50% are White, and the average age is 36.[17] A developing trend is the abuse of narcotics in rural areas. The increase in abuse is significantly higher in rural areas than in metropolitan areas.[18] The percentage of heroin users admitted into treatment who inject the drug has decreased, although it remains the primary mode of use for those in treatment.[19]

During the Vietnam War, U.S. soldiers' use of narcotics generated much concern. Heroin and other drugs were widely available in Southeast Asia. The heroin that service personnel used was 95% pure, inexpensive, and sold openly. Although some soldiers injected heroin, most smoked it after having mixed it with marijuana or tobacco. An estimated 10% to 15% of U.S. troops were addicted to heroin.

To deal with the impending dilemma of massive numbers of addicted service personnel, the military established heroin treatment centers in Vietnam. In conjunction with the military's slogan that addiction "stopped at the South China Sea," every soldier was tested for heroin. This program, called "Operation Golden Flow," required soldiers failing the drug test to attend a treatment program. Ironically, heroin usage was greater in the rehabilitation programs than during active duty.[20]

Only about 1% to 2% of the soldiers continued to use narcotics 8 to 12 months after returning to the United States.[21] In the United States, heroin was perceived as a deleterious substance. In Vietnam, soldiers took heroin as a means of escaping from a situation they saw as intolerable. Heroin simply did not play a role in the life of these soldiers once they returned home. This situation clearly points to the important role of *set* (state of mind) and *setting* to drug-taking behavior.

Worldwide Comparison

Opium production was confined primarily to southeastern and southwestern Asia from the end of World War II until the late 1980s.[22] Since that time, white powder heroin from South America has been the most available in the United States. Afghanistan is the largest heroin producer worldwide, but much of its heroin is consumed by large heroin addict populations in Eurasia, southeastern Asia, and parts of Africa.[23]

On Campus

Among full-time college students, 0.5% reported using heroin at least once, and 0.1% used heroin in the previous 30 days.

Source: *Monitoring the Future,* 2007.

chippers Nickname for individuals who use narcotics occasionally or on weekends

narcotic An opium-based central nervous system depressant used to relieve pain and diarrhea

opiate A class of drugs derived from opium

opioid A family of drugs with characteristics similar to those of opium

opium The plant from which narcotics are derived

morphine An analgesic drug derived from opium; used medically as a painkiller

codeine Mild narcotic that suppresses coughing; a derivative of opium

Exact figures for the extent of heroin addiction in other countries are difficult to obtain, because many countries deny that they have a drug problem. Also, the covert nature of drug addiction obscures the extent of the problem, and in some countries penalties for drug use and drug trafficking are not imposed because these crimes are of low priority.[24]

It is estimated that about 15.5 million people abuse opium and heroin worldwide. It is estimated that nearly 8.5 million people abuse opiates, including heroin, in Asia, although the region with the highest percentage of abusers is Eastern Europe.[25] In North America, it is estimated that 1.3 million people abuse opiates.[26] A major consequence of injecting drugs is the risk of contracting HIV/AIDS. Injection drug use accounts for one-third of new HIV infections; however, injection drug use is responsible for 80% of all HIV cases in Europe and Central Asia.[27]

Characteristics of Narcotics

Opiates are narcotics. Law enforcement personnel often use the term **narcotic** to refer to illegal drugs, although many illegal drugs are chemically different from narcotics. Opiates refer to a family of drugs with characteristics similar to opium. A generic term used interchangeably with **opiate** is **opioid**. These drugs may be natural or synthetic.

Opium

The opium poppy, *Papaver somniferum,* which means "the poppy that brings sleep," has been called "the plant of joy." Cultivated throughout Asia and the Middle East, it grows to a height of 3 to 4 feet and has white, red, or purple flowers. After poppies bloom and the petals fall, an egg-sized, round seedpod remains. A white, milky sap exudes from the seedpod after it is cut open. Once the sap dries, a brown, thick, gummy resin forms. This is **opium**. The opium poppy has only 10 days to manufacture opium.

Many early civilizations, including Sumeria, Assyria, and Egypt, used opium. The Egyptians gave it to infants, the Greeks and Romans held opium in high regard, and the Greeks sold cakes and candies made from opium. Greek physicians Hippocrates and Galen used opium extensively for medical purposes and viewed the drug with much reverence. Thus, recreational use and addiction were not unusual.

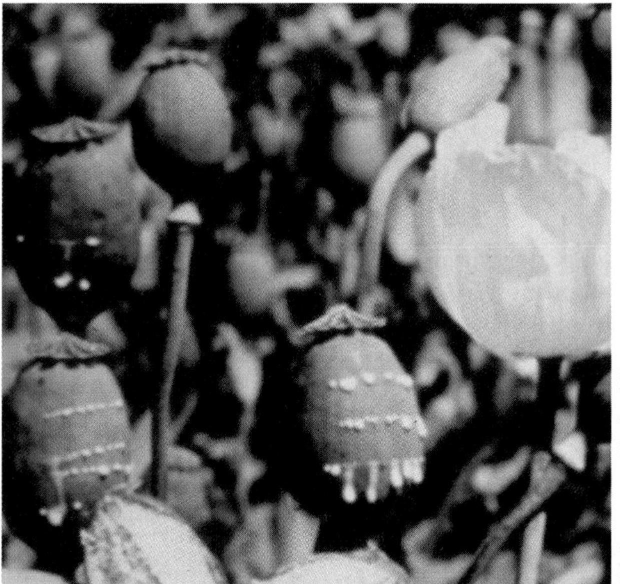

U.S. Department of Justice, DEA.

The milky fluid that oozes from the seedpod of the poppy is opium.

Morphine

In 1803, Friedrich Serturner of Germany synthesized morphine from opium and called his discovery *morphium.* The name **morphine** comes from Morpheus, Greek god of dreams. The effects of morphine occur more rapidly than those of opium. Also, morphine is about 10 times more potent, although physicians accepted it initially as safer and purer than opium. Another alkaloid that was isolated from opium 30 years later is **codeine**. This word comes from the Greek and means "poppy head." Like morphine,

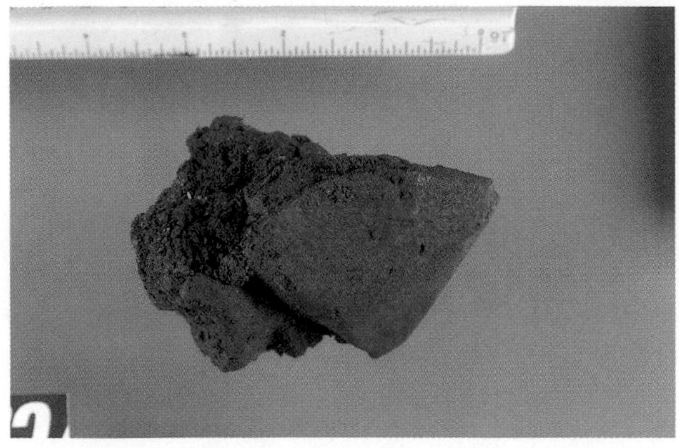

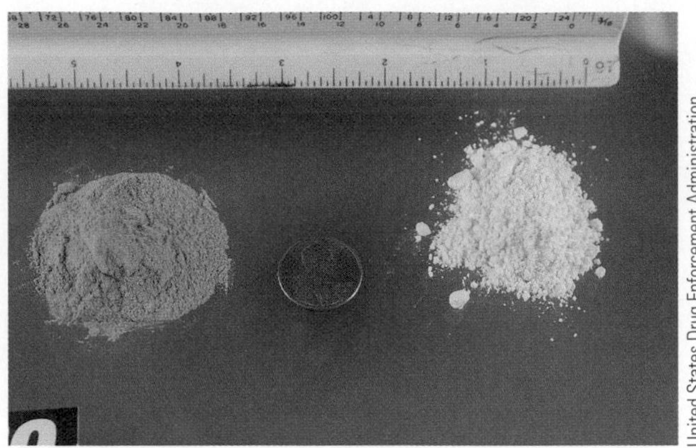

United States Drug Enforcement Administration.

Black tar heroin (left) is darker in color than Asian heroin (right) and comes from Mexico, but is otherwise similar.

codeine can result in dependency. Codeine can be deadly also. In one recent incident, a baby died following being breastfed. The baby's mother had received codeine for pain relief.[28]

How morphine is administered and its dosage have a bearing on its effectiveness. If taken orally, it is not very effective. In therapeutic doses, morphine builds up in the spleen, kidneys, lungs, and liver and binds to blood proteins. Its actions last 4 to 5 hours. Almost all morphine passes through the body within 24 hours, but small amounts can be detected in urine for 2 to 4 days. Morphine can traverse the placenta of a pregnant woman and thereby enter the bloodstream of the fetus. Morphine has a profound effect on psychomotor performance, especially on reaction time.[29]

Heroin

Heroin (diacetylmorphine) was first synthesized from morphine in 1874. The word *heroin* is derived from a German word meaning "heroic." Heroin was promoted originally as a cure for morphine addiction.[30] In a turnabout, morphine later was touted as a cure for heroin addiction.

Heroin was manufactured in 1898 by Bayer, a German pharmaceutical company, which marketed it for ailments ranging from coughs to tuberculosis to bronchitis. Newspaper and magazine advertisements exhorted heroin as a better type of aspirin. When heroin was introduced, it was believed not to be addicting. Now we know, however, that the likelihood of becoming addicted is twice as great for heroin as for morphine.

Heroin can be taken several ways. When smoked, its effects are rapid. Like morphine, it is ineffective when ingested. Individuals who use heroin are more likely to inhale it rather than inject it.[31] One is more likely to become addicted when injecting heroin; however, it is a popular misconception that heroin is not addictive when it is smoked or snorted.[32]

Heroin is 3 to 10 times more powerful than morphine. This greater potency results from heroin being much more lipid-soluble than morphine. Also, heroin reaches the brain more quickly and in higher concentrations.

Fentanyl, Methadone, and Other Synthetic Opiates

Synthetic opiates are chemically constructed rather than naturally produced. They elicit effects that are behaviorally similar to those of morphine but bear little chemical resemblance and relieve less severe pain. They differ in duration of action, potency, intensity, and effectiveness. Examples of synthetic opiates are meperidine (Demerol), methadone (Dolophine), oxycodone (Percodan), pentazocaine (Talwin), and propoxyphene hydrochloride (Darvon). These drugs are available only by prescription.

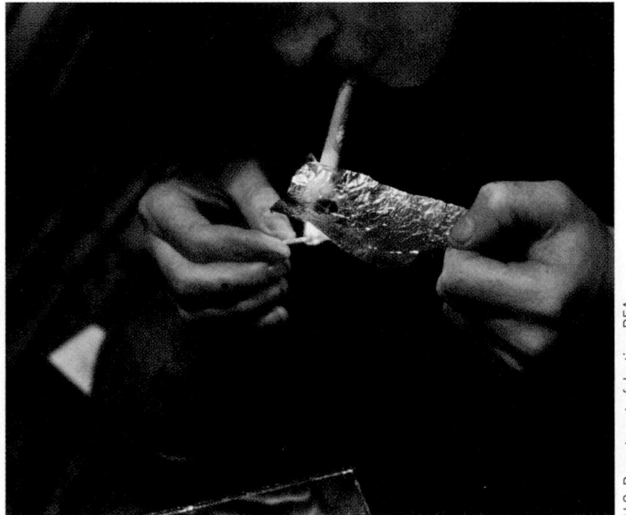

U.S. Department of Justice, DEA.

Synthetic narcotics come in many different shapes and forms.

A powerful synthetic opiate that is considerably stronger than heroin, but with similar analgesic effects, is **fentanyl** (Sublimaze). Known colloquially as **China white**, fentanyl carries a much greater risk of a fatal overdose than heroin does. Fentanyl is not amenable to oral use, but it can be injected or snorted. There are a number of clandestine fentanyl labs throughout the United States, although Mexico is the most likely source for it.[33] Fentanyl is often mixed with other drugs, especially heroin. Because it is extremely potent, a small error in diluting or cutting the drug can result in a fatal overdose.

A synthetic opiate widely used as an analgesic in medicine is **meperidine**. Better known as Demerol, meperidine takes effect within 10 minutes after being injected and remains in effect for 2 to 4 hours. It is considerably less potent than morphine. When a pregnant woman is in labor, this drug is preferred over other analgesics because its side effects, especially respiratory depression in newborns, are milder. At one time, meperidine was erroneously believed to be nonaddicting. Other disadvantages to meperidine are that it is not as effective for relieving pain and has adverse interactions with other drugs that could lead to central nervous system problems, including seizures. Consequently, some hospitals ban its routine use.[34]

Another synthetic narcotic is **propoxyphene hydrochloride** (Darvon). Darvon is related structurally to methadone. It is used primarily to assuage mild pain. At first Darvon was thought to have few side effects and not to cause dependency. We now know that Darvon can result in dependency, affect intellectual and motor abilities, and even be fatal. Because of its potential to be lethal, some groups are trying to have Darvon and similar drugs banned.[35]

Methadone was first synthesized during World War II by scientists in Nazi Germany as a substitute for morphine. Its effects are comparable to those of morphine, but it is more active when taken orally. The potency of methadone when injected subcutaneously (just below the skin) is equivalent to that of morphine. Methadone can be taken with water or alcohol.

heroin (diacetylmorphine) A potent drug that is a derivative of opium

fentanyl A synthetic narcotic that is 1,000 times more potent than heroin

China white A synthetic analgesic drug derived from fentanyl that mimics heroin but is considerably more potent

meperidine A synthetic derivative of morphine

propoxyphene hydrochloride A mild narcotic that has the potential to cause dependence

methadone A drug given to heroin addicts to block withdrawal effects and euphoria

Although methadone is used to lessen severe pain, it is most noted for blocking withdrawal symptoms and euphoric effects from narcotics. Unfortunately, it produces its own euphoria and dependence. There was one instance in which a 22-month-old child died after ingesting methadone.[36] About 5% of infants whose mothers took methadone while pregnant experienced seizures.[37] Table 8.3 lists common narcotics, including their street names.

OxyContin

From 1996 to the present, the number of prescriptions for painkilling drugs grew dramatically. One drug that has gained much attention is OxyContin, a particularly strong painkiller. OxyContin works by blocking the pain signals from nerves. It allows patients to swallow fewer pills, and it offers patients pain relief that lasts three times longer than for other painkillers. It has been shown to be as effective for relieving pain in cancer patients as other pain-killing drugs.[38]

OxyContin is not without its risks. Thousands of people have become addicted to OxyContin. However, one study found that the majority of OxyContin

TABLE 8.3 Common Narcotics

Drug	Common Name	Street Name
Heroin	Diacetylmorphine	Snow, Stuff, Harry, H, White Horse, Horse, Hard Stuff, White Stuff, Joy Powder, Scag, Junk
Morphine	Morphine sulfate	Morpho, Miss Emma, Unkie, Hocus, M
Codeine	Codeine, Empirin with codeine, cough syrups with codeine	Schoolboy
Meperidine	Demerol, Mepergan	Doctors
Methadone	Dolophine	Dollies, Methadose
Oxycodone	Percodan, Talwin, Darvon, Pentazone, Propoxyphyene	—

Source: Health EDCO, a division of WRS Group, Inc.

users admitted into drug treatment obtained the drug illegally and not for medical purposes.[39] Even when the drug is obtained for medical purposes, its users are more likely to use other drugs. In other words, it serves as a gateway drug for many individuals.[40]

The drug's manufacturer, Purdue Pharma, admits that somewhere between dozens and hundreds of people have died from the drug. Purdue Pharma has been trying to address problems with OxyContin through educational sessions with the Drug Enforcement Agency (DEA) and the Food and Drug Administration (FDA). In 2007, Purdue Pharma agreed to pay $634.5 million for understating problems with the drug.

Because OxyContin in combination with other drugs resulted in almost 65,000 emergency room visits in 2006, some people see this dilemma as an opportunity to educate the public about the dangers of prescription drugs.[41] The abuse of OxyContin is especially acute in Appalachia, where the drug is referred to as "hillbilly heroin."[42] The Kentucky attorney general and other officials have sued Purdue Pharma for millions of dollars to recoup expenses for drug programs and law enforcement.[43] Besides illegal diversion, there are numerous accounts of people robbing pharmacies to obtain the drug.[44]

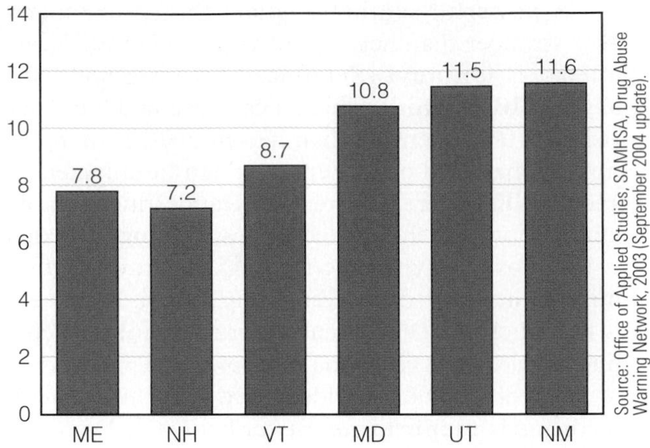

Figure 8.1 Opiate-related Drug Misuse Deaths per 100,000 Population: 2003

Physical and Psychological Effects

The feelings derived from narcotics can be induced naturally by the release of endorphins in the brain. Endorphins help regulate a person's response to stress and pain. These are the same chemicals responsible for the so-called runner's high. Opiates mimic endorphins in the brain.

Many dangers associated with narcotics arise from their illegal status. Physical problems related to narcotics frequently result from using these drugs in unclean, unsafe environments. Because of the types of people associated with illegal narcotics, homicide is a threat. Also, because the unregulated use of narcotics is against the law, they often are contaminated. For instance, heroin may be contaminated with other drugs or with substances such as sugar, starch, powdered milk, quinine, and strychnine.

The peril of narcotics is compounded by how they are administered. Sharing needles is a practice fraught with danger. According to the Centers for Disease Control and Prevention, 2005 data indicate that of 41,897 AIDS cases that were diagnosed, 8,381 were due to injection drug use.[45] Of course, thousands of AIDS cases go undetected and/or unreported.

Medical maladies such as septicemia (blood poisoning), abscesses, hepatitis, HIV/AIDS, and endocarditis (a potentially fatal inflammation of the heart lining) arise from the use of unsterile needles, not from narcotics per se. Death may come within several seconds to users who inadvertently inject air into their veins. Repeated injections into the same vein can lead to its collapse. Figure 8.1 shows the number of opiate misuse deaths per 100,000 population in six states within the United States.

Physical Effects

Narcotics cause drowsiness, vomiting, nausea, and difficulty concentrating. The pupils of the eyes constrict to such an extent that this has given rise to the term "pinpoint pupil." Narcotics lower body temperature, dilate blood vessels in the skin, and lower blood pressure. These effects are manifested in a flushed, warm face and neck.

Opiates impede the ability to urinate, and a common and potentially serious side effect from opiates is constipation. Addicts tend to neglect their diet and engage in other poor health habits. In sum, many addicts simply live unhealthy lifestyles.

Users who inject heroin feel intense, immediate reactions. Euphoria is followed by gradually anesthetizing sensations, then sleep and lethargy. Initial users paint a picture of disorientation and discomfort. Some regular users describe feelings of peace and contentment.

When heroin is injected, initial users describe a "rush" similar to a sexual orgasm. The rush tends to last less than a minute, after which feelings of relaxation take over. Despite the sexual euphoria that accompanies injection, heroin addicts have little, if any, sex drive. Male addicts also have difficulty with achieving an erection.[46] In males, heavy use can retard development of secondary sex characteristics, and in females menstruation may stop, rendering them infertile. Ironically, during withdrawal male users sometimes have a spontaneous erection and ejaculation, and women can experience orgasm.

Infants born to women who took narcotics while pregnant exhibit withdrawal symptoms such as irritability, difficulty in feeding, sweating, tremors, stuffy nose, diarrhea, and vomiting. These infants have a shorter gestation and lower birth weight. One difficulty is that female addicts often lack parenting skills; thus, it is hard to know whether educational difficulties arose from heroin use or parental inability.[47] Interestingly, the babies of heroin-addicted women adopted or placed in foster homes have *not* been found to be intellectually or developmentally impaired despite low birth weight, small head circumference, and withdrawal symptoms.[48] This suggests that environmental deprivation might play a large role in children's development.

One of the most serious consequences of injecting drugs is infection with HIV, which leads to AIDS. The incidence of AIDS among injection drug users is increasing rapidly. Statistics for the past ten years show that injection drug use is the second leading cause for AIDS.[49] The United States is not the only country experiencing an increase in HIV/AIDS. Eastern Europe has experienced a 1,300% increase in HIV/AIDS since 1996, and 90% of infections in Russia can be attributed to needle sharing.[50] AIDS is one of the ten leading causes of death in the United States for adults aged 25 to 44.[51] An encouraging point is that AIDS had been the leading cause of death for this age group in the mid-1990s.[52]

Besides risking infecting their babies, pregnant women who use heroin are more likely to miscarry and deliver prematurely, and the risk of sudden infant death syndrome (SIDS) also increases.[53] One study found that most injection drug users were unable to stop their drug use.[54] In addition, many injection drug users have accompanying psychiatric disorders.[55]

AIDS has become more diffused in the heterosexual population because most injection drug users are heterosexual. Education has reduced the spread of AIDS in the gay population, but injection drug users are more resistant to education.

Emotional and Social Effects

Narcotics affect emotional and social health. They relieve psychic distress arising from anxiety, hostility, feelings of inadequacy, and aggression. However, the stress of rationalizing and defending one's drug use increases emotional discomfort. Heroin addicts lack the ability to control their impulsivity. They have difficulty regulating their inhibitions and in making decisions.[56] Addicts will take more time to make decisions and frequently make risky decisions.[57] In addition, it is not uncommon for seniors with medical problems to use narcotics to commit suicide.[58]

Users sometimes ignore or become alienated and hostile toward friends and family members who previously were important. The lifestyle of a drug addict makes it difficult to maintain intimacy. An Australian study of heroin addicts receiving treatment in prison found that nearly one-half of the addicts had antisocial personalities.[59] Whether heroin use preceded antisocial behavior or vice versa is hard to know.

William Burroughs's autobiographical novel *Junky* describes how narcotics make people feel less sociable. Opiates result in lethargy, and users lack motivation. However, instead of claiming that narcotics produce lethargy, lethargic people simply may be more likely to use narcotics. Likewise, whether addicts use heroin to feel euphoria or to avoid dysphoria is unclear.

Heroin use has been associated with criminal behavior, unemployment, and violence. It is not uncommon for heroin users to engage in prostitution, burglary, and theft. One study revealed that almost 11% of state and local law enforcement officials say that heroin is the drug that contributes most to property crime.[60]

Needle-Exchange Programs

Although unsafe sexual practices is the most common cause of HIV, the second most common HIV risk behavior is injection drug use. One solution is to get people who inject drugs to bleach needles or exchange needles for clean ones. Many health care personnel favor needle-exchange programs (NEPs) or giving hypodermic needles to addicts at no cost. Prominent groups supporting NEPs are the American Medical Association, the American Bar Association, and the U.S. Conference of Mayors. The federal government rejects the NEP concept, preferring a criminal justice approach to a public health approach.

Congress banned federal funding for NEPs in 1988 and has since renewed the ban numerous times.[61] However, in 2007, Congress and the Bush administration approved a measure allowing locally raised tax dollars to be spent on NEPs.[62] Still, it is believed that only a fraction of injection drug users are adequately serviced.[63] One study reported a 5.9% decrease in HIV infection rates in cities with NEPs and a 5.8% increase in cities without NEPs.[64]

Laws regarding the legality of NEPs are unclear, although some programs operate despite the lack of legal authority. Slightly more than half operate legally, about one-fourth operate illegally but are tolerated, and about one-fourth operate illegally and underground.[65] A number of states such as New York, Rhode Island, Illinois, and New Hampshire are considering decriminalizing the possession of needle syringes.[66]

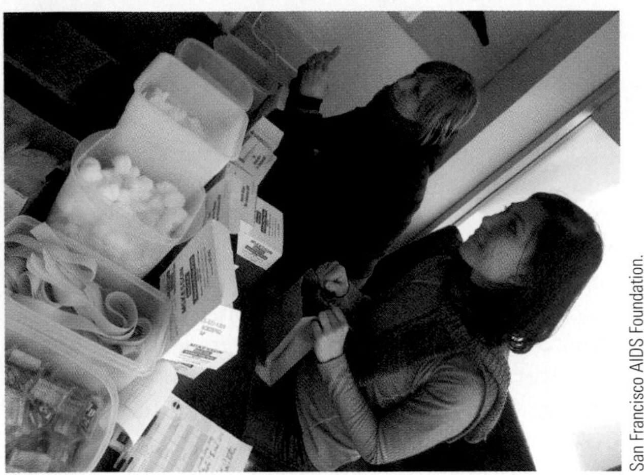

San Francisco AIDS Foundation.

The San Francisco AIDS Foundation's HIV Prevention Project has been disseminating free needles since 1993.

Legally operated programs are more likely to offer services such as HIV counseling, tuberculosis skin testing, and drug treatment.

An argument against NEPs is that they give the appearance of condoning drug use. Also, because addicts do not want to be identified, many do not benefit from NEPs. Youths who use heroin have a high rate of needle sharing. Therefore, services for adolescents who inject drugs might have to be tailored to their needs.[67] Young people who frequent medically supervised injection facilities were more likely to have had medical or legal problems than those who were hesitant to go to such facilities.[68]

The first country to implement an NEP was the Netherlands. Results of NEPs in the Netherlands, Switzerland, and Denmark have been encouraging. Officials in these countries claim that their NEPs have retarded the spread of HIV/AIDS. In Amsterdam, HIV transmission rates were significantly reduced if NEPs were combined with other harm reduction strategies.[69] Besides reduced HIV infections, Australian officials report reduced hepatitis C infections. Also, Australia saved at least $2.4 billion as a result of NEPs.[70]

An 18-month study funded by the U.S. Centers for Disease Control and Prevention found that NEPs are likely to reduce new HIV infections without increasing drug use.[71] Providing clean needles is estimated to save 30 people each day from contracting HIV infection. Another benefit of NEPs is that they serve as gateways for users to access social and medical services.[72]

Dependency

Physical dependence, psychological dependence, and tolerance develop quickly, although the idea that a person is addicted after trying these drugs one time is a myth. However, after several months of intense use, some users are capable of taking 40 to 50 times the amount that would kill the person with less tolerance.[73]

Another myth is that all addicts are moral degenerates. Numerous studies point out that most addicts maintain some ethical responsibility within their social environment.[74] A third myth is that hospitalized patients given opiates in a medically supervised environment will become addicted.[75]

Dependency, though, does produce numerous withdrawal symptoms. After withdrawal, the desire for narcotics sometimes persists for years. Withdrawal symptoms appear 8 to 12 hours after the last injection, peaking in 48 to 72 hours. The symptoms have been compared to a bad case of the flu. Although this "flu" is unpleasant, it is not as severe as typically shown in the media.

Withdrawal symptoms, which subside after several days, include the following:

- diarrhea
- runny nose
- constant yawning
- insomnia
- muscle aches and pains
- dysphoria
- fatigue
- tearing
- perspiration
- restlessness
- anxiety
- irritability
- stomach cramps

The hands and legs shake. The person is literally "kicking the habit."

Factors affecting the difficulty of withdrawal include availability of a social support network, the addict's desire to stop, the physical environment during withdrawal, and the convenience and practicality of alternative opiates. Withdrawal from narcotics is not life-threatening, yet many users avoid going through it out of fear. The anticipation of withdrawal could be worse than the physical act of withdrawing. To avoid withdrawal, an addict uses the drug several times daily. Some people think that addicts are really addicted to the *thought* of being addicted, to actually shooting up, and to the lifestyle of an addict. Heroin addicts do not all follow the same path after becoming addicted. In a 33-year study of heroin addicts, it was found that many quit using after becoming addicted while others quit after an extended time. Yet, some addicts continued using heroin for many years.[76]

People can become drug-dependent in less than 2 weeks if they take increasing amounts of narcotics. About half of narcotic abusers become dependent. The average amount of time a person is addicted is 6 to 8 years. Dependency may develop because of psychological distress, not because of the pharmacological makeup of narcotics themselves. A study of addicts who abstained from narcotics for 3 years after having been removed from the environment in which they used drugs revealed that they relapsed within a month after returning to their original environment.[77] This implies that addiction is more than a physical phenomenon.

Males with eating disorders exhibit personality traits such as anxiety, fearfulness, and antisocial behaviors. Male heroin addicts also display these traits. One study reported similarities between male anorectics and male heroin addicts.[78] Some people use drugs to modulate intense feelings of rage and anger. Psychic or inner pain reflecting depression accounts for some dependencies. People who are dependent on narcotics are depressed at levels significantly higher than occasional narcotics users, who are more depressed than nonusers.[79] Whether depression precedes dependency or dependency precedes depression is unclear. Nonetheless, it is not uncommon for heroin addicts to commit suicide.[80]

Toxicity

Because opiates depress the central nervous system, they lower respiration, pulse rates, and blood pressure. Narcotics are capable of depressing the respiratory system to the point of death. Even when prescribed, narcotics can be fatal.[81] In many cases of deaths from narcotic overdose, another drug such as alcohol is present. The synergistic effect of narcotics and other drugs can be fatal.

Throughout the 1990s to the present, the number of people dying from a heroin overdose has steadily increased.[82] Death from an overdose of heroin is slow. People who die quickly from an overdose are likely to die from **anaphylactic shock**, a condition caused by an allergic reaction to contaminants such as quinine, which are used to cut or dilute the heroin. Sellers increase their profits by cutting heroin with adulterants such as quinine, cornstarch, and lactose.

A study in Australia found that the mortality rate of illicit opiate users was 13 times higher than that for the general population.[83] Data from the U.S. federal government show that narcotics are the most common cause of misuse and abuse deaths in 29 metropolitan areas.[84]

Medical Benefits

The word *narcotic* evokes a highly negative response. People are likely to think of narcotics as completely destructive. In medicine, however, narcotics offer a number of benefits. Narcotics have benefited humankind in important ways. Unfortunately, a practice that has become more common is the illegal diversion of prescribed narcotics.[85]

anaphylactic shock A condition caused by an allergic reaction to contaminants such as quinine, which are used to cut or dilute heroin

analgesics Drugs that relieve pain

Analgesia

Pain relief is a primary benefit of narcotics. Patients receiving morphine, for example, are still aware of pain, but their perception of pain and their response to it are altered in positive ways. Patients experience the discomfort associated with the pain, but they do not lose consciousness. Opiates block the sensation of pain from being transmitted to the brain and reduce negative feelings connected to the pain. Although narcotics alleviate all types of pain, they are more effective with continuous dull pain than with sharp, intermittent pain. Narcotics are favored over other **analgesics** because they have fewer adverse effects on intellectual and motor ability.

Between 1996 and 2002, the pharmaceutical market for painkillers quadrupled to $1.9 billion. Unfortunately, the number of people who have become dependent on those painkillers has risen also. Many people are under the mistaken notion that these drugs are safe. If patients become abusers, the question is raised: Who is at fault if one becomes dependent on painkillers—the doctor or the patient? Yet, according to the United Nations, needless pain is a global tragedy that can be addressed through increasing accessibility to narcotic drugs.[86]

In the United States, morphine is one of the main drugs used for analgesic purposes. It can relieve pain for up to 6 hours.[87] Despite concerns about its potential for addiction, morphine effectively alleviates pain. It is used in hospices without negatively affecting survival rates.[88] In England, heroin is commonly used to relieve severe pain, especially the pain associated with cancer. In the United States, use of heroin for medical purposes is illegal. Because there is much concern about the abuse of narcotics, particularly heroin, many people who could benefit from these drugs do not receive them or receive an inadequate dosage. In medical determinations, the potential benefits of narcotics should be weighed against their potential drawbacks. In addition, research has shown that patients receiving narcotics for pain relief are very unlikely to become dependent on them.[89]

Gastrointestinal Difficulties

A traveler's worry, "Delhi belly" or "Montezuma's revenge" refers to an intestinal disorder that people commonly experience when traveling abroad. In many less-developed countries, diarrhea is a major cause of death among the young and elderly. Because these countries lack good sanitation, food and water supplies become contaminated, leading to serious infections of the gastrointestinal system.

Narcotics are effective in treating diarrhea. Food passes through the intestinal tract as a result of peristaltic contractions. Narcotics slow down these contractions and the speed at which material is removed from the body. A disadvantage is that sometimes the contractions are restricted to point at which spasms occur.

Cough Suppressant

Many people who take medication for coughs have used narcotics without being aware of it. Narcotic agents slow activity of the cough control center, located in the medulla of the brain. The opium derivative codeine has long been used for its **antitussive** properties. Cough medicines with codeine can be obtained on a nonprescription basis, but codeine is now a regulated drug.

Nonopiate drugs such as **dextromethorphan (Delsym)**, which are chemically similar to opiates, often are found in cough preparations today in place of codeine. It is believed that dextromethorphan, also known as DMX, is the fastest growing drug problem in the United States. An estimated 2.4 million teens have gotten high from it.[90] In addition, over 12,000 emergency room visits can be attributed to DMX. Some symptoms of adverse reactions include blurred vision, loss of coordination, stomach pain, and rapid heartbeat.[91] Dextromethorphan also may impair judgment, resulting in injury or fatality.[92]

Treatment and Support Groups

In 2005, 237,000 people were admitted to treatment programs for narcotic abuse.[93] Narcotic addiction is difficult to treat effectively. The **recidivism** (relapse) rate is high, but the longer one is off drugs, the more likely he or she will remain abstinent. One benefit of treatment is that addicts live longer.[94]

Addicts do not have to be consigned to a lifetime of addiction. Many addicts mature or grow out of drug use. Treatment programs range from psychotherapy to behavior modification to acupuncture to medical intervention. The following sections review several types of treatments. Therapeutic communities are covered in Chapter 15.

Detoxification

Withdrawal from narcotics is not as life-threatening or as severe as many people believe. Most addicts are withdrawn from narcotics gradually, although rapid **detoxification** can be just as effective. Unfortunately, most patients undergoing detoxification fail to complete the program. Freeing one's body of drugs does not remove the person's desire to take drugs.

To help addicts in withdrawal, they receive drugs such as clonidine, buprenorphine, naltrexone, naloxone, and the best known, methadone. Clonidine was used to treat hypertension initially, and it was found also to eliminate some drug withdrawal symptoms. Naloxone reduces the amount of time addicts require to undergo withdrawal, but it triggers withdrawal more suddenly.

Typically, detoxification is completed in 10 to 14 days if it is conducted on an inpatient basis. Federal guidelines allow methadone to be administered for up to 30 days on an outpatient basis, although the time can be extended to 180 days if 30 days is found to be insufficient or if the addict is likely to relapse.

Narcotic Antagonists

Drugs that block narcotics from producing their reinforcing effects are called antagonists. **Antagonists** remove the physical need for opiates, but not the psychic need. They complement psychotherapy or group therapy. Examples are naltrexone, buprenorphine, nalorphine, naloxone, and cyclazocine. Nalorphine and cyclazocine were the first antagonists used, but they have been discarded because of their unpleasant side effects. Naloxone (Narcan) subsequently replaced these drugs because it did not produce dysphoria or physical dependence. The effectiveness of naloxone as an antagonist, however, is limited. It works for a short time only. It is used frequently in emergency situations to handle overdoses from narcotics.

Naltrexone (Trexan) is administered orally and is generally effective for a few days. Taking naltrexone negates the effects of heroin injected during the same period. Therefore, naltrexone is useful during detoxification. It is not recommended for people who have acute hepatitis or liver failure, because high doses are linked to hepatic toxicity. In Britain, naltrexone has been shown to be somewhat effective when given to prisoners prior to their release from prison.[95]

Naltrexone is not viewed as a complete form of treatment because addicts crave narcotics after discontinuing medication. Moreover, the dropout rate for individuals receiving naltrexone is substantial.[96] Naltrexone works best when it is used in conjunction with some type of additional reward.[97]

Another drug used to ameliorate withdrawal is **buprenorphine**. The FDA initially approved it to treat pain. It is less addictive than other drugs. Buprenorphine also reduces cocaine use. Its long-term efficacy, however, has not been determined, although buprenorphine was shown to be more effective than other antagonists for treating heroin addiction.[98] Nonetheless, many people receiving buprenorphine found it improved their quality of life.[99] One study found that 75% of patients receiving buprenorphine were still in treatment after 1 year.[100] Another advantage is that it has fewer side effects than other antagonists.[101]

antitussives Drugs that act as cough suppressants

dextromethorphan (Delsym) An over-the-counter nonnarcotic drug found in cough preparations

recidivism Relapse

detoxification Eliminating drugs from the body; usually the initial step in treatment of the effects of alcohol and other drugs

antagonists Drugs that occupy receptor sites and inhibit narcotic activity

naltrexone A narcotic antagonist that blocks the reinforcing effects of narcotics

buprenorphine A synthetic narcotic used to treat narcotic addiction

Methadone and Other Treatments

Since 1960, methadone has been the drug used most frequently to treat heroin addiction. Psychiatrist Marie Nyswander and biochemist Vincent Dole promoted methadone because traditional therapy was ineffective in getting addicts to stop using heroin. Methadone clinics offer individual and group psychotherapy as well as support to addicts. No treatment parallels the effectiveness of methadone. Relative to other forms of treatment, it has been found that methadone maintenance is more cost effective.[102]

People in methadone maintenance programs reduce their use of illegal drugs, especially heroin, and fewer people become HIV-positive while receiving methadone. Prisoners given methadone prior to their release are less likely to use heroin.[103] Similar results have been found for others.[104] One study indicated that parents in methadone maintenance and a program to address parenting skills are less likely to engage in child abuse.[105] On the other hand, fathers receiving methadone without further help have not been shown to improve parenting skills.[106] Women who take methadone while breastfeeding will secrete methadone in breast milk but their infants have not been shown to have greater neurobehavioral problems than infants whose mothers were not on methadone.[107]

Methadone maintenance programs constitute the single most acceptable treatment for heroin addicts by preventing these addicts from getting high.[108] Methadone is highly specific to opiate addiction. It does not alter the effects of cocaine, alcohol, benzodiazepines, and other drugs. Methadone maintenance programs have other problems, though. Many addicts resist coming for treatment. Methadone is euphoric for people who are not addicted to heroin. It leads to addiction, though many people consider addiction to methadone preferable to addiction to heroin. Another issue is whether methadone should be a step toward eventual abstinence or whether it is an acceptable lifelong treatment.

The life of a methadone patient is not easy. Methadone has to be administered daily to avert withdrawal symptoms. Methadone patients face discrimination in housing, insurance, and employment. Methadone produces side effects ranging from hallucinations to sexual dysfunction, insomnia, muscle pain, profuse perspiration, frequent urination, nausea, numbness in the extremities, and constipation. Methadone programs have been accused of controlling population growth because the drug has been linked to sexual impotence, and most patients are from disadvantaged backgrounds. Signs and symptoms that the dosage of methadone is too high include drowsiness, euphoria, respiratory depression, pinpoint pupils, and skin flush.

Despite its limitations, methadone maintenance has several advantages. Methadone can be orally administered, it is easy to monitor, it eliminates the need for needles, and it reduces the risk of overdosing. Withdrawal symptoms are prevented for up to 24 hours. Euphoric effects from heroin are blocked for the same amount of time, and patients experience no sedation from methadone. Methadone patients who abuse cocaine reduce their cocaine use while in treatment.

The longer patients stay in treatment, regardless of the type of substance abuse treatment, the more likely treatment will be successful. Another benefit is that patients are less apt to be hospitalized, saving thousands of dollars.

The FDA monitors methadone maintenance programs closely. Addicts are screened to ensure that they are physiologically dependent on heroin. Adolescent addicts are not eligible to receive methadone except under special circumstances. Addicts can obtain methadone only by enrolling in a maintenance program; no one can receive methadone from private physicians.

One drawback to having a centralized location for receiving methadone is that addicts often congregate at that location—a situation that is not well accepted by people living near the clinic. This concern by neighbors has some justification because drug dealing and alcohol consumption are common around the treatment centers.

Methadone maintenance does not constitute a complete treatment. Rather, it should be viewed as part of a larger treatment. Methadone maintenance

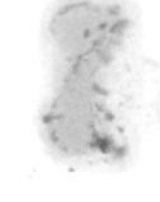

does not address the social and psychological factors leading to addiction in the first place. During rehabilitation, patients are advised to participate in constructive activities such as employment, vocational training, volunteer work, or homemaking. A stable source of legal income reduces the likelihood that patients will resort to drug dealing or other criminal activities.

Only a minority of people successfully withdraw from methadone. Individuals who drop out of treatment or who are discharged unfavorably from treatment have a higher rate of death. According to 2006 data from the Drug Abuse Warning Network (DAWN), 45,130 people went to emergency rooms due to methadone.[109] One factor that has reduced relapse is emphasis on abstaining from heroin. Methadone patients who use marijuana during treatment, however, were more likely to relapse.[110]

An alternative drug approved by the FDA in 1993 is **levo-alpha-acetylmethadol (LAAM)**. One advantage of LAAM over methadone is that it blocks withdrawal symptoms for up to 3 days. In 2000, 5,715 people were treated with LAAM.[111] Since that time, concerns have been raised about the safety of LAAM. Hence, the federal government has added restrictions to its use.[112]

Heroin addicts treated with methadone prefer LAAM to methadone. LAAM produces fewer significant withdrawal symptoms than methadone, and LAAM could be an effective alternative for patients who do not benefit from methadone. One study found that individuals taking LAAM are more likely to stay in treatment, have lower arrest rates, and are less likely to use drugs than individuals in methadone maintenance programs.[113] With LAAM, addicts are not locked into a routine of daily treatment, though some addicts could be allergic to it.

Narcotics Anonymous

Modeled on the principles of Alcoholics Anonymous, Narcotics Anonymous (NA) is a self-help group that was formed in 1953. It is designed to help people who are addicted to heroin and medically prescribed narcotics. The number of NA group meetings proliferated from 5 in 1964 to more than 25,000 by 2007.[114] Of its members, 55% are male, 70% are Caucasian, 72% are employed full-time, and 71% are between the ages of 31 and 50.[115]

Like Alcoholics Anonymous, NA is based on a 12-step model, but the groups are distinctly different. Some people are members of both groups. One difference between the groups is that to members of NA, the problem is not chemical but, rather, the result of one's behavior. Alcoholics Anonymous deals exclusively with alcohol, whereas NA addresses all drugs including alcohol.

Summary

Opium and its derivatives are painkilling, sleep-inducing drugs. Narcotic use increased dramatically in the United States in the 1800s because of the Civil War, immigration of Chinese workers, invention of the hypodermic needle, inclusion of opiates in patent medicines, and their easy accessibility. By the end of the 19th century, the typical opiate user was White, middle-class, middle-aged, and female. In 1914, federal legislation made nonmedical use of narcotics illegal. The typical addict changed to a young, lower-class male. By the 1960s, the cost of heroin escalated, and its purity went down. In the 1970s, narcotic abuse declined. The trend has changed since the 1980s, and the availability and purity of heroin have increased.

Not all users become dependent. Some people are chippers—occasional users who can control their use. During the Vietnam War, thousands of service personnel smoked opium, and nearly all ceased using opium after they returned to the United States.

Early civilizations used opium extensively. Morphine, synthesized from opium in the early 1800s, acts more quickly and powerfully and is more toxic. In the late 1800s, heroin was developed as a cure for morphine addiction and other medical maladies. Synthetic opiates produce behavioral effects similar to those of narcotics. They differ in effectiveness, potency, and intensity. One common potent and dangerous synthetic narcotic is fentanyl.

Users describe the rush from injecting narcotics in glowing terms. Among the many side effects, however, are vomiting, drowsiness, contraction of the pupils, and constipation. Some users claim to feel less psychic distress, although they still have difficulty relating to others. Physical problems that often accompany association with people in the drug trade arise from drug impurities, unsterile needles, and a generally unhealthy lifestyle. One of the most serious concerns resulting from the injection of drugs is contracting HIV infection, which leads to AIDS.

Although drugs can lead to physical dependency, people have little chance of developing dependency from using a drug just once. Some people become dependent as a means of dealing with distress, rage, and psychic pain.

One reason for addicts not seeking treatment is the fear of withdrawal, characterized by insomnia, diarrhea, irritability, and aches and pains. Addicts are not likely to die during withdrawal, though. If they do, it may be due to anaphylactic shock caused by an allergic reaction from contaminants in heroin.

Despite their drawbacks, narcotics have medical uses. They are effective analgesics, especially for continuous dull pain. Also, they stop diarrhea and suppress coughing.

A powerful narcotic is OxyContin. This drug has resulted in numerous deaths, and its manufacturer is reformulating the drug so that its effects will be less lethal.

Treating narcotic addiction has not been especially successful. Recidivism is high. The first step in treatment is detoxification. Ridding the body of narcotics is relatively easy, but the desire to continue drug use remains intense. Narcotic antagonists such as naloxone, naltrexone, buprenorphine, nalorphine, and cyclazocine block the reinforcing effects of narcotics. These drugs complement therapy rather than replace it. LAAM is effective for 3 days rather than for 1 day.

Methadone is the drug most often used to treat narcotic addiction. It blocks the effects of heroin for up to 24 hours. The effectiveness of methadone is questioned, though, because many patients are addicted to drugs other than narcotics and methadone does not block the effects of other drugs. During treatment, addicts are offered social, vocational, and psychological support. Methadone programs are criticized because one addicting drug is replaced by another addicting drug. Moreover, these programs do not reach the root of addiction.

A support group is Narcotics Anonymous (NA). NA is modeled after Alcoholics Anonymous, although NA deals with the process of addiction and not with the chemical as such.

levo-alpha-acetylmethadol (LAAM) An experimental drug that prevents narcotic withdrawal symptoms for about 3 days

Thinking Critically

1. Heroin is one of the most effective painkilling drugs available today, yet in the United States it is not legal for physicians and hospitals to administer it. Do you think that physicians and hospitals should have the right to administer heroin if conditions warrant? Why or why not?
2. The plots of many movies revolve around illegal trade in narcotics and other drugs. How did you derive your image of narcotics? Do you think young people's image of narcotics is affected by how the media depict narcotics?
3. NEPs are controversial. Some people think these programs condone drug use. On the other hand, these programs may reduce the spread of HIV. Who should decide if an NEP is to be implemented? Should the decision be made by elected officials, health care personnel, clergy, or someone else?
4. Concern has been raised over using methadone as a substitute for heroin, as both are addictive. Methadone given in a clinical setting, however, is pure, and addicts do not have to engage in illegal activity to afford their drugs. Is using drugs as therapy for other drugs a wise practice?

Web Resources

Narcotics Anonymous
http://www.na.org/
This site provides information on Narcotics Anonymous groups, which are structured similar to the 12-step model of Alcoholics Anonymous.

National Institute on Drug Abuse
http://www.nida.nih.gov/ResearchReports/Heroin/heroin.html
This site provides complete information about the effects of heroin and other narcotics.

Notes

1. "Morphine Daze," *Current Events*, 106 (March 5, 2007): 5.
2. M. Keire, "Dope Fiends and Degenerates: The Gendering of Addiction in the Early Twentieth Century," in *The American Drug Scene,* edited by J. A. Inciardi and K. McElrath (Los Angeles: Roxbury Publishing Company, 2004).
3. S. J. Gould, "Taxonomy as Politics," *Harper's* (April 1990): 24–26.
4. D. T. Courtwright, *Dark Paradise: Opiate Addiction in America Before 1900* (Cambridge, MA: Harvard University Press, 1992).
5. J. P. Hoffman, "The Historical Shift in the Perception of Opiates: From Medicine to Social Menace," *Journal of Psychoactive Drugs,* 22 (1990): 53–62.
6. Substance Abuse and Mental Health Services Administration, *Results from the 2006 National Survey on Drug Use and Health: National Findings* (Rockville, MD: Office of Applied Studies, 2007).
7. *World Drug Report 2007* (New York: United Nations Office of Drugs and Crime, 2007).
8. "National Trends in Drug Abuse," *Pulse Check* (Washington, DC: Office of National Drug Control Policy, 2004).
9. United Nations Office of Drugs and Crime, supra note 7.
10. ONDCP *Fact Sheet: Breaking Heroin Sources of Supply* (Rockville, MD: Office of National Drug Control Policy, 2004).
11. *National Drug Threat Assessment 2008* (Johnstown, PA: National Drug Intelligence Center, 2007).
12. Substance Abuse and Mental Health Services

Administration, *Drug Abuse Warning Network, 2006: National Estimates of Drug-Related Emergency Room Visits* (Rockville, MD: Office of Applied Studies, 2008).
13. "Buprenorphine: A New Treatment for Opioid Addiction," *Harvard Mental Health Newsletter*, 17 (February 2001): 8–11.
14. Substance Abuse and Mental Health Services Administration, supra note 6.
15. "National Trends in Drug Abuse," supra note 8.
16. N. E. Zinberg, *Drug Set and Setting: The Basis for Controlled Intoxicant Use* (New Haven, CT: Yale University Press, 1984).
17. Substance Abuse and Mental Health Services Administration, *Treatment Episode Data Set (TEDS): 1995–2005. National Admissions to Substance Abuse Treatment Services* (Rockkville, MD: Office of Applied Studies, 2007).
18. "Narcotic Painkiller Abuse Rises Sharply in Rural Areas," *Alcoholism and Drug Abuse Weekly,* 16 (August 30, 2004): 3–5.
19. Substance Abuse and Mental Health Services Administration, supra note 6.
20. N. E. Zinberg, "Heroin Use in Vietnam and the United States: A Contrast and a Critique," *Archives of General Psychiatry,* 26 (1972): 486–488.
21. J. R. Robins, J. E. Helzer, M. Hesselbrock, and E. Wish, "Vietnam Veterans Three Years After Vietnam," in *Yearbook of Substance Abuse,* edited by L. Brill and C. Winick (New York: Human Sciences Press, 1979).
22. ONDCP Fact Sheet: Breaking Heroin Sources of Supply, supra note 10.
23. National Drug Intelligence Center, *The Availability of Southwest Asian Heroin in the United States: A Market Analysis* (Johnstown, PA: National Drug Intelligence Center, March 2007).
24. R. W. Lee and S. B. MacDonald, "Drugs in the East," *Foreign Policy,* 90 (1993): 89–107.
25. *World Drug Report 2007* (New York: United Nations Office of Drugs and Crime, 2007).
26. Ibid.
27. The United Nations, *2006 Report on the Global AIDS Epidemic* (Switzerland: UNAIDS, 2006).
28. "A Caution about Breastfeeding While Using Codeine," *Child Health Alert* (November 2006): 4.
29. *Drugs and Human Performance Fact Sheets, Morphine (and Heroin)* (Washington, DC: National Highway Traffic Safety Administration, April 2004).
30. D. Newnham, "Historic Blunders," *Times Educational Supplement*, June 23, 2006: 5.
31. The DASIS Report, *Heroin—Changes in How It Is Used: 1995–2005* (Rockville, MD: Substance Abuse and Mental Health Services Administration, April 26, 2007).
32. Drug Policy Information Clearinghouse, *Heroin* (Washington, DC: Office of National Drug Control Policy, December 2007).
33. National Drug Intelligence Report, *Fentanyl: Situation Report* (U. S. Department of Justice, June 5, 2006).
34. S. M. Adams, "Meperidine to Manage Pain Related to Diverticular Disease," *American Family Physician*, 73 (June 15, 2006): 2123.
35. "Group Seeks Ban on Some Painkillers," *New York Times*, 155 (March 1, 2006): 15.
36. R. Riascos, P. Kumfa, R. Rojas, H. Cuellar, and F. Descartes, "Fatal Methadone Intoxication in a Child," *Emergency Radiology*, 15 (January 2008): 67–70.
37. S. R. Kendall, "Treatment Options for Drug-Exposed Infants," in *Medications Development for the Treatment of Pregnant Addicts and Their Infants,* edited by C. N. Chiang and L. P. Finnegan (NIDA Research Monograph 149) (Washington, DC: Government Printing Office, 1995).
38. C. M. Reid, R. M. Martin, and J. A. Sterne, "Oxycodone for Cancer-Related Pain: Meta-Analysis of Randomized Controlled Trials," *Archives of Internal Medicine*, 166 (April 24, 2006): 837–843.
39. D. Carise, K. L. Dugosh, A. T. McLellan, A. Camilleri, G. E. Woody, and K. G. Lynch, "Prescription OxyContin Abuse Among Patients Entering Addiction Treatment," *American Journal of Psychiatry*, 164 (November 2004): 1750–1756.
40. M. Wunsch, K. Nakamoto, A. Goswami, and S. H. Schnoll, "Prescription Drug Abuse Among Prisoners in Rural Southwestern Virginia," *Journal of Addictive Diseases*, 26 (2007): 15–22.
41. "Trial of OxyContin: An Opportunity for Treatment Field to Educate," *Alcoholism and Drug Abuse Weekly*, 19 (June 25, 2007): 1–4.
42. *The Double Life of OxyContin: Miracle Painkiller and Illicit Street Drug* (Washington, DC: National Conference of State Legislatures, May 2002).
43. Associated Press, "Kentucky: State Sues OxyContin Maker," *New York Times*, October 5, 2007: 19.
44. *Drug Facts, OxyContin* (Washington DC: Office of National Drug Control Policy, March 5, 2004).
45. *HIV/AIDS Surveillance Report: HIV Infection and AIDS in the United States and Dependent Areas, 2005* (Atlanta: Centers for Disease Control, 2007).
46. O. Al-Gommer, S. George, S. Haque, H. Moselhy, and T. Saravanappa, "Sexual Dysfunction in Male Opiate Users: A Comparative Study of Heroin, Methadone, and Buprenorphine," *Addictive Disorders and Their Treatment*, 6 (September 2007): 137–143.
47. J. Topley, D. Windsor, and R. Williams, "Behavioural, Developmental and Child Protection Outcomes Following Exposure to Class A Drugs in Pregnancy," *Child: Care, Health and Development*, 34 (January 2008): 71–76.
48. R. H. Fishman, "Normal Development After Prenatal Heroin," *Lancet*, 347 (1996): 1397.
49. *HIV/AIDS Surveillance Report: HIV Infection and AIDS in the United States and Dependent Areas, 2005,* supra note 45.
50. P. A. Selwyn, "Medical and Health Consequences of HIV/AIDS and Drug Abuse," in *Drug Addiction Research and the Health of Women,* edited by C. L. Wetherington and A. B. Roman (Rockville, MD: National Institute on Drug Abuse, 1998).
51. M. Heron, "Deaths: Leading Causes for 2004," *National Vital Statistics Reports*, 56 (November 20, 2007).
52. Ibid.
53. *ONDCP Fact Sheet, Heroin,* supra note 10.
54. N. Galai, M. Safacian, D. Vlahov, A. Bolotin, and D. D. Celéntano, "Longitudinal Patterns of Drug Injection Behavior in the ALIVE Study Cohort, 1988–2000," *American Journal of Epidemiology,* 158 (2003): 695–704.
55. M. Kidorf, E. R. Disney, V. L. King, K. Neufeld, P. L. Beilenson, and R. K. Brooner, "Prevalence of Psychiatric and Substance Abuse Disorders in Opioid Abusers in a Community Syringe Exchange Program," *Drug and Alcohol Dependence,* 74 (2004): 115–122.
56. A. J. Verdejo-Garcia, J. C. Perales, and M. Perez-Garcia, "Cognitive Impulsivity in Cocaine and Heroin Polysubstance Abusers," *Addictive Behaviors*, 32 (May 2007): 950–966.
57. D.H. Fishbein, et al., "Neurocognitive Characterizations of Russian Heroin Addicts Without a Significant History of Other Drug Use," *Drug and Alcohol Dependence,* 90 (September 6, 2007): 25–38.
58. D. C. Voaklander, et al., "Medical Illness, Medication Use and Suicide in Seniors: A Population-Based Case-Control Study," *Journal of Epidemiology and Community*

Health, 62 (February 2008): 138–146.
59. S. Darke, S. Kaye, and R. Finlay-Jones, "Antisocial Personality Disorder, Psychopathy, and Injecting Heroin Use," *Drug and Alcohol Dependence,* 52 (1998): 63–69.
60. *National Drug Threat Assessment 2008,* supra note 11.
61. K. Krajick, "Damage Control: Needle Exchange Programs Make Sense and Save Lives," *Ford Foundation Report,* Summer 2002.
62. "Preventing AIDS Prevention," *New York Times,* December 28, 2007.
63. J. McNeely, J. H. Arnsten, and M. Gourevitch, "Improving Access to Sterile Syringes and Safe Syringe Disposal for Injection Drug Users in Methadone Maintenance Treatment," *Journal of Substance Abuse Treatment,* 31 (2006): 51–57.
64. K. Patel, "Research Note: Drug Consumption Rooms and Needle and Syringe Exchange Programs," *Journal of Drug Issues,* 37 (Summer 2007): 737–747.
65. D. Paone, "DPF Funds D.C. Syringe Exchange Programs," *Drug Policy Letter* (January/February 1999).
66. "Syringe Laws More Likely Than Controversial Needle Exchange Programs," *AIDS Alert,* 15 (July 2000): 73–79.
67. M. D. Kipke, J. B. Unger, R. F. Palmer, and R. Edgington, "Drug Use, Needle Sharing, and HIV Risk Among Injection Drug-Using Street Youth," *Substance Use and Misuse,* 31 (1996): 1167–1187.
68. J. M. Stoltz, et al., "Characteristics of Young Illicit Drug Injectors Who Use North America's First Medically Supervised Safer Injecting Facility," *Addiction Research and Theory,* 15 (February 2007): 63–69.
69. C. Van Den Berg, C. Smit, G. V. Brussel, R. Coutinho, and M. Prins, "Full Participation in Harm Reduction Programmes Is Associated with Decreased Risk for Human Immunodeficiency Virus and Hepatitis C Virus: Evidence from the Amsterdam Cohort Studies Among Drug Users," *Addiction,* 102 (2007): 1454–1462.
70. M. G. Law and R. G. Batey, "Injecting Drug Use in Australia: Needle/Syringe Programs Prove Their Worth, but Hepatitis C Still on the Increase," *The Medical Journal of Australia,* 178 (March 3, 2003): 197–198.
71. "Briefing Science and Health: Report Backs Needle Exchanges," *New York Times,* May 18, 2001.
72. Patel, supra note 64.
73. D. M. Grilly, *Drugs and Human Behavior,* 5th ed. (Boston: Allyn & Bacon, 2006).
74. J. Sullum, "H: The Surprising Truth about Heroin and Addiction," *Reason,* 35 (June 2003): 32–40.
75. P. J. Goldstein, H. H. Brownstein, P. J. Ryan, and P. A. Bellucci, "Crack and Homicide in New York City: A Case Study in the Epidemiology of Violence," in *Crack in America: Demon Drugs and Social Justice,* edited by C. Reinarman and H. G. Levine (Berkeley: University of California Press, 1997).
76. H. Yih-Ing, D. Huang, C. Chih-Ping, and M. D. Anglin, "Trajectories of Heroin Addiction," *Evaluation Review,* 31 (December 2007): 548–563.
77. J. F. Maddux and D. P Desmond, "Residence Relocation Inhibits Opiate Dependence," *Archives of General Psychiatry,* 39 (1982): 1313–1317.
78. L. Bradvir, A. Frank, P. Hulenvik, A. Medvedeo, and M. Berglund, "Heroin Addicts Reporting Previous Heroin Overdoses Also Report Suicide Attempts," *Suicide and Life-Threatening Behavior,* 37 (August 2007): 475–481.
79. Maddux and Desmond, supra note 77.
80. G. Abbate-Daga, F. Amianto, and L. Rogna, "Do Anorectic Men Share Personality Traits with Opiate Dependent Men? A Case-Control Study," *Addictive Behaviors,* 32 (January 2007): 170–174.
81. "Prescription Opioids in the News in 2007," *Alcoholism and Drug Abuse Weekly,* 20 (January 17, 2008): 1–8.
82. Substance Abuse and Mental Health Services Administration, *Mortality Data from the Drug Abuse Warning Network 2002* (Rockville, MD: U.S. Department of Health and Human Services, 2004).
83. G. K. Hulse, D. R. English, E. Milne, and C. D. J. Holman, "The Quantification of Mortality Resulting from the Regular Use of Illicit Opiates," *Addiction,* 94 (1999): 221–229.
84. Substance Abuse and Mental Health Services Administration, *Drug Abuse Warning Network, 2006: National Estimates of Drug-Related Emergency Room Visits,* supra note 12.
85. W. R. Davis and B.D. Johnson, "Prescription Opioid Use, Misuse, and Diversion Among Street Drug Users in New York City," *Drug and Alcohol Dependence,* 92 (January 1, 2008): 267–276.
86. A. L. Taylor, "Addressing the Global tragedy of Needless Pain: Rethinking the United Nations Single Convention on Narcotic Drugs," *Journal of Law, Medicine and Ethics,* 35 (December 2007): 556–570.
87. *National Drug Threat Assessment 2008,* supra note 11.
88. N. P. Sykes, "Morphine Kills the Pain, Not the Patient," *Lancet,* 369 (April 21–27, 2007): 1325–1326.
89. R. Mathias, "Research Eases Concerns About Use of Opioids to Relieve Pain," *NIDA Notes,* 15 (March 2000): 12–13.
90. J. Consiglio, "Legal and Lethal," *Choices* (February/March, 2008): 10–12.
91. "Visits for Cough Medicine ODs Dramatically Rising: Monitor for Life-Threatening Conditions," *ED Nursing,* 10 (March 2007): 57–58.
92. D. A. Levine, "Pharming: The Abuse of Prescription and Over-the-Counter Drugs in Teens," *Current Opinion in Pediatrics,* 19 (June 2007): 270–274.
93. The DASIS Report, *Facilities Operating Opioid Treatment Programs: 2005* (Rockville, MD: Substance Abuse and Mental Health Services Administration, 2006).
94. A. Gibson, L. Degenhardt, R. P. Mattick, R. Ali, J. White, and S. O'Brien, "Exposure to Opioid Maintenance Treatment Reduces Long-Term Mortality," *Addiction,* 103 (March 2008): 462–468.
95. W. Mistral, S. Wilkinson, C. Mastache, S. Midgley, and F. Law, "Efficacy of Naltrexone Treatment with Combined Crack and Opiate Users: A Descriptive Study of a New Treatment Service in Bristol, UK," *Drugs: Education, Prevention and Policy,* 15 (February 2008): 107–109.
96. E. V. Nunes, J. L. Rothenberg, M. A. Sullivan, K. M. Carpenter, and H.D. Kleber, "Behavioral Therapy to Augment Oral Naltrexone for Opioid Dependence: A Ceiling on Effectiveness?" *The American Journal of Drugs and Alcohol Abuse,* 32 (2006): 503–517.
97. R. Mathias, "New Approaches Seek to Expand Naltrexone Use in Heroin Treatment," *NIDA Notes,* 17 (March 2003): 8–11.
98. R. E. Johnson, M. A. Chutuape, E. C. Strain, S L. Walsh, M. L. Stitzer, and G. E. Bigelow, "A Comparison of Levomethadyl Acetate, Buprenorphine, and Methadone for Opioid Dependence," *New England Journal of Medicine,* 343 (2000): 1290–1297.
99. A. M. Ponizovsky and A. Grinspoon, "Quality of Life Among Heroin Users on Buprenorphine versus Methadone Maintenance," *American Journal of Drugs and Alcohol Abuse,* 33 (September 2007): 631–642.
100. "Buprenorphine Now Available for Treating Heroin Dependence in U.S.," (College Park, MD: CESAR: Center

for Substance Abuse Research, March 31, 2003).

101. A. Ponizovsky, A. Grinspoon, and A. Margolis, "Well-Being, Psychosocial Factors, and Side-Effects Among Heroin-Dependent Inpatients After Detoxification Using Buprenorphine versus Clonidine," *Addictive Behaviors*, 31 (November 2006): 2002–2013.

102. R. Schilling, K. Dornig, and L Lundgren, "Treatment of Heroin Dependence: Effectiveness, Costs, and Benefits of Methadone Maintenance," *Research on Social Work Practice*, 16 (January 2006): 48–56.

103. T. W. Kinlock, et al., "A Randomized Clinical Trial of Methadone Maintenance for Prisoners: Results at 1-Month Post-Release," *Drug and Alcohol Dependence*, 91 (December 1, 2007): 220–227.

104. G. W. Joe, P. M. Flynn, and K. M. Broome, "Patterns of Drug Use and Expectations in Methadone Patients," *Addictive Behaviors*, 32 (August 2007): 1640–1656.

105. R. Reading, "Reducing Potential for Child Abuse Among Methadone-Maintained Parents: Results from a Randomized Controlled Trial," *Child: Care, Health and Development*, 34 (January 2008): 134–135.

106. T. J. McMahon, J. D. Winkel, and B. J. Rounsaville, "Drug Abuse and Responsible Fathering: A Comparative Study of Men Enrolled in Methadone Maintenance Treatment," *Addiction*, 103 (February 2008): 269–283.

107. L. M. Jansson, et al., "Methadone Maintenance and Breastfeeding in the Neonatal Period," *Pediatrics*, 121 (January 2008): 106–114.

108. J. F. Kauffman and G. E. Woody, *Matching Treatment to Patient Needs in Opioid Substitution Therapy* (Treatment Improvement Protocol, TIP Series 20) (Rockville, MD: U.S. Department of Health and Human Services, 1995).

109. Substance Abuse and Mental Health Services Administration, supra note 12.

110. D. A. Wasserman, M. G. Weinstein, B. E. Havassy, and S. M. Hall, "Factors Associated with Lapses to Heroin Use During Methadone Maintenance," *Drug and Alcohol Dependence*, 52 (1998): 183–192.

111. "Facilities Providing Methadone/LAAM Treatment to Clients with Opiate Addiction," *The DASIS Report*, December 6, 2002.

112. J. H. Jaffe, "Can LAAM, Like Lazarus, Come Back from the Dead?" *Addiction*, 102 (September 2007): 1342–1343.

113. M. D. Anglin, B. T. Conner, J. Annon, and D. Longshore, "Levo-alpha-acetylmethadol (LAAM) Versus Methadone Maintenance: 1-Year Treatment Retention, Outcomes, and Status," *Addiction*, 102 (September 2007): 1432–1442.

114. *Information about NA* (Van Nuys, CA: NA World Services, 2007).

115. Ibid.

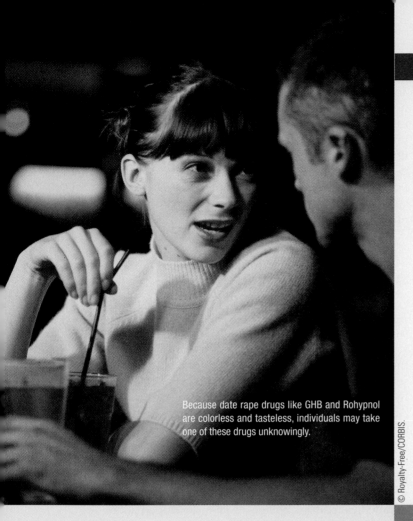

Because date rape drugs like GHB and Rohypnol are colorless and tasteless, individuals may take one of these drugs unknowingly.

FACT OR FICTION?

1. It is possible to buy prescription drugs through the Internet, although it is illegal to buy them without a prescription.
2. Those who enter treatment for abuse of prescription drugs are better educated than people abusing other types of drugs.
3. Doctors are more likely to prescribe barbiturates for sleep now than they were 20 years ago.
4. Withdrawal from sedatives can be life-threatening.
5. The illegal use of methaqualone (Quaalude) has grown in popularity in the last decade.
6. People who enter treatment for benzodiazepine abuse are likely to be older than people who enter treatment for abuse of other illegal drugs.
7. When it is used in conjunction with alcohol, the effects of Rohypnol can be fatal.
8. The highest rate of inhalant use by youths occurs among Asians.
9. More people die from inhaling air fresheners than from inhaling gasoline.
10. Nitrous oxide has been used as an anesthetic by dentists.

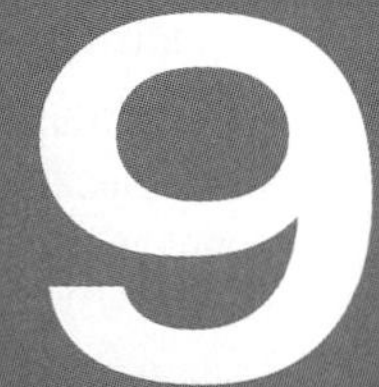
Turn the page to check your answers

9

Sedative-Hypnotic Drugs

Chapter Objectives

After completing this chapter, the reader should be able to describe:

- The original purposes for which barbiturates were developed
- The differences between ultra-short-acting, short-acting, intermediate-acting, and long-acting barbiturates
- The medical applications of barbiturates and their potential side effects
- The effectiveness of sedative-hypnotic drugs
- The physical and psychological effects of methaqualone
- The medical uses of benzodiazepines and their side effects
- The various drugs associated with "date rape"
- The extent of inhalant use among adolescents
- Side effects associated with inhalants

FACT OR FICTION?

1. **Fact:** Despite the illegality of buying prescription drugs through the Internet without a prescription, such a practice occurs.
2. **Fact:** People who abuse prescription drugs have higher levels of education than people abusing other types of drugs.
3. **Fiction:** The fact is—because sleeping pills interfere with the quality of one's sleep, doctors are less likely to prescribe them today.
4. **Fact:** Even though sedatives are frequently prescribed, withdrawal without medical supervision can be life-threatening.
5. **Fiction:** The fact is—about the same percentage of people use methaqualone today as they did 10 years ago.
6. **Fact:** The average age for admission to treatment for benzodiazepine abuse is 37 compared with 34 for other illegal drugs. People admitted for treatment for benzodiazepines are older than people admitted into treatment for other illegal drugs.
7. **Fact:** The effects of the depressant action of Rohypnol increase when used with alcohol.
8. **Fiction:** The fact is—White youths are most likely to use inhalants, followed by Hispanics, Asians, and Blacks.
9. **Fiction:** The fact is—one study showed that gasoline accounted for more fatalities than air fresheners.
10. **Fact:** Nitrous oxide has been given to dental patients as an anesthetic, although its use has declined in recent years.

Sedative-hypnotic drugs derive their name from the relaxing, calming effect they produce in low doses and their sleep-inducing (soporific), hypnotic effect when taken in high doses. Sedative-hypnotic drugs are central nervous system depressants, though some users believe they have a stimulating effect because these people become less inhibited after ingesting them.

The three main types of sedative-hypnotic drugs are barbiturates, nonbarbiturate sedatives, and minor tranquilizers. Side effects of these drugs include nausea, lethargy, vomiting, skin rashes, and upset stomach. Other effects are hangover, fever, blurred vision, facial numbness, impaired judgment, poor motor coordination, and a condition resembling dementia. Women are particularly vulnerable to these drugs. Fifty-six percent of people treated for dependence on sedatives are women and 55% of emergency room visits involving prescription drug abuse cases involve women.[1]

As the dosage increases, so does the likelihood of a fatal overdose. Also, people can become physically and psychologically dependent. Once a person stops using the drug, the withdrawal symptoms can be life-threatening. An unfortunate consequence of some prescription drugs in this class is that they may be used to commit suicide. One Canadian study of older people who committed suicide revealed that 21% died from self-poisoning.[2] In this chapter we will examine various categories of sedative-hypnotic drugs, date-rape drugs, and inhalants.

Adolescents and Prescription Drugs

In 2007, the Office of National Drug Control Policy (ONDCP) initiated a media campaign addressing the increase in young people who are diverting prescribed medicines, including sedative-hypnotic drugs, for nonmedical purposes. In 2006, over 5 million Americans ages 12 and older had used a pain reliever at least once in the previous 30 days.[3] An important point is that the younger one is when first using prescription drugs for nonmedical purposes, the more likely one is to later abuse drugs. It is estimated that 42% of individuals who used prescription drugs for nonmedical reasons by age 13 later developed abuse of prescription drugs.[4]

After marijuana, prescription drugs are the most commonly used illegal drugs. (Though prescription drugs are legal when approved by a physician, they are illegal when taken without a doctor's approval.) In 2007, 6.2% of high school seniors had used a sedative for nonmedical purposes within the previous 12 months.[5] Adolescents in western and southeastern states have higher rates of abuse. Girls are more likely to intentionally abuse prescription drugs than boys. Not surprisingly, more girls than boys develop dependency. One misconception among adolescents is that these drugs provide a medically safe high, and one-third believe there is nothing wrong with using prescription drugs without a prescription occasionally. Almost one-half of adolescents state that they obtain the drugs from a friend or relative.

Between 1995 and 2005 admissions into substance abuse treatment for abuse of prescription pain relievers increased 300%. In addition, unintentional poisoning deaths from sedative-hypnotic drugs and antidepressants increased 84% over a recent 5-year time span. Adolescents report that parents do not care as much if they are caught using prescription medications as opposed to other drugs. These parents feel that prescription drugs, even when used for nonmedical purposes, are much safer than street drugs.

It should not be surprising that adolescents feel less shame when caught using these drugs and that parents are less likely to talk to their children about prescription drugs.[6]

sedative-hypnotic Class of drugs that produce relaxing to sleep-inducing effects depending on dosage

barbital A sedative-hypnotic drug used to treat anxiety and nervousness; the original barbiturate

Veronal Brand name for barbital

phenobarbital Second barbiturate developed; produces relaxation and relieves anxiety

Barbiturates

In the early 1860s, Germany's Bayer laboratories developed the first barbiturate, although it was not introduced into general medicine until 1903. This depressant, synthesized from chemicals in urine, was initially called **barbital** (all barbiturates in the United States end with the letters *al*). Originally, barbital was effective for inducing sleep. When barbital was introduced in 1903, its brand name was **Veronal**. A second barbiturate, **phenobarbital**, was marketed for medical use in 1912. It produced relaxation and relief from anxiety.

TABLE 9.1 Selected Barbiturates

Generic Name	Trade/Brand Name	Type of Barbiturate
pentobarbital sodium	Nembutal	Short-acting
secobarbital	Seconal	Short-acting
talbutal	Lotusate	Short-acting
amobarbital	Amytal	Intermediate-acting
butabarbital	Butisol	Intermediate-acting
phenobarbital	Luminal	Long-acting

Types of Barbiturates

Based on their potency and the length of time they act, barbiturates are classified as ultra-short-acting, short-acting (less than 4 hours), intermediate-acting (4 to 6 hours), or long-acting (more than 6 hours). Short-acting barbiturates require less time to take effect than long-acting barbiturates, and their effects do not last as long. Because they act more quickly, short-acting barbiturates are more likely than long-acting barbiturates to be abused. Drugs that take effect rapidly have a higher abuse potential than slow-acting drugs. The length of time that barbiturates act depends on dose, differences among users, and method of administration. A list of selected barbiturates is presented in Table 9.1.

Effects of Barbiturates

Like alcohol, barbiturates produce a depressed, mood-altering action on the central nervous system. They also affect activity of the muscle tissue, the heart, and respiration. In a manner similar to the effects of alcohol, barbiturates can cause confusion, shorter attention span, impaired cognitive functioning, inadequate emotional control, slurred speech, poor judgment, hangovers, and intoxication. Activities such as driving an automobile are ill-advised while a person is using barbiturates because reaction time, hand-eye coordination, and energy levels are affected adversely. Hostility and rage commonly surface after taking barbiturates. As with other drugs, the extent to which barbiturates affect users depends on one's state of mind, the setting in which the drug is used, and the individual's previous experiences with the drug.

Barbiturates sometimes are ingested to ameliorate the effects of amphetamines or to allay the effects of heroin withdrawal. A typical scenario consists of taking amphetamines ("speed") during the day to get

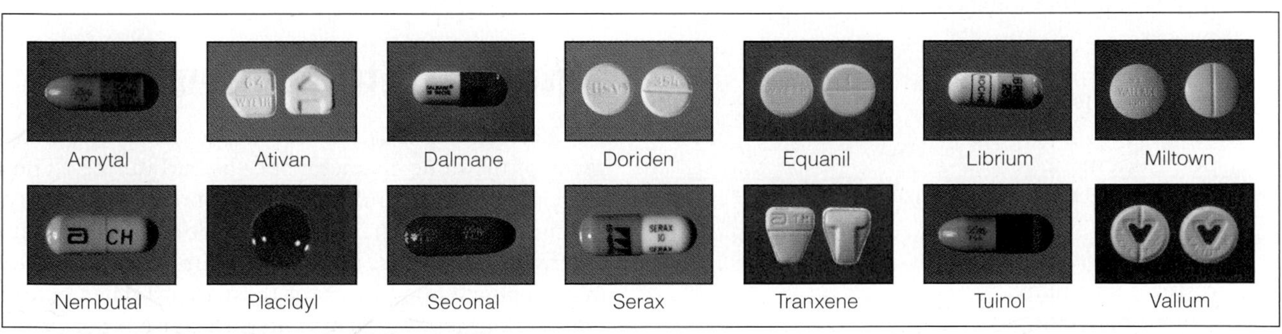

Depressants come in different shapes and forms.

charged up ("wired") and barbiturates at night to go to sleep. People who take barbiturates chronically develop a tolerance to them. Also, people develop a cross-tolerance to chemically similar drugs such as alcohol and minor tranquilizers. If large quantities (800 to 1,000 mg) of barbiturates are taken daily, dependence can result in 4 to 6 weeks.

Potential Hazards

Dangers associated with barbiturates range from fatigue to fatal overdose. Moderate side effects include emotional upset, nausea, vertigo, vomiting, and diarrhea. One study of college students found that those who used sedatives were more likely to experience panic attacks than those who did not use sedatives.[7] Barbiturates can depress breathing, resulting in insufficient oxygen in the blood. Because the heartbeat is depressed, the blood pressure drops. A person can go into shock and fall into a coma or die.

Infants of women who took barbiturates during pregnancy can be born with congenital dependency. As these babies go through withdrawal, they exhibit symptoms similar to those of adults. Barbiturates taken during pregnancy can cause birth defects, brain damage, or death to the fetus because of oxygen deficiency.

When taken with other depressants, especially alcohol, barbiturates have a synergistic effect. The combination of alcohol and barbiturates can lead to accidental or intentional death. Another concern is that withdrawal is life-threatening without medical supervision. Withdrawal is marked by profuse sweating, insomnia, muscular twitching, paranoia, vomiting, aches and pains, cramps, quick temper, and, in severe instances, nightmares, hallucinations, and seizures. From 2004 to 2005, there was an increase of 19% in the number of people going to emergency rooms due to barbiturates.[8] Possible side effects of barbiturates include the following:

- reduced attention span
- impaired cognitive functioning
- diminished hand-eye coordination
- inadequate emotional control
- nausea
- vomiting
- birth defects
- confusion
- poor judgment
- slurred speech
- vertigo
- diarrhea
- respiratory failure
- violent behavior

On Campus

Among individuals between ages 18 and 25, more than 2% have used sedatives illegally.

Substance Abuse and Mental Health Services Administration, *Results from the 2006 National Survey on Drug Use and Health: National Findings* (Rockville, MD: Office of Applied Studies, 2007).

Medical Uses

During the 1960s, barbiturates were overprescribed, and thousands of people became dependent on them. Despite the consequences, barbiturates serve several medical functions. They are used primarily as sleeping pills, as well as for certain convulsive disorders and, to a limited extent, for anxiety. The group for whom these drugs are most prescribed is the elderly, although the long-term benefits of these drugs are not well-studied.[9] The percentage of hospitalized older patients who are given sedative-hypnotic drugs to treat insomnia ranges from 31% to 88%.[10] Among hospitalized children, 3% to 6% are given sleep medications.[11]

Short-acting barbiturates continue to be used for anesthetic purposes. During surgery the barbiturate **thiopental (pentothal)** reduces brain swelling and cerebral pressure and improves blood circulation. In recent years the number of prescriptions for barbiturates has declined because other drugs are less toxic and less likely to result in dependency.

About one-third of adults report difficulties either falling asleep or staying asleep. The effectiveness of barbiturates as sleep agents is questionable, because they interfere with **rapid eye movement (REM)**, which is necessary for a restful sleep. People deprived of REM have difficulty concentrating and can hallucinate. Barbiturate users may experience **rebound insomnia**, because one symptom of barbiturate withdrawal is insomnia. People who take sleeping pills often wake up more tired than when they went to sleep. An analogous phenomenon is waking up the morning after consuming too much alcohol. A person might sleep for hours but wake up exhausted. Therefore, barbiturates are counterproductive to sleep over time.

Nonbarbiturate Sedatives

Nonbarbiturate sedatives are depressants that share many of the same characteristics as barbiturates. They increase sedation and sleep while reducing anxiety. Examples of these drugs include chloral hydrate, paraldehyde, bromides, and meprobamate. Except for meprobamate, the history of these drugs dates before the development of barbiturates. Because other drugs are safer than nonbarbiturate sedatives, the latter are rarely used today.

Chloral Hydrate

When used to induce sleep, **chloral hydrate** works rapidly. With a typical dose (1 to 2 g), sleep usually comes in less than an hour, for 8 to 11 hours. Unfortunately, the margin between an effective dose (ED) and a lethal dose (LD) is slight. One study that compared chloral hydrate and music therapy on inducing sleep and sedation in children undergoing EEG testing found that music therapy was a better alternative.[12]

In addition to inducing sleep, chloral hydrate formerly was given to opiate addicts to enable them to overcome addiction and to alcoholics to help them deal with potentially fatal withdrawal symptoms. Chloral hydrate causes less cardiovascular and respiratory depression than barbiturates at comparable doses. Use of chloral hydrate fell into disfavor because it produces gastric distress, vomiting, and flatulence. Other side effects are unsteadiness, nightmares, and dependency. Chloral hydrate is better known as Mickey Finn or "knockout drops."

thiopental (pentothal) A barbiturate that is used as a general anesthetic

rapid eye movement (REM) A stage during sleep that is needed for the sleep to be restful

rebound insomnia A side effect of sleeping pills in which falling asleep becomes more difficult rather than less difficult

chloral hydrate A nonbarbiturate sedative; also called "knockout drops" or Mickey Finns; induces sleep

paraldehyde A nonbarbiturate, sedative-hypnotic drug used with severely disturbed mental patients

bromides Nonbarbiturate sedatives used to treat epileptic convulsions

meprobamate A minor tranquilizer marketed under the trade names of Miltown and Equanil; also used for treating psychosomatic conditions

Miltown Brand name for meprobamate

minor tranquilizer Drug used primarily to relieve anxiety

anxiolytic Refers to anxiety-reducing drugs

Equanil The first modern drug developed to relieve anxiety

methaqualone A sedative-hypnotic drug that relieves tension and anxiety without barbiturate-like aftereffects

Paraldehyde

Paraldehyde has been around for more than 100 years. It is an effective, yet safe, central nervous system depressant. Unlike other depressants, it causes little respiratory depression. In the 1950s it was given to severely disturbed patients in mental hospitals.

Like chloral hydrate, paraldehyde used to be provided to alcoholics to help manage their withdrawal symptoms. Its biggest drawback was that it produced a terrible smell and taste. Consequently, people who took paraldehyde had extremely bad breath. It is no longer used.

Bromides

The discovery of **bromides** dates back to 1826. In the past, they were administered to treat schizophrenia and epilepsy. Bromides proved to be unsuccessful. Currently, they are rarely provided as sleep agents, because they build up in the user's body, cause depression, and can be highly toxic. Other side effects include constipation, sedation, violent delirium, mental confusion, headache, dermatitis, psychomotor difficulties, and psychosis.

Meprobamate

Meprobamate was first marketed in 1955 under the brand name **Miltown**. The drug, which is classified as a **minor tranquilizer**, was derived from a muscle relaxant and was one of the first **anxiolytic** drugs, used to relieve anxiety. In addition to treating anxiety, meprobamate was prescribed for psychosomatic conditions. One article written in 1957 discussed concerns about the widespread prescribing of meprobamate and other tranquilizers.[13]

The United States clearly was ready for drugs to relieve anxiety because meprobamate was immediately popular. Medical practitioners promptly accepted and prescribed it as a safe alternative to barbiturates. Sales of Miltown, also known as **Equanil**, exceeded $500,000 in its initial year.

It was reported to cause physical and psychological dependence. At a rate of slightly more than twice the recommended dosage, a person can become physically dependent on meprobamate. Withdrawal from meprobamate is quite severe. Consequently, by 1970, the drug was listed as a controlled substance and the number of refills was regulated. Because of its low margin of safety and the availability of acceptable alternatives, meprobamate is rarely prescribed today.

Methaqualone

In an effort to find a desirable alternative to barbiturates—a drug that would relieve nervous tension and anxiety and promote sleep, yet not produce barbiturate-like hangovers—the pharmaceutical company W. H. Rorer introduced **methaqualone** in 1965.

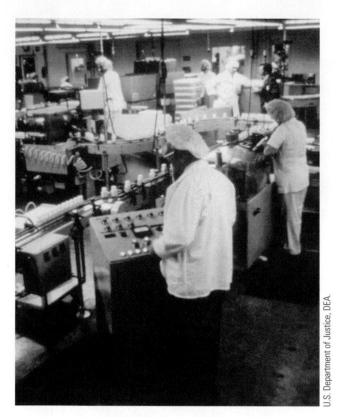

U.S. Department of Justice, DEA.

Depressants found on the illicit market are usually legitimately manufactured pharmaceuticals that have been diverted for illegal use.

Initially marketed under the brand name **Quaalude**, it also has been called Optimal, Sopor, Parest, Somnafac, and Bi-Phetamine T.

Methaqualone originally was tested in India to treat malaria but was found to be ineffective. Two common street terms for it are "Disco-Biscuits" and "Ludes." Methaqualone gained popularity as a recreational drug and illegal use escalated. Much of the methaqualone bought on the street was manufactured legally but diverted illegally.

Misconceptions

Methaqualone had a reputation as an aphrodisiac because of its disinhibiting effect. It was presumed that decreasing inhibition would increase sexual desire. Yet, the drug has no properties that increase the desire to have sex. With a little imagination, nearly any drug can be perceived as an aphrodisiac (just about every drug has been). Methaqualone is no more disinhibiting than alcohol or other central nervous depressants and it actually interferes with sexual behavior.

When it was approved for medical use, the U.S. Food and Drug Administration (FDA) did not closely monitor methaqualone, because it was thought to be safer than barbiturates and nonaddictive. The FDA was wrong, and the misconception was potentially hazardous. The drug is quite harmful and just as addictive. Withdrawal symptoms, which can be extremely severe, include mania, seizures, vomiting, convulsions, and death. During the 1970s, dozens of people, including the popular musician Jimi Hendrix, overdosed on methaqualone, and thousands were treated in emergency rooms.

Effects

Besides lowering inhibitions, methaqualone induces dreamlike moods at dosage levels of 75 mg. At higher doses, 130 to 300 mg, one might feel anesthetized and fall to sleep—sometimes permanently! Additional effects include the following:

reduced inhibitions	disorientation
diarrhea	drowsiness
menstrual irregularities	headache
depersonalization	pain in extremities
restlessness	anxiety
dry mouth	hangover
paranoia	nosebleeds
anorexia	memory loss

Memory is affected, and this lack of recall may account for some of the accidental overdoses. A person may not remember taking the drug and, subsequently, ingest more.

In combination with alcohol, methaqualone is especially lethal because these two drugs are synergistic. The number of emergency room visits because of methaqualone overdoses has declined sharply since the late 1970s. In 1983, the major manufacturer of methaqualone, Lemmon Pharmaceutical Company, stopped production. Since 1985, prescriptions for the drug have not been allowed in the United States. Although methaqualone use and abuse have declined in the United States, it remains a problem in South Africa, other parts of Africa, and India.[14]

Minor Tranquilizers

Minor tranquilizers were first developed in the 1950s, but the most popular type, called **benzodiazepines**, was not developed until the early 1960s. Also known as anxiolytics, these drugs are used primarily to treat anxiety although they are also effective as anticonvulsant drugs. Today, most users are women, because they are more likely than men to be diagnosed with anxiety disorders. An unfortunate consequence is that anxiety can promote the abuse of mind-altering substances such as minor tranquilizers, alcohol, and other prescribed medications.

Benzodiazepines

Quaalude Brand name for methaqualone

benzodiazepines A type of minor tranquilizer; examples are Librium and Valium

Valium (diazepam) A minor tranquilizer

fetal benzodiazepine syndrome A condition of infants caused by the mother's use of benzodiazepine during pregnancy; affected children have malformed face, poor muscle tone, tremors, poor coordination, delayed mental development, and learning disabilities

Despite their decline in popularity, benzodiazepines are one of the most commonly used drugs in Western societies.[15] Besides reducing anxiety, these minor tranquilizers induce sleep, reduce panic attacks and epilepsy, and control petit mal seizures. In the 1950s they were used in place of barbiturates for treating anxiety and sleep disorders. They are effective as anti-anxiety and sleep aids on a short-term basis only.

When first developed, these drugs were not thought to cause physical dependency (except in rare instances), withdrawal symptoms, or fatal overdoses. However, benzodiazepines are addictive and produce tolerance and withdrawal symptoms comparable to those for alcohol and barbiturates. Between 15% and 44% of long-term users become dependent on them.[16] One concern is that substance abusers who are given benzodiazepines for a medical problem may become dependent on these drugs.[17] Most people admitted into treatment for benzodiazepine abuse are female (59%) and White (88%).[18] One Australian study reported that a significant percentage of police detainees were dependent on benzodiazepines.[19]

Taking benzodiazepines at levels higher than recommended causes withdrawal symptoms to appear within a few days after abstinence, and symptoms can occur within 6 months after daily use. These symptoms include anxiety, muscle tension, and insomnia. Ironically, benzodiazepines are taken to reduce anxiety and improve sleep.

Despite their potential harm, benzodiazepines have a wider margin of safety, fewer side effects, and less severe side effects than barbiturates. When taken with barbiturates or alcohol, however, the risk of a fatal overdose increases. Benzodiazepines have been a factor in a number of suicides. A list of commonly prescribed benzodiazepines and their purposes is provided in Table 9.2

Because benzodiazepines have muscle-relaxing properties, they are prescribed for backache, muscle strain, multiple sclerosis, and Parkinson's disease.

TABLE 9.2 Selected Benzodiazepines

Generic Name	Brand Name	Medical Purpose
alprazolam	Xanax	Tranquilizer
chlordiazepoxide	Librium	Tranquilizer
clonazepam	Klonopin	Anticonvulsant
clorazepate	Tranxene	Tranquilizer
diazepam	Valium	Tranquilizer
flurazepam	Dalmane	Insomnia
oxazepam	Serax	Tranquilizer
triazolam	Halcion	Insomnia

Benzodiazepines are given to veterans suffering from posttraumatic stress disorder (PTSD).[20] They reportedly lead to weight gain by increasing the appetite. Though they enable people to fall asleep, the quality of sleep is affected adversely by reducing REM.

Although the number of prescriptions for these drugs has declined, their abuse is one of the most serious forms of drug abuse in the elderly population, especially women. A recent study conducted in France noted that benzodiazepines may be responsible for as many as 20,000 injurious falls and 1,800 deaths among people over age 80.[21] Dialysis patients taking benzodiazepines also experience a higher mortality rate.[22] Another group that is especially vulnerable to the sedating effects of benzodiazepines consists of people who have liver damage. A report from the United Nations states that these drugs are prescribed inappropriately to deal with social problems such as unemployment and relationship difficulties.[23]

Research on the psychological effects of benzodiazepines is inconsistent. Some research has found that they cause rage, hostility, and aggression, but other research points to a decrease in aggression among users. Benzodiazepines interfere with men's ability to attain an erection and achieve orgasm. Women experience less vaginal secretion, although they can be sexually aroused.

The fetus is affected by the mother's use of these drugs. Some children of women who took **Valium (diazepam)** in the first 3 months of pregnancy were more likely to have cleft palates, though subsequent studies contradict this finding. Within hours after delivery, withdrawal symptoms appeared in infants whose mothers used recommended, normal levels of Valium.

Similar to fetal alcohol syndrome, some women who took Valium while pregnant had children with **fetal benzodiazepine syndrome**, a condition marked by tremors, a malformed and expressionless face, learning disabilities, poor muscle tone, delayed hand-eye coordination and mental development, hyperactivity, and irritability. The validity of this condition is questioned because many women who take these drugs while pregnant also may be consuming other drugs.

Halcion (triazolam) is another benzodiazepine prescribed for sleep. It has also been used to sedate patients receiving dental implants.[24] It is a highly controversial drug because it reportedly produces a number of distressing side effects. Writer William Styron described how Halcion exacerbated his depression and how he contemplated suicide while taking the drug.[25] Others report similar experiences. Many people have filed lawsuits against its manufacturer, Upjohn Pharmaceuticals, claiming it caused adverse reactions. There have been reports of people on Halcion and similar drugs eating, making telephone phone calls, and driving while sleeping.[26]

Because Halcion interferes with memory, it can lead to accidental overdose. The ability to recall previously learned information is not affected adversely, but learning new information is temporarily more difficult. Other effects include nausea, paradoxical excitement, constipation, and dizziness. Because minor tranquilizers can cause confusion, ataxia (a lack of coordination), and fatigue lasting 1 to 3 hours, operating motor vehicles, using power tools, or running marathons while taking the drug is not advised. Halcion and other sedative-hypnotic drugs increase the risks of accidents because they produce a "hangover" effect after their use.[27] The FDA continues to allow Halcion to be prescribed, although it has been banned in more than a dozen countries.

"Date Rape" Drugs

Rohypnol

A powerful drug related to Valium is **Rohypnol**. Also known as "roofies," "rope," and "roche," Rohypnol (flunitrazepam) has been used in Europe since the 1970s. It gained a reputation as a "date rape" drug because women are unknowingly given this colorless, odorless, tasteless drug (usually in alcohol) and then raped. It leaves its victims disinhibited, helpless, and vulnerable. In efforts to help women avoid unwitting ingestion, coasters have been developed to detect drinks spiked with Rohypnol, and three Scottish students have developed a drinking straw that detects date-rape drugs like Rohypnol.[28]

Rohypnol is 5 to 10 times more powerful than Valium. On the college campus, Rohypnol sometimes is added to punch during parties. The effects of Rohypnol are greatly enhanced and more dangerous in combination with alcohol. This mixture can cause sedation, muscle relaxation, blackouts, addiction, complete memory loss, and even death. Many Rohypnol users experience amnesia, respiratory depression or arrest, and discoordination, and they have a higher rate of automobile accidents. The number of adolescents who have ever knowingly taken Rohypnol is about 1%.[29] Rohypnol use has been popular at raves.[30]

The drug takes effect 20 to 30 minutes after ingestion, and the effects last for 2 to 10 hours, depending on the dosage. When one stops using Rohypnol, dependency and withdrawal symptoms include headache, anxiety, muscle pain, confusion, irritability, hallucinations, delirium, convulsions, shock, and even death. Rohypnol is inexpensive and readily available. Two common misconceptions about Rohypnol are that (a) it cannot be detected by urine testing and (b) it is free of adulterants because it comes in sealed packages.

Physicians in the United States had been prescribing Rohypnol for insomnia, but in 1996 the federal government passed legislation banning its legal use. Because of its sedative-hypnotic effect, Rohypnol is legally prescribed in 60 countries around the world. As a result, Rohypnol is accessible for illegal use in the United States. Rohypnol, as well as Valium and other prescription drugs, is transported legally across the Mexican border and then illegally diverted.

To address concerns posed by Rohypnol, the Drug Enforcement Agency is trying to reschedule it as a Schedule I drug, which would increase penalties for its use. The drug's manufacturer, Hoffman-LaRoche, opposes the rescheduling of Rohypnol. Criminal penalties for its use while committing a crime are severe. Anyone using Rohypnol or other controlled substances for the purpose of facilitating a crime of violence, including rape, can be sentenced to up to 20 years in prison.

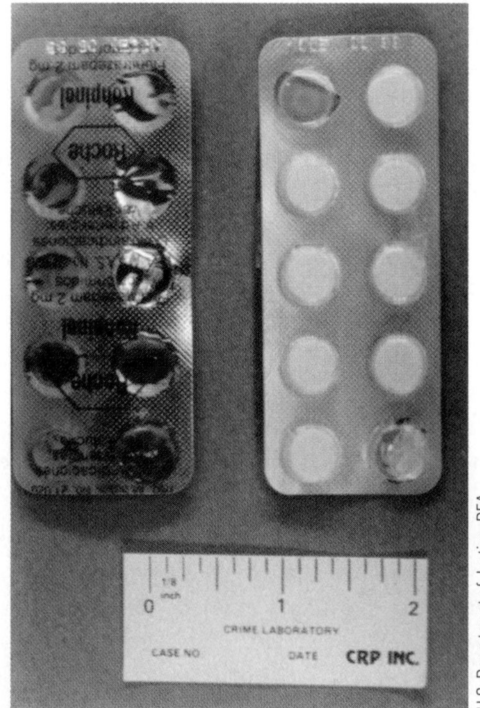

U.S. Department of Justice, DEA.

Rohypnol, a "date rape" drug, is sold inexpensively in Mexico and smuggled into the United States.

Gamma-Hydroxybutyrate (GHB)

Another drug referred to as a "date rape" drug is **gamma-hydroxybutyrate**, or **GHB**. Nicknames for GHB include Easy Lay, Grievous Bodily Harm, Gook, and Gamma 10. Like Rohypnol, GHB is odorless, tasteless, and easy to produce. The use of GHB has grown, especially in western states.

GHB has a reputation as an aphrodisiac because it is believed to enhance the sense of touch and sexual prowess. One study reported that 18% of users took GHB to enhance sex while 13% took it to be sociable and another 13% took the drug to alter their consciousness.[31] GHB use is not uncommon among gay men. A survey found that 29% of gay men indicated that they had taken GHB recently while at a club.[32] Some bodybuilders use GHB illicitly as a growth hormone stimulant.

Medically, GHB has been shown to be useful in opiate detoxification. It has been used experimentally to treat narcolepsy. In addition, it has been hypothesized that GHB may be helpful for treating alcohol dependence.[33]

Based on data collected from various emergency rooms around the United States, GHB was involved in 1,861 emergency room visits in 2005.[34] In 1994, GHB was involved in only 56 visits. GHB has the potential to be deadly, because it causes the respiratory system to shut down. When GHB is mixed with alcohol, the person may lose memory and consciousness. Other effects are vomiting, nausea, seizures, hallucinations, coma, and respiratory distress. When GHB is combined with alcohol and other central nervous system depressants, the potential for death escalates.

Halcion A drug used to induce sleep

Rohypnol A powerful depressant; one of the "date rape" drugs

gamma-hydroxybutyrate (GHB) A type of neurotransmitter that produces relaxation and sleepiness; one of the "date rape" drugs

gateway drugs Substances that are used before use of more dangerous drugs; alcohol, marijuana, tobacco, and inhalants are considered gateway drugs

Inhalants

Inhalant abuse, also called "huffing," was noted during World War I. Compared with many other drugs of abuse, inhalants receive little attention by researchers. Therefore, in-depth knowledge about inhalants is limited. The lack of research regarding inhalants could reflect the fact that many inhalant abusers are not in treatment. Studying inhalants is important, because they serve as **gateway drugs**. Also, inhalant abusers are more likely to abuse additional drugs.

Among adolescents ages 12 and 13, inhalants are the most frequently used class of illegal drugs. Inhalants were used by 3.4% of 12-year-olds and 4.8% of 13-year-olds. The popularity of inhalants with teens is attributed to their low cost, availability, and size. (Because inhalants come in small packages, they are easily concealed.) An interesting point is that 12- and 13-year-olds are more likely to use inhalants than older adolescents.[35] Moreover, the number of girls who have used inhalants has surpassed the number of boys.[36] Among incarcerated adolescents, more than one-third have used inhalants.[37] One in ten adults have used inhalants at least one time.[38] Within the military, inhalants are the third most commonly abused class of drugs.[39]

Although many inhalants have anesthetic-like properties, they are not considered sedative-hypnotic drugs. Inhalants are classified by how they are used rather than by their effects on the central nervous system. Inhalants are grouped into three classes: volatile hydrocarbon solvents, aerosols, and anesthetics. Inhalants such as gasoline, paint thinners, plastic cement, Magic Markers, cleaning supplies, glue, and nail polish remover have no known medical use. Indications of inhalant abuse include one's breath or clothing having a chemical odor or the appearance of disorientation.[40]

Short-term effects include drooling, nausea, sneezing, hypersensitivity, loss of coordination, and coughing. Long-term effects include frequent nosebleeds; liver and kidney damage; sores around the mouth, throat, and nose; weight loss; depression, irritability, and disorientation; paranoia; hostility; and bone marrow abnormalities. Inhalants accounted for 4,312 emergency room visits in 2005.[41]

Abuse of solvents is strongly related to antisocial disorders. Gasoline sniffing by children is a prominent factor in lead poisoning, which adversely affects physical and mental growth.

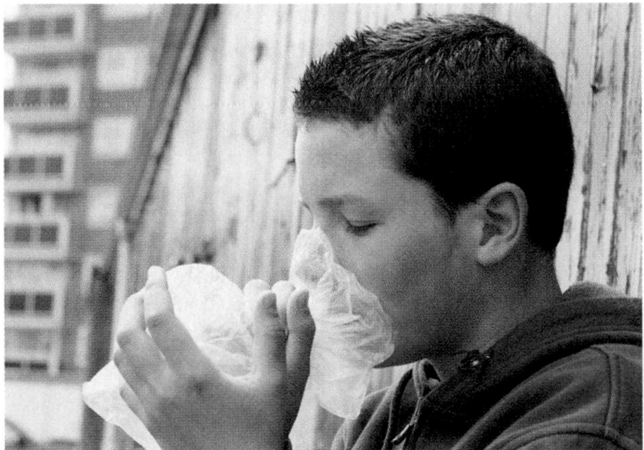

Sniffing an inhalant-soaked rag from a bag is a form of "huffing."

Glue and Other Solvents

Glue and other solvents are squeezed into paper bags, handkerchiefs, or rags, placed over the nose, and inhaled. The psychoactive agent in glue is **toluene**, which is found in unleaded gasoline and the glue used for building model airplanes.

Glue sniffing was given scant attention until the 1960s, at which time reports of glue sniffing appeared in newspapers throughout the United States. By warning readers of the dangers of sniffing glue, newspaper articles turned an obscure problem into a major problem. The number of teens inhaling glue increased greatly.

Inhalants are considered gateway drugs. Among inner-city Chicago youths, those who used inhalants by age 16 were much more likely to use heroin than those who used inhalants at a later age.[42] Inhalants often are the first drug abused by children, especially those in poor or rural areas. Some individuals continue to use inhalants as long as 15 years.

Inhalant users describe the effects as a hazy euphoria, comparable to alcohol intoxication. Some users have violent outbursts, delusions, double vision, disinhibition, ringing in the ears, speech impairment, hallucinations, muscle weakness, disorientation, vomiting, and nausea. These effects are temporary and disappear following exposure to air. A more serious physical threat is immediate cardiorespiratory arrest. Also, solvent sniffing can lead to physical and emotional damage resulting from the lead found in glue and gasoline.

Although solvents do not produce withdrawal symptoms or physical dependence, use of solvents has been implicated in kidney damage, respiratory system depression, irregularities in the heart (cardiac arrhythmias), and possibly liver damage. Another concern about solvent inhalation is brain damage, although the evidence is inconclusive.

Solvent users can develop anemia and bone marrow damage. Seizures can result from inhaling solvents, and the user may die from heart failure or suffocation. Because inhalants are put into bags and sniffed, the user can pass out and accidentally suffocate.

Anesthetic Inhalants

Ether was marketed commercially in the 18th century as an industrial solvent and an anesthetic. Although the purpose of ether was to eliminate pain during surgery, it was an attractive alternative to alcohol, because it produced intoxication and was less expensive than alcohol. Upper-class Europeans and Americans were the first to use the drug recreationally, but individuals in lower socioeconomic classes soon followed.

Nitrous oxide, a colorless gas with a sweet taste and odor, was discovered by Joseph Priestly and synthesized by Humphrey Davy. A Connecticut dentist, Horace Wells, noted the anesthetic properties of nitrous oxide and incorporated it into his dental practice. When it was given for the first time during surgery, it was considered a dismal failure, because the person to whom the gas was given woke up during the operation and screamed in agony. Despite this early setback, nitrous oxide found its way into medicine. One person who experimented with nitrous oxide was psychologist William James, who contended that it altered his consciousness and that he experienced mystic revelations.

Anesthetic gases render pharmacological effects similar to barbiturates. They provide sedation, pain relief, anxiety relief, and sleep. If people use nitrous oxide in conjunction with alcohol, they receive no greater analgesic effect from this combination. If a patient is given nitrous oxide during surgery, an adequate supply of oxygen is necessary because the decreased oxygen level in the blood can cause irreparable brain damage, a condition called **hypoxia**. Nonmedical use of nitrous oxide (and other inhalants) can lead to hypoxia.

A popular source for nitrous oxide is whippets, small cartridges designed for whipped cream containers. The immediate effects of inhaling nitrous oxide are euphoria, hallucinations, giddiness, and reduced inhibitions. These effects contributed to its nickname, "laughing gas." Also, nitrous oxide impairs cognitive and psychomotor performance. It interferes with memory and concentration. Nitrous oxide may cause death.

Nitrite Inhalants

The final classification of inhalants, the nitrite group, is used for both medical and nonmedical purposes. The three types of nitrites are **amyl nitrite**, **butyl nitrite**, and **isobutyl**. The benefits of nitrites were established more than 150 years ago. In the mid-1800s, amyl nitrite was used as a vasodilator; it relaxed the muscles in the walls of the blood vessels. Subsequently, the drug was used to relieve angina pectoris and to treat congestive heart failure. Also, amyl nitrite is given as an antidote for cyanide poisoning. When inhaled, amyl nitrite alters consciousness and intensifies the sexual experience.

Originally, amyl nitrite came in mesh-enclosed glass ampules called "pearls." As the glass ampules were crushed by the fingers, they emitted a popping sound—hence the nickname "poppers." Nitrites increase intracranial pressure by dilating cerebral blood vessels, producing euphoria.

Like amyl nitrite, butyl nitrite and isobutyl nitrite dilate the blood vessels, but they are not used therapeutically. Butyl nitrite is found in many commercial products such as perfume and antifreeze.

The popularity of inhaling nitrites for sexual purposes—heightened libido, aphrodisiac properties, and prevention of premature ejaculation—escalated in the mid-1970s. At one time, sales of nonprescription nitrites totaled $50 million. One group noted for its use of nitrites is gay males, although use by this group has declined. Among high school seniors, less than 1% abused nitrites in the most recent surveys.[43]

Despite the claims of improved sexual performance, no research indicates that nitrites have any direct effect on sexual ability. A real danger, however, is that brief exposure to nitrites at moderate dosages suppresses the immune system. Therefore, they have been linked to HIV and AIDS. Animal studies have linked nitrite inhalation with infectious diseases and the development of tumors.

Side effects of nitrites include pounding headache, nausea, feelings of warmth, drop in blood pressure, throbbing sensations, rapid pulse, and sometimes loss of consciousness. Additional effects are blurred vision, eye irritation, and eye pressure. Crusty lesions may appear where the skin comes into contact with butyl nitrite, suggesting a possible allergic reaction. These lesions can form on the nose, lip, scrotum, and penis. Because nitrites are flammable and explosive, burns are another potential hazard. Trade names of products containing nitrites, which typically are found in adult bookstores, head shops, and mail order catalogs, include the following:

Aroma of Men	Heart On
Ban Apple Gas	High Ball
Bang	Jac Aroma
Bolt	Liquid Increase
Bullet	Locker Room
Climax	Mama Poppers
Crypt Tonight	Oz
Cum	RUSH
Discorama	Satan's Scent
Hardware	Toilet Water

Summary

Just as their name suggests, sedative-hypnotic drugs produce relaxation, and sometimes sleep, depending on the dosage. The three classes of sedative-hypnotic drugs are barbiturates, nonbarbiturate sedatives, and minor tranquilizers. Side effects associated with sedative-hypnotic drugs include nausea, lethargy, vomiting, upset stomach, blurred vision, hangover, fever, and impaired judgment. These drugs can cause physical dependency and severe withdrawal symptoms. The margin of safety between an effective dose and lethal dose is minimal.

A problem that has arisen in recent years is the illegal use of prescription drugs by adolescents. Although prescription drugs can be obtained legally, many adolescents are getting them illegally. Adolescents perceive prescription drugs to be safer than traditional illegal drugs.

Barbiturates, developed in Germany in the 19th century and marketed in the early 1900s, are categorized by how long they act and how quickly they work. They are prescribed primarily for sleep, although they also are used to treat convulsions, diabetes, and anxiety, as well as serving as anesthetics. Because of overprescribing during the 1960s, barbiturate dependency markedly increased.

Their effects are modified by differences in users, previous experience with the drugs, dosage, set and setting, and method of administration. Barbiturates have adverse effects on coordination, attention span, and reaction time. Moreover, they can be fatal, because they alter heart rate, respiration, and blood pressure. Withdrawal can be life-threatening, too. Babies of women who took barbiturates while pregnant are more likely to be born with congenital dependency, birth defects, and brain damage.

Nonbarbiturate sedatives are chemically different from barbiturates but produce similar effects. Examples are chloral hydrate, paraldehyde, bromides, meprobamate, and methaqualone. Chloral hydrate formerly was used to induce sleep and to overcome the addiction to opiates and alcohol. Because of unpleasant side effects, it is no longer prescribed.

Paraldehyde was given to severely disturbed mental patients but fell into disfavor because of its terrible

toluene The psychoactive agent in glue

ether An inhalant dating back to the late 1700s

nitrous oxide An inhalant also known as laughing gas

hypoxia A lack of oxygen within body tissues; hypoxia can lead to brain damage resulting from an inadequate supply of oxygen to the brain

amyl nitrite An inhalant used to treat angina pectoris and congestive heart failure

butyl nitrite An inhalant no longer used for medical purposes but found in products such as perfume and antifreeze

isobutyl One type of nitrite that is used to treat angina pain; also causes vasodilation, flushing, and warmth

taste and smell. Bromides were used in the treatment of schizophrenia and epilepsy but proved to be ineffective.

Meprobamate (Miltown) was one of the first drugs prescribed specifically to relieve anxiety. The medical community quickly accepted it, though the drug produced psychological and physical dependence and severe withdrawal symptoms. Methaqualone, which was viewed as a safe alternative to other sedative-hypnotic drugs, was incorrectly perceived to be nonaddictive and an aphrodisiac. Side effects include restlessness, depersonalization, a dream-like state, an anesthetized feeling, and sleep. Withdrawal symptoms are vomiting, seizures, and possibly death.

Benzodiazepines are the drugs most commonly prescribed to relieve anxiety. They are effective for only a short time because they produce a rebound effect, causing individuals to feel less rested after use. They are prescribed for backaches, multiple sclerosis, muscle strain, and Parkinson's disease. Initially, these drugs were believed to be safe, but now it is known that they lead to tolerance and physical dependency. Although a person can become dependent in 4 to 6 weeks of taking normal doses, these drugs are safer than barbiturates. The elderly and people with liver damage are vulnerable to the effects of benzodiazepines. Babies exposed to these drugs during their mother's pregnancy have a greater incidence of cleft palate and are likely to undergo withdrawal symptoms.

Two well-known date rape drugs are Rohypnol and GHB. GHB has been implicated in an increasing number of fatalities. Rohypnol and GHB are given to unknowing individuals, resulting in numerous cases of sexual abuse.

Inhalants with sedative-hypnotic properties are classified as hydrocarbon solvents, aerosols, and anesthetics. Teenagers, the primary users of inhalants, take them because they are easy to obtain and conceal, work quickly, and are relatively inexpensive. Glue is considered a gateway drug for teenage boys, although an increasing number of girls have begun abusing inhalants. Its effects last about 45 minutes and include intoxication, hallucinations, violent outbursts, seizures, and even cardiorespiratory arrest. Solvents can produce irregular heartbeat, respiratory system depression, anemia, kidney damage, seizures, and death. Some cases of lead poisoning in children have been attributed to solvents.

Two examples of anesthetic inhalants are ether and nitrous oxide. At one time, people used ether as an inexpensive substitute for alcohol. Nitrous oxide eventually found its way into medicine. If it is used during surgery, it is necessary to provide adequate oxygen or patients will suffer from hypoxia. Nitrous oxide also interferes with memory and concentration.

The three types of nitrites are amyl nitrite, butyl nitrite, and isobutyl nitrite. They dilate blood vessels and relax the muscles. Amyl nitrite is available only by prescription. The most common use of nitrites—especially in the 1970s—has been to intensify sexual experiences. Research, however, has not supported this effect. Nitrites can affect the immune system and are linked to HIV. Other effects of nitrites include eye irritation and lesions on the nose, lip, and genitalia.

Thinking Critically

1. Physicians are aware of the potential for dependency on barbiturates. Should they be more careful when writing prescriptions for barbiturates? If a patient becomes dependent on barbiturates, is that the responsibility of the doctor or the patient?
2. A prescribed drug for sleep is Halcion. In one case, a woman taking Halcion killed her mother and blamed the drug and its manufacturer. She was acquitted. Do you think a bad reaction to a prescribed drug is a reasonable defense? Should a person be acquitted for a crime committed while under the influence of a prescribed drug?
3. Newspapers and magazines publish many articles about drugs and drug use. These articles about drugs might have the effect of increasing their use. What are the advantages and disadvantages of newspapers and magazines publishing articles about drugs?
4. Nonprescribed nitrites have been linked to the Kaposi's sarcoma virus, a form of cancer prevalent in AIDS patients. Should nitrites be more strongly regulated?

Web Resources

American Medical Association
http://www.ama-assn.org
This site includes information regarding the development and promotion of standards in medical practice, research, and education.

Consumer Reports
http://www.consumerreports.org/health/home.htm
This site provides help in assessing the effective and safety of various prescription drugs. It enables consumers to talk to their physicians more knowledgeably about prescription drugs.

Notes

1. Office of National Drug Control Policy, *Women and Prescription Drugs* (Washington, D.C.: ONDCP, April, 2007).
2. D. C. Voaklander, B. H. Rowe, D. M. Dryden, J. Pahal, P. Saar, and P. Kelly, "Medical Illness, Medication Use and Suicide in Seniors: A Population-Based Case-Control Study," *Journal of Epidemiology and Community Health*, 62 (February 2008): 138–146.
3. Substance Abuse and Mental Health Services Administration, *Results from the 2006 National Survey on Drug Use and Health: National Findings* (Rockville, MD: U.S. Department of Health and Human Services, 2007).
4. S. E. McCabe, B. T. West, M. Morales, J. A. Cranford, and C. J. Boyd, "Does Early Onset of Non-Medical Use of Prescription Drugs Predict Subsequent Prescription Drug Abuse and Dependence? Results from a National Study," *Addiction*, 102 (2007): 1920–1930.
5. L. D. Johnston, P. M. O'Malley, J. G. Bachman, and J. E. Schulenberg, *Monitoring the Future: National Results on Adolescent Drug Use, Overview of Key Findings, 2007* (Bethesda, MD: National Institute on Drug Abuse, 2008).
6. Office of National Drug Control Policy (ONDCP), *Prescription for Danger: A Report on the Troubling Trend of Prescription and Over-the-Counter Drug Abuse Among the Nation's Teens* (Washington, D.C.: ONDCP, January 2008).
7. B. J. Deacon and D. P. Valentiner, "Substance Use and Non-Clinical Panic Attacks in a Young Adult Population," *Journal of Substance Abuse,* 11 (2000): 7–15.
8. Substance Abuse and Mental Health Services Administration, *Drug Abuse Warning Network, 2005: National Estimates of Drug-Related Emergency Room Visits* (Rockville, MD: Office of Applied Studies, 2007).
9. S. H. Tariq and S. Pulisetty, "Pharmacotherapy for Insomnia," *Clinics in Geriatric Medicine*, 24 (February 2008): 93–105.
10. J. H. Flaherty, "Insomnia among Hospitalized Older Persons," *Clinics in Geriatric Medicine*, 24 (February 2008): 51–67.
11. L. J. Meltzer, J. A. Mindell, J. A. Owens, and K. C. Byars, "Use of Sleep Medications in Hospitalized Pediatric Patients," *Pediatrics*, 119 (June 2007): 1047–1055.
12. J. Loewy, C. Hallan, E. Friedman, and C. Martinez, "Sleep/Sedation in Children Undergoing EEG Testing: A Comparison of Chloral Hydrate and Music Therapy," *American Journal of Electroneurodiagnostic Technology*, 46 (December 2006): 343–355.
13. "This Week 50 Years Ago," *New Scientist*, 195 (September 29, 2007): 14.
14. G. McCarthy, B. Myers, and N. Siegfried, "Treatment for Methaqualone Dependence in Adults," *Cochrane Database of Systematic Reviews* (2007).
15. M. G. Sim, E. Khong, and T. D. Wain, "The Prescribing Dilemma of Benzodiazepines," *Australian Family Physician*, 36 (November 2007): 923–926.
16. A. Chetley, *Problem Drugs* (Amsterdam: Health Action International, 1995).
17. D. A. Ciraulo and A. P. Nace, "Benzodiazepine Treatment of Anxiety or Insomnia in Substance Abuse Patients," *The American Journal of Addictions,* 9 (2000): 276–284.
18. "Characteristics of Primary Benzodiazepine Admissions: 2000," *The DASIS Report,* November 21, 2003.
19. W. Loxley, "Benzodiazepine Use and Harms among Police Detainees in Australia," *Trends and Issues in Crime and Criminal Justice*, 336 (May 2007).
20. J. A. Hermos, M. M. Young, E. V. Lawler, D. Rosenbloom, and L.D. Fiore, "Long-Term, High-Dose Benzodiazepine Prescriptions in Veteran Patients with PTSD: Influence of Preexisting Alcoholism and Drug-Abuse Diagnoses," *Journal of Traumatic Stress*, 20 (October 2007): 909–914.
21. A. Pariente, et al., "Benzodiazepines and Injurious Falls in Community Dwelling Elders," *Drugs and Aging*, 25 (2008): 61–70.
22. W. C. Winkelmayer, J. Mehta, and P. S. Wang, "Benzodiazepine Use and Mortality of Incident Dialysis Patients in the United States," *Kidney International*, 72 (December 2007): 1388–1393.
23. "UN Warns on Lifestyle Drugs," *Chemist and Druggist* (March 3, 2001): 7.
24. D. Flanagan, "Oral Triazolam Sedation in Implant Dentistry," *The Journal of Oral Implantology*, 30 (2004): 93–97.
25. W. Stryon, "Prozac Days, Halcion Nights," *Nation* (January 4, 1993): 11.
26. R. Sandroff, "Sleeping-Pill Warnings," *Consumer Reports on Health*, 19 (May 2007): 1–2.
27. A. Vermeeren, "Residual Effects of Hypnotics: Epidemiology and Clinical Implications," *CNS Drugs*, 18 (2004): 297–328.
28. A. Labi, "Date Rape's Last Straw," *Chronicle of Higher Education*, 53 (February 2, 2007): 5.
29. Johnston et al., supra note 5.
30. "Rave Realities: The Truth about Club Drugs," *Science World,* 60 (January 12, 2004): 8.
31. H. R. Sumnall, K. Woolfall, S. Edwards, J. C. Cole, and C. M. Benyon, "Use, Function, and Subjective Experiences of Gamma-hydroxybutyrate (GHB)," *Drug and Alcohol Dependence*, 92 (January 1, 2008): 286–290.
32. P. N. Halkitis, "GHB Use Among Gay and Bisexual Men," *Addictive Behaviors*, 31 (November 2006): 2135–2139.
33. O. Ameisen, "Are the Effects of Gamma-hydroxybutarate (GHB) Partly Physiological in Alcohol Dependence?" *American Journal of Drug and Alcohol Abuse*, 34 (February 2008): 235–236.
34. Substance Abuse and Mental Health Services Administration, supra note 8.
35. The NSDUH Report, *Inhalant Use across the Adolescent Years* (Rockville, MD.: Substance Abuse and Mental Health Services Administration, March 13, 2008).
36. "Girls Surpass Boys in Deadly Practice," *USA Today Magazine*, 136 (October 2007): 15.
37. M. O. Howard, R. L. Balster, L. B. Cottler, L. Wu, and M. G. Vaughn, "Inhalant Use Among Incarcerated Adolescents in the United States: Prevalence, Characteristics, and Correlates of Use," *Drug and Alcohol Dependence*, 93 (March 2008): 197–209.
38. L. Wu and C. L. Ringwalt, "Inhalant Use and Disorders Among Adults in the United States," *Drug and Alcohol Dependence,* 85 (2006): 1–11.
39. "Inhalant Abuse in the Military: An Unrecognized Threat," *Military Medicine*, 172 (April 2007): 388–392.
40. "Getting High on Household Products," *Nursing*, 37 (November 2007): 66.
41. Substance Abuse and Mental Health Services Administration, supra note 3.
42. E. O. Johnson, C. G. Schultz, J. C. Anthony, and M. E. Ensminger, "Inhalants to Heroin: A Prospective Analysis from Adolescence to Adulthood," *Drug and Alcohol Dependence,* 40 (1995): 159–164.
43. Johnston et al., supra note 5.

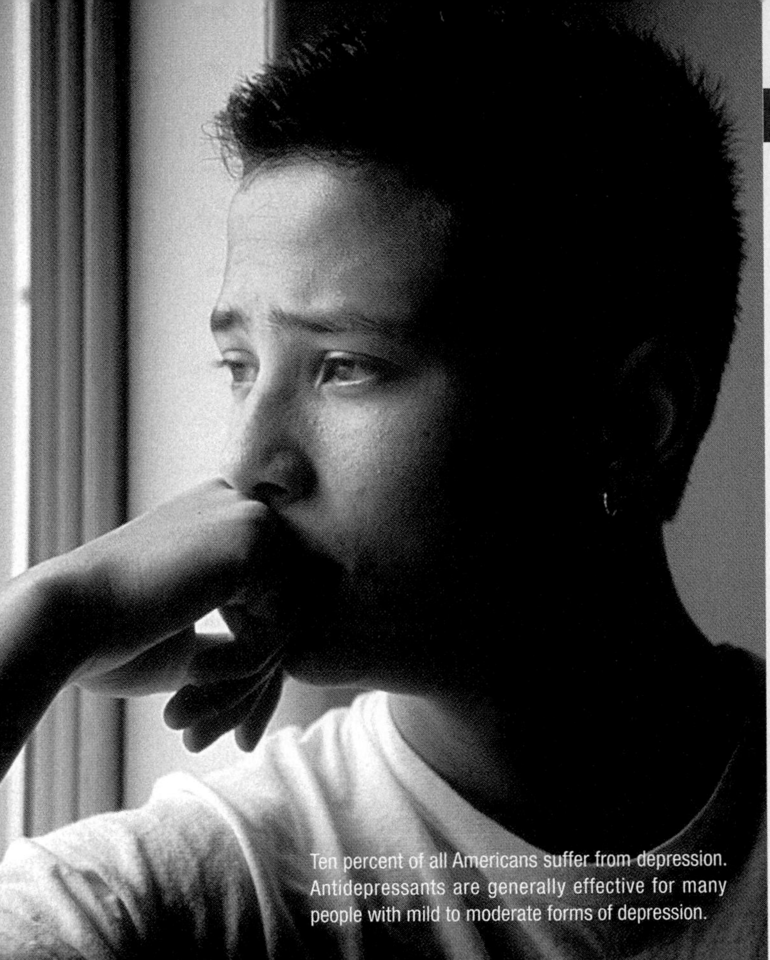

Ten percent of all Americans suffer from depression. Antidepressants are generally effective for many people with mild to moderate forms of depression.

FACT OR FICTION?

1. Most people with a mental illness seek professional help for their illness.
2. The highest rate of depressive episodes occurs among individuals who work full-time and are personal-care and service workers.
3. One side effect associated with antidepressants is sudden weight loss.
4. Most people who seek a mental health therapist obtained that person's name from a friend or family member.
5. The number of children receiving antidepressant drugs has decreased since 2000.
6. Although the effectiveness of antidepressant drugs is questionable, most patients believe they are helped by these drugs.
7. Before antidepressants were given to children, they were tested thoroughly for side effects and for effectiveness for depression.
8. Although the number of children in the United States taking antipsychotic drugs has increased, the number of children in other countries taking these drugs has decreased.

Turn the page to check your answers

10 Psychotherapeutic Drugs

Chapter Objectives

After completing this chapter, the reader should be able to describe:

- Difficulties in defining what is meant by mental illness
- The various types of mood disorders
- The difference between psychosis and neurosis
- Early treatments used with mentally ill patients
- Advantages and disadvantages of the various types of antidepressants
- The benefits and limitations of Prozac, Zoloft, and Paxil
- The conditions for which lithium is most effective
- The effectiveness of antipsychotic drugs

FACT OR FICTION?

1. **Fiction:** The fact is—it is estimated that only about 10% of people with mental illness seek professional help.
2. **Fact:** Government data indicate that over 10% of personal-care and service workers had a major depressive episode in the previous year.
3. **Fiction:** The fact is—weight gain rather than weight loss is a common side effect associated with antidepressants.
4. **Fiction:** The fact is—a study from *Consumer Reports* found that only 20% of patients received a therapist's name from a friend or family member.
5. **Fiction:** The fact is—the number of children receiving antidepressant drugs has increased significantly over the last several years.
6. **Fact:** Most people who take antidepressant drugs feel that they benefit from them.
7. **Fiction:** The fact is—one major concern regarding antidepressant drugs is that they were not tested for their effects on children.
8. **Fiction:** The fact is—the rate of children receiving antipsychotic drugs has more than doubled in some European countries.

A growing problem in people of all ages is mental illness. Pinpointing precise factors that contribute to the emotional adversities people face is difficult. Possible causes range from childrearing practices, to heredity, to biochemical imbalances, to our fast-paced and get-ahead-at-any-cost mentality. Compounding the problem is the fact that the meaning of *mental illness* is unclear. In this chapter, we will examine the concept of mental illness and the drugs used to treat its various forms.

Understanding Mental Illness

In a literal sense, one could say that **mental illness** means an illness of the mind. In this sense, mental illness would be the result of a brain disease or a biochemical imbalance. The famous U.S. physician Benjamin Rush, who lived two centuries ago, speculated that mental illness arises from problems with the blood vessels in the brain. Mental illness, however, involves much more than anatomical structures and hormones. It implies inappropriate thinking and behavior as well. The word *inappropriate* is subject to individual interpretation. Even if we agree that a person's behavior or thinking may exceed a socially acceptable range, who is to determine what is appropriate? One definition of a mental disorder is "an abnormal state of mind (whether of a continuous or an intermittent nature), characterized by delusions, or by disorders of mood or perception or volition or cognition."[1] Many people contend that the distinction between mental health and mental illness is fuzzy.[2]

Mental Illness and Medicine

Identifying people as mentally ill frequently is left to the judgment of medical personnel, who view illness, regardless of whether it is physical or mental, from a disease perspective. This implies that illness results from a **pathogen**—suggesting that mental illness is a disease that has symptoms and a cure. This approach involving symptoms, diagnosis, and cure is the basis for the **medical model**.

The application of the medical model to emotional problems gives rise to some concern. For one thing, behaviors deemed inappropriate or unacceptable might not be the result of any given disease. Many people have difficulties adjusting to the stresses and problems of life. Should they be labeled mentally ill?

A critic of the medical model is psychiatrist Thomas Szasz, who says that the concept of mental illness is a myth.[3] He argues that most people identified as mentally ill do not have any type of disease. If mental illness is a myth, as Szasz contends, should drugs be administered to individuals to regulate their behaviors? The use of drugs in treating mental illness dates back many centuries, although drugs used in the past and present to treat mental illness do not *cure* it. Instead, drugs treat symptoms related to mental illness and moderate people's behavior.

Mental Illness and Special Populations

No group of people is immune to the possibility of mental illness. American adolescents appear to be experiencing major depressive episodes at an increasing rate. Nearly 12% of 16- and 17-year-olds had a major depressive episode within the previous 12 months. Also, 70% of these adolescents indicated that the episode was either severe or very severe.[4] According to the World Health Organization, 20% of all children and adolescents suffer from a disabling mental illness, and 50% of all adult mental illness started during adolescence.[5] Depression in adolescents has been shown to be associated with family history of depression.[6]

Another group affected by depression is postpartum women. The U.S. Centers for Disease Control and Prevention (CDC) reports that 10% to 15% of mothers are affected by postpartum depression within the first 12 months following birth. Rates of postpartum depression are greater among women who are younger or experience partner-related stress or physical abuse. Also, women with less education and who receive Medicaid benefits are more likely to experience postpartum depression.[7]

Besides adolescents and birthing mothers, the elderly are increasingly susceptible to mental illness. Among North Americans, the rate of suicide among people ages 50 and older has continued to escalate.[8]

mental illness A condition caused by a mood disorder or by disorganized thinking

pathogen Any organism that produces disease

medical model The premise that a pathogen is responsible for a person's illness or disease

psychosis A severe mental condition marked by loss of contact with reality

schizophrenia A type of functional psychosis; literally, "split mind"

mood disorder A form of psychosis that affects the person's emotions; can be depression or mania

depression Dejection characterized by withdrawal or lack of response to stimulation

mania A mood disorder characterized by inappropriate elation, an irrepressible mood, and extreme cheerfulness

Types of Disorders

Emotional problems range from anxiety to psychosis. Anxiety and worry are common, normal experiences. When they become disproportionate and interfere with daily life, however, problems arise. When discomfort turns to panic, skepticism turns to fear, and concern turns to unrealistic worry, the person has to deal with these barriers to everyday functioning. Obsessive-compulsive behaviors, psychosomatic ailments, phobias, and panic attacks are examples. Anxiety typically is treated with antianxiety drugs. (A review of antianxiety drugs is included in Chapter 9.)

Psychosis

A **psychosis** is a condition in which the person loses contact with reality. Psychoses are divided into two categories: organic and functional. "Organic" refers to physical causes. Some causes of organic psychoses are excessive use of drugs such as cocaine and alcohol, brain infections, metabolic or endocrine disorders, brain tumors, and neurological diseases.

Functional psychoses are those that have no known or apparent cause. One type is **schizophrenia**. This term, which literally means "split mind," is a misnomer because a schizophrenic does not have two or more personalities. Three symptoms mark schizophrenia: delusions, hallucinations, and a restricted range of emotions.

An estimated 1% of the population is schizophrenic, with women and men being affected about equally. It is believed that the number of people ages 55 and older who will be diagnosed with schizophrenia will double in the next 20 years.[9] Although heredity is a major factor, schizophrenia may arise from an interaction of environment and heredity. Parents, social factors, nutrition, and environmental chemicals may play a role. Years of alcohol abuse also can lead to schizophrenia-like psychosis.

Mood disorders are typified by **depression** at one extreme and **mania** at the other. Depression is highly correlated with substance abuse.[10] Similarly, alcohol use and depression are strongly linked. Although alcohol use and depression are associated, it is conceivable that this is because alcohol is used to deal with one's depression.[11] A relationship also was found between smoking and depression, especially among female smokers.[12] Depressed people may smoke as a form of self-medication. It has been reported that many smokers who successfully complete a smoking cessation program become less depressed.[13] Women are more likely than men to have depression, but men have higher rates of substance abuse disorders and antisocial personality disorder.[14] Unfortunately, only one of three people who need it seek help for depression.[15]

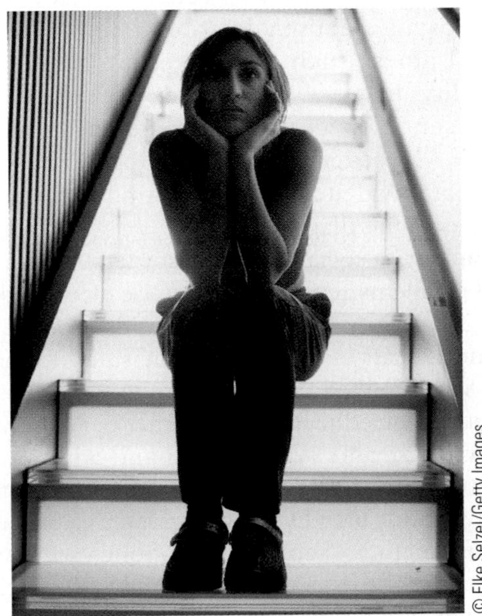

Depression is a type of mood disorder.

Some people alternate between mania and depression. This is called **bipolar affective disorder**. Other people have only mania or depression. About 10% of people develop **unipolar depression**, the most common form.[16] An estimated 5% of children experience depression before they reach adolescence. Symptoms of depression include feelings of worthlessness, shortened attention span, less pleasure from activities that had been enjoyable, sleep and appetite disturbances, diminished ability to concentrate, and possibly suicidal thoughts. Approximately 15% of depressed individuals commit suicide.[17]

Bipolar affective disorder, formerly called manic-depression, is marked by alternating periods of mania, depression, and normalcy. It is estimated that 1 in 5 patients with depression have bipolar disorder.[18] Some individuals with substance abuse problems are misdiagnosed with bipolar illness.[19] A factor contributing to misdiagnosis is that some people who experience a manic episode have hallucinations or delusions. Mania, which can arise suddenly and last for days or months, is characterized by inappropriate elation, an irrepressible mood, and extreme cheerfulness and enthusiasm. A frequent problem among people with bipolar disorder is noncompliance with medications. One study found that more than 60% do not always adhere to taking medications.[20]

Dual Diagnosis (Co-Occurring Disorders)

Dual diagnosis, more commonly referred to today as *co-occurring disorders*, describes a person with two or more existing mental illnesses, each of which can be diagnosed independent of the others. According to substance-abuse expert Tracy Wallace, "the symptoms are not just a clutter resulting from one disorder."[21] Common co-occurring disorders include substance abuse/addiction or alcoholism and a mental illness such as depression, anxiety, or a personality disorder. Individuals with these disorders present a special challenge to treatment personnel.[22] Moreover, some mental health personnel express ambivalence about working with patients who have a dual diagnosis.[23]

People with social anxiety disorder who also have alcohol problems report that they use alcohol to cope with their anxiety.[24] The treatment dropout rate for these individuals is quite high. One study found that people who smoked, had recent mood episodes, and lacked a college education had higher dropout rates.[25] A study of cocaine addicts with and without post-traumatic stress disorder (PTSD) noted that cocaine addicts without PTSD showed greater improvement after treatment.[26] Similarly, alcoholics who are bipolar have less success in treatment than individuals with either bipolar disorder or alcoholism only.[27] On a positive note, however, one program in Norway that used a group skills training intervention approach reported that 83% of these patients completed the program.[28]

Treatment of Mental Illness Before 1950

Before 1950, remedies for mental illness were crude, unscientific, and even cruel. Mentally ill people were subjected to bloodletting, were given sneezing powder, were flogged and starved, and had hot irons applied to their bodies. In the 1840s, manic patients were treated with cannabis (marijuana) because it brought about euphoria. This treatment was stopped because its benefits were found to be only temporary. In the 1930s schizophrenic patients were administered insulin to put them into a coma. Insulin treatment might have been effective at first, but subsequent studies indicated a high relapse rate.

Psychoanalysis grew in popularity starting with Sigmund Freud. Today it seldom is used to treat patients with mental problems.

Eventually, scientists such as Kraepelin, Pinel, and Esquirol devised a classification system of mental illnesses. Drugs such as amphetamines were used with depressed patients and inhaled carbon dioxide and antihistamines were given to patients having other classifications. Some patients received barbiturates and other depressants and slept for a week or more. **Electroconvulsive therapy (ECT)**, first developed in 1938, was used to treat depression and psychosis. ECT involves attaching electrodes to one's head and delivering electrical impulses to the brain. Electrical activity in the brain is temporarily interrupted and a seizure within the brain is triggered.[29] After much apprehension regarding the effects of ECT, it is making a comeback in the treatment of depression.

Electroconvulsive therapy has raised several concerns, especially in regard to its effects on memory and cognition. In the past many patients receiving ECT experienced adverse cognitive effects[30] Significant memory loss was not an uncommon effect. One author points out that ECT is unregulated and that many people going through medical school are not informed about ECT.[31] Despite concerns about ECT, it is increasingly used as a treatment option in Canada.[32]

Demographics of Drugs and Mental Disorders

Between 10% and 15% of the general population receives drugs for emotional problems each year. Forty-three percent of all people with mental disorders reside in the United States and Europe.[33] Prescriptions for antidepressants have increased 3- to 5-fold among American youths ages 2 to 19 since the 1990s.[34]

Some people are more likely than others to receive medication. Older people are more likely to be prescribed drugs for emotional disorders. Higher levels of medication use also correlate with more education, living by oneself, and higher income. Also, women are twice as likely as men to use prescribed drugs for mental disorders.

bipolar affective disorder A mental condition characterized by alternating moods of depression and mania; formerly called manic-depression

unipolar depression A mental disorder marked by alternating periods of depression and normalcy

psychoanalysis A form of talk therapy based on Freudian principles

electroconvulsive therapy (ECT) Controlled administration of electric shock as a treatment for mental illness

monoamine oxidase inhibitor (MAO) An antidepressant drug used for acute anxiety, obsessive-compulsive behavior, and phobias

iproniazid A monoamine oxidase inhibitor

Antidepressants

Depression is a primary factor in thousands of suicides each year. In 2004, there was an 18% increase in suicides for adolescents.[35] Yet, treating depression is complicated because almost everyone becomes depressed at some time or another—some for understandable reasons. Distinguishing between a temporary period of depression or a situational depression and depression as an emotional disorder requiring medical intervention is difficult. Moreover, determining which depressed individuals will respond to antidepressant medications poses a challenge.

In the past, stimulants were used to treat depression. Depression now is treated with three major classes of drugs—monoamine oxidase inhibitors, tricyclic antidepressants, and selective serotonin reuptake inhibitors. Although these drugs are effective, some people get discouraged because they sometimes require several weeks to take effect. One study found that counseling was as effective for treating mild to moderate depression, although a combination of counseling *and* antidepressants appeared to work best.[36]

Monoamine Oxidase Inhibitors

Monoamine oxidase (MAO) is an enzyme found on the outer membranes of subcellular particles known as mitochondria. MAO renders inactive the neurotransmitters serotonin, dopamine, and norepinephrine. As antidepressants, MAO inhibitors block the action of monoamine oxidase.

The antidepressant properties of MAO inhibitors were discovered accidentally. First introduced in the 1950s, they were used to treat tuberculosis patients who, on receiving the MAO inhibitor **iproniazid**, became energetic. Subsequently, this drug was used with depressed patients even though it proved to be too toxic for treating tuberculosis. The use of iproniazid as an antidepressant was stopped after it was linked to the deaths of 54 people.

The three principal MAO inhibitors currently utilized in the United States are tranylcypromine (Parnate), phenelize (Nardil), and isocarboxazid (Marplan). MAO inhibitors are effective only in depressed patients who have high levels of MAO activity. Overall, they have a low efficacy rate.

After patients begin to use MAO inhibitors, 2 weeks or more must pass before the drug relieves the symptoms of depression. MAO inhibitors are not the antidepressant of choice. They are given to patients who remain depressed after being given a minimum of two tricyclic drugs. They work best in patients whose depression becomes more acute as the day progresses (in contrast to many depressed people who feel worse in the morning and improve during the day).

On Campus

Nearly 19% of college students reported that they experienced depression within the previous 12 months.

Source: American College Health Association, 2008.

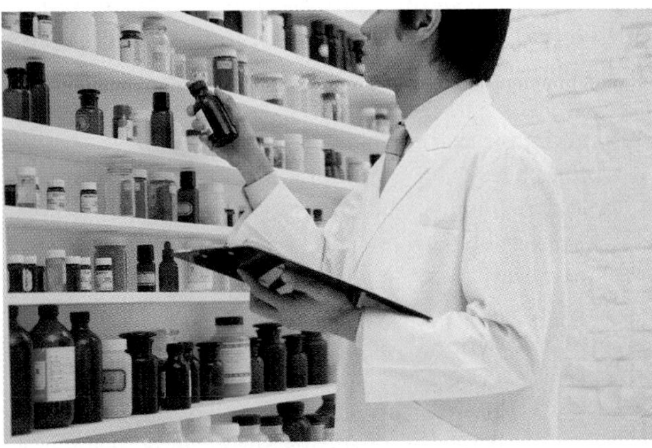

Michael Hitoshi/Getty Images

There are many antidepressant drugs available to effectively treat depression.

People exhibiting neurotic conditions such as acute anxiety, obsessive-compulsive behavior, and phobias respond positively to MAO inhibitors.[37] Also, individuals who have panic attacks respond better to the MAO inhibitor phenelzine than to the tricyclic antidepressant drug imipramine. Rhenelzine also has been used with people who become depressed following romantic rejection—heartbreak. They tend to oversleep, overeat, and have an unstable mood as a result of being rejected.

Another group for which MAO inhibitors seem to work are depressed elderly patients. Elderly patients who cannot tolerate some of the side effects of tricyclics respond favorably to MAO inhibitors.

Side effects of MAO inhibitors include fatigue, dizziness, dry mouth, and drowsiness. Impotence and ejaculatory problems have been reported in men, and some women have difficulty achieving orgasm. A significant and potentially serious side effect of MAO inhibitors is low blood pressure (hypotension). The opposite effect, however, can occur when MAO inhibitors are taken simultaneously with tricyclic drugs, psychostimulants, and L-dopa. This extremely high blood pressure can lead to fever, bleeding in the brain, headaches, and possibly death. Also, dangerous levels of hypertension occur when MAO inhibitors interact with foods containing **tyramine**, an amino acid. The interaction of MAO inhibitors and tyramine produces nausea, a stinging headache, vomiting, palpitations, internal bleeding, skin flush, and death.

One drawback to MAO inhibitors is the strict dietary regimen that patients must follow. People using MAO inhibitors absolutely must avoid foods that contain tyramine. A rise in blood pressure results from the interaction of MAO inhibitors and tyramine, causing the release of catecholamines. This action produces **sympathomimetic effects**, including elevated blood pressure. After a person stops taking MAO inhibitors, the body can take 2 weeks to readjust. Besides high and low blood pressure, other toxic effects include hallucinations, high fever, agitation, and convulsions. Foods rich in tyramine include the following:

- aged cheeses
- blue cheese
- old cheddar
- mozzarella
- Parmesan
- Swiss
- Chianti wine
- sauerkraut
- concentrated yeast extracts
- sausage
- pickled herring brine
- Chinese foods
- beer and ale

MAO inhibitors are dangerous, too, because they interact with certain medications, especially dextromethorphan, found in over-the-counter cough medications, and Demerol. MAO inhibitors are potentially fatal if the individual is taking other antidepressants that affect serotonin, such as Prozac. The recommendation is to wait at least 5 weeks after stopping Prozac before taking MAO inhibitors.

Despite their limitations, MAO inhibitors have some advantages. They do not cause tolerance, psychological dependence, or withdrawal symptoms after their use is discontinued. They are not likely to be abused because they have little effect on people who are not depressed.

Tricyclic Antidepressants

The term *tricyclic* is derived from the chemical structure of **tricyclic antidepressants**, which are shaped like three-ringed compounds. First introduced in the 1950s, originally these drugs were used with psychotic patients, and it was noted that they had an antidepressant effect. They relieve the primary symptoms of depression, though different tricyclics are used depending on symptoms.

Amitriptyline (Elavil) is used for depression accompanied by agitation. Imipramine (Tofranil) is given for depression involving psychomotor retardation, as well as for agoraphobia, panic attacks, and obsessive-compulsive behavior. Clomipramine (Anafranil) has been used to treat obsessive-compulsive behaviors also.

Tricyclics are superior to MAO inhibitors. The antidepressant action of tricyclics, however, takes three to four weeks to attain a therapeutic level.[38] These drugs accumulate in fatty areas of the body such as the brain and lungs, are excreted primarily in the urine, and are metabolized by the liver. Features of common tricyclic antidepressants are outlined in Table 10.1.

TABLE 10.1 Tricyclic Antidepressants

Generic Name	Brand Names	Type of Depression
imipramine	Tofranil Janimine Presamine SK-Pramine	Psychomatic retardation
amitriptyline	Elavil Endep	Agoraphobia, panic attacks, obsessive-compulsive behavior
clomipramine	Anafranil Aventyl Pamelor	Obsessive-compulsive behavior
desipramine	Norpramin Pertofrane Adapin Sinequan	Anxiety, panic disorder

Effectiveness

Symptoms of acute depression are effectively removed in most cases in which the proper dosage of tricyclic antidepressants is taken and adequate time is allowed for the drugs to take effect. Imipramine helped to relieve symptoms of depression including insomnia, listlessness, and loss of appetite in 60% to 70% of patients in one study. In general, antidepressant drugs are 60% to 70% effective for treating major depression.[39] The mood and confidence of patients improve and suicidal thoughts are eliminated.

Tricyclics work best with severe unipolar depression. Patients with bipolar depression who are given tricyclics sometimes go from being depressed to being manic. Consequently, these drugs are not recommended for use in bipolar depression.

Tricyclics seem to be successful in treating a number of disorders besides depression. For patients whose primary symptoms are related to phobias, some tricyclic drugs help facilitate behavioral treatment. Tricyclics also are effective in moderating pain.[40] Moreover, they can be beneficial in treatment of the eating disorder bulimia. Because these drugs do not produce euphoria, they are not used for recreational purposes.

Side Effects

Common side effects of tricyclics are distorted vision, **tachycardia**, dry mouth, constipation, sleepiness, and urinary retention. On standing up, the blood pressure can drop significantly. Confusion and disorientation are other typical effects. Less frequent side effects are rashes (especially in the elderly), jaundice, glaucoma, tremors, and impotence. Another side effect is the development of type 2 diabetes, especially when tricyclics are taken with the newer antidepressants.[41]

When tricyclic antidepressants are used in combination with alcohol, the risk of a deadly reaction increases. An overdose can result in coma, cardiac difficulties, and respiratory problems. Because another concern is suicide, patients who are contemplating suicide should be assessed before tricyclics are prescribed.

Patients frequently experience side effects during the period before antidepressants take effect. Therefore, many discontinue taking the medication before it has a chance to act. Generally, these patients did not receive more than a 2-week supply of tricyclics.

If patients cease taking tricyclics abruptly, they demonstrate withdrawal symptoms such as chills, muscle aches, and malaise. Tolerance to tricyclics does not develop, and psychological dependency is minimal. People who are not depressed are unlikely to take tricyclics because of the undesirable side effects.

tyramine An amino acid that interacts with monoamine oxidase inhibitors to cause very high levels of hypertension

sympathomimetic effects An increase of blood to the brain and muscle, allowing the body to flee or fight

tricyclic antidepressants Drugs that effectively remove the symptoms of acute depression

tachycardia Faster than normal heart rate

Toxicity

Even at low dosage levels, tricyclics can be toxic, and excessive levels of tricyclic antidepressant drugs can be fatal. A therapeutic dosage of imipramine is about 300 mg a day, and a lethal dose is about 2,000 mg. Early warning signs of toxicity include low blood pressure, low body temperature, excitement, seizures, restlessness, reduced breathing, dry skin, flushed face, and coma. The coma can last 1 to 3 days and is followed by confusion and disorientation. Death, which occurs within 24 hours of ingestion, usually results from irregular heart rate (arrhythmia) or from the heart simply no longer working.

Selective Serotonin Reuptake Inhibitors

A newer family of antidepressants was developed in the 1980s. Known as selective serotonin reuptake inhibitors (SSRIs), these drugs include Prozac, Zoloft, Paxil, and others. These drugs are widely promoted for treating depression and have other benefits such as reducing aggressive and violent behavior[42] and agoraphobia.[43] Yet, there are several concerns regarding these drugs. The first concern deals with their efficacy. Some studies suggest that pharmaceutical companies exaggerate their effectiveness. In England the government wants 3,600 more psychotherapists to be trained as an alternative to drug therapy.[44] Adverse effects of SSRIs include sexual dysfunction, increase in weight, and altered sleep patterns.[45] Another concern is that these drugs may increase the likelihood

Side Effects of Tricyclic Antidepressants

- Tachycardia
- Dry mouth
- Confusion
- Hypotension
- Disorientation
- Impotence
- Glaucoma
- Distorted vision
- Sleepiness
- Constipation
- Urinary retention
- Tremors
- Rashes
- Jaundice
- Respiratory problems
- Coma
- Death

of youth suicide, although the evidence indicates that the risk of youth suicide is overstated.[46] Pediatric depression is a national problem. Many children who commit suicide suffer from depression. It is reported that antidepressants, especially in conjunction with cognitive behavior therapy, actually reduce the risk of pediatric suicide.[47]

Prozac

Every so often a "wonder drug" appears that is supposed to be more effective and less toxic than existing drugs. The antidepressant **Prozac (fluoxetine)** is such a drug.

Contributing to the popularity of Prozac is the fact that it has fewer unpleasant and serious side effects than other antidepressant drugs. The efficacy of Prozac in treating symptoms related to depression, however, does not exceed that of other antidepressants. Overall, it has been shown that antidepressant drugs are not much better than placebos.[48]

In addition to being prescribed for depression, Prozac is used for bulimia and obesity, anxiety, and obsessive-compulsive disorders. Higher doses are required for obsessive-compulsive disorders than for depression.

Prozac reduces symptoms of tension, irritability, and dysphoria in women. It curtails the rate of panic attacks. It does not cause the hypotension, weight gain, or irregular heart rhythms that are common with other treatments. Side effects include headaches, sweating, fatigue, jitteriness, anxiety, stomach upset, nausea, insomnia, dizziness, sexual dysfunction, and reduced appetite. Long-term side effects have not been determined; however, Prozac and similar antidepressants may weaken bones by reducing bone density.[49] The use of Prozac has not been limited to humans. It has been given to dogs to help relieve canine depression and compulsive licking. One study, in which rats were given Prozac and other antidepressants, showed that these drugs actually stimulated the growth of new brain cells.[50]

Prozac has sparked several legal issues. Unhappy consumers have filed lawsuits against the drug's manufacturer, Eli Lilly. One critic, author William Styron, says, "It is Lilly's concerted efforts to minimize such sinister side effects that remain even now indefensible."[51] Because Prozac has been linked to violent behavior, some people have used this information as a criminal defense, claiming they cannot be held responsible for crimes committed while on the drug.

Prozac has been implicated in a number of suicides, but it is unclear if Prozac *causes* violent behavior toward self or others. The issue may hinge on how one views the evidence. Depression can lead to suicide or violence whether or not a person is receiving treatment.

Zoloft

Another popular SSRI is Zoloft (sertraline). Zoloft seems to be as effective as tricyclic antidepressants for treating moderate to severe depression. It is especially effective with elderly patients. Increasing numbers of children, as young as age 5, are given Zoloft and other antidepressants, despite a lack of scientific proof that these drugs are safe and effective for children.[52] Zoloft is the most commonly prescribed antidepressant for patients with acute coronary syndrome. Like Prozac, Zoloft is used to treat obsessive-compulsive disorders. However, there is a small risk that Zoloft and other antidepressants may contribute to birth defects.[53]

Paxil

One of the newest antidepressant drugs is Paxil (paroxetine). It was the most heavily advertised antidepressant between 1999 and 2003.[54] Like the other SSRIs, Paxil increases brain levels of serotonin, the neurotransmitter that affects mood and alertness. In one survey of Paxil users, it was reported that 59% believed that the drug was beneficial, though 21% felt drowsiness or disorientation, 53% experienced decreased sexual interest or performance, and 22% gained weight.[55] The American College of Obstetricians and Gynecologists reports that Paxil taken during pregnancy increases the risk of cardiac malformations and neonatal complications.[56]

The U.S. Food and Drug Administration (FDA) recommended that Paxil not be prescribed for children and adolescents because of the increased risk of suicides. One study indicated that teens and children taking Paxil are 3.2 times more likely to attempt suicide than others taking placebos.[57] GlaxoSmithKline, the company that manufactures Paxil, allegedly failed to disclose data regarding the drug's side effects.[58] GlaxoSmithKline agreed to pay the state of New York $2.5 million to avoid an extended lawsuit.

GlaxoSmithKline recently distributed a derivative of Paxil known as PaxilCR. This new version has several advantages over Paxil. First, it is well tolerated by users and has a low patient dropout rate. Besides being used for depression, PaxilCR has been approved for the treatment of social anxiety disorder.[59] In addition, PaxilCR is prescribed for panic disorder and premenstrual syndrome.[60] One other advantage of PaxilCR is that it is sold at 31% of the cost of Paxil.[61]

Wellbutrin

Wellbutrin, also known as bupropion, is one of the more recent antidepressants to be marketed. Wellbutrin comes in different versions: It can be taken once a day, twice a day, or three times a day. All three formulae are equally effective.[62] Wellbutrin acts by inhibiting the uptake of dopamine and norepinephrine. Besides its use for depression, the drug, under the name Zyban, is used for smoking cessation. It is estimated that 25% of individuals are initially prescribed Zyban to stop smoking. Except in rare instances, people who used Zyban for smoking cessation did not experience adverse side effects.[63]

Wellbutrin has been approved for seasonal affective disorder also. Seasonal affective disorder affects about 5% of all Americans, three-fourths of whom are women.[64] One study found that it helped reduce the risk of depression by 44% if it is taken in the fall prior to symptoms appearing.[65] Unlike other antidepressant drugs, Wellbutrin has not been shown to cause weight gain.

A generic version of Wellbutrin, referred to as Wellbutrin XL, was approved in 2006. In the previous year it was the highest selling brand name drug in the United States, totaling $1.3 billion.[66] According to the U.S. FDA, this generic version of Wellbutrin is safe although its manufacturer, Teva Pharmaceutical Industries, came under review for numerous complaints against the drug.[67] The drug is well tolerated by most people, and its side effects are usually mild and temporary. They include loss of appetite, weight loss, dry mouth, skin rash, perspiration, insomnia, ringing in the ears, anxiety, nausea, agitation, and stomach pain.[68] The drug should not be used by people with a history of seizures or eating disorders, or by those who are taking MAOI antidepressants.

Prozac (fluoxetine) An antidepressant drug

Wellbutrin An antidepressant drug that is used to help people stop smoking

lithium A psychotherapeutic drug used to treat symptoms associated with mania

chlorpromazine An antipsychotic drug

Lithium

A drug used to treat manic symptoms is **lithium**. John Cade, an Australian physician, experimented with lithium to reduce kidney damage in animals and observed that it sedated them. Subsequently, he found that lithium had a similar effect on humans.

Before lithium was introduced, patients with mania had recurring episodes of mood swings. Though Cade's research into lithium's antimanic properties was noted in the 1940s, it received little attention in the United States for 20 years because of the drug's high levels of toxicity. The FDA officially approved lithium in 1970, despite many reservations. When lithium was first administered, many individuals with kidney and cardiovascular problems died. Consequently, physicians were reluctant to prescribe it. Moreover, other drugs such as **chlorpromazine**, with antimanic properties but fewer toxic effects, were available.

Lithium is a positively charged ion that is similar to sodium. It typically is taken orally in salt form and is concentrated in the brain but may accumulate in other body parts such as muscle and bone. It is readily absorbed from the gastrointestinal tract within 8 hours and is excreted in urine. The level of lithium in the body is influenced by the body's sodium level. If a person has a high sodium level, lithium will be readily excreted. If an individual has a low sodium level, high levels of lithium will be retained. One's inability to excrete lithium can lead to toxic levels in the body.

Because lithium has a relatively low margin of safety, administration of the drug is monitored carefully. Its side effects include tremors, excessive thirst, frequent urination, fluid retention, and weight gain. An advantage to lithium is that it has no effect on normal individuals at therapeutic levels.

Effectiveness

Lithium is effective for acute mania and for preventing mania and depression from recurring. The maximal benefit is achieved in 1 to 2 weeks, although many patients respond positively in 3 to 4 days. Lithium is especially effective for patients whose manic-depression is genetic. One limitation is that patients have unusually stable moods, even when expressions of emotion are warranted. Lithium typically is prescribed in conjunction with antipsychotic drugs because manic symptoms do not subside for several days.

Lithium prevents symptoms of mania. It is believed that almost two-thirds of patients will relapse into a manic condition within a year of stopping medication.[69] Lithium is effective for people who have unipolar depression and do not respond to tricyclic antidepressant drugs. Its success varies when it is used to treat premenstrual syndrome, hyperactivity in children, and outbursts of aggression or anger. Lithium minimizes impulsivity. Some research shows that it significantly increased the abstinence period of alcoholics, but other research on lithium use with chronic alcoholics is inconclusive. Some evidence suggests that lithium is useful in managing behavioral problems in individuals with an intellectual disability.[70] Also, lithium appears to help reduce the likelihood of suicide among those with bipolar depression.[71]

Side Effects

At therapeutic levels, the side effects of lithium include nausea, thirst, excessive perspiration, and hand tremors. After lithium is administered, the

Side Effects of Lithium

- Nausea
- Excessive perspiration
- Water retention
- Vomiting
- Confusion
- Drowsiness
- Tinnitus
- Kidney dysfunction
- Respiratory depression
- Thirst
- Hand tremors
- Frequent urination
- Diarrhea
- Weight gain
- Muscular weakness
- Distorted vision
- Coma
- Death

body initially loses sodium and potassium; this is followed by sodium and water retention. Lithium users urinate frequently and in large amounts, a condition known as **polyuria**. Also, lithium users consume water frequently and excessively, a condition called **polydipsia**. Polyuria and polydipsia rarely cause significant kidney damage. Additional side effects associated with lithium are vomiting, diarrhea, confusion, weight gain, drowsiness, and muscular weakness.

Side effects that occur less often include **tinnitus** (ringing sounds in the ear), distorted vision, and a metallic taste in the mouth. Increased amounts of lithium can result in impaired kidney function, respiratory depression, coma, and even death. Taking lithium during pregnancy increases the risk of fetal damage. Also, the drug can be passed to the newborn in breast milk. Lithium does not cause physical dependency or severe withdrawal symptoms, but restlessness and irritability follow cessation of use.

Toxicity

The amount needed for therapeutic purposes, the **therapeutic window**, is small. Three to four times the therapeutic level can cause grave consequences. Yet, carefully monitored patients can take the drug for years. Symptoms of lithium toxicity are intense nausea, tremors, irregular heartbeat, lowered blood pressure, abdominal pain, mental confusion, vomiting, diarrhea, and convulsions. Elderly patients may be at greater risk because they excrete lithium at a slower rate than younger patients.[72]

Antipsychotic Drugs

Antipsychotic drugs, also known as **major tranquilizers**, are used to treat and manage psychological disorders ranging from psychosis to violent behavior to schizoprenia. Antipsychotic drugs, called **neuroleptics** in Europe, are pharmacologically different from minor tranquilizers and other sedative-hypnotic drugs. Although antipsychotic drugs have been used to relieve anxiety, that is not their primary purpose. Developed in the mid-1950s, antipsychotic drugs are used especially for schizophrenia. They do not *cure* schizophrenia or other forms of mental illness but, rather, treat symptoms associated with mental illness. A mentally ill or schizophrenic person is able to function normally while taking these drugs.

Like many medications, antipsychotic drugs were discovered by accident. French surgeon Henri Laborit noted the calming effect of chlorpromazine, an anesthetic used to ameliorate anxiety and shock during surgery. Chlorpromazine later was given to psychotic patients at a military hospital in Paris. Patients receiving chlorpromazine appeared calm, and their thinking was less disorganized. Moreover, patients did not lose consciousness.

Chlorpromazine was marketed in 1955 in the United States under the trade name **Thorazine**. It is credited with revolutionizing the treatment of people with mental disorders. Despite the proliferation of people diagnosed as mentally ill beginning in the 1950s, the number of hospitalized mental patients in the United States dramatically declined from 600,000 in 1955 to about 150,000 by the mid-1980s, because their illnesses could be better managed by drugs. Newer antipsychotic drugs are not necessarily any more effective, but they may have fewer adverse effects.[73]

Well-known antipsychotic drugs include haloperidol (Haldol), trifluoperazine (Stelazine), flu-phenazine (Prolixin), olanzipine (Zyprexa), quetiapine (Seroquel), promazine (Sparine), and thioridazine (Mellaril). To obtain maximum effectiveness, schizophrenic patients have to take antipsychotic drugs for 4 to 6 weeks, although some symptoms of schizophrenia decline within the first week of treatment. The results of recent studies investigating whether antipsychotic drugs are effective for treating the symptoms of anorexia nervosa are inconclusive.[74]

Although antipsychotic drugs can be administered by injection, they usually are ingested. Injecting antipsychotic drugs does not offer much of an advantage because they require several days to take effect. Some patients receive injections of antipsychotic drugs so the drug can be released slowly into the bloodstream.

One problem with antipsychotic drugs is that they are absorbed erratically; thus, it is difficult to determine an effective dose precisely. These drugs build up in fatty areas in the brain and lungs. Because of their high affinity for lipids, they cross the placenta easily and affect the fetus.

Children and Antipsychotic Drugs

An increasing number of children are being prescribed antipsychotic medications. More children in the United States are prescribed antipsychotic drugs more frequently than children in other developed countries. Nonetheless, the use of antipsychotic drugs by children is growing in other countries as well. In Great Britain, three times as many children ages 7 to 12 were prescribed antipsychotic drugs in 2005 as compared to 1992.[75] Similarly, the number of Dutch youth who were prescribed antipsychotic drugs more than doubled from 1997 to 2005. Moreover, the length of time these drugs were prescribed increased.[76] They are beneficial for treating antipsychotic conditions; however, they also produce adverse effects in children. Some of the adverse effects include excessive weight gain, type 2 diabetes, neurological symptoms, digestive problems, and cardiovascular conditions. These effects are more prevalent in females.[77]

polyuria Frequent urination

polydipsia Frequent and excessive consumption of water

tinnitus A condition marked by constant ringing in the ears

therapeutic window The amount of drug needed for therapeutic purposes

major tranquilizers Antipsychotic drugs

neuroleptics The European term for antipsychotic drugs

Thorazine Major tranquilizer used to treat psychosis

extrapyramidal symptoms Neurological symptoms characterized by difficulty walking, shuffling, and inflexible joints

acute dyskinesia Inappropriate motor movements as a side effect of antipsychotic drugs

Parkinsonism A form of acute dyskinesia marked by tremors, weakness in the extremities, and muscle rigidity

bradykinesia Motor movements that are slow and limited

dystonia A type of dyskinesia marked by involuntary and inappropriate postures and muscle tones

akathesia Jerky, uncontrollable constant motion, motor restlessness, occasional protruding tongue, and facial grimace

tardive dyskinesia A side effect of antipsychotic drugs marked by involuntary repetitive facial movements and involuntary movement of the trunk and limbs

Effectiveness

Although schizophrenics receiving antipsychotic drugs almost always show improvement, a small percentage gets worse. While the extent to which patients improve varies widely, symptoms of schizophrenia are greatly reduced in the majority of patients.[78] Patients taking antipsychotic drugs become less belligerent, agitated, and impulsive. Autistic or withdrawn patients sometimes become more responsive and communicative. Delusions, disorganized thinking, and hallucinations disappear, and insight, memory, judgment, appetite, and sleep improve. Improvement is most rapid during the first several weeks of treatment.

Although many people taking antipsychotic drugs relapse, it appears that these drugs reduce violent behavior.[79] For patients having a relapse, psychosocial factors may be the root cause. Stress, interpersonal problems, and overly critical and intrusive relatives increase the risk of relapse. Despite the effectiveness of antipsychotic drugs and the fact that newer antipsychotic drugs have fewer side effects, the rate of noncompliance is very high.[80]

Side Effects

Antipsychotic drugs produce many undesirable motor problems, called **extrapyramidal symptoms**. Inappropriate motor movements—**acute dyskinesias**—sometimes appear within a year after treatment begins. Acute dyskinesias take several forms, which follow:

1. **Parkinsonism:** A condition marked by a dull facial expression, weakness in the extremities, tremors, rigidity, and extremely slow and limited movements (**bradykinesia**). These symptoms, resembling Parkinson's disease, appear in about 40% of patients.
2. **Dystonia:** Sudden and involuntary muscle spasms of the head, neck, lips, and tongue. Slurred speech and eyes deviated up are common also.
3. **Akathesia:** Characterized by jerky and uncontrollable constant motion, motor restlessness, and an occasional protruding tongue and facial grimace. This condition is exhibited in about 20% of patients.

Another major side effect, **tardive dyskinesia**, is marked by motor disorders such as involuntary repetitive facial movements, lip smacking, involuntary movement of the trunk and limbs, and twitching. Newer antipsychotic drugs produce fewer side effects. The incidence of tardive dyskinesia varies considerably, although it is more likely to occur with patients who develop their psychosis after age 50 and among females. Symptoms of tardive dyskinesia appear within a year after initiation of antipsychotic drug treatment and sometimes are irreversible.

Tardive dyskinesia may arise as a function of the length of time a person takes antipsychotic drugs rather than the amount taken. In one study, after treatment ceased, tardive dyskinesia reversed itself in 55% of patients, although symptoms related to tardive dyskinesia worsened initially.[81] Another study revealed that symptoms took up to 5 years to disappear after treatment was stopped.[82]

Numerous, less severe side effects are associated with antipsychotic drugs. Some of these are difficulty urinating, constipation, dry mouth, altered skin pigmentation, changes in heart rate, jaundice, and extreme sensitivity to sunlight and an allergic response in which the patient sunburns easily. Other effects are cessation of menstruation (amenorrhea), weight gain, breast development, milk production (even in males), sedation, and hypotension. Other possible side effects are autism, dementia, diabetes, and high cholesterol.[83] Many of these side effects are less common with newer antipsychotic drugs. Patients sometimes sleep more at first, but sleep cycles or REM sleep are not altered. Susceptible patients experience an increase in epileptic seizures after taking antipsychotic drugs.

Patients develop tolerance to the side effects of these drugs but do not develop tolerance to therapeutic dosages. Therefore, patients do not have to increase the dosage to benefit from the drug. A patient can take antipsychotic drugs for years without having to increase the dosage. The difference between a therapeutic and a toxic level of antipsychotic drugs is considerable. Hence, the risk of a fatal overdose, either accidental or intentional, is low. Antipsychotic drugs do not cause physical dependency, and people do not use them for nonmedical or recreational purposes.

Summary

Mental illness is a vague, ill-defined problem that is increasing in the general population. Its causes can be social, genetic, biochemical, or some combination of these. Mental illness encompasses more than diseases of the brain and central nervous system; it entails behavior or thinking that is considered inappropriate. Social norms often serve as the basis to determine whether a given behavior exceeds what is considered acceptable. Traditionally, mental illness has been based on a medical (disease) model.

Two common mental disorders are depression/mania and schizophrenia. The latter is a psychotic illness marked by hallucinations, delusions, and a restricted range of emotions. A disorder that is often misdiagnosed as schizophrenia is bipolar affective disorder, a mental condition in which the person alternates between depression *and* mania. Unipolar major depression refers to depression only. Between 10% and 15% of the U.S. population receives medication for a mental or emotional problem. Increasingly, more individuals are presenting more than one type of disorder. This is referred to as dual diagnosis.

Antidepressant drugs are effective for mild to moderate cases of depression, but most people suffering from depression do not seek help for their condition. Three types of drugs used to treat depression are monoamine oxidase (MAO) inhibitors, tricyclic antidepressants, and selective serotonin reuptake inhibitors (SSRIs). MAO inhibitors repress the activity of certain neurotransmitters in the brain. They have been found to be largely ineffective and are used only after other antidepressant drugs have failed. They are more effective in elderly patients and in patients who suffer from anxiety, obsessive-compulsive behavior, and panic attacks. One serious side effect is high blood pressure resulting when foods containing tyramine are consumed concurrently with MAO inhibitors.

Tricyclic drugs are more effective in removing symptoms of acute depression and about 60% effective in eliminating symptoms of chronic depression. Tricyclics also are used for treating phobias, chronic pain, and bulimia. Some side effects are irregular heartbeat, confusion, constipation, disorientation, hypotension, and coma. Tolerance and physical dependence do not occur with tricyclic antidepressants, but malaise, muscle aches, and chills appear when treatment is stopped.

Prozac is part of the family of SSRIs that also include Zoloft and Paxil, and is reportedly more effective and less toxic than other antidepressants. Preliminary research indicates that Prozac is about 60% effective for depression. It also is used for anxiety, eating disorders, and obsessive-compulsive behaviors. Long-term effects have not been established. Another antidepressant drug, Wellbutrin, is used increasingly.

Lithium is administered primarily to treat mania. When given initially, it caused a number of deaths in people with kidney and cardiovascular problems. Its effects are altered by the level of sodium in the body. Lithium not only ameliorates the symptoms of mania and depression but also prevents these symptoms from recurring. It is especially effective with individuals whose mania and depression are genetic. Lithium also is used to treat premenstrual syndrome, hyperactivity, and aggression. It can cause kidney damage, respiratory depression, coma, and death, and taking lithium during the first trimester of pregnancy increases the risk of a birth defect.

Antipsychotic drugs are particularly helpful in treating symptoms of schizophrenia in adults as well as children. They reduce symptoms in the majority of schizophrenics. As a side effect, some patients exhibit symptoms similar to those of Parkinson's disease. Another side effect, tardive dyskinesia, is marked by involuntary facial movements, which may be irreversible, although one study found that the symptoms were reversed in more than one-half of the patients. Less severe effects include dry mouth, weight gain, constipation, breast development, amenorrhea, sensitivity to light, epilepsy, and sleepiness. Tolerance to and physical dependence on antipsychotic drugs do not develop.

Thinking Critically

1. A century ago, mentally ill people were called crazy or lunatics. Today we are more sophisticated and refer to these people as mentally ill. Did the change in terminology alter people's attitudes? When you think of a person labeled as mentally ill, what comes to mind?
2. Some people who have committed crimes claim that a prescription drug caused their behavior. Do you think this is a reasonable defense? Why?
3. Antipsychotic drugs often are effective in reducing symptoms associated with schizophrenia. Not everyone with schizophrenia, however, wants to take the medication. Should people be required to take antipsychotic drugs against their will? Or should they have the choice to decline treatment, even though the drugs may help?

Web Resources

American Psychological Association
http://www.apa.org/
This site provides information and research concerning psychological disorders.

Internet Mental Health
http://www.mentalhealth.com/
This site provides descriptions of the 54 most common mental disorders, including diagnosis and treatments.

Notes

1. J. Dawson, "Judicial Review of the Meaning of Mental Disorder," *Psychiatry, Psychology and Law,* 10 (2003): 164–170.
2. P. Vineis, "Methodological Insights: Fuzzy Sets in Medicine," *Journal of Epidemiology and Community Health,* 62 (March 2008): 273–278.
3. Thomas Szasz, *The Myth of Mental Illness* (New York: Hoeber-Harper, 1961).
4. Substance Abuse and Mental Health Services Administration. *Major Depressive Episode among Youths Aged 12 to 17 in the United States: 2004 to 2006* (Rockville, MD: NSDUH Report , May 13, 2008).
5. M. L. Belfer, "Child and Adolescent Mental Disorders: The Magnitude of the Problem Across the Globe," *Journal of Child Psychology and Psychiatry,* 49 (March 2008): 226–236.
6. F. Tozzi, et al., "Family History of Depression Is Associated with Younger Age of Onset in Patients with Recurrent Depression," *Psychological Medicine,* 38 (May 2008): 641–649.
7. U.S. Centers for Disease Control and Prevention, "Prevalence of Self-Reported Postpartum Depressive Symptoms—17 States, 2004–2005," *MMWR: Morbidity and Mortality Weekly Report,* 57 (April 11, 2008): 361–366.
8. D. C. Voaklander, et al., "Medical Illness, Medication Use and Suicide in Seniors: A Population-Based Case Control Study," *Journal of Epidemiology and Community Health,* (February 2008): 138–146.
9. C. I. Cohen, et al., "Focus on Geriatric Psychiatry. Schizophrenia in Later Life: Clinical Symptoms and Social Well-Being," *Psychiatric Services,* 59 (March 2008): 232–234.
10. K. S. Griswold, H. Aronoff, J. B. Kernan, and L. S. Kahn, "Adolescent Substance Use and Abuse: Recognition and Management," *American Family Physician,* 77 (February 1, 2008): 331–336.
11. C. G. Brown and S. H. Stewart, "Exploring Perceptions of Alcohol Use as Self-Medication for Depression among Women Receiving Community-Based Treatment for Alcohol Problems," *Journal of Prevention and Intervention in the Community,* 35 (2008): 33–47.
12. M. M. Husky, C. M. Mazure, P. Paliwal, and S. A. McKee, "Gender Differences in the Comorbidity of Smoking Behavior and Major Depression," *Drug and Alcohol Dependence,* 93 (January 11, 2008): 176–179.
13. J. J. Prochaska, et al., "Treating Tobacco Dependence in Clinically Depressed Smokers: Effect of Smoking Cessation on Mental Health Functioning," *American Journal of Public Health,* 98 (March 2008): 446–448.
14. A. J. Zautra, *Emotions, Stress, and Health* (New York: Oxford University Press, 2003).
15. R. Fields, *Drugs in Perspective* (New York: McGraw-Hill, 2001).
16. Zautra, supra note 14.
17. R. M. Julien, *A Primer of Drug Action,* 9th ed. (New York: W. H. Freeman, 2001).
18. R. M. Hirschfeld, "Screening for Bipolar Disorder," *American Journal of Managed Care,* 13 (November 2007): 164–169.
19. C. Stewart and R. S. El-Mallakh, "Is Bipolar Disorder Overdiagnosed among Patients with Substance Abuse?" *Bipolar Disorders,* 9 (September 2007): 646–648.
20. B. A. Gaudiano, L. M. Weinstock, and I. W. Miller, "Improving Treatment Adherence in Bipolar Disorder: A Review of Current Psychosocial Treatment Efficacy and Recommendations for Future Treatment Development," *Behavior Modification,* 32 (May 2008): 267–301.
21. Tracy Wallace, personal communication (2008).
22. J. Askey, "Dual Diagnosis: A Challenging

Therapeutic Issue of Our Time," *Drugs and Alcohol Today*, 7 (December 2007): 33–39.
23. M. W. Adams, "Comorbidity of Mental Health and Substance Misuse Problems: A Review of Workers' Reported Attitudes and Perceptions," *Journal of Psychiatric and Mental Health Nursing,* 15 (March 2008): 101–108.
24. S. E. Thomas, P. K. Randall, S. W. Book, and C. L. Randall, "A Complex Relationship Between Co-occurring Social Anxiety and Alcohol Use Disorders: What Effect Does Treating Social Anxiety Have on Drinking?" *Alcoholism: Clinical and Experimental Research*, 32 (January 2008): 77–84.
25. F. S. Graff, M. L. Griffin, and R. D. Weiss, "Predictors of Dropout from Group Therapy among Patients with Bipolar and Substance Abuse Disorders," *Drug and Alcohol Dependence*, 94 (April 2008): 272–275.
26. L. M. Najavits, et al., "Six-Month Treatment Outcomes of Cocaine-Dependent Patients with and without PTSD in Multisite National Trial," *Journal of Studies on Alcohol and Drug Studies,* 68 (May 2007): 353–361.
27. C. K. Farren and S. McElroy, "Treatment Response of Bipolar and Unipolar Alcoholics to an Inpatient Dual Diagnosis Program," *Journal of Affective Disorders*, 106 (March 2008): 265–272.
28. R. W. Grawe, R. Hagen, B. Espeland, and K. T. Mueser, "The Better Life Program: Effects of Group Skills Training for Persons with Severe Mental Illness and Substance Use Disorders," *Journal of Mental Health*, 16 (October 2007): 625–634.
29. G. Uko-Ekpenyong, "What You Should Know About Electroconvulsive Therapy," *Nursing,* 37 (August 2007): 57–60.
30. J. Prudic, "Strategies to Minimize Cognitive Side Effects with ECT: Aspects of ECT Technique," *Journal of ECT*, 24 (March 2008): 46–51.
31. M. Fink and M. A. Taylor, "Electroconvulsive Therapy," *JAMA: Journal of the American Medical Association*, 298 (July 18, 2007): 330–332.
32. H. Hoag, "Inducing Seizures among Seniors," *CMAJ: Canadian Medical Association Journal*, 178 (May 6, 2008): 1264–1266.
33. "Key Developments in Psychiatry," *The Practitioner* (September 3, 2003): 656.
34. J. F. Leckman and R. A. King, "A Developmental Perspective on the Controversy Surrounding the Use of SSRIs to Treat Pediatric Depression," *American Journal of Psychiatry*, 164 (September 2007): 1304–1306.
35. "Antidepressants and Suicidal Behavior: Cause or Cure?" *American Journal of Psychiatry*, 164 (July 2007): 989–990.
36. "Drugs vs Talk Therapy," *Consumer Reports,* 69 (October 10, 2004): 22–29.
37. T. Blake, "Tracking Down the Ups and Downs of Antidepressants," *Nursing*, 37 (April 2007): 49–51.
38. Ibid.
39. M. E. Thase, J. C. Papakostas, and M. J. Gitlin, "Augmentation Strategies in the Treatment of Major Depressive Disorder," *Primary Psychiatry*, 14 (December 2007): 1–19.
40. G. McCleane, "Antidepressants as Analgesics," *CNS Drugs*, 22 (2008): 139–156.
41. L. C. Brown, S. R. Majumdar, and J. A. Johnson, "Type of Antidepressant Therapy and Risk of Type 2 Diabetes in People with Depression," *Diabetes Research and Clinical Practice*, 79 (January 2008): 61–67.
42. L. J. Siever, "Neurobiology of Aggression and Violence," *American Journal of Psychiatry*, 165 (April 2008): 429–442.
43. "Antidepressants Have the Central Role in the Pharmacological Treatment of Agoraphobia with Panic Disorder," *Drugs and Therapy Perspectives*, 24 (April 2008): 13–16.
44. A. C. Grayling, "Mindfields: Talking Down Antidepressants," *New Scientist*, 197 (March 8, 2008): 49.
45. N. Sussman, "Medical Complications of SSRI and SNRI Treatment," *Primary Psychiatry,* 15 (February 2008): 37–41.
46. S. Kutcher and D. M. Gardner, "Use of Selective Serotonin Reuptake Inhibitors and Youth Suicides: Making Sense from a Confusing Story," *Current Opinion in Psychiatry,* 21 (January 2008): 65–69.
47. "The FDA Pediatric Advisories and Changes in Diagnosis and Treatment of Pediatric Depression," *American Journal of Psychiatry*, 164 (June 2007): 843–845.
48. B. Bower, "Drug or No Drug," *Science News*, 173 (March 1, 2008): 132–133.
49. G. Isaacson, "A Bone to Pick with Prozac," *Psychology Today*, 40 (September/October 2007) 23.
50. "Growing Hope; Depression; How Antidepressant Drugs Work," *Economist* (December 9, 2000): 3.
51. William Styron, "Prozac Days, Halcion Nights," *Nation* (January 4, 1993): 11.
52. C. L. Whitfield, *The Truth about Depression: Choices for Healing* (Deerfield Beach, FL: Health Communications, 2003).
53. D. Gellene, "The Nation; Small Link Found between Antidepressants, Birth Defects," *Los Angeles Times*, June 28, 2007: 10.
54. "Drugs vs Talk Therapy," supra note 36.
55. Ibid.
56. S. Damlo, "ACOG Releases Guidelines on the Use of SSRIs during Pregnancy," *American Family Physician*, 76 (August 15, 2007): 587.
57. S. H. Jurand, "New Data Show Paxil May Increase Suicide Risk in Children," *Trial,* 39 (October 2003): 75–76.
58. J. Giles, "Did GlaxoSmithKline Trial Data Mask Paxil Suicide Risk?" *New Scientist*, 197 (February 9, 2008): 12.
59. "PaxilCR Well Tolerated and Effective for Social Anxiety Disorder," *Biotech Business Week* (March 15, 2004): 176.
60. "FDA Approves PaxilCR for New Indication," *Mental Health Weekly Digest* (November 10, 2003): 32.
61. "Paxil Alternative Available," *Psychopharmacology Update,* 15 (June 2004): 7.
62. S. Dhillon, L. P. Yang, and M. P. Curran, "Bupropion: A Review of Its Use in the Management of Major Depressive Disorder," *Drugs*, 68 (2008): 653–658.
63. F. Humayun, T. M. Shebab, J. A. Tworek, and R. J. Fontana, "A Fatal Case of Bupropion (Zyban) Hepatotoxicity with Autoimmune Features: Case Report," *Journal of Medical Case Reports* (September 18, 2007): 88–96.
64. "Winter Blues: When to Consider Drugs," *Consumer Reports*, 72 (November 2007): 52.
65. P. Greenfield, "A Dose of Your Own Medicine," *Women's Health*, 4 (November 2007): 102.
66. "Generic Version of Wellbutrin XL," *FDA Consumer* (March–April, 2007): 4.
67. A. Georgiades, "FDA Deems Generic Wellbutrin XL to Be Safe," *Wall Street Journal—Eastern Edition*, 251 (April 17, 2008): D5.
68. S. Dhillon, P. H. Yang, and M. P. Curran, "Bupropion: A Review of Its Use in the Management of Major Depressive Disorder," *Adis Drug Evaluation*, 68 (2008): 653–689.
69. "Pharmacy Update: Bipolar Disorder," *Chemist and Druggist* (May 10, 2008): 18.
70. S. Deb, et al., "The Effectiveness of Modd Stabilizers and Antiepileptic Medication for the Management of Behaviour Problems in Adults with Intellectual Disability: A Systematic Review," *Journal of Intellectual Disability Research,* 52 (February 2008): 107–113.

71. K. N. Fountoulakis, H. Grunze, P. Panagiotidis, and G. Kaprinis, "Treatment of Bipolar Depression: An Update," *Journal of Affective Disorders*, 109 (July 2008): 21–34.
72. M. Casher and J. Bostwick, "Lithium: Using the Comeback Drug," *Current Psychiatry*, 7 (May 2008): 59–60.
73. J. Bhattacharjee and H. G. G. El-Sayeh, "Aripiprazole Versus Typicals for Schizophrenia," *Cochrane Database of Systematic Reviews*, 2008.
74. A. Court, C. Mulder, S. E. Hetrick, R. Purcell, and P. D. McGorry, "What Is the Scientific Evidence for the Use of Antipsychotic Medication in Anorexia Nervosa?" *Eating Disorders*, 16 (May/June 2008): 217–223.
75. F. Rani, M. L. Murray, P. J. Byrne, and I. C. Wong, "Epidemiologic Features of Antipsychotic Prescribing to Children and Adolescents in Primary Care in the United Kingdom," *Pediatrics*, 121 (May 2008): 1002–1009.
76. L. J. Kalverdijk, et al., "Use of Antipsychotic Drugs among Dutch Youths between 1997 and 2005," *Psychiatric Services*, 59 (May 2008): 554–560.
77. J. M. Jerrell and R. S. McIntyre, "Adverse Events in Children and Adolescents Treated with Antipsychotic Medications," *Human Psychopharmacology: Clinical and Experimental*, 23 (June 2008): 283–290.
78. D. M. Grilly, *Drugs and Human Behavior*, 5th ed. (Boston: Allyn & Bacon, 2005).
79. "Newer Antipsychotics Appear to Stem Violent Behavior," *Ascribe Health News Service*, April 11, 2004.
80. K. Duckworth and M. J. Fitzpatrick, "Special Section on Implications of CATIE: NAMI Perspective on CATIE: Policy and Research Implications," *Psychiatric Services*, 59 (May 2008): 537–539.
81. D. V. Jeste, J. B. Lohr, K. Clark, and R. J. Wyatt, "Pharmacological Treatments of Tardive Dyskinesia in the 1980s," *Journal of Clinical Psychopharmacology*, 8 (1988): 38S–48S.
82. H. L. Klawans, C. M. Tabner, and A. Barr, "The Reversibility of 'Permanent' Tardive Dyskinesia," *Clinical Neuropharmacology*, 7 (1984): 153–159.
83. "Possible Link Explored between Antipsychotics and Several Conditions," *RN*, 67 (June 2004): 76.

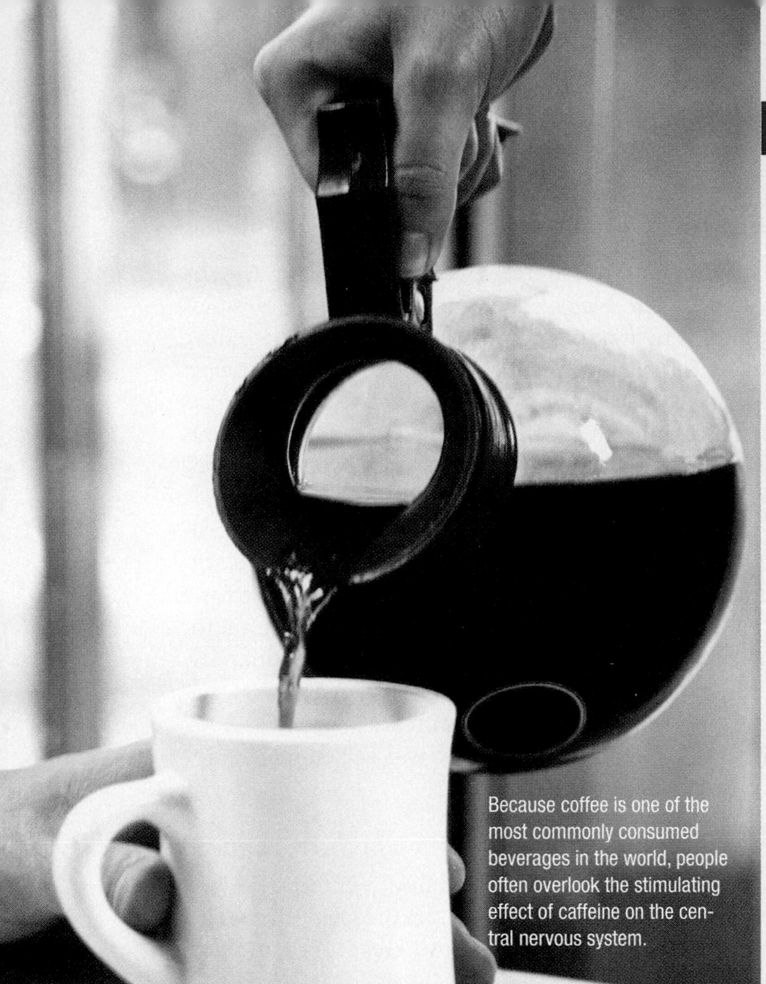

Because coffee is one of the most commonly consumed beverages in the world, people often overlook the stimulating effect of caffeine on the central nervous system.

FACT OR FICTION?

1. Cocaine accounts for twice as many emergency room visits as heroin.
2. Among 12th-grade students, cocaine is more likely to be used today than in the 1980s.
3. As many people go to emergency rooms for crack cocaine as for powder cocaine.
4. Previously, cocaine was used medicinally as a local anesthetic.
5. The depressant effects of alcohol reduce the stimulating effects of cocaine, making serious side effects less likely to occur.
6. The majority of powder cocaine users who enter treatment are White, and the majority of crack cocaine users who enter treatment are Black.
7. Attention deficit/hyperactivity disorder is limited to children and teenagers. Very few adults have this condition.
8. After Mexico, the largest producer of methamphetamines is Canada.
9. Boys are more than twice as likely as girls to be identified with attention deficit/hyperactivity disorder (ADHD).
10. Moderate amounts of caffeine can increase cardiovascular endurance.

Turn the page to check your answers

11

Stimulants: Cocaine, Amphetamines, Methamphetamines, and Caffeine

Chapter Objectives

After completing this chapter, the reader should be able to describe:

- The extent of illegal stimulant use in the United States
- Factors contributing to the popularity of cocaine in the 1980s
- Reasons "crack" is considered an evil drug
- How the method of administering of cocaine alters its effects
- The impact of stimulants on prenatally exposed children
- The medical consequences of amphetamines
- The connection between amphetamines and attention deficit/hyperactivity disorder (ADHD)
- The physical and psychological effects of methamphetamines
- Whether caffeine is a physically harmful drug

FACT OR FICTION?

1. **Fact:** Cocaine accounts for nearly 450,000 emergency room visits.
2. **Fiction:** The fact is—about twice as many high school seniors tried cocaine in the mid-1980s than today.
3. **Fiction:** The fact is—powder cocaine accounts for more than three times as many people going to the emergency room as crack cocaine.
4. **Fact:** Although other drugs have replaced cocaine for medical purposes, it has been used as a local anesthetic.
5. **Fiction:** The fact is—alcohol exacerbates the effects of cocaine, increasing the risk of a fatal overdose.
6. **Fact:** Forty-seven percent of people seeking treatment for powder cocaine use are White and 59% of people seeking treatment for crack cocaine use are Black.
7. **Fiction:** The fact is—an estimated 8 million adults in the United States have attention deficit/hyperactivity disorder.
8. **Fiction:** The fact is—after Mexico, countries in Southeast Asia are the largest methamphetamine producers. Canada's production is nil.
9. **Fact:** For every 4 girls identified with ADHD, 10 boys are identified with it.
10. **Fact:** Caffeine improves work output marginally.

During times of fatigue and lethargy, people sometimes look for substances that will elevate their mood and make them energetic. Stimulants provide these effects. They are capable of modifying a person's activity level, mood, and central nervous system. Some stimulants, such as cocaine and methamphetamines, are illegal. Others, such as amphetamines, require a prescription. In addition, legal stimulants such as caffeine and nicotine are among the most widely used drugs in the world. This chapter covers all of the major legal and illegal stimulants except nicotine, which is discussed in Chapter 7.

Cocaine

In 2008, 4.4% of high school seniors in the United States reported having used cocaine at least one time during the past year. Among 8th-grade students, 1.8% reported having used cocaine, and 3.0% of 10th-grade students indicated having used cocaine at least one time in the previous 12 months.[1] The percentage of high school seniors who have ever used cocaine has declined since the 1980s, when it was the most popular of the illegal stimulants.[2] Nonetheless, more drug-related emergency room visits result from cocaine use than from use of any other illegal drug. In 2005, nearly 450,000 emergency room visits were due to cocaine.[3]

Background

Cocaine comes from the leaves of the coca plant, ***Erythroxylon coca***. Natives living in the Andes Mountains typically chew the leaves of the coca plant to relieve fatigue, for spiritual reasons, or to enhance well-being. Chewing coca leaves does not seem to cause dependence, possibly because the leaves contain less than 1% cocaine. Also, when coca leaves are chewed or brewed in tea, they do not cause biological harm or social dysfunction.[4]

The largest producer of cocaine is Colombia, although its production of cocaine has decreased significantly since 2000. Bolivia and Peru account for a small percentage of cocaine production. One factor that resulted in Colombia's decrease was the increase in spraying to eradicate the coca plant. In addition, seizures of cocaine increased significantly between 2002 and 2005, although less cocaine was seized in 2006.

Properties

Cocaine is an odorless, crystalline, white powder. It produces intense euphoria, alertness, and energy, as well as inhibited appetite and sleep. As a medical

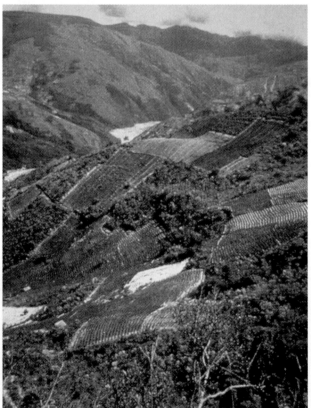

U.S. Department of Justice, DEA.

The Upper Huallaga Valley of Peru is one of the primary sources of the coca leaf.

use, cocaine sometimes is put into a mixture called a **Brompton's cocktail**, which is used to manage cancer pain. Also, cocaine is used in surgical procedures on the facial area because that area has many blood vessels and cocaine constricts blood flow and blood vessels. The anesthetizing action takes effect within a minute and lasts up to 2 hours. At one time cocaine was used to allay withdrawal symptoms from narcotic addiction and to treat depression.

Erythroxylon coca Coca plant from which cocaine is derived

Brompton's cocktail A combination of heroin and cocaine sometimes used to treat terminally ill patients

crack cocaine A variation of cocaine made by heating cocaine after mixing it with baking soda and water

freebase A variation of cocaine in which cocaine is separated from its hydrochloride salt by heating, using a volatile chemical such as ether

Mode of Intake

Cocaine can be snorted, smoked, or injected. The mode of intake has a bearing on its potential to cause addiction. The more quickly one gets high, the more likely addiction will occur. Injected cocaine reaches the brain the fastest, and euphoria is rapid and intense. Snorted cocaine is absorbed into the bloodstream through the nasal mucous membranes. Most recreational or experimental users snort cocaine initially. It reaches the brain in 10 to 15 minutes, resulting in a "high."

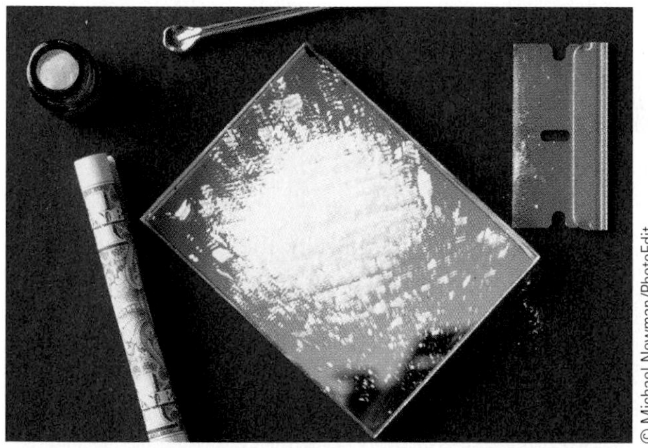

© Michael Newman/PhotoEdit.

Cocaine paraphernalia includes mirrors, razor blades, and scales used by drug dealers.

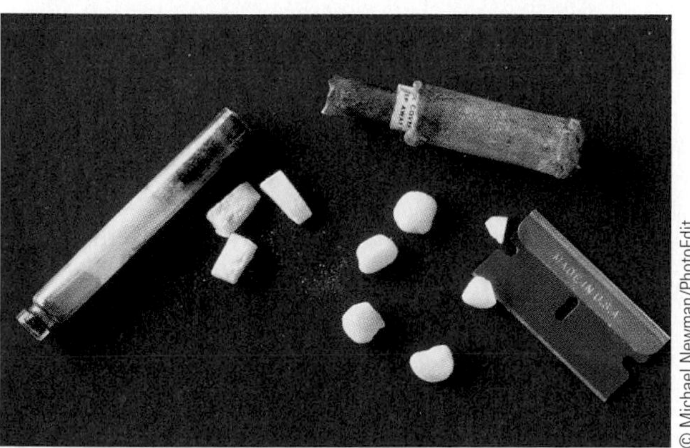

© Michael Newman/PhotoEdit.

Crack pipes are often homemade.

Like injected cocaine, **crack cocaine** reaches the brain in seconds. The immediate reinforcement or reward is critical to addiction. In 2005, 73% of people admitted into treatment for cocaine abuse smoked the drug. This percentage is a slight decrease from 1995.[5]

Freebasing cocaine started in the mid-1960s. In the **freebase** process, cocaine is treated with an alkaloid to separate it from its hydrochloride salt. Then it is mixed with ether to remove the impurities. Although the euphoria derived from freebasing cocaine is intense and fast, it is brief. The user is getting high quickly at twice the cost for a relatively shorter time. Figure 11.1 depicts different forms of cocaine.

Historical Use

The history of cocaine as a medicinal agent dates back more than 100 years. Cocaine originally was isolated from coca leaves by the German scientist Niemann

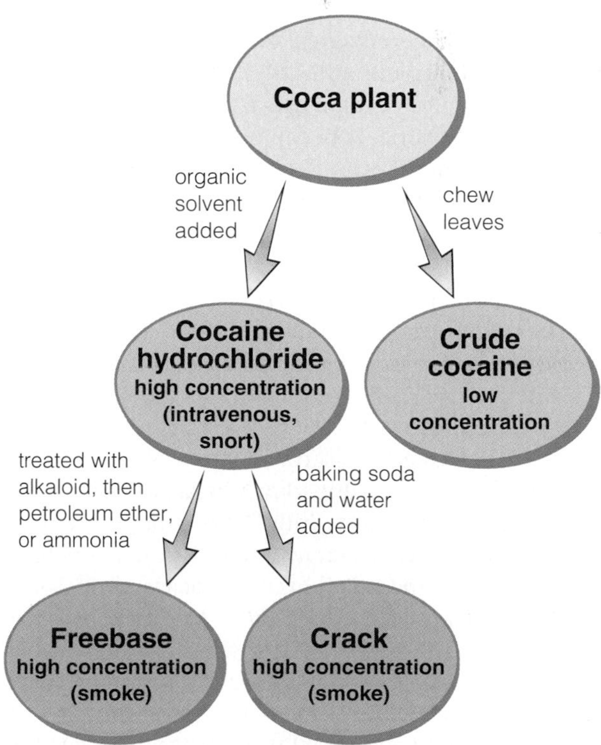

Figure 11.1 Forms of Cocaine

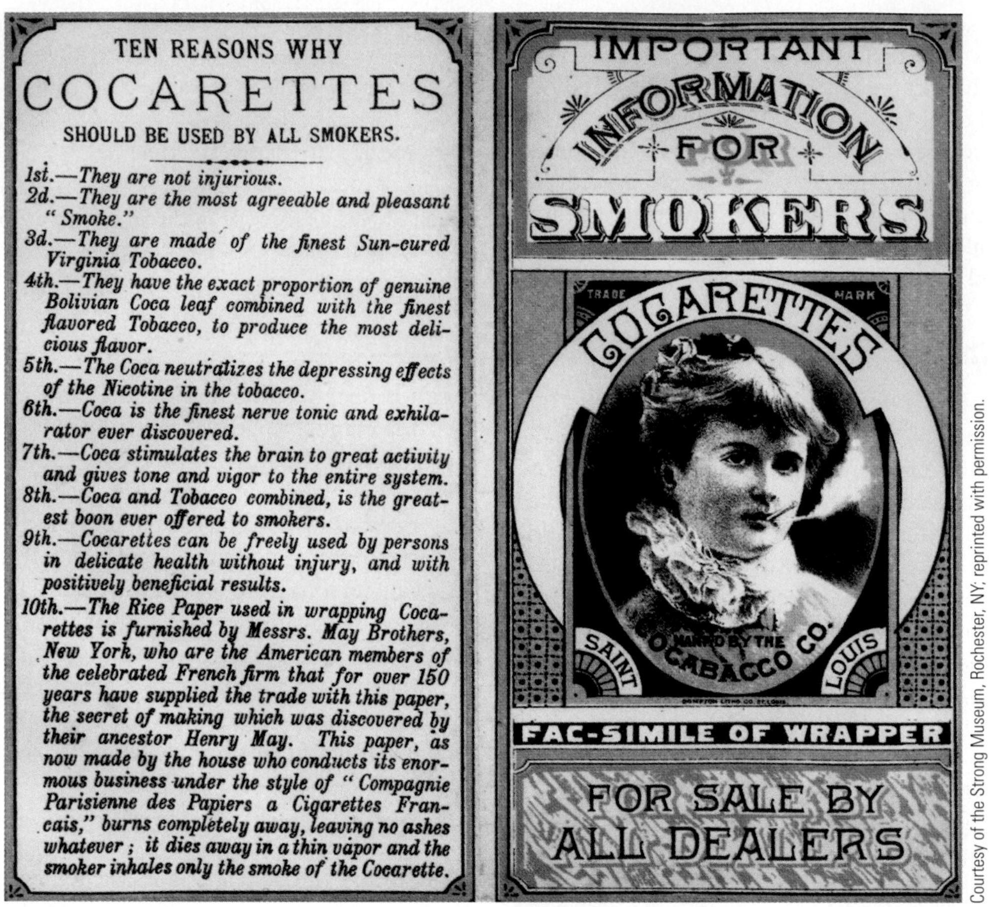

In the late 1800s the Cocabacco Company manufactured cocarettes.

around 1859. Within several years, Sigmund Freud spoke of cocaine in magical terms and recommended it to alleviate opiate addiction, depression, and fatigue. Eventually, cocaine use and dependence spread throughout Europe. It became so popular that luminaries including Ulysses S. Grant, Pope Leo XIII, and Sarah Bernhardt touted it. Freud later was held responsible for the "third scourge of humanity" (the first two were alcohol and opiate addiction), whereupon he stopped recommending the drug.

Cocaine was originally included in one of the world's most popular beverages, Coca-Cola. (Coca-Cola derived its name from two of its ingredients: kola nuts and cocaine.) For people opposed to alcohol, Coca-Cola was advertised as a "temperance drink." Coca leaves were also added to a bordeaux wine called Vin Mariani. Even John Stith Pemberton, the original developer of Coca-Cola, invented his own version of cocaine-laced wine called French Coca Wine in 1884.[6] In 1898, druggist Caleb Davis Bradham invented Pepsi-Cola in New Bern, North Carolina, to compete against Coca-Cola. Like Pemberton, Bradham developed the beverage for its medicinal properties.[7]

Despite the widespread use of cocaine by the turn of the 20th century, many people condemned it because it led to dependency. Ironically, the individuals speaking out against cocaine were the same individuals who had promoted it—physicians. By 1914 almost every state in the United States had passed laws to control cocaine use. Finally, with passage of the Harrison Narcotic Act of 1914, the federal government officially (although erroneously) designated cocaine as a narcotic.

After the Harrison Act was enacted and nonmedical use of cocaine became illegal, its use declined. When amphetamines were introduced in 1927, its use declined further. But in the 1970s, its use reemerged. In the succeeding decade cocaine use increased in Europe and in countries where it had been almost nonexistent. The increase in cocaine use was accompanied by an increase in cocaine-related deaths.

Partly responsible for the rise of cocaine use in the 1970s was the declining popularity of amphetamines and the increased availability of cocaine. During the 1960s amphetamines had been the drugs of choice. The desire for amphetamines, however, decreased as media campaigns warned people that "Speed kills." Cocaine was seen as a safer alternative. Moreover, pharmaceutical manufacturers were limiting supplies of amphetamines.

Also contributing to the interest in cocaine in the 1980s was the fact that movie stars, musicians, and professional athletes reportedly used it. These celebrities established the groundwork for making cocaine glamorous, and it became the "champagne" of drugs. Another factor that furthered the popularity of cocaine was the rejection of the traditional work ethic and middle-class values of the 1950s and 1960s, replaced by a laid-back, relaxed lifestyle; people "mellowed out" and "did their own thing."

A parallel set of values emerged out of the 1970s, with an emphasis on getting ahead, making it to the top, striving to be the best, and being successful. Cocaine delivered feelings of being masterful, competent, and invincible. Thus, it satisfied the mood of the time and became the drug of choice for many people.

U.S. Department of Justice, DEA.

The effects of crack are quick and brief.

Current Use

In 2006, an estimated 2.4 million Americans ages 12 and older were current cocaine users, the majority of them between 18 and 25 years of age.[8] Figure 11.2 shows the age that cocaine was first used in contrast to when other drugs were first used. Chronic, hardcore drug users—who represent about 20% of drug users—account for two-thirds of the total amount of cocaine used in the United States. Also, males are more likely to use cocaine than women, in greater amounts, and for a longer duration, and women are not as likely to inject it.[9] Of cocaine abusers seeking treatment, a significant percentage meet the criteria for attention deficit/hyperactivity disorder (ADHD) as children and as adults.[10]

Crack

Crack cocaine emerged in the 1980s, though accounts of its use were noted as far back as the early 1970s. It is the product of mixing cocaine with baking soda and water and then heating the mixture. This simple process produces small chunks or rocks, which can be smoked. Smoking the chunks or rocks produces a crackling sound—hence, the term *crack*. Crack is usually smoked, but it can also be injected. Because it comes in small units, the cost is low. The euphoria from crack is brief (about 10 to 20 minutes), and the desire to repeat usage is high. Most people who have used crack, however, do not continue to use it.

Crack use is a problem among impoverished, inner-city adolescents. Before the less expensive crack form was available, fewer people used cocaine. But even poor people can afford to buy crack. In one encouraging development, more than 82% of secondary students disapprove of crack use even though many state that the drug is not difficult to obtain.[11]

Crack use may be correlated with other problems. In one study, more than 60% of women addicted to crack had been sexually abused, and 70% had symptoms of depression.[12] In 2003, 30% of state and local

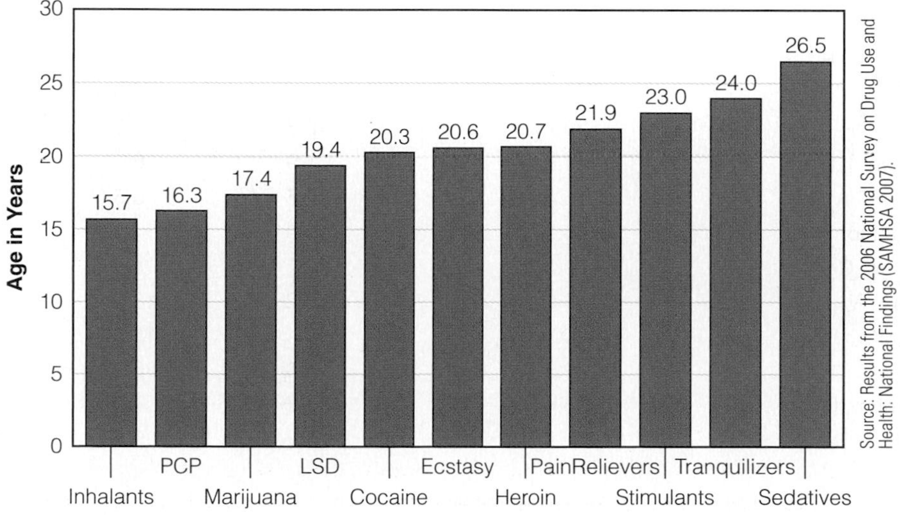

Figure 11.2 Mean Age at First Use for Specific Illicit Drugs among Past Year Initiates Ages 12 to 49: 2006

law enforcement agencies nationwide listed crack cocaine as their greatest drug threat.[13] Between October 1, 2004, and September 30, 2005, 6,282 people were sentenced in federal courts on crack cocaine–related charges. Approximately 95% of the cases involved trafficking.[14] The connection between crack use and violence, then, might be related to the drug trade and not solely to the use of crack. The percentage of adult arrestees in various American cities testing positive for crack or powder cocaine is shown in Table 11.1.

In a study of 300 gang members in San Francisco, the gang members had a rule against using crack, even though they sold it to others. Use by gang members was deemed bad for business.[15]

The crack trade has contributed to a sharp increase in inner-city murders. Gang members kill each other (and innocent bystanders) to gain control of the crack market. Couriers often are children who are known as *mules*, used because they are subject to less severe penalties if caught. Some schools ban pupils from carrying paging devices or cellular telephones because they may be used to sell drugs.

Crack is costly not only to users but to society as well. In a study of crack addicts, many female addicts

TABLE 11.1 Use and Acquisition of Powder Cocaine among Adult Male Arrestees, 2003

Primary City	Arrestees Testing Positive for Cocaine* (%)	Arrestees Reporting Powder Cocaine Use (%)		
		Past 7 Days	Past 30 Days	Past Year
Albuquerque, NM	35.0	12.4	15.3	22.9
Anchorage, AK	25.4	8.3	11.6	17.6
Atlanta, GA	49.8	8.5	10.1	15.5
Boston, MA	31.8	6.9	10.1	20.8
Charlotte, NC	35.2	5.8	7.8	12.6
Chicago, IL	50.6	6.7	8.3	11.0
Cleveland, OH	39.0	2.5	4.5	8.5
Dallas, TX	32.7	8.3	11.2	15.5
Denver, CO	38.3	8.8	10.8	16.5
Honolulu, HI	11.6	1.3	2.3	5.7
Houston, TX	22.6	19.6	24.0	27.2
Indianapolis, IN	35.3	5.1	8.6	13.3
Las Vegas, NV	21.9	7.2	9.6	14.1
Los Angeles, CA	23.5	10.1	11.4	17.6
Miami, FL	47.1	17.7	22.3	28.4
Minneapolis, MN	28.4	4.7	6.5	11.4
New Orleans, LA	47.6	8.3	9.8	12.7
New York, NY	35.7	8.3	10.2	12.1
Omaha, NE	20.5	1.7	3.4	8.3
Philadelphia, PA	30.3	7.6	10.7	14.8
Phoenix, AZ	23.4	5.5	7.6	12.9
Portland, OR	29.7	10.6	14.5	20.4
Sacramento, CA	21.6	4.9	6.1	9.6
Salt Lake City, UT	15.4	7.5	9.5	16.5
San Antonio, TX	30.5	12.0	14.8	21.2
San Diego, CA	10.3	3.2	4.2	8.4
Seattle, WA	36.6	8.2	13.0	21.6
Tampa, FL	30.1	8.4	11.5	17.0
Tucson, AZ	42.5	18.0	23.9	30.7
Washington, DC	26.5	2.7	4.2	5.8
Median	30.1	7.2	9.6	13.6

* Arrestee tested positive for either crack or powder cocaine.

Source: *Drug and Alcohol Use and Related Matters among Arrestees 2003.* Table 5. National Institute of Justice.

traded sex for crack, and male addicts traded crack for sex. Also, condoms were used only "sometimes." This has led to high rates of AIDS and associated costs of treatment.

speedball Injectable combination of heroin and cocaine

Cocaine and the Media

Jazz musicians commonly used cocaine during the 1930s and 1940s. One song that referred to cocaine was Cole Porter's "I Get a Kick Out of You," popular in 1934. The lyrics include the following:

> I get no kick from cocaine.
> I'm sure that if I took even one sniff
> It would bore me terrifically too,
> But I still get a kick out of you.

Starting in the 1960s, references to drugs in music were conspicuous. The Grateful Dead's "Casey Jones" (1970), "Let It Bleed" (1969) and "Sister Morphine" (1971) by the Rolling Stones, and more recently "Girl on LSD" (1994) by Tom Petty and the Heartbreakers alluded to cocaine. In the early 1990s, rap musicians promoted cocaine use. Their message in popular music has since changed, so at present, cocaine use is maligned and discouraged.

Accounts of cocaine use also are found in literature. Sir Arthur Conan Doyle's fictional detective Sherlock Holmes was a noted recreational user of cocaine for mental stimulation. Robert Louis Stevenson is believed to have written *Dr. Jekyll and Mr. Hyde* while receiving cocaine treatments for tuberculosis. John Belushi's life and ultimate death from a mixture of cocaine and heroin are chronicled in Robert Woodward's book *Wired: The Short Life and Fast Times of John Belushi. Snowblind,* by Robert Sabbag, describes cocaine as integral to a world of glamour, status, and intrigue. References to cocaine are found in comic books, particularly the action-adventure type of comic.

The media offer a paradoxical view of cocaine. The drug is connected with high status, yet the messages often carry a negative connotation. Stories presenting negative images of cocaine appear regularly in newspapers and popular magazines such as *Sports Illustrated, Newsweek,* and *Time.*

Effects

Cocaine can produce a myriad of effects. One area that is affected by cocaine use is educational achievement. It has been shown that as cocaine use went down in the 1990s, educational achievement went up.[16]

The physical effects of cocaine depend on how the drug enters the body. Some cocaine users place the drug under their tongue, allowing quick absorption of the cocaine. When it is snorted, cocaine is absorbed readily through the mucous membranes of the nose (which have a rich supply of blood vessels) and quickly enters the bloodstream. The peak phase of a cocaine high when taken in this way occurs in 10 to 20 minutes. Intravenous injection produces a high in about 30 seconds and lasts about 10 minutes. Injection, however, is the least common method of taking cocaine.

A variation is the **speedball**, an injected mixture of cocaine and heroin. This mixture carries a higher risk of dependency and overdose, and speedball users have higher rates of psychopathology and HIV infection than other cocaine abusers. Also, when cocaine is used in conjunction with fentanyl, a narcotic more powerful than heroin, there is an increased likelihood of a fatal overdose.[17] In Scotland, the number of deaths resulting from using cocaine and alcohol together has increased despite an overall decrease in drug-related deaths.[18]

Physical Consequences

When cocaine is snorted, irritations to the nasal membranes, hoarseness, sore throat, and inflamed sinuses are common. Because cocaine is an anesthetic, the nasal passages, throat, and palate become numb from frequent snorting. Snorting leads to sneezing, congestion, burns, sores, and upper respiratory infections including pulmonary congestion, bronchitis, and pneumonia. In extreme cases, people who chronically snort cocaine

Physical Effects of Cocaine

- Elevated blood pressure
- Excessive perspiration
- Nausea, vomiting, abdominal pain
- Headache
- Tightened muscles (including muscles controlling bowel movements)
- Slower digestive process
- Anorexia
- Nutritional deficiencies
- Rapid pulse
- Faster breathing rate
- Increased body temperature
- Urge to urinate, defecate, belch
- Inflammation of trachea and bronchi
- Hoarseness or laryngitis
- Chronic wheezing and heavy coughing
- Coughing up pus, mucus, blood
- Seizures
- Hallucinations

incur septal necrosis, in which the cartilage separating the two nostrils is destroyed. In a study of female inmates it was found that those women who used cocaine were four times more likely to experience tooth decay compared to inmates who were not drug users.[19]

When the effects of cocaine wear off, blood pressure and respiration descend below normal levels, precipitating withdrawal symptoms and an increased desire to take more cocaine. Malnutrition is a problem because cocaine users have less interest in food. Babies born to women who used cocaine during pregnancy are more likely to have growth deficiencies than those of nonusers.

People who smoke freebase cocaine often cough up a tarry residue. Freebasing cocaine can cause significant lung damage such as acute bronchoconstriction.[20] Smoked cocaine, especially crack, can produce chest pain, rapid heart rate, irregular heart contractions, circulatory failure, blood pressure that increases to the point of hemorrhaging, or congestive heart failure and death. Injected cocaine carries different risks than snorted cocaine. Besides AIDS, injected cocaine has been linked to inflammation of the heart lining (endocarditis) and liver (hepatitis).

Cocaine accounts for more than one half of all people going to emergency rooms for drug-related incidents even though the number of emergency room visits because of cocaine has decreased. Figure 11.3 illustrates the fact that cocaine causes more emergency room visits than heroin and marijuana.[21]

Cocaine-related crime, abuse rates, and numerous overdose incidents continue to be a burden. Cocaine is believed to be responsible for more violent crime and property crime than any other drug.[22] An encouraging point is that the number of people testing positive for cocaine in the workplace has declined. This may be the result of reduced cocaine availability.[23]

Psychological Effects

Because the psychological effects of cocaine are subjective, they are open to interpretation. Descriptions of the psychological effects of cocaine are based on interviews with users whose objectivity is questionable. The psychological mosaic of cocaine abusers includes frenzied mood swings, delusions of extraordinary abilities, distortions of perspective, and impaired memory and mental functioning. Because their perspective of the world is dramatically altered, cocaine users claim they are in control, exhilarated, and confident. These delusionary reactions have prompted people to call cocaine "the big lie."

People under the influence of cocaine manifest many social deviations. Some cocaine users become engrossed in repetitive, compulsive behaviors without being aware of what they are doing. Users become detached and neglect personal hygiene, friends, jobs, and schoolwork.

Some cocaine users describe the pleasure they derive from cocaine use as orgasmic. Cocaine often is used as a prelude to romance. Ironically, excessive use actually interferes with sexual pleasure. Like alcohol, it might increase the desire for sex but diminish the ability to perform.

Men and women have different reasons for using cocaine. Women are more likely to use cocaine for depression and stress and have more difficulty

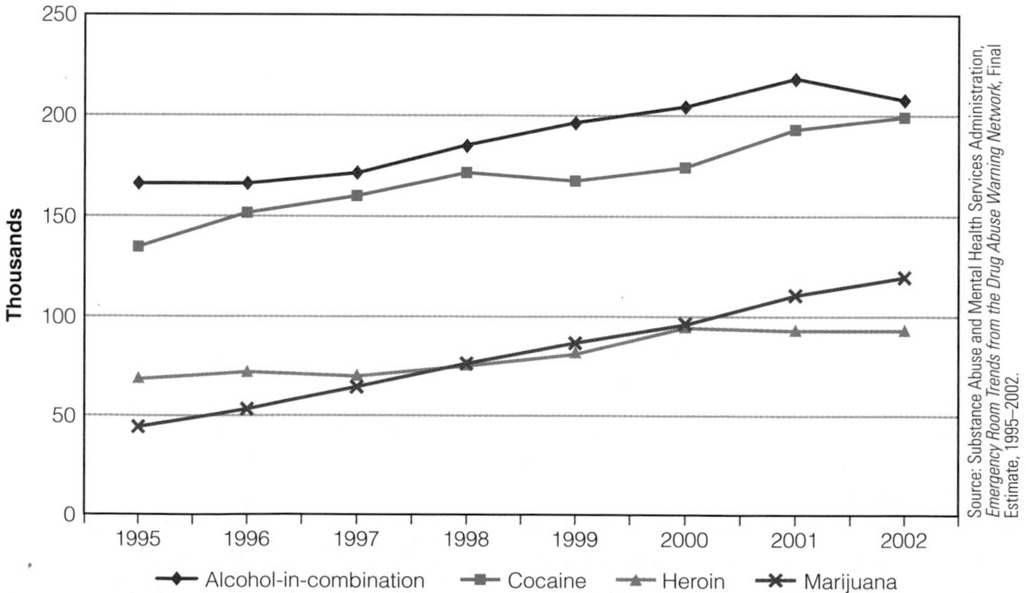

Source: Substance Abuse and Mental Health Services Administration, *Emergency Room Trends from the Drug Abuse Warning Network*, Final Estimate, 1995–2002.

Figure 11.3 Emergency Room Mentions of Alcohol-in-Combination, Cocaine, Heroin, and Marijuana: 1995 through 2002

Psychological Effects of Cocaine

- Talkativeness
- Mood swings
- Hallucinations
- Repetitive behaviors
- Extreme depression
- Neglect of personal hygiene
- Rage and violent behavior
- Delusions
- Distorted perceptions
- Depersonalization
- Suicidal ideation
- Paranoia

overcoming addiction. Women are also more likely to use cocaine to feel sociable, whereas men use it for physical energy.[24]

In the extreme, cocaine psychosis is marked by severe depression, paranoia, rage, thoughts of suicide, and aggressive and violent behavior. Psychiatric patients who abuse cocaine and alcohol together have a higher likelihood of homicidal behavior than those who abuse only cocaine or only alcohol. Also, cocaine use can exacerbate the symptoms of post-traumatic stress disorders.[25]

Feelings of paranoia can trigger bizarre behavior that mimics schizophrenia. Some users hallucinate that their arms and legs are getting longer or think they are having an out-of-body experience.

Cocaine diminishes one's need for sleep and the ability to go to sleep. Changes in perception occur, distance becomes distorted, and colors intensify. The user may feel bugs crawling on or under the skin, called *cocaine bugs* or formication. People reportedly have tried to rid themselves of these bugs by burning their arms and legs with cigarettes or matches or by scratching themselves constantly.

Dependence

Not all cocaine users, even those who have taken cocaine over several years, experience dependence and withdrawal. Research has not found a "cocaine personality" that accounts for dependency. Nevertheless, cocaine users build up tolerance to effects of the drug. Unfortunately, users do not develop tolerance to health risks such as seizures, heart attacks, or strokes. The pleasure derived from cocaine use is self-reinforcing, and some users go on "coke runs," or binges. Perhaps dependency arises not from the desire to feel euphoric but, rather, from the desire not to feel dysphoric.

Cocaine users do not have the classic withdrawal symptoms that narcotic addicts exhibit. Moreover, the withdrawal symptoms associated with cocaine are not life-threatening. Symptoms following cessation of cocaine use include depression, lack of energy, poor appetite, less pleasure from activities, restlessness, and agitation. Scientists are working on the development of a vaccine for preventing addiction to cocaine and other drugs. The concept is to train one's immune system to extinguish the drugs prior to their affect on the nervous system.[26]

ibogaine A hallucinogen that is used to treat cocaine dependence

Chronic cocaine users demonstrate three phases following abstinence[27]:

1. Intense craving, agitation, anorexia, and deep depression (the "crash"), which can last from 9 hours to 4 days.
2. Withdrawal, during which the person is incapable of feeling normal pleasure, but depression moderates and sleeping becomes easier; can last up to 10 weeks, although signs and symptoms of moderate cocaine withdrawal tend to stabilize over 7 to 10 days.
3. Extinction, during which improvement is considerable, but periods of depression and occasional craving can last for months and even years.

A controversial drug given to cocaine addicts is the African hallucinogen **ibogaine**, which allegedly works by blocking withdrawal symptoms while suppressing the craving for drugs. Evidence of its effectiveness is limited to animal studies and unconfirmed reports from individuals. In addition to research regarding cocaine, ibogaine is being tested to determine whether it is effective for treating narcotic, alcohol, and tobacco dependence. The National Institute on Drug Abuse states there is no long-term proof that it works.

Ibogaine is illegal in the United States, but it is used in Holland. Some drug-dependent Americans have gone abroad to use ibogaine.

Propranolol, a drug used to treat high blood pressure, has shown promise in helping cocaine addicts. Propranolol eases withdrawal symptoms, making it easier for cocaine addicts to remain in treatment.[28] Disulfiram, a drug used to treat alcoholism, has also shown potential as a treatment for cocaine addicts. Typically cocaine addicts are given antidepressants to lessen withdrawal symptoms.[29]

Death from Cocaine

Because cocaine can cause irregular heartbeat (cardiac arrhythmias), high blood pressure, and chest pains, it can trigger heart attacks. It is capable of destroying the heart muscle by disrupting its blood supply (myocardial infarctions). Coronary artery disease leading to death is relatively common in cocaine users; in fact, cocaine has been shown to increase calcium deposits in the body, resulting in an increase in cocaine-related coronary deaths.[30] Some deaths result from "body packing," a method of smuggling cocaine by which it is placed in condoms or plastic bags and swallowed. Often the bags break and the cocaine leaks into the intestines.

Some fatalities from cocaine use result from uncontrolled seizures, strokes, or paralysis of breathing muscles. A lethal dose of cocaine has not been determined precisely. Some people die from relatively low levels.

When death strikes, it tends to come quickly. Some victims do not reach medical facilities in time to receive medical attention. Data from the most recent Drug Abuse Warning Network profile showed that during one year 111 people died from cocaine overdose in Miami, 216 in Boston, 108 in Atlanta, 289 in Detroit, and 521 in New York City.[31] Males make up the majority (68%) of fatal overdoses. Though the majority of deaths from cocaine overdose occur among people between the ages 35 and 54, a recent University of Florida study found that the number of college students dying from cocaine use is increasing.[32]

People who inject cocaine are in danger of contracting HIV infection and the eventually fatal AIDS. A person with a weakened immune system is more susceptible to bacterial or viral infections such as pneumonia and meningitis, as well as cancer. In some cities cocaine and other drugs are injected in places called **shooting galleries**. Because of the illegal status of cocaine and the clandestine nature of shooting galleries, educating addicts about the need to discard needles safely or how to clean needles properly is not easy.

Cocaine and Pregnancy

It is estimated that one out of every 25 women will use an illegal drug while pregnant.[33] Compared with other pregnant women, those who use cocaine drink more, smoke more, have worse nutritional intake, and generally are in poorer overall health. Of women giving birth, 8% to 10% had exposed their fetuses to cocaine in one study.[34] Blood flowing through the placenta delivers oxygen to the fetus. Cocaine constricts blood vessels and thereby blood flow and oxygen. Also, cocaine can cause detachment of the placenta, as well as premature labor, by stimulating uterine contractions, and women who use cocaine during pregnancy have higher rates of spontaneous abortion.

Some babies of women who use cocaine while they are pregnant have neurological problems, perhaps caused by strokes before birth. Cocaine-exposed babies have higher rates of congenital heart defects, lower birth weights, and seizures, and they are more at risk for sudden infant death. Cocaine-exposed babies tend to be born with smaller heads, which often reflect smaller brains. Also, these babies are more prone to urinary tract problems.[35] Determining whether these effects result from the mother's cocaine use or from poor prenatal care is difficult. Also, fetal development can be affected by alcohol consumption, cigarette smoking, and other drugs, as well as environmental factors such as poverty, poor nutrition, homelessness, violence, and crime.

Media articles have warned that social and psychological consequences will surface as prenatally exposed children enter school. These children were expected to be irritable, hyperactive, and difficult to console. Such dire forecasts, however, may be unfounded.[36] Prenatal exposure also has little impact on infant growth[37]:

> Condemning these drug-exposed children with labels indicating a permanent handicap is premature. Such prophecies of doom lead researchers to overlook what has long been known about the remediating effects of early intervention.[38]

In a study of women who used cocaine, infants' cognitive development was affected by the mothers' postnatal drug use and poor maternal interaction. The cognitive development of infants whose mothers stopped using cocaine after giving birth was higher than for infants whose mothers continued to use drugs.[39] One study found that the average IQ score of cocaine-exposed four-year-old children was 79 and the IQ scores of other four-year-old children from the same impoverished environment averaged 82.[40] Home environments that are mentally stimulating lessen the prenatal effects of cocaine.[41]

Amphetamines

Amphetamines have played an important role since first marketed in 1927. During World War II, they were given to American soldiers to help them overcome fatigue, heighten their mood, and improve their endurance. They do, however, produce side effects that are disadvantageous in combat. Hitler's bizarre behavior near the end of World War II, in which he was alternately depressed and happy, is speculated to have been caused by amphetamines.

Early Applications

When amphetamines were developed, they were effective in treating asthma. Under the name **Benzedrine**, amphetamine was sold in inhalers. The user would open the inhaler, put the concentrated amphetamine liquid on a cloth, and inhale it. Eventually, the inhalers were used nonmedically, and the U.S. Food and Drug Administration banned amphetamines in inhalers in 1959.

Amphetamines were used for treating depression, for increasing work capacity, and for treating **narcolepsy**.

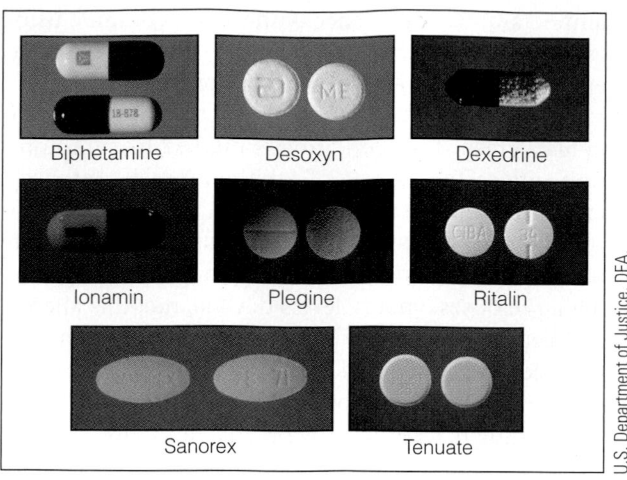

U.S. Department of Justice, DEA.

There are a variety of amphetamines on the market today.

shooting gallery A place to buy and inject drugs

Benzedrine An amphetamine used to treat nasal congestion and asthma

narcolepsy Condition in which the person involuntarily falls asleep; commonly called sleeping sickness

Narcoleptics fall asleep spontaneously and sometimes sleep for long periods. It was noted that narcoleptic patients given amphetamines were not hungry. The drug then was used to suppress appetite and ward off fatigue. Beginning in the late 1930s, it was given to hyperactive children. During World War II, American airmen in Great Britain often took Benzedrine pills. In the 1960s there were 20 million prescriptions written for amphetamines for weight-loss purposes.[42] Amphetamines and amphetamine-like drugs are still used to treat obesity.[43]

Pharmacology

Amphetamines can be administered by ingestion, injection, snorting, or inhalation. When taken orally, they produce peak effects in 2 to 3 hours. The half-life is 10 to 12 hours and they are not totally eliminated from the body for about 2 days.

The effects are felt more quickly—usually within 5 minutes—when they are injected. Because tolerance to amphetamines develops quickly, many users do not derive pleasure from the drug. Therefore, they increase the dosage or go on binges to maintain their high. Among users who prefer methamphetamines, a stronger form of amphetamine, injection is preferred to snorting.

Smoking methamphetamine is growing in popularity. Crystals of methamphetamine, known as "ice," are put into the glass bowl of a pipe and heated from below. The vapors then are inhaled. When methamphetamines are taken like this, the person feels the effects in a few seconds.

Because amphetamines increase activity of the sympathetic nervous system, they are classified as sympathomimetic drugs. Their physiological effects are similar to those in people who are emotionally aroused: increased respiration and perspiration, higher blood pressure and body temperature, increased blood flow to the extremities, and dilation of the pupils.

Amphetamines are absorbed by the blood and distributed rapidly. Their chemical structure is similar to that of the neurotransmitters norepinephrine and dopamine. Amphetamines stimulate receptor sites for these neurotransmitters. Another explanation for their stimulating action is that they send norepinephrine and dopamine back to their presynaptic sites by blocking their uptake. By stimulating norepinephrine receptors, the drug makes the individual feel more alert. When dopamine receptors are stimulated, the person becomes euphoric and more active.

Amphetamines are removed from the body in two ways:

1. They are excreted through urine after being transformed by liver enzymes.
2. They are deactivated and removed by adding molecules to the amphetamine compound.

Potential psychological effects of amphetamines include paranoia, violence, restlessness, agitation, hallucinations, confusion, and anxiety. Possible physical effects are tremors, tinnitus (ringing in ears), dry mouth, excessive perspiration, increased blood pressure, poor coordination, and convulsions. Amphetamines are especially harmful to the cardiovascular system and can cause cardiac arrest. Recent evidence indicates that amphetamine use increases the risk of a stroke five-fold.[44]

Effects of Amphetamines

Psychological
- Paranoia
- Violent behavior
- Restlessness
- Agitation
- Confusion
- Anxiety
- Hallucinations

Physical
- Tremors
- Tinnitus
- Dry mouth
- Excessive sweating
- High blood pressure
- Poor coordination
- Convulsions
- Cardiac arrest

The Amphetamine Trade

Japan and Sweden have had far more severe problems with amphetamine abuse than the United States has. To maintain production during World War II, Japanese workers were given amphetamines. As the war ended, massive amounts of the drug remained. To reduce this surplus, pharmaceutical companies sold amphetamines without prescription. This led to amphetamine abuse and medical problems. About 2% of Japan's population was abusing the drug. By the mid-1950s, the Japanese government curtailed production of the drug and provided more treatment, education, and punitive measures. This effort helped to reduce abuse.

Amphetamine abuse was a serious problem in Sweden in the 1940s, necessitating stringent regulations. Although the abuse of orally ingested amphetamines declined, a segment of hardcore users began injecting amphetamines intravenously. The Swedish government dealt with this dilemma by providing narcotics and stimulants to abusers. Within 2 years, this program was considered a failure. By 1968, Sweden had banned amphetamines and other stimulants. More recently, Poland became one of the largest amphetamine producers for the European market.

Although people in the United States could legally obtain amphetamines in the 1930s, they also were available illegally. The main users were truck drivers and college students. Truck stops often served as distribution sites. In addition, amphetamines were obtained easily by prescription to treat depression or obesity. Hospital emergency rooms would administer amphetamines to people who had overdosed on sleeping pills. Because of indiscriminate prescribing, the federal government imposed regulations in 1965 to limit their access.

Amphetamines had been so available that every man, woman, and child could be supplied several times daily. They represented about 8% of prescriptions in 1970. By this time, the drug subculture was in place, especially in San Francisco, and drug use flourished for several years before it began to decline.

During the well-known "Summer of Love" in San Francisco in 1967, young people gathered to protest the Vietnam War, decry prejudice and poverty, engage in "free love," and take mind-altering drugs, primarily marijuana and LSD. Within a short time, heroin and amphetamines replaced marijuana and LSD as the drugs of choice. The "flower child" was supplanted by the "speed freak." In some locations, such as Hawaii, amphetamines have remained the drug of choice.

Consequences of Amphetamine Use

Like cocaine, amphetamines do not produce classic withdrawal symptoms similar to those with narcotics or barbiturates. Still, most people who are dependent on amphetamines experience withdrawal, continue using them despite problems, cannot stop, develop tolerance, and give up other activities to use amphetamines.[45]

After several days of moderate to heavy use, individuals crash. This condition is marked by symptoms opposite to the effects of amphetamines—lethargy, exhaustion, depression, and hunger. Symptoms of amphetamine withdrawal, though not life-threatening, are undeniable. Within hours after an individual stops taking large doses, energy levels decline, mood is altered, and sleep may follow, for up to 24 hours. On waking, the user feels depressed. One study found that nearly 4% of suicide victims tested positive for amphetamines.[46]

Stimulants can improve mental and physical performance. For simple tasks amphetamines are effective, but for tasks requiring complex thinking, such as problem-solving and decision-making, they are counterproductive. Because high doses affect judgment and decision-making skills negatively, they can cause severe behavioral problems. In the District of Columbia in 2007, 3.7% of all adult arrestees tested positive for amphetamines. This is an increase from the 2.5% who tested positive in 2006.[47]

One way in which amphetamines have been shown to influence judgment is that users are less likely to use condoms when engaging in sexual behavior.[48] An Australian study found that a significant number of adolescents who used amphetamines displayed mental health problems.[49]

In some instances, users act compulsively and repetitiously. Laboratory animals given high doses have been known to turn in circles continuously or gnaw at the bars of their cages. Gross motor skills improve at the same time as fine motor skills are impaired. Athletes who need speed and strength benefit more from amphetamines than athletes who have to be accurate, although the risks outweigh the benefits. One group of people who are currently using amphetamines is professional baseball players. Although Major League Baseball is concerned about players using steroids, an increasing number are taking amphetamines. However, many players are obtaining prescriptions to take the drugs legally. In 2006, 28 players received amphetamines because they were diagnosed with attention deficit disorder. In 2007, that number jumped to 103. In essence, 7.6% of professional baseball players received amphetamines for therapeutic purposes.[50]

Amphetamine psychosis, a condition marked by paranoia, aggressiveness, fearfulness, disordered thinking, mania, and hallucinations, is a significant problem related to chronic use. Suspicion and paranoia often lead to hostile and violent behaviors. Actually, the violent behavior might be caused by sleep deprivation, which also can result in suspiciousness and paranoia. Some evidence suggests that use of amphetamines can cause brain damage and exacerbate Tourette's syndrome and tardive dyskinesia.

The dosage of amphetamines required to generate side effects varies among individuals, though beginning users are more likely to have side effects because they have less tolerance. As little as 2 mg can produce negative side effects in some people, whereas other people can take 15 mg before having adverse effects.

"Speed kills," a popular slogan of the 1960s, alluded to the potential consequences of taking amphetamines. Amphetamine abusers can die from their risk-taking behavior while under the drug's influence, from suicide resulting from the severe depression following a "run," or from the associated unhealthy lifestyle in which nutrition and health are neglected. Few people actually die from an overdose, although people can incur irregular heartbeat, heart stoppage, and strokes during heavy usage.

Methamphetamines

After World War II, **methamphetamines**, popularly known as **speed**, began to be widely abused in the United States. In 2003, more than 12 million Americans tried methamphetamines at least once.[51] Like amphetamines, this more potent version was used to treat narcolepsy, suppress appetite, and relieve the symptoms of Parkinson's disease. Methamphetamines, however, are more likely than amphetamines to be used for nonmedical purposes. **"Speed freaks"** go on binges, shooting up every few hours over a 5- or 6-day period before crashing and then sleeping from 12 hours to 4 days. Problems of methamphetamines are not limited to the United States. The number of methamphetamine labs is increasing greatly in Central Europe.[52]

methamphetamine A more potent form of amphetamine

speed A stimulant drug; another name for methamphetamine

"speed freak" Someone who uses methamphetamines over a period of time

Clandestine Methamphetamine Laboratories

The three main types of harm associated with methamphetamine labs are (1) physical injury from explosions, fires, chemical burns, and toxic fumes; (2) environmental hazards; and (3) child endangerment.[53] Methamphetamine labs can explode due to the processing of chemicals at extremely high temperatures. Moreover, safety procedures and adequate ventilation are often overlooked. Not only is the lab a danger to the people making the drug, but police sometimes will trigger explosions when entering a lab. A common way for methamphetamine labs to be discovered is that a fire or explosion occurs.

As indicated, methamphetamine labs pose environmental hazards. For every pound of manufactured methamphetamine, 5 to 6 pounds of hazardous waste are produced.[54] The waste may be disposed of by pouring it down the drain, dumping it along roads, placing it in streams or lakes, or by burning it. Sanitation workers can experience adverse reactions due to their exposure to the hazardous waste. Contamination from hazardous waste can remain in the soil or water supply for many years.

Children are endangered by methamphetamine labs because they are commonly exposed to the chemicals at these labs. It has been reported that police found more than 3,000 children at methamphetamine labs in 2003.[55] Approximately two-thirds tested positive for toxic levels of chemicals. Children are also at risk for burn injuries when a lab explodes. It is not uncommon for children at labs to be neglected or abused. Additionally, guard dogs are subject to many of the same dangers.

In the United States, methamphetamines have become the number-one drug problem in rural areas according to the Drug Enforcement Agency. Over 9,300 methamphetamine laboratories were raided nationally in 2003.[56] There are two types of methamphetamine labs: super labs and small-time labs. The majority of the super labs, where large quantities of methamphetamines are produced, are located in California. The federal government's strategy for reducing the methamphetamine supply is to curtail access to the chemicals used to make the drug.[57] Besides production in clandestine laboratories in the United States, however, Mexico has become a major source for the drug.

Nicknames for Methamphetamines

- Speed
- Ice
- Crystal
- Meth
- Chicken powder
- Go-fast
- Glass
- Crank
- Christy
- Crystal-meth
- Chalk
- Peanut butter-crank
- Shabu-shabu
- Zip

Methamphetamine's Effects

Methamphetamine-related emergency room visits, admissions to publicly funded treatment facilities, and deaths have increased significantly. In 2005, 108,905 individuals visited emergency rooms as a result of methamphetamines. This is an increase of 35,000 people over the previous years. In addition, among those individuals going to emergency rooms, over 15,000 went there to be detoxified.[58] Methamphetamines or amphetamines are responsible for 12% of all people admitted to publicly funded substance abuse facilities. More people sought treatment from smaller metropolitan areas than from large metropolitan areas. Moreover, a higher percentage of Caucasians sought treatment than Blacks or Hispanics.[59]

Since the mid-1990s, methamphetamine abuse has spread from the West to cities in the Midwest and Southeast.[60] Methamphetamine users in the Midwest are more likely to take the drug intravenously, and consequently are at a higher risk for medical complications.[61] One encouraging note is that the number of "new" methamphetamine users has declined from previous years.[62]

The abuse of methamphetamines is not limited to any one group of people. Females and adolescents who report low religiosity, binge drinking, and selling drugs had higher rates of methamphetamine abuse.[63] One group that has been especially affected is Native Americans. The number of Native Americans being treated for methamphetamine abuse doubled from 2,167 in 2000 to 4,077 in 2004.[64] Among the general population, treatment admissions for methamphetamine abuse grew exponentially from 14,570 in 1992 to 129,079 in 2004.[65] This latter number represents 7% of all admissions for drug abuse. It is relevant to note that about one-half of all treatment admissions for methamphetamine abuse were referred by the criminal justice system.

Many users take methamphetamines in conjunction with other drugs such as cocaine and marijuana. Methamphetamines are the drug of choice for many young people because of the relatively low cost, and the high can last up to 14 hours. Methamphetamines produce many adverse effects, including slurred speech, loss of appetite, excitement, increased blood pressure and heart rate, irregular heartbeat, a pounding heart sensation, severe chest pain, hot flashes, excessive perspiration, anxiety, tremors, confusion, insomnia, convulsions, memory loss, violent behavior, elevated body temperature, paranoia, auditory hallucinations, and death. Recent research shows that methamphetamines can cause irreversible damage to blood vessels in the brain.

An emerging problem is methamphetamine-related identity theft. In 2006, there were 246,035 identity thefts reported. It is believed that an increasing number of identity thefts are committed by methamphetamine abusers.[66] The states with the highest rates of identity thefts are Arizona, Nevada, California, Texas, and Florida.

In the late 1970s, **ice** entered the drug scene. Named for its clear crystal form, ice is also called **crystal meth** and **crank**. Ice has been produced largely in Far Eastern countries, primarily Korea, Taiwan, and the Philippines, and transported to the United States, most commonly into Hawaii.

The increase in the amount of ice available can be attributed to the proliferation of clandestine laboratories. Ice can be manufactured from chemicals purchased legally from chemical supply stores. The percentage of

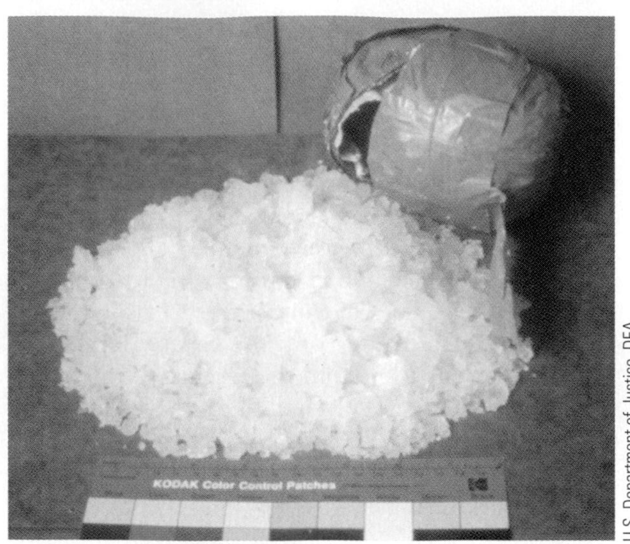

U.S. Department of Justice, DEA.

"Ice," so named because of its appearance, is a smokable form of methamphetamine.

adult arrestees in various American cities testing positive for methamphetamine and other drugs is shown in Table 11.1.

Ice can be injected or smoked. When it is smoked, the user feels profound emotional and physical arousal in a few seconds. Ice often is used compulsively, and users do not eat or rest for days. The dangers from ice possibly exceed those of other stimulants because its effects last 12 or more hours. (In contrast, the effects from crack last several minutes.) Ice poses numerous problems: Users are less resistant to illness. The liver, kidneys, and lungs are especially vulnerable. Babies born to pregnant women who have taken ice tend to be asocial and incapable of bonding. Ice causes psychological dependence and withdrawal symptoms including anxiety, intense depression, fatigue, insomnia, paranoia, and delusions.

Ritalin

Stimulants have been used to treat children's behavioral problems since 1937. The most prescribed drug for **attention deficit/hyperactivity disorder (ADHD)** is **Ritalin** (methylphenidate). ADHD usually begins in childhood and is characterized by developmentally inappropriate hyperactivity, impulsivity, and inattention. Changes in the criteria and their interpretation have broadened, allowing more individuals to be diagnosed with ADHD. Now ADHD is the number-one identified childhood psychiatric disorder in the United States. Because diagnosis of ADHD is imprecise, some parents and physicians are questioning whether Ritalin is overprescribed. In the United Kingdom, per capita use of Ritalin is $1/10$ of the amount used in the United States. Also, per capita Ritalin use in France and Italy is

$^{1}/_{20}$ of the amount prescribed in the United States.[67] In one study of college students about 30% reported using Ritalin illegally in the past year.[68]

The number of children treated with Ritalin is unprecedented. Americans consume more than 80% of the world's Ritalin.[69] More than 4 million children in the United States take Ritalin.[70] The increase in the diagnosis of ADHD is partly attributable to heightened public awareness and changes in educational policy in which schools are obliged to identify children with the disorder. Interestingly, one study found that children who took Ritalin were less likely to abuse illegal drugs as they aged.[71]

Ritalin has a good safety record with school-aged children. Increasingly, however, toddlers ages 2 to 4 are being given Ritalin, and its safety with this age group has not been determined.[72] Compared with amphetamines and cocaine, Ritalin is milder and causes fewer side effects. Because the high from Ritalin is brief, it is not as likely as cocaine to be abused. The typical dose is 10 to 30 mg in the morning and at midday.

Using Ritalin to treat children exhibiting ADHD is paradoxical. Logically, if a child is hyperactive, Ritalin should increase activity. Instead, the drug helps moderate a child's activity level. A low dosage of Ritalin helps children's cognitive processing, whereas a high dosage helps children with severe ADHD. Ritalin and other stimulants enhance the functioning of the reticular activating system, which helps children focus attention and filter out extraneous stimuli.

It is estimated that Ritalin and other stimulants are effective with 80% to 90% of children with ADHD.[73]

Many adverse effects have been associated with Ritalin. These include insomnia, weight loss, headaches, irritability, nausea, and dizziness. Research into whether Ritalin affects a child's growth is inconclusive. Several studies have found that 10% to 15% of children experience weight loss.[74] Ritalin does not cause physical dependency in children, although psychological dependence is possible. A rare problem is facial tics. If tics appear, they tend to subside once the person stops taking Ritalin.

Caffeine

Caffeine is the world's most frequently consumed stimulant. In the United States, about 90% of people drink caffeinated beverages.[75] Many people get their stimulation through tea, which contains caffeine and **theophylline**, a stimulant from the same chemical family as caffeine. Theophylline is less potent than caffeine, but the caffeine content is greater in some types of tea than in some coffees. Theophylline acts as a bronchodilator and is effective for treating asthma. Used since the 1970s, theophylline is a safe drug that actually increases the growth rate of asthmatic children and does not interfere with sleep.

Products containing caffeine extend beyond beverages to gum, mints, beer, candy, sunflower seeds, and soap.[76] Caffeine is found in many over-the-counter and prescription medicines and chocolate. Because caffeine is so ubiquitous, many children are receiving it unknowingly. Many experts recommend that children under age six avoid caffeinated beverages altogether.[77] A glass of chocolate milk has about 5 mg of caffeine. A stimulant in chocolate, **theobromine**, is related chemically to caffeine but is less powerful. Theobromine is more plentiful in cocoa than is caffeine.

Because millions of people consume caffeine, they may not want to believe that the legal substances they are consuming have psychological, pharmacological, and physiological properties similar to those of illegal drugs. The difference is a matter of degree. Caffeine is milder than amphetamines and cocaine. The amount of caffeine in various soft drinks is shown in Table 11.2.

ice Crystals of methamphetamine that are smoked, inhaled, or injected

crystal meth A variation of methamphetamine; one example is ice

crank A term for methamphetamines

attention deficit/hyperactivity disorder (ADHD) A condition in which the individual is hyperactive and easily distracted, which inhibits learning

Ritalin A mild stimulant used to treat attention deficit/hyperactivity disorder (ADHD)

theophylline A stimulant found in tea; in the same chemical family as caffeine

theobromine A stimulant found in chocolate; chemically related to caffeine

High-Energy Caffeinated Beverages

Increasingly, beverage companies are trying to boost the sale of soft drinks by adding more caffeine to new products. It is estimated that U.S. residents, especially adolescents, spent $3.4 billion last year on high-energy drinks.[78] The U.S. Food and Drug Administration does not regulate caffeine in food and drinks. However, its guidelines suggest that a safe level of caffeine is 72 milligrams per 12 ounces. Many beverages such as Red Bull, Monster, and Rock Star exceed that level.

To counter the sedating effects of alcohol, some individuals alternate with these high-energy drinks when drinking alcohol. There are reports of young people ending up in the emergency room for rapid heartbeat and nausea following consumption of energy drinks.[79] One high-energy drink that has received much criticism for its name is Cocaine. This drink is marketed as an alternative to the illegal drug.

TABLE 11.2 Caffeine Content in Selected Soft Drinks and Energy Drinks

Drink	Company	Milligrams of Caffeine in 12 oz.
Soft Drinks		
JOLT	Wet Planet	72
Mountain Dew Code Red	PepsiCo	55
Mountain Dew	PepsiCo	55
Mello Yello	Coca-Cola	51
Diet Coke	Coca-Cola	45
Dr Pepper	Cadbury	41
Pepsi-Cola	PepsiCo	38
Energy Drinks		
Redline Power Rush	Vital Pharmaceuticals	1680
JOLT Endurance Shot	Wet Planet	900
Cocaine Energy Drink	Redux Beverages	400
Blow (Energy Drink Mix)	Kingpin Concepts	360
Monster	Monster Beverage	120
Red Bull	Red Bull	116

Pharmacology

Although most people who use caffeine do so orally, it can be administered rectally or by injection. Like that of other drugs, the onset of its actions occurs quickly when it is injected. Caffeine acts as an antagonist to receptors for the inhibitory neurotransmitter **adenosine**. Therefore, the action of caffeine as a stimulant arises from its inhibitory effect. Caffeine obstructs adenosine's inhibition of brain cells, heightening alertness and mood.

When two negative numbers are multiplied together, the product is positive. This is exactly how caffeine works. By reducing inhibition, the effect is stimulation. Peak effects from caffeine occur 30 to 45 minutes after consumption. One study found that college students were able to maintain more attention during a 75-minute lecture if they consumed caffeine an hour prior to the lecture.[80]

Caffeine use by well-conditioned athletes has been found to improve their endurance on a short-term basis. Caffeine, at a high level of intake, has been placed on the International Olympic Committee's list of banned substances.[81] Extreme caffeine intake, however, has been linked to a low blood sugar condition called **hypoglycemia**. Excessive sweating, feelings of tiredness, fainting, and weakness are characteristics of low blood sugar.

Caffeine is metabolized by liver enzymes. The kidneys excrete almost all the caffeine ingested, but tiny amounts are eliminated through saliva, feces, semen, and breast milk. Women should be cautioned that oral contraceptives and pregnancy slow the metabolism and excretion of caffeine. Cigarette smoking increases the metabolism of caffeine.[82]

Properties and Risks

Caffeine is a member of the **xanthine** family. Xanthines are stimulants that improve work capacity, alertness, and motor performance while curbing fatigue. Another benefit is that caffeine widens air passages in the lungs, enabling asthmatics to breathe easier and deeper. There is some evidence to suggest that moderate amounts of caffeine may reduce the risk of type 2 diabetes in younger and middle-aged women.[83]

If caffeine is taken on an empty stomach, it releases stomach acids and digestive enzymes, causing an upset stomach. Caffeine increases the need to urinate and can cause dehydration. Both caffeinated and decaffeinated drinks produce a laxative effect. Other effects include nervousness, anxiety, insomnia, heartburn, and symptoms of premenstrual syndrome. Although caffeine can improve motor performance, it adversely affects motor coordination.

Caffeine has been implicated in a wide array of cardiovascular conditions from heart disease to hypertension, although it should be noted that studies examining the role of caffeine in these diseases are contradictory and do not yield definitive results.[84] However, a study in the *Journal of the American Dietetic Association* demonstrated that caffeine may raise blood pressure levels in some people who are prone to hypertension.[85]

Caffeine might contribute to breast lumps, breast tenderness, and cysts. The American Cancer Institute, however, states that there is no association between fibrocystic breast disease and caffeine. Studies conducted in the 1990s found no conclusive evidence linking breast cancer to caffeine. In sum, other than aggravating gastrointestinal problems and causing jitteriness, caffeine has not been found to have a cause-and-effect relationship on health. At the level at which most people consume caffeine, it is considered safe.

Effects of Caffeine

The effects of caffeine on wakefulness, coordination, and mood vary considerably among individuals. At moderate levels, caffeine increases blood pressure, body temperature, blood sugar levels, metabolism, urination, and hand tremors, and decreases appetite and coordination. In large amounts, it causes nausea, diarrhea, shaking, headache, and nervousness. At its worst, caffeine can cause convulsions, respiratory failure, and, if one drinks 70 to 100 cups of coffee, death.

Because caffeine stimulates the cortex of the brain, thought processes quickly improve, becoming more efficient, albeit temporarily. Memory improves and reaction time decreases. Other benefits include easing of asthma, relieving of painful bouts of gallstones, and weight loss.[86] Past studies reveal, though, that college students who consumed the most coffee had lower grades and more psychological and physiological problems.[87] This research does *not* suggest a cause-and-effect relationship. One could reason that students who drink a lot of coffee happen to be students who do more poorly in school.

Heavy caffeine use also affects the developing fetus, because caffeine crosses the placenta easily. In numerous studies, women who used moderate amounts—3 cups of coffee daily—were *not* likely to have miscarriages, nor were their babies likely to be of low birth weight or have any fetal abnormalities. One Danish study that followed 1,200 women who drank at least 3 cups of coffee daily reported no effect on infant length or gestation.[88] Numerous studies are inconclusive regarding whether caffeine use affects rates of miscarriage.[89] However, infants can receive caffeine through breast milk. Children nursed by mothers who drink caffeinated beverages appear more nervous or agitated. The effects of caffeine are greater in newborns and infants because they cannot metabolize and eliminate caffeine as readily as adults.

Caffeine users seem to need the drug to achieve alertness and to eliminate withdrawal symptoms, which appear in people who consume $2\frac{1}{2}$ cups of coffee or more daily. Withdrawal symptoms become apparent about 12 to 16 hours after the last caffeine intake. Headache is the most commonly reported withdrawal symptom. Others include depression, lethargy, lower energy level, sleepiness/drowsiness, and irritability.

Decaffeinated Coffee

Because of the adverse publicity surrounding caffeine use, many people are drinking decaffeinated coffee, in which the caffeine has been displaced from the coffee bean using a hot water solution. The caffeine then is taken out of the water with the aid of an organic solvent. The National Cancer Institute identified the original solvent, trichloroethylene, as potentially carcinogenic. Subsequently, methylene chloride, a substance used in paint remover, was substituted. Methylene chloride also might contribute to cancer. A survey conducted by *Consumer Reports* found that decaffeinated coffee has some degree of caffeine. In six different locations where decaffeinated coffee was purchased, levels of caffeine varied from 5 milligrams to 32 milligrams per 10 to 12 ounces.[90] About 100 milligrams is considered normal in a typical cup of coffee.

adenosine A neurotransmitter for which caffeine acts as an antagonist

hypoglycemia A condition of low levels of sugar in the blood

xanthine A type of stimulant; caffeine is an example

caffeinism Excessive caffeine consumption resulting in caffeine dependency

On Campus

Ostensibly to protect students from the "dangers of caffeine," student Andrew Epstein pulled a hoax at Amherst College with the announcement that coffee would be hereafter banned on campus. Although the ban lasted only 1 day (the Day of No Joe), Epstein's aim was to draw attention to the hypocrisy of drug laws.

Source: Chronicle of Higher Education (July 2001).

Caffeinism

Dependency on caffeine is called **caffeinism**. More than one-half of moderate coffee drinkers who stop drinking it experience moderate to severe headaches. Most caffeine users acknowledge that they are dependent on it and that they have difficulty stopping. Caffeinism is marked by irritability, depression, and insomnia. One study reported that caffeine withdrawal may occur in people who drink as little as 1 cup of coffee or 2 cups of tea daily.[91]

Despite the fact that caffeine cessation may result in withdrawal symptoms, some people contend that it is not addictive and should not be used in the same sentence as cocaine or heroin addiction.[92] Others maintain that the withdrawal symptoms do not endanger one's health.[93] About one-fourth of users experience withdrawal symptoms when they discontinue drinking it.[94] Also, people are more accident-prone during withdrawal.

Summary

Stimulant drugs increase activity levels and alter mood. Cocaine is the most commonly used illegal stimulant. Derived from the coca plant, cocaine is a colorless, crystalline powder after it is refined. It was included in many over-the-counter products until the Harrison Narcotic Act was passed in 1914.

A variation, freebase, appeared in the 1960s. The popularity of cocaine rose in the 1970s, accompanied by an increase in cocaine-related deaths. In the 1980s the more affordable crack cocaine emerged. Its effects are short-lived but profound.

Snorting is the most common mode of intake; the peak effects are felt in 10 to 15 minutes. The peak effects from injected cocaine are felt in 30 seconds and last about 10 minutes.

When it is smoked, cocaine can cause nasal, pulmonary, and cardiovascular problems and even death. Injected cocaine can lead to HIV/AIDS, inflammation of the heart lining, and hepatitis. Psychological effects include mood swings, distortions, and delusions. Users report feeling confident, in control, and exhilarated. Cocaine impairs sexual performance and, in high doses, can induce depression, thoughts of suicide, and violent behavior.

Cocaine abstinence has three phases: (1) the *crash*, marked by intense craving and deep depression; (2) *withdrawal*, when depression moderates but the person is incapable of feeling normal pleasure; and (3) *extinction*, when depression and craving subside but may reappear. Although cocaine withdrawal is unlikely to be fatal, using the drug itself can have tragic consequences because it can produce an irregular heartbeat or heart attack.

The use of cocaine during pregnancy is related to a higher incidence of miscarriages and premature deliveries. Cocaine-exposed newborns are more likely to have congenital heart defects and seizures. The impact of cocaine on the school performance of cocaine-exposed children is being questioned and is not clear.

Amphetamines, another type of stimulant, have been used to treat asthma, narcolepsy, fatigue, and hyperactivity and to promote weight loss. When ingested, the peak effects are felt in 2 to 3 hours. When injected, the peak effects occur in less than 5 minutes. A stronger methamphetamine, crystal-meth, or ice, is smoked and takes effect in a few seconds.

Beginning in the 1940s, amphetamines and methamphetamines, also known as speed, were a problem in the United States. As weight-reducing agents, amphetamines have limited success because people eat for reasons other than hunger and users develop tolerance.

Stimulants are used with children who have attention deficit/hyperactivity disorder (ADHD). Though it may seem paradoxical, treating hyperactivity with stimulants can be effective when it is prescribed appropriately. A drawback is that they might inhibit growth.

Medically unsupervised use of amphetamines can lead to mania, aggressiveness, paranoia, and violent behavior. Fatal overdoses are not likely, but people have died from their behaviors while they are taking amphetamines. Whether the psychotic-like effects that amphetamines produce are the result of the drugs or sleep deprivation is not clear.

Methamphetamines entered the drug scene in the 1980s. Their effects can last 12 hours or more, and their use has been linked to liver, kidney, and lung damage. Babies born to women who took methamphetamines while pregnant show signs of being asocial and incapable of bonding.

Caffeine, a member of the xanthine family, is the most widely used drug in the United States. Theophylline and theobromine, found in tea and chocolate, respectively, also are in the xanthine family. Both are less potent than caffeine. Caffeine is included in many over-the-counter medications and prescriptions. Its peak effects appear 15 to 45 minutes after ingestion. Side effects are upset stomach, excessive urination, heartburn, anxiety, insomnia, and symptoms of premenstrual syndrome. It also impairs motor coordination.

At moderate doses caffeine is considered safe, but at extremely high doses caffeine can be fatal. Heavy caffeine use during pregnancy has been related to complications at birth and higher rates of miscarriage. Daily caffeine use of 600 mg for 6 to 15 days can lead to caffeinism. Cessation of caffeine use produces withdrawal symptoms including headaches, low energy levels, depression, drowsiness, and irritability. Many people have switched to decaffeinated beverages. The process of decaffeination, however, utilizes organic solvents that may be carcinogenic.

Thinking Critically

1. Cocaine use can be reduced by reducing the amount of cocaine entering the country or by reducing demand for the drug. Do you favor putting more tax dollars into stopping drugs from coming into the United States or into persuading people not to take drugs?

2. HIV infection can be transmitted through unclean needles. If a person knowingly is infected with HIV and gives an unclean needle to another person, should that person be prosecuted for a criminal offense if the second person gets infected?

3. Society is concerned with child abuse. Do you consider cocaine use during pregnancy to be a form of child abuse? If so, do you also consider alcohol or tobacco use during pregnancy as forms of abuse? Elaborate.

4. Although caffeine is a psychoactive drug, it usually is not viewed as such. If the word *drug* were placed on containers with caffeine in them, would that alter your view or use of caffeine?

5. Many people have switched to decaffeinated beverages. Their reasons are not always based on

fact. There are many misconceptions regarding caffeine. Ask people you know who drink decaffeinated drinks why they do so.

Web Resources

DrugHelp
http://www.drughelp.org
This site, a service of the American Council for Drug Education (an affiliate of Phoenix House Foundation), provides information, counsel, and referral to treatment centers.

Cocaine Anonymous World Services
http://www.ca.org/
This site provides support to people who have a desire to stop using cocaine as well as other mind-altering substances.

Notes

1. L. D. Johnston, P. M. O'Malley, J. G. Bachman, and J. E. Schulenberg, *Monitoring the Future, National Results on Adolescent Drug Use: Overview of Key Findings* (Bethesda, MD: National Institute on Drug Abuse, 2008).
2. Ibid.
3. Substance Abuse and Mental Health Services Administration, *Drug Abuse Warning Network, 2005: National Estimates of Drug-Related Emergency Room Visits* (Rockville, MD: Office of Applied Studies, 2007).
4. R. D. Weiss, S. T. Mirin, and R. B. Bartel, *Cocaine* (Washington, DC: American Psychiatric Press, 1994).
5. Substance Abuse and Mental Health Services Administration, *The DASIS Report: Cocaine Route of Administration Trends: 1995–2005* (Rockville, MD: Office of Applied Studies, February 2007).
6. M. M. Cohen, "Jim Crow's Drug War: Race, Coca Cola, and the Southern Origins of Drug Prohibition," *Southern Cultures*, 12 (Fall 2006): 55–80.
7. B. Stoddard, *The Big Nickle Drink* (Claremont, CA: Double Dot Enterprises, 2003).
8. Substance Abuse and Mental Health Services Administration, *Results from the 2006 National Survey on Drug Use and Health: National Findings* (Rockville, MD: Office of Applied Studies, 2007).
9. B. Powis, P. Griffiths, M. Gossop, and J. Strang, "The Differences Between Male and Female Drug Users: Community Samples of Heroin and Cocaine Users Compared," *Substance Use and Misuse*, 31 (1996): 529–543.
10. F. R. Levin, S. M. Evans, and H. D. Kleber, "Prevalence of Adult Attention-Deficit Hyperactivity Disorder Among Cocaine Abusers Seeking Treatment," *Drug and Alcohol Dependence*, 52 (1998): 15–25.
11. Johnston et al., supra note 1.
12. C. J. Boyd, "Antecedents of Women's Crack Cocaine Abuse: Family Substance Abuse, Sexual Abuse, Depression and Illicit Drug Use," *Journal of Substance Abuse Treatment*, 10 (1993): 433–438.
13. *National Drug Threat Assessment 2007* (Johnstown, PA: National Drug Intelligence Center, 2007).
14. *Facts and Figures: Crack* (Rockville, MD: Office of National Drug Control Policy, 2006).
15. D. Waldorf, "Don't Be Your Own Best Customer—Drug Use of San Francisco Gang Drug Sellers," *Crime, Law and Social Change*, 19 (1993): 1–15.
16. V. S. Harder and H. D. Chilcoat, "Cocaine Use and Educational Achievement: Understanding a Changing Association Over the Past 2 Decades," *American Journal of Public Health*, 97 (October 2007): 1790–1793.
17. M. J. Hull, M. Juhascik, F. Mazur, M. A. Flomenbaum, and G. S. Behonick, "Fatalities Associated with Fentanyl and Co-administered Cocaine or Opiates," *Journal of Forensic Sciences*, 52 (November 2007): 1383.
18. "Scotland Cites Hike in Cocaine-Related Deaths," *Narcotics Enforcement and Prevention Digest*, 12 (October 16, 2007): 4.
19. A. N. Morton, "The Oral Health Effects of Illegal Drug Abuse," *Corrections Today*, 69 (October 2007): 54–56.
20. *Drug Facts* (Rockville, MD: Office of National Drug Control Policy, 2008).
21. Substance Abuse and Mental Health Services Administration, supra note 3.
22. *National Drug Threat Assessment*, supra note 13.
23. Ibid.
24. P. G. Erickson, E. M. Adlaf, R. G. Smart, and G. F. Murray, *The Steel Drug: Cocaine and Crack in Perspective* (New York: Lexington Books, 1994).
25. H. E. Doweiko, *Concepts of Chemical Dependence*, 7th ed. (Belmont, CA: Thomson/Wadsworth, 2008).
26. J. Interlandi, "Are Vaccines the Answer to Addiction?" *Newsweek*, 151 (January 14, 2008): 17.
27. F. H. Gawin, "Cocaine Addiction: Psychology and Neurophysiology," *Science*, 251 (1991): 1580–1586.
28. E. Nagourney, "Vital Signs: Treatment; A New Tool to Resist the Pull of Cocaine," *New York Times*, April 17, 2001.
29. ONDCP Drug Policy Information Clearinghouse, *Cocaine* (Rockville, MD: Office of National Drug Control Policy, 2003).
30. L. Whitten, "Cocaine Abuse and HIV Are Linked with Coronary Calcification," *NIDA Notes*, 20 (April 2006): 8–9.
31. Substance Abuse and Mental Health Services Administration. *Drug Abuse Warning Network, 2003: Area Profiles of Drug-Related Mortality* (Rockville, MD: 2005).
32. "Florida College Student Deaths from Cocaine on Rise," *Narcotics Enforcement and Prevention Digest*, 12 (November 17, 2006): 7.
33. Substance Abuse and Mental Health Services Administration, supra note 8.
34. W. Y. Sun and W. Chen, "The Impact of Maternal Cocaine Use on Neonates in Socioeconomic Disadvantaged Population, *Journal of Drug Education*, 27 (1997): 389–396.
35. March of Dimes Foundation. *Illicit Drug Use during Pregnancy*. 2008.
36. H. L. Surratt and J. A. Inciardi, "Cocaine-Exposed Infants and the Criminalization of Pregnancy," in *The American Drug Scene*, edited by J. A. Inciardi and K. McElrath (Los Angeles: Roxbury Publishing Company, 2004).
37. Ibid.
38. B. Zuckerman, D. Frank, and E. Brown, "Overview of the Effects of Abuse and Drugs on Pregnancy and Offspring," in *Medications Development for the Treatment of Pregnant Addicts and Their Infants*, edited by C. N. Chiang and L. P. Finnegan (NIDA Research Monograph

149) (Washington, DC: Government Printing Office, 1995).
39. P. Blackwell, K. Kirkhart, D. Schmitt, and M. Kaiser, "Cocaine/Polydrug-Affected Dyads: Implications for Infant Cognitive and Mother-Infant Interaction during the First Six Postnatal Months," *Journal of Applied Developmental Psychology,* 19 (1998): 235–248.
40. Weiss et al., supra note 4.
41. "Environment Lessons Impact of Prenatal Cocaine Exposure," *Alcoholism and Drug Abuse Weekly,* 16 (June 7, 2004): 3–4.
42. M. A. Miller, "History and Epidemiology of Amphetamine Abuse in the United States," in *The American Drug Scene,* edited by J. A. Inciardi and K. McElrath (Los Angeles: Roxbury Publishing Company, 2004).
43. *Speed Fast Facts*. Do It Now Foundation, June 1, 2007.
44. J. Cromley, "High Life, High Risk," *Los Angeles Times*, April 9, 2007.
45. L. Topp and S. Drake, "The Applicability of the Dependence Syndrome to Amphetamines," *Drug and Alcohol Dependence,* 48 (1997): 113–118.
46. D. Karch, A. Crosby, and T. Simon, "Toxicology Testing and Results for Suicide Victims—13 States, 2004," *MMWR Weekly*, 55 (November 24, 2006): 1245–1248.
47. District of Columbia Pretrial Services Agency (November, 2007). Available online at http://www.dcpsa.gov/foia/foiaERRpsa.htm.
48. B. C. Leigh, S. L. Ames, and A.W. Stacy, "Alcohol, Drugs, and Condom Use Among Drug Offenders: An Event-Based Analysis," *Drug and Alcohol Dependence*, 93 (January, 2008): 38–42.
49. L. Degenhardt, C. Coffey, P. Moran, J. B. Carlin, and G. C. Patton, "The Predictors and Consequences of Adolescent Amphetamine Use: Findings from the Victoria Adolescent Health Cohort Study," *Addiction*, 102 (July 2007): 1076–1084.
50. M. S. Schmidt, "Baseball Is Challenged on Rise in Stimulant Use," *New York Times*, January 16, 2008.
51. Johnston et al., supra note 1.
52. N. Kulish, "Europe Fears Meth Foothold Is Spreading," *New York Times*, November 23, 2007.
53. M. S. Scott and K. Dedel, *Clandestine Methamphetamine Labs* (U.S. Department of Justice, August 2006).
54. Ibid.
55. Ibid.
56. D. Johnson, "Policing a Rural Plague," *Newsweek* (March 8, 2004): 41.
57. *Synthetic Drug Control Strategy* (Rockville, MD: Office of National Drug Control Policy, 2006).
58. Substance Abuse and Mental Health Services Administration, supra note 3.
59. Substance Abuse and Mental Health Services Administration, *The DASIS Report: Methamphetamine/Amphetamine Treatment Admissions in Urban and Rural Areas: 2004* (Rockville, MD: Office of Applied Studies, 2007).
60. G. Hargreaves, "Clandestine Drug Labs," *FBI Law Enforcement Bulletin* (April 2000): 1–6.
61. K. M. Grant, S. S. Kelley, S. Agrawal, J. L. Meza, J. R. Meyer, and D. J. Romberger, "Methamphetamine Use in Rural Midwesterners," *The American Journal on Addictions*, 16 (2007): 79–84.
62. Substance Abuse and Mental Health Services Administration, "Methamphetamine Use," *The NSDUH Report* (Rockville, MD: Office of Applied Studies, 2007).
63. M. A. Herman-Stahl, C. P. Krebs, L. A. Kroutil, and D. C. Heller, "Risk and Protective Factors for Nonmedical Use of Prescription Stimulants and Methamphetamine among Adolescents," *Journal of Adolescent Health*, 39 (2006): 374–380.
64. A. Murr, "A New Menace on the Rez," *Newsweek* (September 27, 2004): 30.
65. Substance Abuse and Mental Health Services Administration (June 2, 2006). Available online at http://www.icpsr.umich.edu/SAMHDA.
66. "Methamphetamine-Related Identity Theft," *Intelligence Bulletin* (Department of Justice: May 2007).
67. C. Marwick, "U.S. Doctor Warns of Misuse of Prescribed Stimulant," *British Medical Journal,* 326 (January 11, 2003): 67.
68. C. Teter, S. Esteban, C. Boyd, and S. Guthrie, "Illicit Methylphenidate Use in an Undergraduate Student Sample: Prevalence and Risk Factors," *Pharmacotherapy,* 23 (2003): 609–617.
69. Marwick, supra note 67.
70. J. C. Anderson, "Back to School Health Tips: Expert Available to Comment on ADHD," *Ascribe Health News Service,* August 31, 2004.
71. J. Evans, "ADHD Medications Affect School Attendance and Substance Abuse: Retrospective Studies," *Family Practice News,* 34 (April 1, 2004): 75.
72. C. Kolb, "Drugged-Out Toddlers," *Newsweek,* March 6, 2000.
73. L. Scahill, D. Carroll, and K. Burke, "Methylphenidate: Mechanism of Actions and Clinical Update," *Journal of Child and Adolescent Psychiatric Nursing,* 17 (April–June 2004): 85–86.
74. J. Elia, P. J. Ambrosini, and J. L. Rapoport, "Treatment of Attention-Deficit-Hyperactivity Disorder," *New England Journal of Medicine,* 340 (1999): 780–788.
75. R. Goldberg, *Taking Sides: Clashing Views on Controversial Issues in Drugs and Society* (Guilford, CT: McGraw-Hill/Dushkin, 2008).
76. S. Gupta, "The Caffeine Habit," *Time,* 170 (October 1, 2007): 62.
77. J. Abbasi, "Is Coffee Okay for Kids?" *Parenting,* 22 (February 2008).
78. K. Barrow, "Wired Nation," *Science World,* 64 (November 12, 2007): 22–23.
79. N. Shute, "Over the Limit," *U.S. News and World Report,* 142 (April 23, 2007): 60+.
80. P. Peeling and B. Dawson, "Influence of Caffeine Ingestion on Perceived Mood States, Concentration, and Arousal Levels During a 75-mm University Lecture," *Advances in Physiology Education,* 31 (December 2007): 332–335.
81. J. Berning, "Caffeine and Athletic Performance," *Clinical Reference Systems,* May 24, 2006.
82. "Caffeine Fix?" *Choice* (June 2000): 29–36.
83. R. M. van Dam, W. C. Willett, J. E. Manson, and F. B. Hu, "Coffee, Caffeine, and Risk of Type 2 Diabetes: A Prospective Cohort Study in Younger and Middle-Aged U.S. Women," *Diabetes Care,* 29 (February 2006): 398–403.
84. H. L. Muncie, "The Safety of Caffeine Consumption," *American Family Physician,* 76 (November 1, 2007): 1284–1285.
85. "Coffee, Caffeine, and Blood Pressure," *Journal of the American Dietetic Association,* 100 (May 2000): 598.
86. L. Mooney, "Should You Decaf Your Life?" *Prevention,* 52 (July 2000): 131–140.
87. K. Gilliland and D. Andress, "Ad Lib Caffeine Consumption, Symptoms of Caffeinism, and Academic Performance," *American Journal of Psychiatry,* 138 (1981): 180.
88. "Good News: Caffeine in Pregnancy Doesn't Affect the Baby's Growth," *Child Health Alert,* 25 (March, 2007): 5.
89. D. Grady, "Pregnancy Problems Tied to Caffeine," *New York Times,* January 21, 2008.
90. "Is It Really Decaf?" *Consumer Reports,* November 2007: 7.
91. N. Boyce, "Storm in a Coffee Cup," *New Scientist* (January 2000): 28–31.
92. C. K. Erickson, "Addicted to Speculation about Caffeine," *Addiction Professional,* 4 (March–April 2004): 9.
93. S. Satel, "Is Caffeine Addictive? A Review of the Literature," *American Journal of Drug and Alcohol Abuse,* 32 (November 2006): 493–502.
94. J. R. Hughes, A. H. Oliveto, A. Ligouri, J. Carpenter, and T. Howard, "Endorsement of DSM-IV Dependence Criteria Among Caffeine Users," *Drug and Alcohol Dependence,* 52 (1998): 99–107.

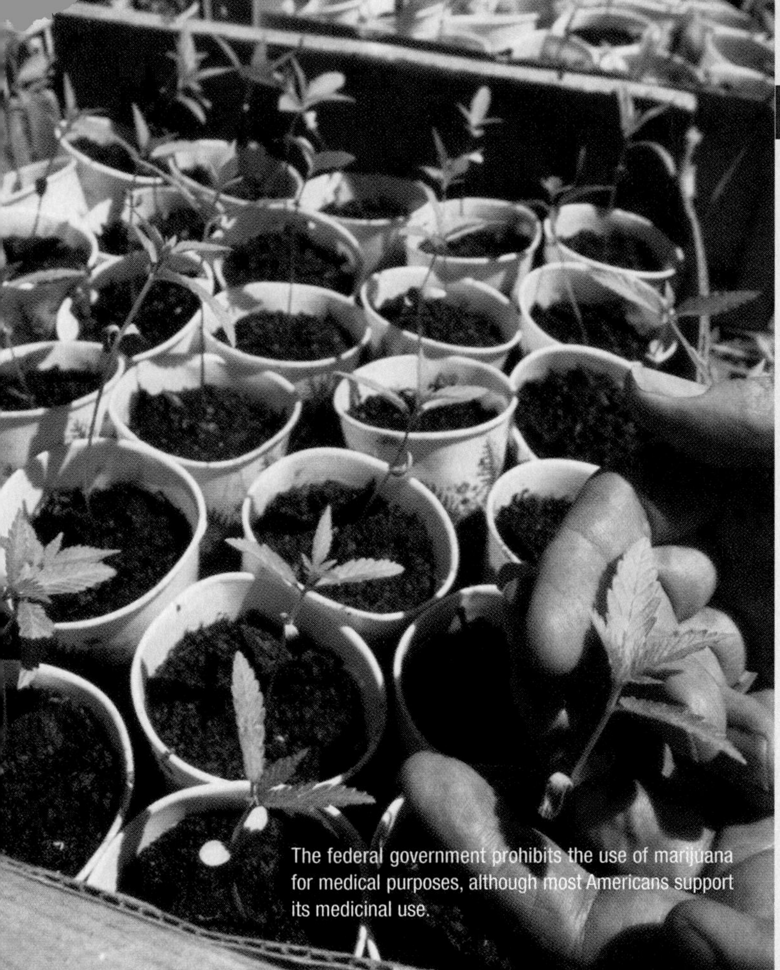

The federal government prohibits the use of marijuana for medical purposes, although most Americans support its medicinal use.

© Roger Ressmeyer/CORBIS.

FACT OR FICTION?

1. The word *canvas* is derived from the word *cannabis*, and many famous paintings are on marijuana fibers.
2. A higher percentage of high school seniors used marijuana in 1975 than in 2008.
3. Despite the availability of marijuana, the number of adults dependent on marijuana has decreased.
4. About 30% of high school seniors have been exposed to a drugged or drinking driver.
5. Most young people who try marijuana for the first time do so during the winter months.
6. At one time, marijuana seeds were put into birdseed.
7. The early Colonial settlers planted marijuana because they recognized its medicinal value.
8. The federal government owns a farm in Mississippi where it grows marijuana to be used for research purposes.
9. Public opinion polls reveal that the majority of Americans favor legalizing marijuana.
10. The federal government allows the medical use of marijuana only to treat the side effects of chemotherapy on cancer patients.

Turn the page to check your answers

12 Marijuana

Chapter Objectives

After completing this chapter, the reader should be able to describe:

- The origin of marijuana in the United States
- The different species of marijuana
- The extent of marijuana use
- The effects of marijuana on various systems in the body
- Whether marijuana contributes to mental illness
- The effects of marijuana on academic performance
- Medical conditions for which marijuana is prescribed
- Whether marijuana use leads to the use of other drugs
- Arguments for and against the legalization of marijuana

FACT OR FICTION?

1. **Fact:** The word *canvas* comes from *cannabis* and many famous paintings were done on fibers made from marijuana.
2. **Fact:** Although the use of marijuana is cyclical, more high school seniors used marijuana in 1975 than in 2008.
3. **Fiction:** The fact is—from the early 1990s to the early 2000s, marijuana dependence among adults increased 22%.
4. **Fact:** One national study found that 30% of high school seniors were exposed to a drugged or drinking driver within the past two weeks.
5. **Fiction:** The fact is—because of less supervision, June and July are the most common months for a young person to use marijuana for the first time.
6. **Fact:** Even after marijuana was made illegal in 1937, birdseed manufacturers were allowed to include marijuana seeds in birdseed.
7. **Fiction:** The fact is—marijuana was not used for medicinal purposes in the United States until the early 1990s.
8. **Fact:** The federal government grows marijuana on a well-guarded farm in Mississippi.
9. **Fiction:** The fact is—the majority of Americans favor keeping marijuana illegal according to national public opinion polls.
10. **Fiction:** The fact is—the federal government does not allow marijuana to be used for any medical purpose.

Marijuana, or **cannabis**, is one of the world's oldest known drugs. The medicinal value of marijuana was described by the ancient Chinese, Greeks, Persians, Romans, East Indians, and Assyrians. Marijuana was used to regulate muscle spasms, lessen pain, and combat indigestion. Marijuana, too, is an important part of early U.S. history. Physicians used it to treat migraine headaches and as an anticonvulsant. In the late 1800s, marijuana was used to treat menstrual cramps, labor pains, spastic conditions, and insomnia.

The early settlers in Jamestown, Virginia, planted marijuana for its fiber, which was used for making rope. Called **hemp**, it was a prominent crop during the Civil War and also was used during World War II. Today, the commercial growing of hemp is forbidden by the Drug Enforcement Administration. However, in 2007, North Dakota State University filed a lawsuit supporting farmers' rights to grow hemp for legal products in order to help the agricultural community.[1]

Not until the 20th century was marijuana used for its euphoric effect. Marijuana was used in the early 1900s by Mexican farm workers and Caribbean dockworkers. After coming to the United States, many of these immigrants lived in the Southwest. New Orleans was a central site for marijuana distribution because of its location on the Mississippi River. Marijuana use spread quickly. People living in the North and East started smoking it during the 1920s, coinciding with alcohol prohibition.

As more people smoked marijuana, articles appeared in magazines and newspapers denigrating its effects. It was linked to crime and violence, especially in Blacks and Mexican Americans. The film *Reefer Madness* depicted marijuana use as causing the moral decay of young people, brain damage, and mental illness. Despite the American Medical Association's support of the medicinal use of marijuana, politicians and the general public presented marijuana as a heinous drug. Marijuana use was restricted, even for medical purposes, and it was banned altogether after the Marijuana Tax Act was enacted in 1937. Despite its legal status, the federal government estimates that 3,577 American adolescents will use marijuana for the first time on an average day.[2]

Characteristics

Derived from the hemp plant, the most common strain of marijuana in the United States is *Cannabis sativa*. The primary mood-altering, psychoactive agent in marijuana is **delta-9-tetrahydrocannabinol**, or THC. The hemp plant is hardy and grows throughout the world.

The original hemp plants were cultivated in the United States for rope and contained low levels of

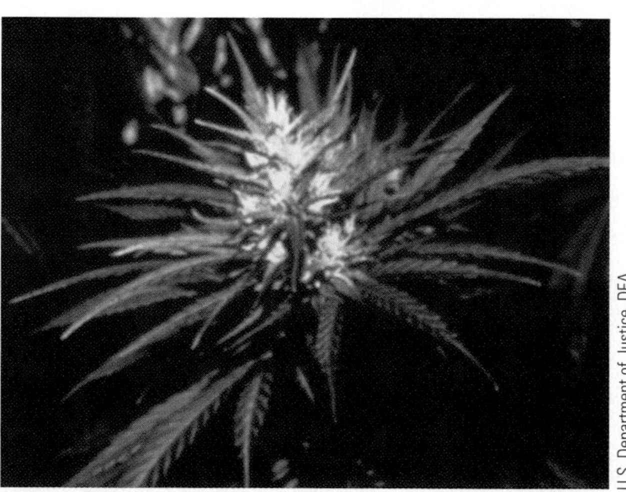

U.S. Department of Justice, DEA.

Marijuana is made from the dried leaves and flowering tops of Cannabis sativa.

THC, seldom exceeding 1%. Several factors influence THC levels: the plant's sex, soil and climate conditions, the part of the plant that is used, and how the plant is harvested, prepared, and stored. Marijuana contains more than 500 chemicals, 60 of which are unique to the plant. The chemicals in the plant are called **cannabinoids**. One carcinogenic compound in marijuana smoke and tobacco smoke is **benzopyrene**. Marijuana smoke contains 70% more benzopyrene and 50% more tar than tobacco smoke, and marijuana releases five times as much tar into the lungs as cigarettes.[3] This is noteworthy because marijuana smokers keep the smoke in their lungs for an extended time, inhale more deeply, and take in more smoke.

cannabis A genus of plant that is also known as marijuana

hemp Marijuana plant that may be used to make rope, clothing, and paper

delta-9-tetrahydrocannabinol (THC) The psychoactive agent in marijuana

cannabinoids Chemicals found in marijuana plants

benzopyrene Carcinogenic compound found in marijuana and tobacco

ganja Tops and flowers of the cannabis plant

bhang Lower leaves, stems, and seeds of the cannabis plant

sinsemilla Seedless marijuana; derived from unfertilized female cannabis plants

hashish A potent form of marijuana taken from resin of the cannabis plant

charas A potent form of marijuana also known as hashish

hash oil Substance made by separating resin from the cannabis plant by boiling the plant in alcohol; it has a very high THC content

Species and Forms of Marijuana

Among the several species of cannabis plants are the following:

1. *Cannabis sativa*, the most widespread, used primarily to make rope. George Washington's Mount Vernon farm grew it for that purpose. *Cannabis sativa* has a tall, woody stem and can reach a height of 20 feet.
2. *Cannabis indica*, from India originally, grown for its psychoactive properties. This species grows to a height of only 3 to 4 feet.
3. *Cannabis ruderalis*, found mainly in northern Europe and parts of Asia. It is marked by a short growing season and low potency.

Ganja, consisting of the tops and flowers of the female cannabis plant, is considered the best quality marijuana. **Bhang** consists of the lower leaves, stems, and seeds of the cannabis plant and is regarded as poor quality marijuana. Ganja is several times more potent than bhang.

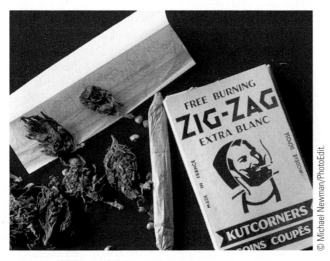

© Michael Newman/PhotoEdit.

Marijuana paraphernalia includes rolling papers, clips, and pipes.

Another type of marijuana is **sinsemilla**, which means "without seeds." It is derived from the unfertilized female cannabis plant. THC levels in sinsemilla are greater than those in other types of marijuana. Female marijuana plants produce more resin and flowers, which contain higher THC concentrations.

Two other forms of marijuana are **hashish**, known in India as **charas**, and **hash oil**. Although the THC content of hashish and hash oil varies, these forms of marijuana are more potent than *Cannabis sativa*. Hashish, taken from the resin of the cannabis plant, usually is smoked in a pipe, though it can be eaten. Hash oil is made by separating the resin from the cannabis plant by boiling it in alcohol. Hash oil, with a THC content of 60%, is mixed with cigarette tobacco and smoked.

THC levels of marijuana smoked in the United States range from 2% to 5%. Today, marijuana is reportedly stronger (THC levels of 8% to 16%) than it was in the 1960s and 1970s. According to a Dutch study, potency affects usage. For example, younger smokers preferred more potent marijuana and smoked more frequently than older marijuana users.[4]

Points of Origin

Because the cannabis plant is resilient, it can be grown almost anywhere. Marijuana production is especially high in Colombia and Mexico. Other countries in

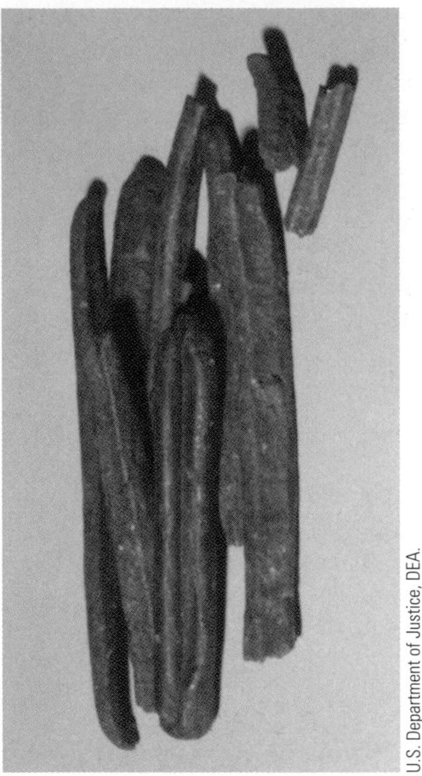

U.S. Department of Justice, DEA.

Hashish is available in resinous sticks.

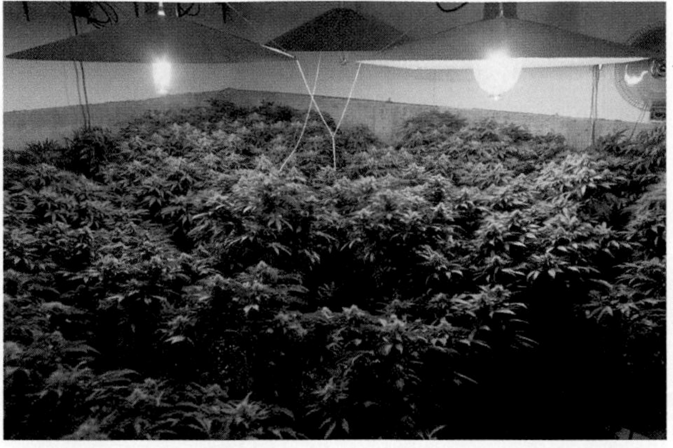

© Dan Lamont/CORBIS.

Indoor marijuana cultivation has become more prevalent in recent years, as producers attempt to avoid detection while increasing crop yields.

Latin America, and in Asia and the Caribbean, also produce marijuana. Because of their lack of government control and political instability, Lebanon, Morocco, Pakistan, and Thailand also are known for producing much marijuana. Over 1.1 million kilograms of marijuana were seized on the Mexican border in 2006 and over 4,100 kilograms were seized on the Canadian border in the same year.[5]

Indoor Cultivation

The indoor cultivation of marijuana has escalated in recent years. There are several reasons for this development. First, it is easier to avoid eradication, especially in view of the fact that federal, state, and local law enforcement have vigorously increased their efforts to eradicate marijuana plants. Secondly, indoor cultivation has allowed for production of marijuana with a higher THC content. Also, the profits of indoor cultivation are higher because marijuana plants can be harvested four to six times per year. It is estimated that the number of indoor sites increased 38% between 2001 and 2006. The growth of indoor marijuana production is attributed to Mexican and Cuban drug trafficking organizations. States that have seen the largest growth of indoor sites are Florida, Georgia, and North Carolina.[6]

Extent of Use

Worldwide, marijuana is the fourth most commonly used drug, surpassed by nicotine, caffeine, and alcohol. Marijuana is the most commonly used illegal drug in the United States. In 2008, 19.4% of high school seniors had used marijuana within the previous 30 days.[7] In the United States, most users smoke it sporadically. In India, Jamaica, Greece, and Egypt, marijuana is more likely to be smoked daily and in greater quantities. In France, 27.5% of 15-year-olds used marijuana within the previous year, as did 18.3% of 15-year-olds in Ireland and 4.1% of 15-year-olds in Greece.[8]

Participation in athletics does not preclude the use of marijuana. Male high school athletes have higher rates of marijuana use than nonathletes; female high school athletes, however, engage in less use of marijuana than nonathletes.[9]

Although researchers have found correlations among grades, truancy, religious commitment, and marijuana use, the most important reasons that students significantly increased their use of marijuana in the 1990s relate to a reduced perception of risk and less disapproval of its use.[10] Among full-time college students, the percentage who used marijuana during the past 30 days increased from 14.1% in 1991 to 16.8% in 2007.[11]

Marijuana use is associated with alcohol and cigarette use. The Center on Addiction and Substance Abuse has reported that 12-year-olds who drank alcohol and smoked cigarettes within 30 days of a survey were 30 times more likely to use marijuana than young people who did not use alcohol or cigarettes. In addition, the younger one is when first starting marijuana and alcohol use, the more likely it is that one will inject drugs later in life.[12] During the 1990s, the age of first marijuana use deviated only slightly. Figure 12.1 shows the average ages of first use for the years 2002 to 2007.

Approximately 80% of students receive their marijuana from a friend;[13] among young adults, marijuana typically is sold or shared within home, apartment, or dormitory settings (see Figure 12.2). Table 12.1 shows the trends in annual, monthly, and daily use of marijuana and hashish by high school seniors from 1991 to 2008.[14]

Becoming a parent was the most important social variable leading to marijuana cessation in one study.[15] Moreover, people who used marijuana for social reasons rather than to alter their mood were more likely to quit using marijuana. Individuals who started using marijuana early in life were less likely to stop using it

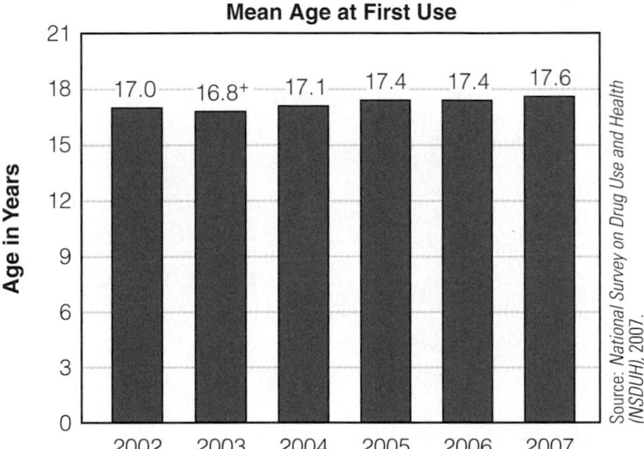

Figure 12.1 Mean Age at First Use of Marijuana among Past Year Marijuana Initiates Aged 12 to 49: 2002–2007

TABLE 12.1 Trends in Marijuana and Hashish Use by High School Seniors

Year	Past 12 Months	Past 30 Days	Daily
1991	23.9%	13.8%	2.0%
1992	21.9	11.9	1.9
1993	26.0	15.5	2.4
1994	30.7	19.0	3.6
1995	34.7	21.2	4.6
1996	35.8	21.9	4.9
1997	38.5	23.7	5.8
1998	37.5	22.8	5.6
1999	37.8	23.1	6.0
2000	36.5	21.6	6.0
2001	37.0	22.4	5.8
2002	36.2	21.5	6.0
2003	34.9	21.2	6.0
2004	34.3	19.9	5.6
2005	33.6	19.8	5.0
2006	31.5	18.3	5.0
2007	31.7	18.8	5.1
2008	32.4	19.4	5.4

Source: *Monitoring the Future: National Results on Adolescent Drug Use, Overview of Key Findings,* 2008.

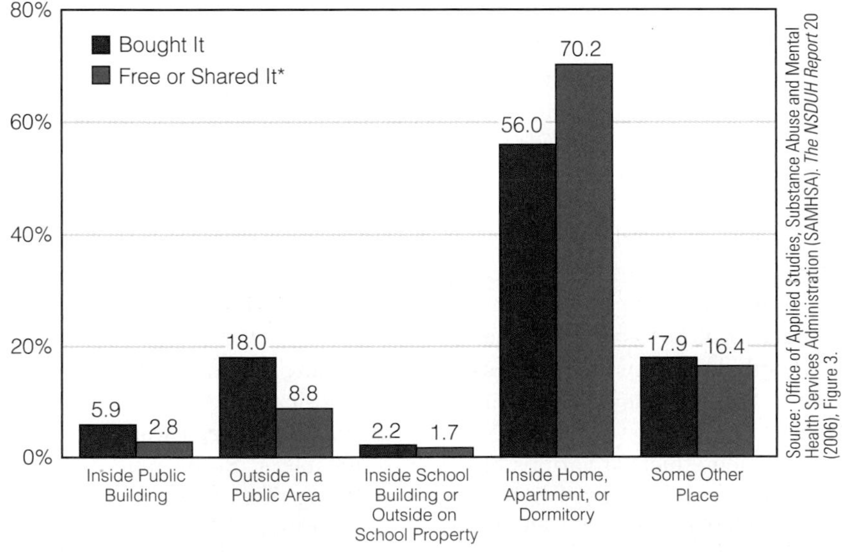

* Persons aged 18 to 25 who had not bought or traded for marijuana in the past year and who obtained their most recently used marijuana for free.

Figure 12.2 Location and Method of Obtaining Marijuana among Past-Year Users Aged 18 to 25

than those who started using it later. Also, continued marijuana use was greater among people who used other illicit drugs as well.

Pharmacology of Marijuana

Methods of Administration

Marijuana can be smoked or ingested. Most users in the United States smoke it, but ingestion is more common in other countries. Marijuana cannot be injected because the resin from the cannabis plant does not dissolve in water. If it is smoked, it takes effect more quickly than if it is ingested. Smoked THC is three times more potent than THC that is ingested. If ingested, marijuana's actions last longer. Generally, effects from smoked marijuana last 2 to 4 hours.

Most marijuana smokers roll the marijuana into a cigarette, although an alternative is to roll marijuana into a **blunt**, a type of cigar in which some of the tobacco is removed and replaced with marijuana. Among adolescents, 3.5% have used cigars with marijuana in them. The more likely one is to use marijuana, the more likely that marijuana will be used in a cigar.[16] Researchers disagree over whether more THC is absorbed through this method. Factors influencing the effects of marijuana include dosage, THC content, depth of inhalation, interval between puffs, and length of time it is held in one's lungs.

Absorption

When marijuana is smoked, THC reaches the brain within a few seconds, and the person experiences the psychological and physiological effects within several minutes. Euphoria can last for a few hours. The most intensive or peak effects are felt in about 30 minutes. When smoked, about half of the THC is absorbed by way of the lungs into the bloodstream. If ingested, the effects may not be felt for a couple of hours because less THC is absorbed. Those effects can last between 3 and 12 hours. Stomach contents also influence the effect of marijuana. People who consume marijuana orally are more likely to feel nausea and discomfort than those who smoke it.

Unlike alcohol, for which effects at various blood alcohol levels have been researched, precise behavioral and psychological effects of varying THC levels have not been determined. Marijuana is fat soluble, and its metabolites can remain in the fatty tissue of heavy users for 2 to 3 weeks after use; casual users can test positive for up to 3 days after use. This does not mean that heavy users feel the effects for 2 to 3 weeks.

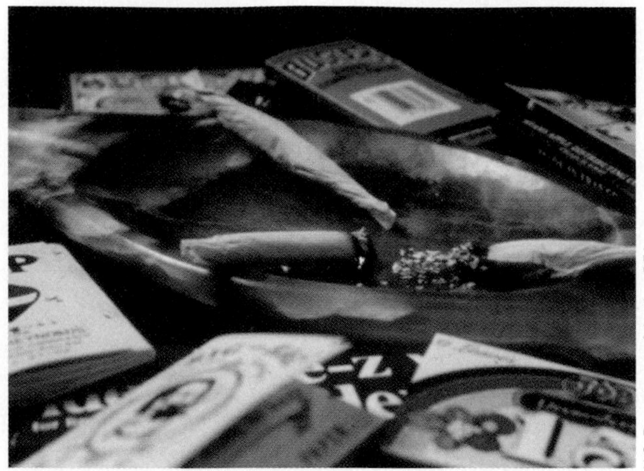

U.S. Department of Justice, DEA.

Marijuana is most often rolled into cigarettes and smoked.

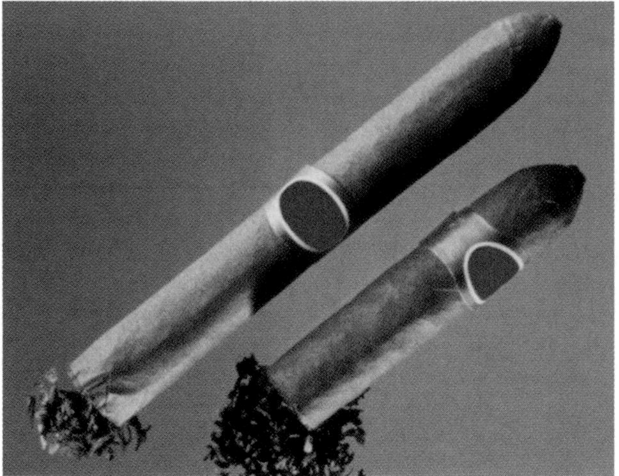

U.S. Department of Justice, DEA.

Hollowed out cigars packed with marijuana, called blunts, are gaining in popularity.

Marijuana smokers feel the effects only while the drug is circulating through the bloodstream. THC initially is detoxified by the liver and is eliminated primarily through the feces.

Tolerance

Animal studies reveal that tolerance to the physiological effects of marijuana develops, but there is dispute regarding whether humans develop pharmacological, or physical, tolerance. In studies proving pharmacological tolerance, it was more likely to develop among daily users. Some evidence, however, shows that smoking three marijuana cigarettes a week can result in tolerance.[17] Many users claim they get high from decreasing doses, though no evidence of **reverse tolerance** exists. If a person gets high more easily with subsequent use, the setting and familiarity might be factors. Euphoria, then, could result from expectations or previous experience. In short, because of previous experience with marijuana, users are able to adjust and respond to its effects. Frequent users also experience less loss of memory, coordination, and concentration.

blunt A marijuana-containing cigar; to create a blunt, tobacco is removed from a regular cigar and marijuana is inserted

reverse tolerance A drug user's experiencing the desired effects from lesser amounts of the same drug

Physical Dependence

One study of twins found that if one twin started smoking marijuana before age 17, the other twin was more likely to initiate marijuana use by that age also. This leads researchers to conclude that marijuana use may be heritable.[18] Although most experts agree that physical dependence on marijuana does *not* occur, whether marijuana causes physical dependency might depend on how dependency is defined. Columbia University drug expert Denise Kandel maintains that young people may develop physical dependency because they are more sensitive to marijuana. One argument against marijuana causing physical dependency is that its use drops dramatically as people age. However, it has been found that marijuana dependency among adults was about the same in the early 2000s as it was in the early 1990s.[19] Also, a study in Germany reported that individuals who smoked marijuana at least five times a week were likely to be marijuana smokers 10 years later.[20] This suggests that either they did not want to stop smoking marijuana or they had difficulty trying to stop. Another study found that monkeys would continue pushing a lever that resulted in their being injected with THC.[21]

One study found that one in every six people who smoked marijuana daily for 70 months experienced withdrawal symptoms of nervousness, tension, restlessness, appetite changes, and sleep disturbances.[22] Another study reported that 60% of regular marijuana smokers experienced significant withdrawal symptoms.[23] Other reported symptoms include irritability, nausea, vomiting, diarrhea, and sweating. Aggressiveness in long-term users seems to increase during withdrawal.[24] (Ironically, one immediate effect of marijuana is reduced aggression.) According to one leading expert, withdrawal is marked by anxiety and insomnia.[25] One study found that withdrawal symptoms following marijuana cessation are comparable to the withdrawal symptoms following cigarette cessation.[26]

Withdrawal Symptoms Associated with Marijuana

- Nausea
- Vomiting
- Perspiration
- Irritability
- Runny nose
- Restlessness
- Diarrhea
- Lack of appetite
- Insomnia
- Hot flashes

Psychological Dependence

Most drug experts think marijuana can result in psychological dependence. Most people who smoke marijuana are occasional users, few of whom become compulsive users. If dependency develops, it is more likely to be motivated by psychosocial than by physiological factors. The drug itself does not necessarily lead to increased use. The perceived need for the drug is believed to be responsible for compulsive use and dependency.

Effects of Marijuana Use

The amount of marijuana that could be fatal has not been established; thus, the margin of safety between effective and lethal doses is wide. Nevertheless, in recent years, the number of marijuana users seen in emergency rooms has increased, along with the number of users seeking treatment. More than 290,000 people went to emergency rooms in 2006 as a result of marijuana use.[27] In a study of first-year college students, it was reported that over 9% had a cannabis use disorder that resulted in concentration problems or missing a number of classes.[28]

Also, one study of adolescents who smoked marijuana at least once a week reported that these adolescents thought about killing themselves three times more often than nonusers, felt more lonely and unloved, were six times more likely to run away from home, were six times more likely to cut classes or skip school, and were five times more likely to steal. In addition, the proportion of admissions for primary marijuana abuse increased from 12% in 1996 to 16% in 2006. Of those admitted primarily for marijuana treatment, the average age for those entering treatment declined significantly to age 24 (the average age for all substance abuse treatment admissions is age 34).[29] The average length of stay in treatment increases when marijuana users also have alcohol or mood disorder problems.[30]

Although determining the specific effects of THC at varying levels is imprecise, driving ability is clearly

Factors Influencing Effects of Marijuana

- Whether it is smoked or ingested
- Dosage
- THC content
- Interval between puffs
- Depth of inhalation
- Length of time in one's lungs
- Set and setting
- Previous experiences

affected by the presence of THC in the bloodstream. Marijuana impairs perceptual and motor skills and the ability to stay awake—skills necessary for driving a car or motorcycle. Marijuana users are overrepresented in driving under the influence statistics; for instance, in Sweden, over a 10-year period, it was found that 18% to 30% of suspects in driving under the influence cases had measureable levels of THC.[31] Marijuana interferes with concentration and the ability to adjust for wind conditions and maintaining a steady speed. Teenagers who smoke marijuana and drive cars are more than twice as likely to be involved in an automobile accident as when they do not smoke. A reported 11% of 16- to 18-year-olds have driven cars within 2 hours of using an illegal substance, primarily marijuana.[32] In Great Britain, about 10% of motorists involved in serious accidents test positive for marijuana. Researchers in Australia found that driving ability was noticeably impaired when THC was in the bloodstream and that as the level of THC increased, the level of impairment increased.[33]

Psychological Effects

Many variables influence the psychological effects of marijuana. Marijuana increases the release of dopamine, a neurotransmitter involved in the experience of euphoria. Therefore, most users report euphoria, as well as relaxation, often followed by sleepiness. Others say they develop insight.

The frequency of and motivations for marijuana use affect its psychological effects. One study found that adolescents who used marijuana experimentally were not as well adjusted as those who abstained from marijuana use. Frequent users demonstrated more psychological problems.[34] Another study noted that marijuana users were no less depressed than nonmarijuana users, although people who took marijuana for medical reasons reportedly were more depressed than nonusers.[35] It has been found also that psychotic individuals were less likely to use marijuana, but when they used it they had more problems.[36] In the publication *The Link between Marijuana and Mental Illness*, the federal government identifies numerous studies supporting the connection between marijuana and mental illness.[37]

Psychological effects are subject to interpretation. What one person may view as desirable or euphoric may be undesirable or dysphoric to another. Although using marijuana to deal with interpersonal dilemmas, stress, and other problems may seem desirable to the user, many mental health experts view this as an inadequate long-term solution to personal problems. Despite the possible connection to interpersonal problems, some researchers maintain that strict enforcement of marijuana is unwarranted.[38]

In terms of interpersonal development, it was reported that those people who used marijuana as they approached adulthood had more relationship difficulties with a partner in their mid- to late 20s.[39] Detrimental psychological reactions to marijuana are the exception rather than the rule, although high doses can induce anxiety, delusions, disorientation, hallucinations, and paranoia. These reactions seem to arise in people who are predisposed to negative reactions. Adverse reactions to marijuana seldom require medical intervention, although this is becoming a more frequent occurrence. If a medical emergency arises, it often occurs with marijuana in combination with other drugs.

Perceptual Effects

Many people report feeling more introspective and sensitive to external stimuli when they are using marijuana. Others claim they are more artistically creative, although objective research does not support this. Marijuana alters perceptions of time and space. Mood changes are marked by anxiety, sadness, laughter, and paranoia. Some people experience panic reactions, which tend to be temporary and often are triggered by a feeling of not being in control. Others use marijuana to cope with social anxiety.[40]

Ascertaining how much perceptual change is attributable to marijuana itself and how much to one's beliefs about its effects is difficult. This point is illustrated in the classic study in which marijuana users were given regular tobacco cigarettes or marijuana cigarettes but did not know which they were given. Marijuana smokers reported being just as high after smoking a regular cigarette as they were after smoking a cigarette with marijuana.[41]

Participants in one study were given Marinol, a prescription drug consisting of capsules containing THC (given to chemotherapy patients to reduce nausea). About half of the subjects said they were drowsy, and one in six said they felt anxiety. Almost as many subjects receiving a placebo reported feeling drowsy, and nearly one in four said they experienced anxiety.[42] In contrast to subjects receiving Marinol, a higher percentage receiving the placebo reported feeling anxiety.

amotivational syndrome A condition characterized by apathy, an inability to concentrate, and little achievement orientation

Cognitive Effects

One reported cognitive effect of marijuana is impairment of short-term memory, although research on this effect is inconsistent. Heavy marijuana users in Costa Rica did not demonstrate cognitive difficulty, but heavy users in Europe, the United States, and India showed memory problems.[43] Many scientists agree that temporary cognitive effects occur, but they do not agree on whether any effects are permanent.

Learning and remembering new information becomes more arduous when using marijuana. Heavy users have more cognitive difficulties than light users. Heavy users were impaired in skills involving expression but were no less capable in vocabulary, mathematics, and reading comprehension. One study reported that frequent users had memory deficits by 12th grade when compared to nonusers. There had been no differences between these students and other students when they were in the fourth grade.[44] Some researchers have found that cognitive deficits persisted for up to 28 days after a person last smoked marijuana.[45]

Because memory is affected adversely, users have difficulty judging time. In numerous studies of marijuana users, the inability to judge time is the psychological effect that is most frequently reported. On the other hand, preliminary research indicates that the drug may be beneficial for individuals suffering from Alzheimer's disease because marijuana blocks an enzyme that leads to a buildup of plaque that is responsible for memory loss.[46]

Amotivational Syndrome

Heavy marijuana users reportedly are unable to concentrate and are unmotivated, apathetic, lacking ambition, and not achievement-oriented. This describes the **amotivational syndrome**. Does marijuana smoking bring about the amotivational syndrome, or are people who frequently smoke marijuana less motivated to start with? One study showed that poor performance in school preceded marijuana use, not that marijuana use preceded poor academic performance.[47] In their review of numerous studies, however, Lynskey and Hall reported that research on marijuana use and amotivational syndrome is inconclusive.[48]

One criterion used to determine motivation is grade point average (GPA). Adolescents who smoke marijuana often are less able to learn and have problems in school and at home. Students who use marijuana weekly, especially younger students, are more likely to drop out of school.[49] Again, people who smoke a great deal might also be predisposed to these problems initially.

The amotivational syndrome is more likely to develop in adolescents than in older people. Older marijuana smokers might view its use in a different context than younger users. For example, a college student might engage in many activities during the course of a day—attend classes, exercise, go to the library, watch a movie, study, smoke a joint. Thus, marijuana may be one small part of that person's day. In contrast, a high school student who smokes marijuana might place more importance on associated factors such as where to smoke, with whom to smoke, and when to smoke. If marijuana assumes an integral role in one's life, the amotivational syndrome is more likely to be present.

Physical Effects

Marijuana affects the body in many ways. A common experience is an increase in appetite. Marijuana acts on the respiratory, cardiovascular, immune, and reproductive systems, as well as on the brain. Some effects are temporary, some can be life-threatening, and others are insignificant.

Short-term effects include increased pulse rate, dilation of the pupils, reddened eyes, and dryness of the mouth and throat. Marijuana poses a greater risk to young people, pregnant and nursing women, and people with cardiovascular problems.

Appetite

Marijuana users consistently report an increase in appetite when they smoke, although no one component of marijuana has been identified as an appetite stimulant. Users indicate that sweet foods are especially appetizing to them. Any drug resulting in the "munchies" has a disadvantage if the user does not want to gain weight. Conversely, one associated factor that may reduce appetite is gum disease. It has been shown that people who use marijuana 3 to 5 times a week are susceptible to gum disease.[50]

The Respiratory System

The THC in marijuana has been used to treat asthma because THC acts as a bronchodilator. Despite this benefit, long-term smoking of marijuana is harmful to the lungs because the smoke contains many respiratory irritants and carcinogens. Daily marijuana smokers who do not use tobacco have more sick days and visits to doctors for respiratory problems than people who do not smoke at all.[51]

Chronic marijuana smoking impairs the flow of air into and out of the lungs. One marijuana cigarette has been reported to equal 20 regular cigarettes in terms of bronchial damage.[52] Some airway obstruction in the lungs might be reversed after abstinence from smoking marijuana.

Marijuana has not been proven definitively to cause lung cancer; however, daily marijuana smokers show damage to the cells lining the airways similar to that seen in cigarette smokers who develop lung cancer. The potential for marijuana smokers to develop lung disease is a concern because marijuana contains 20 times as much ammonia and five times as much hydrogen cyanide as tobacco smoke.[53] It is reported that marijuana smokers will exhibit pathological changes in their lungs 20 years before tobacco smokers.[54]

Because chronic marijuana smokers also tend to be chronic cigarette smokers, ascertaining how much lung damage is from marijuana and how much is from tobacco smoking is difficult. Even so, in one study, people who daily smoked marijuana *only* had significantly higher rates of chronic and acute bronchitis than people who smoked cigarettes only.[55] A review of studies looking at marijuana smoking and lung cancer pointed out that many studies are flawed; thus, some questions remain regarding the substantive damage to one's lungs from marijuana smoking.[56]

The Cardiovascular System

A review of studies over the past three decades indicates that marijuana adversely affects the cardiovascular system.[57] Marijuana smoking, especially by inexperienced smokers, produces tachycardia, a faster heart rate—an increase of an average 14 beats per minute during marijuana use. The acceleration in heart rate is greatest during smoking and for 20 minutes after smoking.

Research on the effects of marijuana on blood pressure is inconsistent. In some instances blood pressure goes up, and in other cases it goes down. Marijuana dilates the peripheral blood vessels, manifested by bloodshot eyes and warm ears.

The Immune System

A properly functioning immune system is essential to ward off infections. Studies involving laboratory animals have consistently demonstrated that marijuana affects the immune system adversely. Though research conducted with humans in the early 1970s indicated that marijuana reduced the immune response, subsequent research has failed to find a consistent relationship between marijuana and immunity.

The Reproductive System

Some users claim that marijuana heightens the sexual experience, and other users claim it makes them less interested in sex. Perhaps people who find marijuana sexually enhancing are predisposed to that effect. Nothing inherent in marijuana justifies its reputation as an aphrodisiac. Feelings of euphoria and increased awareness of stimuli, however, might make a person feel more sexual.

Marijuana has a negative effect on male sexuality because it decreases testosterone levels, sperm count, and libido. It also has been reported that smoking marijuana can reduce the sperm's ability to fertilize an egg.[58] The sperm of frequent marijuana smokers move too fast, decreasing the likelihood of penetration into the egg.[59] Marijuana may affect a woman's reproductive system, too, by inhibiting ovulation. Use of marijuana by pregnant women has been linked to higher rates of miscarriage and ectopic pregnancies.[60] Whether the lower birth weights of infants born to users is attributable to smoking marijuana or to the chemicals in marijuana is unclear. Regardless, it is prudent for women not to use marijuana while they are pregnant.

The Brain

How marijuana interacts with the brain is not entirely clear. Although some past studies reported that marijuana causes serious brain damage, many of these studies were seriously flawed. Subsequent research employing more sophisticated technology has contradicted those findings. Because many marijuana smokers use other drugs, determining the precise effects of marijuana on the brain is difficult. An unpublished report from the World Health Organization suggests that marijuana might produce subtle defects in cognitive functioning, but that the effects are less severe than those produced by alcohol.[61]

Smoking marijuana reduces acetylcholine in the **hippocampus**, the portion of the brain that affects memory. This relationship among marijuana, acetylcholine, and the hippocampus explains how memory is impaired.[62] The activity of the neurotransmitters norepinephrine and dopamine alters the mood, and marijuana affects these as well.

Anticholinergic drugs such as marijuana are believed to be related to schizophrenia, and schizophrenia is more likely to show up in heavy users than in nonusers. People with schizophrenia, however, might be drawn to marijuana to deal with their sense of alienation.[63]

Medical Applications

In the late 1800s, marijuana was used medically to treat convulsions, chronic cough, sleeplessness, gastrointestinal disorders, gonorrhea, and pain. With passage of the Marijuana Tax Act in 1937, physicians in the United States had to stop prescribing preparations made from cannabis, though many of them had cut back already because cannabis was unsuitable for injection and took a long time to take effect when taken orally, and other more effective drugs were available. Also, THC levels in cannabis preparations were not uniform.

After the popularity of recreational marijuana increased in the 1960s, interest in its therapeutic applications likewise surged. Recently, marijuana has been used for treating glaucoma, asthma, nausea and vomiting during cancer chemotherapy, and pain associated with multiple sclerosis. It also has been used to alleviate withdrawal symptoms related to barbiturates, narcotics, and alcohol.

Glaucoma

Glaucoma, caused by pressure building up behind the eye, is the second leading cause of blindness in the United States, afflicting 1.5% of people older than age 50 and about 5% of those older than 70.[64] Although marijuana does not cure blindness, it can reduce the risk by reducing pressure behind the eye. One drawback to marijuana use for glaucoma is the lack of long-term studies.[65]

THC eye drops were developed in 1981. They have not proved to be effective. Because marijuana affects heart rate and blood pressure and causes psychological problems in some patients, its widespread use for glaucoma treatment is unlikely. Moreover, other drugs are effective for treating glaucoma.

Nausea and Vomiting

Marijuana is an effective **anti-emetic** drug to counteract the nausea and vomiting that frequently accompany chemotherapy to treat cancer. Important to the effectiveness of marijuana is the patient's mindset. Those who are uncomfortable taking the drug because of the negative connotations surrounding it might also have difficulty benefiting from it. These people might profit more from medications such as Marinol (THC formulated in sesame oil) or Cesamet (a synthetic cannabinoid), because they do not resemble marijuana.

First marketed in 1986, Marinol was projected to reduce the demand for prescriptive marijuana. Marinol comes in capsule form and produces fewer side effects than marijuana; however, it takes longer to act than smoked marijuana does.[66] Debate continues to swirl around whether Marinol or marijuana is more effective for reducing nausea and vomiting. The reduction in nausea and vomiting could be the result of chemicals other than THC in marijuana. Also, some individuals complain that Marinol is more expensive than marijuana and produces some undesirable side effects.[67]

hippocampus Part of the brain involved with memory; altered by marijuana

anti-emetic A drug that reduces nausea and vomiting; an example is marijuana

More than 40% of oncologists in a survey recommended marijuana to their cancer patients to control nausea and vomiting.[68] The oncologists believed that marijuana and Marinol were equally effective. In 2003, the Canadian government produced marijuana to give to medical patients.[69]

Asthma

Approximately 17 million people in the United States have asthma, of whom about 5,300 die each year.[70] The THC in marijuana is helpful in expanding lung capacity because it dilates the bronchial tubes. Paradoxically, whether smoke goes into the lungs from a marijuana cigarette or a regular tobacco cigarette, lung capacity decreases. Because of this limitation and the availability of other bronchodilators that are more effective and do not produce as many side effects, marijuana is not the drug of choice for treating asthma.

Additional Medical Uses

Marijuana stimulates the appetite. Although this might be undesirable for a dieter, weight gain is beneficial for people with AIDS and those receiving chemotherapy. When receiving chemotherapy, many people lose weight because their appetite diminishes. Marijuana can help these people regain their appetite and put on needed weight. One Australian study reported that nearly 60% of men and women living with HIV/AIDS used marijuana. Although many used the drug recreationally, over 40% believed it helped with their condition.[71] It has been noted that marijuana in moderate amounts relieves pain.[72]

Marijuana has been recommended for partially or completely paralyzed individuals because it acts as a muscle relaxant and relieves pain more safely than narcotics.[73] Marijuana alleviates muscle spasms and tremors; consequently, it may prove to be beneficial to people with multiple sclerosis.[74]

Marijuana is recommended for epilepsy, insomnia, rheumatoid arthritis, and chronic pain conditions. Anecdotal evidence suggests that it helps people with bipolar disorders. Finally, marijuana might be beneficial in treating premenstrual syndrome and menstrual cramps. In the late 1800s, Queen Victoria used marijuana for these purposes.

Decriminalization and Legalization

In 1972, the Presidential Commission on Marijuana and Drug Abuse recommended the decriminalization of marijuana. Between 1973 and 1978, 11 states (Oregon being the first) decriminalized marijuana, making possession a minor offense punishable by a $100 fine. Marijuana was illegal in every state except Alaska, where up to 4 ounces could be grown. In 1990, however, voters in Alaska approved recriminalizing marijuana. In 1998, the Oregon legislature introduced a referendum to recriminalize marijuana. It appeared on the November 2000 ballot, but by a 2-to-1 margin the voters defeated the measure. In 2008, Michigan became the 13th state to approve the medical use of marijuana, while Massachusetts became the 13th state to reduce the possession of marijuana to a misdemeanor.[75] However, in a case in California, it was ruled that employers are allowed to fire a worker who tests positive for marijuana, even if given it for medical reasons.[76]

Perhaps no drug has generated as much discussion regarding decriminalization and legalization as marijuana. Many people believe it is a *relatively* safe drug, although few people are in favor of anyone smoking marijuana before flying an airplane or operating a motor vehicle or heavy equipment. Concern has been voiced that relaxing marijuana laws would give young people the impression that using marijuana is acceptable.

Another argument against marijuana is that it is a gateway drug, leading to the use of more dangerous drugs. How valid is this **steppingstone theory**? Most people who have taken heroin, cocaine, and other illegal drugs have smoked marijuana. Yet, most marijuana smokers do not proceed to use other drugs. Those marijuana smokers who proceed to other drugs start their use at earlier ages and smoke more frequently. The pharmacological properties of marijuana have not been proved to increase the desire to progress to other drugs. Thus, other factors are implicated if other drugs are used. One study found that the increase in the use of hard drugs after using marijuana is greatly overstated for people born since the beginning of the 1970s.[77] Alcohol and cigarettes are better predictors of involvement with illegal drugs.

To illustrate, probably most heroin users have consumed soft drinks. Yet soft drinks are not seen as steppingstone drugs. If a marijuana user progresses to other drugs, factors such as availability and desire may also be relevant.

Many marijuana proponents do not contend that the drug is harmless, only that marijuana laws present a greater danger. Which is the greater problem—marijuana or laws against marijuana? One group that lobbies for a change in marijuana laws is the National Organization for the Reform of Marijuana Laws (NORML). NORML contends that the quality of marijuana would be controlled more effectively if it were legal. Marijuana has medical benefits, and legalization would allow people who would benefit from it to obtain it more easily. The opposing argument is that if marijuana could be easily obtained for medical reasons, what might start out as medical use could become personal, recreational use.

When the legalization of marijuana is debated, marijuana inevitably is compared to tobacco and alcohol. It is argued that marijuana wreaks less havoc on families and society than tobacco and alcohol do. Tobacco is connected more definitively to heart disease and lung cancer than marijuana is. The links between marijuana and heart disease and between marijuana and lung cancer have not been established. Nonetheless, if marijuana were as readily available as alcohol and tobacco, usage rates might rival those of alcohol and tobacco, and problems with marijuana conceivably could become commensurate with those of alcohol and tobacco.

In the Netherlands, marijuana use is not legal, but it is tolerated. The Dutch government takes a pragmatic approach, believing that if it has better control over marijuana use, the risks are reduced. It is estimated that 13% of Dutch high school students have used marijuana compared to 28% of American high school students.[78] It is apparent that widespread marijuana availability does not necessarily result in its widespread use.[79]

A number of European countries such as Belgium, Britain, and Luxembourg have also adopted a less stringent view on marijuana use. Not all European countries have maintained a low level of marijuana use, however. In the Czech Republic, marijuana use increased significantly from 1995 to 2003. It is believed that this increase will affect health care and social services.[80]

Legalization of Marijuana for Medical Uses

Whether marijuana should be legal for medical purposes is hotly debated. One argument in favor is that marijuana has a long history of medical use and is reasonably safe. Opponents of medical marijuana use believe that if marijuana were available for medical use, its nonmedical use would increase dramatically.

The federal government maintains that most evidence showing that marijuana works is anecdotal and is not based on solid scientific research. It has, however, begun to fund research into the efficacy of medicinal uses of marijuana. At the same time, some scientists maintain that the federal government is hindering research into marijuana's medicinal benefits by making it difficult to receive permission to conduct these studies.[81]

In November 1996, California voters passed Proposition 215, eliminating state penalties for medical uses of marijuana. Despite passage of Proposition 215, federal law takes precedence over state law, and the vast majority of politicians at the national level oppose making marijuana medically legal. In June 2001, Nevada state lawmakers approved marijuana use for seriously ill individuals. In the month preceding this approval, however, the U.S. Supreme Court reaffirmed its stance opposing medicinal use of marijuana.[82]

Initiatives to legalize marijuana for medical purposes were on the ballots of numerous states and the District of Columbia. In every instance except in Missouri, voters approved allowing doctors to prescribe marijuana to treat terminal or debilitating illnesses. In Alaska, 58% of voters approved the initiative; in Washington State, 59% of voters approved it; in Oregon, 55%; and in Nevada, 59%.

The Institute of Medicine (IOM) was asked by the federal government to review the research on marijuana's medicinal benefits. The IOM did not conclude that marijuana was beneficial, but it stated that marijuana has "potential for therapeutic use."[83] Despite its stance on the possibility that marijuana may have some medicinal benefit, the IOM has not come out in favor of using marijuana medicinally.

In 1988, Francis Young, the chief administrative law judge for the Drug Enforcement Agency (DEA), recommended that the DEA change marijuana from Schedule I to Schedule II to give support to medical patients who would benefit from it. The DEA refused to accept the recommendation because it questioned the medical value of marijuana. Ironically, morphine and cocaine, drugs with stronger psychoactive effects, currently are used in medicine. In April 2006, the Food and Drug Administration reaffirmed its position that marijuana should remain a Schedule I drug, asserting that marijuana has a high potential for abuse, has no currently accepted medical use in treatment in the United States, and has a lack of accepted safety for use under medical supervision.[84]

Besides the federal government, other organizations who oppose medical marijuana include the American Academy for Ophthalmology, the American Medical Association, the National Multiple Sclerosis Society, and, as noted above, the Institute of Medicine.[85] Despite the position of the federal government, other groups support the use of marijuana for medical purposes. The American College of Physicians, the nation's largest organization of internal medicine doctors, calls for the use of medical marijuana.[86]

One state that is noted for its prescription of medical marijuana is California. However, after the FDA's ruling that marijuana will remain a Schedule I drug, 70 establishments that dispensed marijuana closed.[87] In an interesting twist, medical marijuana vending machines have been set up in several stores in Los Angeles for individuals who carry cards authorizing marijuana use. As the inventor of the marijuana vending machine said, they provide lower prices, convenient access, safety, and anonymity. The DEA is trying to prevent the use of these machines.[88]

steppingstone theory Hypothesis holding that use of soft drugs such as marijuana and alcohol leads to use of harder drugs such as heroin and cocaine

The debate over whether marijuana should be medically legal raises several interesting questions[89]:

- If physicians believe marijuana could be beneficial, do they have a moral obligation to inform their patients of this possibility?
- Should physicians be prosecuted if they recommend marijuana use to their patients?
- What constitutes a legitimate medical use?
- Is improving the quality of mental health a legitimate medical use for marijuana?

Cost

Drug reform advocate Ethan Nadelmann contends that treating drug offenders is much cheaper than incarcerating them.[90] Moreover, legalizing marijuana and other drugs would stem the rise in violence and criminal activity.[91] In the United States, of the 1.8 million people arrested for marijuana possession, about 40% were arrested for possessing very small quantities.[92] According to 2006 data from the FBI, 830,000 people were arrested on marijuana charges. Since 1990, marijuana arrests have gone up more than 150%. Interestingly, the increase in arrest rates has had no impact on marijuana's rate of use.[93]

Most people supporting legalization favor some form of regulation. Nadelmann recommends that buyers show legal proof of age, that package labels reflect THC content, and that health warnings be included. In opposition, Mathea Falco contends that prohibition should be the goal. She maintains that marijuana is unhealthy and the only viable option is elimination of its use.[94] If marijuana were legalized, problems might increase dramatically because of the way in which products would be advertised and marketed.

Crime and Violence

The reputation of marijuana as a cause of violence dates back to Hassan, an Arabian politico who lived during the Middle Ages, and his cult, who purportedly

On Campus

College students convicted of a drug offense, including marijuana possession, are in jeopardy of losing federal financial loans or scholarships based on federal laws.

Source: Anti-Drug Abuse Act (1988).

used hashish in preparation for aggressive acts against others. Still, whether Hassan and his followers actually consumed hashish is unclear. The 1930s film *Reefer Madness* also depicted marijuana as a drug that caused users to become violent.

What effect would legalization of marijuana have on aggression and crime? No one can say for sure. Legalization might result in one set of problems replacing another. The incidence of criminal and violent behavior might go down, whereas interpersonal and intrapersonal problems might escalate. One historical precedent is alcohol prohibition. When alcohol was legally prohibited, alcohol-related arrests dropped by half, but the law laid the groundwork for organized crime, which took over the manufacture and distribution of alcohol.

Because of the illegality of drugs, the cost is high. After the federal government stepped up efforts to stop marijuana growing in Hawaii, its price tripled.

An argument for legalization is that it would remove much of the profit motive.[95] Whether marijuana use causes people to engage in crime is not known. Perhaps the types of people who traffic in drugs would be more likely to be involved with crime and violence initially. Most people who abuse drugs and commit crimes began criminal activity *before* they started to use drugs.

Although marijuana use and crime have a positive connection, a cause-and-effect relationship has *not* been established. Critical factors in crime statistics include unemployment, poverty, illiteracy, inadequate health care, and substandard housing. One study of children in the fourth to ninth grades found that those who reacted to situations with aggression were more likely to use marijuana than those youngsters who did not react with aggression.[96] Another study of adults reported that marijuana use was a factor in partner aggression.[97]

Summary

Marijuana has an extensive history. It was medically important in many countries and was economically essential to the United States in its infancy for the hemp used in making rope. Not until the 1900s was marijuana used for recreational reasons. Early users in the United States were Mexican and Caribbean immigrants who settled in the Southwest. Stories of marijuana causing mental illness, violent behavior, and immorality eventually resulted in passage of the Marijuana Tax Act of 1937.

Marijuana comes from the *Cannabis sativa* plant, and its primary psychoactive agent is delta-9-tetrahydrocannabinol, THC. Levels of THC are affected by the plant's sex, the part of the plant used, soil and climate conditions, and how the plant is stored. *Cannabis indica* and *Cannabis ruderalis* contain smaller amounts of THC.

Variations of marijuana include sinsemilla, hashish, and hash oil. Of these, sinsemilla, which is seedless marijuana, is most potent. The THC content in marijuana might have increased in recent years because of improved cultivation. Major producers are Colombia and Mexico. The amount of marijuana produced in the United States is escalating; about one-fourth of the marijuana currently used in the United States is domestic.

Marijuana works more quickly and more intensely when it is smoked than when it is ingested. THC reaches the brain within seconds after smoking, peak effects occur in about one-half hour, and the high lasts several hours. Influencing the effects of marijuana are THC levels, intervals between puffs, and depth and length of inhalation. Although animal studies show that pharmacological tolerance to marijuana develops, similar studies on humans are inconsistent. Behavioral and psychological tolerance seems to occur in humans, but reverse tolerance—in which users achieve the desired effects with decreasing dosages—has not been proved. Physical dependency on marijuana is not evident, although many young people are seeking treatment for marijuana abuse.

The psychological effects of marijuana vary among users. It can affect mood, sensitivity to external stimuli, and perception of time and space. High doses can lead to panic reactions, anxiety, and paranoia. These effects are more likely in people who are predisposed to these reactions. Appetite, concentration, and memory also are affected. Marijuana reportedly reduces motivation, but this may be a function of the user. This amotivational syndrome is more prevalent in adolescents who smoke marijuana than in older people who do.

Much of the research on the long-term effects of marijuana use has been poorly conducted. Evidence regarding the respiratory system, however, is clear. Marijuana smoke damages lung tissue and impairs lung function. Also, marijuana smoke contains carcinogenic chemicals. Marijuana has not been shown to cause heart attacks in people with a healthy heart, but it could precipitate heart conditions in people who already have coronary heart disease. Marijuana weakens the immune system in animals; similar research on humans is inconsistent. In males, testosterone levels, sperm production, sperm structure, and sperm motility are affected adversely. Women who smoke marijuana might not ovulate. Also, pregnant women who use marijuana give birth to lower-birth-weight babies on average.

Marijuana has been used to treat asthma, glaucoma, and multiple sclerosis. Its use in treating glaucoma has declined because other drugs have proved to be more effective. Because THC expands lung capacity, it formerly was used for asthma, although its benefit was limited. Marijuana seems to be effective in alleviating the nausea and vomiting associated with chemotherapy. About a dozen states have passed referenda approving the use of marijuana for medical purposes, although federal law overrides the state laws.

Many people consider marijuana a relatively safe drug and believe that problems stem from its illegal status. Proponents of legalization argue that it would allow for more control over the distribution and use of the drug, that marijuana causes less physical harm than alcohol and tobacco, and that treating marijuana users is cheaper than incarcerating them. Opponents argue that liberalizing marijuana laws would trigger an increase in personal use, leading to increased expenses of treatment programs. These people believe illegality prevents a number of people from using a drug that may result in negative long-term consequences.

Thinking Critically

1. If the THC content of marijuana has increased over the past two decades, previous research on the effects of marijuana is questionable. How much credence should research be given?
2. Government officials talk about the "War on Drugs." Yet, what this phrase actually means is unclear. Does it refer to stopping the importation of drugs, the use of drugs, or something else? What does "War on Drugs" mean to you?
3. Because marijuana alters consciousness, it has a negative effect on driving ability. Still, some marijuana smokers claim they drive more safely, because their senses are more acute after using marijuana. Can a substance alter consciousness, yet improve the ability to operate a car?
4. Because marijuana may result in babies with lower birth weight, smoking during pregnancy is unwise. If birth difficulties were proven definitely to be caused by marijuana use, would it affect your decision to smoke or not smoke marijuana during pregnancy? Should pregnant women who smoke marijuana be penalized in some way? If so, how?
5. Whether marijuana should be used in the treatment of medical problems is the topic of an ongoing debate. Should the decision to use marijuana for medical purposes be made by government officials or by medical personnel?
6. One argument for legalizing drugs is that the black market in drugs would be reduced. Do you think legalization would reduce the black market? Would you be more tempted to try drugs if you could get them legally? Would the cost of obtaining marijuana affect your decision to use or not to use it? How does legality affect use?

Web Resources

National Institute on Drug Abuse: Marijuana Information
http://www.nida.nih.gov/MarijBroch/Marijintro.html
This site presents information regarding trends in marijuana use.

National Organization for the Reform of Marijuana Laws
http://www.norml.org
This site contains information regarding the legalization of marijuana.

Notes

1. J. Brainard, "University Fights Ban on Growing of Hemp," *Chronicle of Higher Education,* 54 (October 5, 2007).
2. The OAS Report, *A Day in the Life of American Adolescents* (Rockville, MD: Substance Abuse and Mental Health Services Administration, October 18, 2007).
3. "Cannabits (Facts about Marijuana)," *Forbes,* 172 (November 10, 2003): 146.
4. D. J. Korf, A. Benschop, and M. Wouters, "Differential Responses to Cannabis Potency: A Typology of Users Based on Self-Reported Consumption Behaviour," *International Journal of Drug Policy,* 18 (May 2007): 168–176.
5. *National Drug Threat Assessment 2008* (Johnstown, PA: National Drug Intelligence Center, 2007).
6. Ibid.
7. L. D. Johnston, P. M. O'Malley, J. G. Bachman, and J. E. Schulenberg, *Monitoring the Future: National Results on Adolescent Drug Use, Overview of Key Findings, 2006* (Bethesda, MD: National Institute on Drug Abuse, 2007).
8. A. Kokkevi, S. N. Gabhainn, and M. Spyropoulou, "Early Initiation of Cannabis Use: A Cross-National European Perspective,"

Journal of Adolescent Health, 39 (2006): 712–719.

9. B. T. Ewing, "High School Athletes and Marijuana Use," *Journal of Drug Education,* 28 (1998): 147–157.
10. J. G. Bachman, L. D. Johnston, and P. M. O'Malley, "Explaining Recent Increases in Students' Marijuana Use: Impacts of Perceived Risks and Disapproval, 1976 through 1996," *American Journal of Public Health,* 88 (1998): 887–892.
11. L. D. Johnston, P. M. O'Malley, J. G. Bachman, and J. E. Schulenberg, *Monitoring the Future National Survey Results on Drug Use, 1975–2007. Volume II: College Students and Adults Ages 19–45, 2007* (Bethesda, MD: National Institute on Drug Abuse, 2008).
12. K. Corsi, P. Winch, C. Kwiatkowski, and R. Booth, "Childhood Factors That Precede Drug Injection: Is There a Link?" *Journal of Child and Family Studies,* 16 (December 2007): 808–818.
13. The NSDUH Report, *How Youths Obtain Marijuana* (Rockville, MD: U.S. Department of Health and Human Services, September 19, 2003).
14. L. D. Johnston, P. M. O'Malley, J. G. Bachman, and J. G. Schulenberg, *Monitoring the Future Study: National Results on Adolescent Drug Use, Overview of Key Findings, 2007* (Rockville, MD: National Institute on Drug Abuse, 2008).
15. D. B. Kandel and K. Chen, "Predictors of Cessation of Marijuana Use," in *Problems of Drug Dependence, 1997,* edited by L. S. Harris (Proceedings of the 59th Annual Scientific Meeting, NIDA Research Monograph 178) (Rockville, MD: National Institute on Drug Abuse, 1997).
16. The NSDUH Report, *Use of Marijuana and Blunts among Adolescents: 2005* (Rockville, MD: U.S. Department of Health and Human Services, March 9, 2007).
17. H. E. Doweiko, *Concepts of Chemical Dependence,* 6th ed. (Pacific Grove, CA: Brooks/Cole, 2005).
18. M. T. Lynskey, A. C. Heath, K. K. Bucholz, W. S. Slutske, P. A. Madden, E. C. Nelson, D. J. Stratham, and N. G. Martin, "Escalation of Drug Use in Early-Onset Cannabis Users vs. Co-twin Controls," *Journal of the American Medical Association,* 289 (2003): 427–433.
19. W. M. Compton, B. F. Grant, J. D. Colliver, M. D. Glomtz, and F. S. Stinson, "Prevalence of Marijuana Use Disorders in the United States: 1991–1992 and 2001–2002," *Journal of the American Medical Association,* 291 (May 5, 2004): 2114–2121.
20. A. Perkonigg et al., "The Natural Course of Cannabis Use, Abuse and Dependence During the First Decades of Life," *Addiction,* 103 (March 2008): 439–449.
21. A. Berger, "Marijuana Has Potential for Misuse," *British Medical Journal,* 321 (October 21, 2000): 979–981.
22. R. Fortgang, "Is Pot Bad for You? Six Questions Answered," *Rolling Stone* (March 4, 1999): 53.
23. E. Nagourney, "Realities of Breaking a Marijuana Habit," *New York Times,* November 28, 2000.
24. E. M. Kouri, E. G. Pope, and S. E. Lukas, "Changes in Aggressive Behavior Following Discontinuation from Long-Term Marihuana Use," in *Problems of Drug Dependence, 1997,* edited by L. S. Harris (Proceedings of the 59th Annual Scientific Meeting, NIDA Research Monograph 178) (Rockville, MD: National Institute on Drug Abuse, 1997).
25. "Marijuana: A Safe High?" *New Scientist,* 127 (1998): 24–29.
26. R. G. Vandrey, A. J. Budney, J. R. Hughes, and A. Liguori, "A Within-Subject Comparison of Withdrawal Symptoms During Abstinence from Cannabis, Tobacco and Both Substances," *Drug and Alcohol Dependence,* 92 (January 2008): 48–54.
27. Substance Abuse and Mental Health Services Administration, *Drug Abuse Warning Network, 2006: National Estimates of Drug-Related Emergency Department Visits* (Rockville, MD: Office of Applied Studies, 2008).
28. K. M. Caldeira, A. M. Arria, K. E. O'Grady, K. B. Vincent, and E. D. Wish, "The Occurrence of Cannabis Use Disorders and Other Cannabis-Related Problems Among First-Year College Students," *Addictive Behaviors,* 33 (March, 2008): 397–411.
29. Substance Abuse and Mental Health Services Administration, *Treatment Episode Data Set (TEDS) Highlights—2006 National Admissions to Substance Abuse Treatment Services* (Rockville, MD: Office of Applied Studies, 2007).
30. R. L. Pacula, J. Ringer, C. Dobkins, and K. Truong, "The Incremental Inpatient Costs Associated with Marijuana Comorbidity," *Drug and Alcohol Dependence,* 92 (January 2008): 248–257.
31. A. W. Jones, A. Holmgren, and F. C. Kugelberg, "Driving Under the Influence of Cannabis: A 10-Year Study of Age and Gender Differences in the Concentrations of Tetrahydrocannabinol in Blood," *Addiction,* 103 (March 2008): 452–461.
32. J. C. Greenblatt, "Adolescent Self-Reported Behaviors and Their Association with Marijuana Use," in *Analyses of Substance Abuse and Treatment Need Issues* (Rockville, MD: Substance Abuse and Mental Health Services Administration, Office of Applied Studies, 1998).
33. C. Stough, M. Boorman, E. Ogden, and K. Papafotiou, *An Evaluation of the Standardised Field Sobriety Tests for the Detection of Impairment Associated with Cannabis with and without Alcohol* (Australia: National Drug Law Enforcement Research Fund, 2006).
34. J. S. Tucker, P. L. Ellickson, R. L. Collins, and D. J. Klein, "Are Drug Experimenters Better Adjusted Than Abstainers and Users? A Longitudinal Study of Adolescent Marijuana Use," *Journal of Adolescent Health,* 39 (October 2006): 488–494.
35. T. F. Denson and M. Earleywine, "Decreased Depression in Marijuana Users," *Addictive Behaviors,* 31 (2006): 738–742.
36. B. Green, D. J. Kavanaugh, and R. Young, "Predictors of Cannabis Use in Men with and without Psychosis," *Addictive Behaviors,* 32 (December 2007): 2879–2887.
37. Office of National Drug Control Policy, *The Link Between Marijuana and Mental Illness* (Rockville, MD: Office of National Drug Control Policy, 2005).
38. H. A. Pollack and P. Reuter, "The Implications of Recent Findings on the Link Between Cannabis and Psychosis," *Addiction,* 102 (February 2007): 173–176.
39. J. Brooks, K. Pahl, and P. Cohen, "Associations between Marijuana Use During Emerging Adulthood and Aspects of the Significant Other Relationships in Young Adulthood," *Journal of Child and Family Studies,* 17 (February 2008): 1–12.
40. J. D. Buckner, M. O. Bonn-Miller, M. J. Zvolensky, and N. B. Schmidt, "Marijuana Use Motives and Social Anxiety among Marijuana-Using Adults," *Addictive Behaviors,* 32 (October 2007): 2238–2252.
41. R. T. Jones, "Tetrahydrocannabinol and the Marijuana-Induced Social 'High,' or the Effects of the Mind on Marijuana," in *Marijuana: Chemistry, Pharmacology, and Patterns of Social Use,* edited

by A. J. Singer (New York: New York Academy of Sciences, 1971).
42. *Physician's Desk Reference* (Montvale, NJ: Medical Economics Data, 1987), 1760–1762.
43. Fortgang, supra note 22.
44. *Marijuana* (Rockville, MD: Office of National Drug Control Policy, 2007).
45. J. S. Williams, "Cognitive Deficits in Marijuana Smokers Persist After Use Stops," *NIDA Notes,* 18 (December 2003): 8.
46. A. G. King, "Marijuana Component May Offer Hope for Alzheimer's Disease Treatment," *Journal of Chemical Education*, 83 (March 2007): 378–380.
47. K. L. Henry, E. A. Schmidt, and L. L. Caldwell, "Deterioration of Academic Achievement and Marijuana Use Onset among Rural Adolescents," *Health Education Research*, 22 (June 2007): 372–384.
48. M. Lynskey and W. Hall, "The Effects of Adolescent Cannabis Use on Educational Attainment: A Review," *Addiction,* 95 (2000): 1621–1630.
49. M. T. Lynskey, C. Coffey, L. Degenhardt, J. B. Caplin, and G. Patton, "A Longitudinal Study of the Effects of Cannabis on High School Completion," *Addiction,* 98 (2003): 685–692.
50. N. Seppa, "Pot Downer," *Science News*, 173 (February 9, 2008).
51. Greenblatt, supra note 32.
52. D. P. Tashkin, S. Fliegiel, W. Tzu-Chin, H. Gong, R. G. Barbers, A. H. Coulson, M. S. Simmons, and T. F. Beals, "Effects of Habitual Use of Marijuana and/or Cocaine on the Lung," in *Research Findings on Smoking of Abused Substances*, edited by C. N. Chiang and R. L. Hawks (NIDA Research Monograph 99) (Washington, DC: Department of Health and Human Services, 1990).
53. J. Palmer, "Cannabis Smoke Beats Tobacco for Toxic Chemicals," *New Scientist*, 196 (December 12, 2007), 35–36.
54. S. W. Hii, J. D. Tam, B. R. Thompson, and M. T. Naughton, "Bullous Lung Disease Due to Marijuana," *Respirology*, 13 (January 2008): 122–127.
55. Tashkin et al., supra-note 52.
56. R. Mehra, B. A. Moore, K. Crothers, J. Tetrault, and D. A. Fiellin, "The Association Between Marijuana Smoking and Lung Cancer," *Archives of Internal Medicine,* 166 (2006): 1359–1367.
57. A. Aryana, "Marijuana as a Trigger of Cardiovascular Events: Speculation or Scientific Certainty?" *International Journal of Cardiology*, 118 (May 2007): 141–144.
58. "Marijuana and the Single Sperm," *Vibrant Life,* 17 (March 2001): 8.
59. "Stoned Sperm Too Speedy Too Soon," *Chemistry and Industry,* 20 (October 20, 2003): 8.
60. "Behind the Headlines: Does Cannabis Make You Infertile?" *GP* (August 2006): 10.
61. D. Concar, "High Anxieties: What the WHO Doesn't Want You to Know About Cannabis," *New Scientist*, 157 (February 21, 1998): 4.
62. Office of National Drug Control Policy, supranote 37.
63. "Marijuana: A Safe High?" supra note 25.
64. L. Grinspoon and J. B. Bakalar, *Marihuana: The Forbidden Medicine* (New Haven, CT: Yale University Press, 1997).
65. A. G. Kabat and J. W. Sowka, "Just Say No," *Review of Optometry* (February 15, 2007): 138–139.
66. G. Stix, "Herb Remedy: Exploring Ways to Administer Marijuana as Medicine," *Scientific American,* September 18, 1998.
67. "Reefer Madness," *The Economist*, 379 (April 29, 2006): 83–84.
68. R. E. Doblin and M. A. Kleiman, "Marijuana as Medicine: A Survey of Oncologists," in *New Frontiers in Drug Policy,* edited by A. S. Trebach and K. B. Zeese (Washington, DC: Drug Policy Foundation, 1991).
69. "Medicinal Marijuana Officially Available in Canada; U.S. Officials Steaming," *Drug Policy Alliance Newsletter* (August 28, 2003): 8
70. U.S. Centers for Disease Control and Prevention. "Forecasted State-Specific Estimates for Self-Reported Asthma Prevalence," *Morbidity and Mortality Weekly Report* (December 4, 1998): 1022–1025.
71. A. Fogarty et al., "Marijuana as Therapy for People Living with HIV/AIDS: Social and Health Aspects," *AIDS Care,* 19 (February 2007): 295–301.
72. "Marijuana Can Relieve Pain," *Consumer Reports on Health* (February 2008): 10.
73. U. Hagenbach et al., "The Treatment of Spasticity with Delta9-Tetrahydrocannabinol in Persons with Spinal Cord Injury," *Spinal Cord,* 45 (August 2007): 551–562.
74. M. Iskedjian, B. Bereza, A. Gordon, C. Piwko, and T. R. Einarson, "Meta-Analysis of Cannabis Based Treatments for Neuropathic and Multiple Sclerosis–Related Pain," *Current Medical Research and Opinion,* 23 (January 2007): 17–24.
75. P. Armentano, "Working to Reform Marijuana Laws: Truth Prevails," *NORML BLOG,* November 5, 2008 [Accessed December 18, 2008]. Available from http://blog.norml.org/2008/11/05/truth-prevails/.
76. J. McKinley, "Ruling Puts Workplace Limits on California Marijuana Law," *New York Times,* January 25, 2008.
77. A. Golub and B. D. Johnson, "Variation in Youthful Risks of Progression from Alcohol and Tobacco to Marijuana and to Hard Drugs Across Generations," *American Journal of Public Health,* 91 (2001): 225–232.
78. S. Tan-Torres, Amsterdam, *The Prague Journal of Central European Affairs*, 9 (Spring 2007): 59.
79. G. S. Yacoubian, "Assessing the Relationship between Marijuana Availability and Marijuana Use: A Legal and Sociological Comparison between the United States and the Netherlands," *Journal of Alcohol and Drug Education*, 51 (December 2007): 17–34.
80. L. Csemy, P. Lejckova, and P. Sadilek, "Substance Use among Czech Adolescents: An Overview of Trends in the International Context," *Journal of Drug Issues*, 37 (Winter 2007): 119–132.
81. L. Guterman, "The Dope on Medical Marijuana," *Chronicle of Higher Education* (June 2, 2000): A21–A22.
82. "Nevada Moves to Allow Medical Marijuana," *New York Times,* June 5, 2001.
83. J. R. McDonough, "Marijuana on the Ballot," *Policy Review* (April/May 2000): 51–61.
84. "Inter-Agency Advisory Regarding Claims That Smoked Marijuana is a Medicine," *U.S. Food and Drug Administration Press Release*, April 20, 2006.
85. *Medical Marijuana Reality Check* (Washington, D.C.: Office of National Drug Control Policy, February, 2007).
86. E. Bailey, "Doctors Urge Easing of Marijuana Ban," *Los Angeles Times*, February 15, 2008.
87. H. W. Tesorierro, "Backlash Endangers California Pot Dispensaries," *Wall Street Journal*, December 20, 2007.
88. D. Nguyen, "Vending Machines Dispense Pot in LA," *Associated Press*, January 30, 2008.
89. R. Goldberg, *Taking Sides: Clashing Views on Controversial Issues in Drugs and Society*, 8th ed. (McGraw-Hill/Dushkin, 2008).
90. E. A. Nadelmann, "Commonsense Drug Policy," in *The American Drug Scene*, edited by J. A. Inciardi and K. McElrath

(Los Angeles: Roxbury Publishing Company, 2004).
91. Ibid.
92. E. Nadelmann, "Drugs: The War on Drugs Can Be Won," *Foreign Policy,* 162 (September/October 2007): 24–30.
93. J. Sullum, "High Risk," *Reason,* 39 (January 2008).
94. M. Falco, "To Legalize, or Not to Legalize?" *Foreign Policy,* 163 (September/October 2007): 6.
95. P. Reuter, "Why Can't We Make Prohibition Work Better," in *The American Drug Scene,* edited by J. A. Inciardi and K. McElrath (Los Angeles: Roxbury Publishing Company, 2004).
96. P. J. Fite, C. R. Colder, J. E. Lochman, and K. C. Wells, "The Relation Between Childhood Proactive and Reactive Aggression and Substance Use Initiation," *Journal of Abnormal Child Psychology,* 36 (April 2008): 261–271.
97. T. M. Moore et al., "Drug Abuse and Aggression between Intimate Partners: A Meta-Analytic Review," *Clinical Psychology Review,* 28 (February 2008): 248–275.

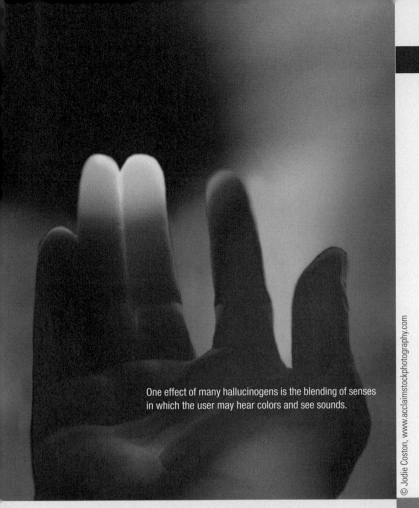

One effect of many hallucinogens is the blending of senses in which the user may hear colors and see sounds.

FACT OR FICTION?

1. Hallucinogens act as stimulants on the central nervous system.
2. Besides the U.S. military, the Russian military is also believed to have experimented with hallucinogens.
3. LSD has been shown to be as addictive as heroin.
4. Among adolescents, the ethnic group most likely to use hallucinogens is Asian.
5. At twice its normal dosage, LSD is fatal.
6. At one time hallucinogenic drugs were associated with witchcraft and sorcery.
7. The psychological effects of psilocybin are more powerful than the psychological effects of LSD.
8. Jimsonweed, which can result in poisoning, is illegal throughout the United States.
9. The effects of PCP are very similar to the effects of ketamine (Special K).
10. More high school seniors use PCP than ketamine annually.

Turn the page to check your answers

13 Hallucinogens

Chapter Objectives

After completing this chapter, the reader should be able to describe:

- Events that led to the popularization of LSD
- Whether LSD affects creativity
- Experiments with LSD conducted by the U.S. government
- The physiological and psychological effects of LSD
- Side effects associated with mescaline and psilocybin
- How various hallucinogenic drugs affect pregnancy
- The role of hallucinogens during the Middle Ages
- How hallucinogens were used for medical purposes
- The emergence of Salvinorin A
- Physiological and psychological effects of ketamine (Special K) and PCP

FACT OR FICTION?

1. **Fiction:** The fact is—hallucinogens do not increase or decrease central nervous system activity.
2. **Fact:** Although the evidence is not conclusive, it appears as though the Russian military gave hallucinogens to prisoners.
3. **Fiction:** The fact is—despite its powerful effects, LSD does not result in addiction.
4. **Fiction:** The fact is—White adolescents are more likely to use hallucinogens than Asian, Black, or Hispanic adolescents.
5. **Fiction:** The fact is—although one may die from behaviors while under the influence of LSD, one does not die from the pharmacological effects of LSD.
6. **Fact:** Numerous hallucinogenic drugs have been applied to the practices of witchcraft and sorcery.
7. **Fiction:** The fact is—LSD's psychological effects are more potent than the psychological effects of psilocybin.
8. **Fiction:** The fact is—currently, jimsonweed is illegal in several states, but the U.S. government has not declared jimsonweed illegal.
9. **Fact:** The chemical structure and the effects of PCP and ketamine are very similar.
10. **Fiction:** The fact is—in 2008 1.1% of high school seniors used PCP and 1.5% of high school seniors used ketamine.

Ever since the beginning of time, humans have sought ways to alter their consciousness. Through trial and error, certain plants were identified as having mind-altering properties. The efforts of early humans were simplified in that an estimated 6,000 different types of plants are capable of altering consciousness.[1] Today about 150 plants are used for hallucinogenic purposes. Although it is not a plant, lysergic acid diethylamide (LSD) is one of the most potent hallucinogens. Scientific interest in hallucinogenic drugs increased after World War II. The availability of mind-altering drugs was (and still is) vast.

Terminology

Terms referring to hallucinogens can be confusing because many terms have been used to describe drugs with hallucinogenic characteristics. The word **hallucinogen** refers to drugs that have the potential to produce hallucinations. Generally, these are chemicals that alter thoughts, feelings, and perceptions. Many of these result in hallucinations only when they are taken in large quantities. Some drugs classified as hallucinogens produce no hallucinations; conversely, some drugs not classified as hallucinogens can induce hallucinations.

Terms Describing Hallucinogens

- **phantasticants**: Drugs having stimulating and inebriating properties
- **psychedelic:** Mind-manifesting
- **psychotomimetic**: Psychotic-like
- **psychotogenic**: Psychosis-generating

Lewis Lewin called hallucinogens **phantasticants** because of their "stimulating and inebriating properties" and their importance to research and science.[2] During the era of tie-dyed shirts, antiwar protests, flower power, Woodstock, acid rock, and political activism, the term **psychedelic**, or "mind-manifesting," was in vogue. Coined by British psychiatrist Humphrey Osmond in 1956, the word referred to the mind-altering properties of naturally occurring hallucinogenic plant substances.[3]

Because hallucinogens reportedly produced psychotic-like symptoms, they also were called **psychotomimetic**. *Psychoto* means "psychosis," and *mimetic* translates into "acting-like." Another term used to describe these drugs is **psychotogenic**, meaning "psychosis-generating." Current research is examining the role of LSD and other drugs as a cause of schizophrenia.[4] Ironically, LSD is now also being studied as a treatment for schizophrenia.[5]

The Origin of Hallucinogens

Almost all drugs that have hallucinogenic properties are derived from plants. Two exceptions are LSD and methylene-dioxymethamphetamine (MDMA), which are produced synthetically. Swiss chemist Albert Hofmann developed LSD as a possible headache remedy in 1938 and discovered its hallucinogenic capabilities accidentally 5 years later. The following passage is the chemist's description of his own initial experience with LSD.

Last Friday, April 16, 1943, I was forced to interrupt my work in the laboratory in the middle of the afternoon and proceed home, being affected by a remarkable restlessness, combined with a slight dizziness. At home I lay down and sank into a not unpleasant intoxicated-like condition, characterized by an extremely stimulated imagination. In a dreamlike state, with eyes closed (I found the daylight to be unpleasantly glaring), I perceived an uninterrupted stream of fantastic pictures, extraordinary shapes with intense, kaleidoscopic play of colors. After some two hours this condition faded away.[6]

The Search for Hallucinogens

Humans' early search for mind-altering drugs has been described in the following way:

> Agents that cause visual, auditory, tactile, taste and other hallucinations or that induce artificial psychoses have been undoubtedly used since earliest human experimentation with the vegetal environment.[7]

These drugs were thought to be consumed primarily for their psychic, not their physical, effects. People took them to escape their everyday existence, to commune with a higher order.

Psychic, sacred, and medicinal powers were attributed to these drugs. Hallucinogens change awareness of reality. They alter perceptions of time, spirituality, and the universe, helping people transcend boundaries of time and space. Mind-altering drugs were central in many Eastern religions, where they were used to achieve religious revelations. Hallucinogenic drugs were used throughout Central and South America, as well as by the ancient Greeks and Romans. More recently, methods of altering one's concepts of time and space involve activities that do not use drugs—such as music, chanting, meditation, and computer games.

Amanita muscaria

One of the earliest and most common hallucinogens is the mushroom ***Amanita muscaria***, also called **fly agaric**. In India 3,500 years ago, the *Rig Veda,* an ancient Hindu book, contained an elaborate description of a drug called **soma**. Soma, which was highly praised and used in religious ceremonies, was actually *Amanita muscaria.* To make them feel more fierce, Viking warriors ingested *Amanita muscaria.*[8] When traveling through Siberia, Europeans noticed villagers ingesting these mushrooms. Within an hour, the villagers would twitch, tremble, feel happy, hallucinate, dance, and then fall into a deep sleep.

Other effects of *Amanita muscaria* include lower heart rate, elevated blood pressure, constriction of pupils of the eye, and excessive perspiration and salivation. This mushroom grows throughout the United States, and it can be lethal.[9] A unique characteristic of *Amanita muscaria* is that it passes through the body and into the urine unchanged. Hence, it can be used more than once.

hallucinogens A class of drugs that induce perceived distortions in time and space

phantasticants A term used to describe hallucinogenic drugs

psychedelic A term used to describe hallucinogenic drugs; means "mind-manifesting"

psychotomimetic Refers to drugs that produce psychotic-like symptoms

psychotogenic Refers to drugs that generate psychosis

Amanita muscaria One of the oldest and most common hallucinogens; derived from the fly agaric mushroom

fly agaric Another name for the hallucinogenic mushroom *Amanita muscaria*

soma From the Greek; literally means "body"

ergotism A condition resulting from ingesting a fungus that grows on grains; marked by muscle tremors, burning, mania, delirium, hallucinations, and eventual gangrene

St. Anthony's fire Burning sensations caused by ergot poisoning; people during the Middle Ages would visit the shrine of St. Anthony in an attempt to cure it

Saint Anthony's Fire

A plant with hallucinogenic properties that was used by ancient Greeks in religious rituals is a fungus of the genus *Claviceps,* which grows on certain cereals, especially rye. One species implicated in deadly epidemics in Europe and elsewhere was *Claviceps purpurea,* the ergot of rye.[10] Reports of ergot poisoning—**ergotism**—killing thousands of people surfaced during the Middle Ages. Ergotism is marked by hallucinations, convulsions, epileptic symptoms, and delirium; gangrene leading to occasional loss of nose, ears, fingers, toes, and feet; and possible death. Pregnant women would miscarry after ingesting this poisonous fungus.

The epidemic was called the "Holy Fire," because people had burning sensations in their hands and feet. To end the destruction, people went on pilgrimages to the shrine of Saint Anthony, the patron saint of fire, epilepsy, and infection. The epidemics, which came to be known as **St. Anthony's fire**, ended with a change in diet that excluded rye. Incidents of ergotism have been reported as recently as 1953.

Ergot poisoning might have played a role in allegations of witchcraft in colonial New England. Young girls who appeared to be suffering from a witch's *spell* may have ingested the ergot fungus. The inability to explain the source of the girls' odd behavior led to accusations of witchcraft in Salem in the 1690s. It was from this fungus that Albert Hofmann extracted LSD in 1938.

The U.S. Experience

LSD did not reach the United States until 1949, when it was used initially to study mental illness, then later used by psychotherapists with their patients, by musicians and artists to enhance their creativity, and by government officials to determine its effectiveness as a mind-control agent.

Later, the drug was woven into certain segments of society. The nonmedical, unregulated use of LSD and the illicit use that followed began to cause much concern. We will look first at mental health uses and the related study of LSD, then its use to enhance creativity, and finally the governmental interventions and impact on the culture.

LSD and Mental Health

In 1953, the U.S. Food and Drug Administration (FDA) approved a request by the Sandoz Pharmaceutical Company to register LSD as a new drug for investigative purposes. One of the first uses of LSD was to study mental illness, especially schizophrenia. Because LSD causes hallucinations, and people with schizophrenia hallucinate, the researchers believed that studying the effects of LSD on the brain would be helpful. Patients under the influence of LSD would serve as models for studying schizophrenia. This line of research was abandoned because people who were given LSD did not have the disordered thinking pattern found in schizophrenics, and LSD produces visual hallucinations, whereas schizophrenics have auditory hallucinations.

Many psychiatrists gave their patients LSD and other hallucinogens to help them develop personal insight and to recall forgotten or repressed experiences. Initial results were promising. Some patients credited LSD with giving them peace of mind after taking it during therapy. Patients who took LSD were less defensive, responded more effectively to their counselors, and exhibited positive emotional responses.

LSD was given to terminally ill cancer patients to help them cope with the specter of death and to other patients to alleviate stress and psychosomatic illnesses. Studies in the 1960s reported that LSD helped terminally ill patients adjust to their impending death and enabled them to be more responsive to their families.[11] LSD was also used in the treatment of autism from 1959 to 1974, although the research was inconclusive.[12] In addition, LSD was used to treat heroin addiction, sexual deviance, sexual dysfunction, and alcoholism. Despite the early studies demonstrating that LSD was helpful in treating alcoholism, subsequent studies found it to be ineffective; after LSD treatment ended, many alcoholics returned to active drinking.[13]

By 1965, an estimated 40,000 patients in psychotherapy had received LSD.[14] Despite indications that LSD could benefit individuals in psychotherapy and terminally ill patients, its use was discontinued because of negative publicity. In the mid-1960s the number of research projects examining the therapeutic uses of LSD dropped from more than 70 to 6.[15] The political climate and potential risks deterred psychiatrists from using LSD in therapy, and Sandoz Pharmaceutical Company ended its production of LSD.

Presently, LSD and other hallucinogens have no accepted medical uses. However, there is ongoing research into whether LSD and other hallucinogens are effective with obsessive-compulsive behaviors, post-traumatic stress disorder, and addiction to narcotics.[16] Other research is focusing on the use of hallucinogens for alcoholism and for anxiety in individuals dying from cancer.[17] The basis for using hallucinogens for studying mental illness is that the drugs may help an individual to lose control of typical thought patterns, enabling the person to work through thoughts of depression and obsessiveness.[18]

LSD and Creativity

Because LSD affects perception strongly, some people, especially artists, believe it enhances creativity. A limitation in determining whether LSD has such effects is that creativity is subjective and thus difficult to measure (one person's scribbling may be another person's masterpiece): "Capturing the elusive elements of a creative act is like trying to weigh a pound of leaping mice."[19]

Objectively, LSD does not seem to improve creativity, although artists who take it largely seem to enjoy its effects. Although LSD will not make a good artist a great artist, it might make that artist more capable of expanding his or her creativity. Artists believe that the perceptual changes from LSD have a profound, positive effect, creating a sense of confusion and disorganization that they view as desirable.[20] In another study, though, many artists believed that their drawing skills vastly diminished while they were under the influence of LSD.[21]

LSD and Government Experiments

Research with LSD and other hallucinogens was conducted at the Edgewood Arsenal in Maryland in the early 1950s. Mind-control experiments by the Russians and Chinese prompted the U.S. Central Intelligence Agency (CIA) and other agencies to conduct their own experiments to assess whether LSD could control the mind and serve as a truth serum. The CIA gave LSD to about 1,500 military personnel.[22] These experiments were not always performed on willing participants, and sometimes the results were tragic.

LSD (lysergic acid diethylamide) A powerful hallucinogen derived from a fungus

psilocybin A hallucinogen found in certain mushrooms in Central America

One unfortunate incident involved a government scientist named Frank Olson. In 1953, the CIA gave LSD to Olson without his knowledge. He experienced a psychotic response and was transported from Maryland to New York City to be hospitalized. The evening before he was to be hospitalized, Olson jumped to his death from a hotel's 10th-story window. The circumstances of Olson's death were not disclosed until 1975, whereupon his family was awarded $750,000. (Similarly, the British government agreed to compensate many of its servicemen who were given LSD without their consent in the 1950s.[23])

In another project, prostitutes in San Francisco were given LSD unknowingly to evaluate the drug's effect on their sexual activities and experiences and on their patrons. The prostitutes and their customers were watched through a two-way mirror.[24] LSD was given to drug addicts also, but the treatment was proven not to be effective.

LSD and the U.S. Culture

Beginning in the early 1960s, hallucinogens became more integrated into American society. Nonmedical interest in LSD was not spurred simply by the desire to achieve euphoria; people took drugs such as LSD as a means of dealing with society and its inherent problems. In his book *LSD: My Problem Child*, Hofmann stated that the appeal of the drug stemmed from

> . . . materialism, alienation from nature through industrialization and increasing urbanization, lack of satisfaction in professional employment in a mechanized, lifeless working world, ennui and purposelessness in a wealthy, saturated society, and lack of a religious, nurturing, and meaningful philosophical foundation of life.[25]

As a result of research by Timothy Leary at Harvard University, interest in hallucinogens grew. While vacationing in Mexico, Leary and some colleagues took "magic mushrooms" and found the experience enlightening. After this experience, Leary and his associate Richard Alpert studied the psychological effects of **psilocybin**, a hallucinogenic mushroom, on humans. They later examined the effects of LSD on humans.

Leary and Alpert believed that LSD and other hallucinogens were psychologically and spiritually beneficial. They gave these drugs to convicts reentering society, to students, and to theologians. Some people thought their research lost its scientific objectivity, and the two subsequently were fired from Harvard. Leary went on to form the League of Spiritual Discovery, whose acronym is LSD.

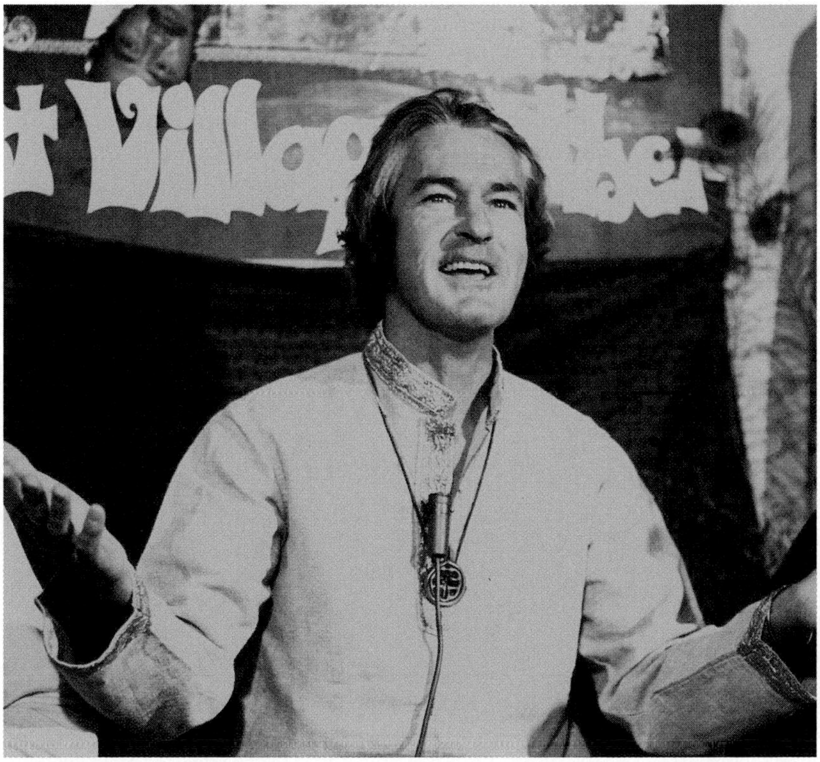

Around the time Leary was involved with LSD, a young writer on the West Coast named Ken Kesey was experimenting with LSD, too. As a graduate student at Stanford University, Kesey participated in research at a nearby hospital in which he was paid to take various hallucinogens. At the same time, Kesey was working at a mental hospital. During the time he was participating in the research and working at the mental hospital, Kesey wrote the critically acclaimed book *One Flew over the Cuckoo's Nest.* He and a group of friends, the "Merry Pranksters," traveled around the United States promoting drugs such as LSD and marijuana.

As the popularity of LSD grew, so did the negative publicity.

Timothy Leary helped to popularize the use of LSD in the early 1960s.

LSD was linked to chromosome damage, brain damage, insanity, suicide, homicide, and other acts of violence. By the end of the 1960s, interest in LSD had waned. In 1965 LSD became an illegal drug.

Review of Major Hallucinogens

The number of hallucinogenic drugs is quite extensive. People go to considerable lengths to find new ways to alter their consciousness. For example, some people in the United States, Canada, Australia, and South and Central America engage in "toad licking," an activity in which they orally ingest glandular secretions or smoke the dried skin of the **bufo** toad. Prior research into the hallucinogenic effects of licking the bufo toad and other toads indicated that it had little effect.

In this section we will review the better-known hallucinogens, with emphasis on their psychological and physiological effects. Notwithstanding the scarcity of clinical research into the effects of hallucinogens on humans, a review of the studies found little evidence of long-term neuropsychological deficits.[26] The research, however, has not been conducted over a long time. Also, people who use hallucinogens tend to use other drugs as well, confounding the research results. Most of the research on humans took place before the mid-1960s, when Congress prohibited the public use and sale of LSD, peyote, mescaline, and similar drugs.

LSD

Of all known hallucinogens, none is more powerful than LSD. Whereas dosages of most drugs are measured in milligrams, or one-thousandth of a gram, dosages of LSD are measured in micrograms, or one-millionth of a gram. LSD produces profound effects on perception and mood.

Tolerance develops rapidly. Thus, people cannot experience the effects of LSD if they have taken it within the previous 3 or 4 days. Also, cross-tolerance between LSD and other hallucinogens occurs.[27] LSD, which is consumed orally, is absorbed through the gastrointestinal tract, metabolized by the liver, and quickly excreted. LSD has no taste, color, or odor.

LSD is taken differently today than when it was first introduced. In the 1960s, it came in the form of a cube or tablet. Today it consists of microdots, or diluted drops that typically are placed on blotter paper and licked. Its effects begin within an hour. Behavioral effects last 6 to 8 hours, but LSD has a half-life of only 3 hours. Hence, the effects last longer than the drug is active. LSD is detectable in urine up to 72 hours after ingestion. Despite adverse publicity, no fatal overdoses are documented. People have died as a result of their behavior while on LSD, such as jumping out of windows, but not from its pharmacological effects.

Since 1997, the use of LSD and other hallucinogens by secondary school students has declined, although there was a slight increase from 2007 to 2008. Figure 13.1 shows the percentage of high school seniors who used LSD during the past year and past month.[28] The U.S. Department of Defense recently decided to cease testing service members for LSD because so few were testing positive, suggesting a low rate of use in this population as well.[29]

LSD operates on the neurotransmitter serotonin in the brain, but little is known about its precise actions. Serotonin plays a role in sensory perception and mood. As potent as LSD is, its physiological effects, which begin about 20 minutes after ingestion, are rather mild and brief. These effects include dilation of the pupils of the eye, tachycardia, a slight rise in blood pressure and body temperature, dry mouth, slight tremors, increased salivation, fatigue, stimulation of uterine contractions, muscle weakness, twitching, numbness, dizziness, and occasionally nausea. Because LSD can stimulate uterine contractions, pregnant women should avoid it.

Although LSD causes chromosome damage, it is just one of the many drugs, including aspirin, that do so. On closer examination, study subjects who have taken LSD have been found to have taken amphetamines, tranquilizers, or heroin at the same time. Thus, to identify LSD as the drug responsible for chromosome damage is not possible. The same is true with studies claiming that women taking LSD gave birth to highly deformed babies and had a higher rate of miscarriage and premature delivery. These women

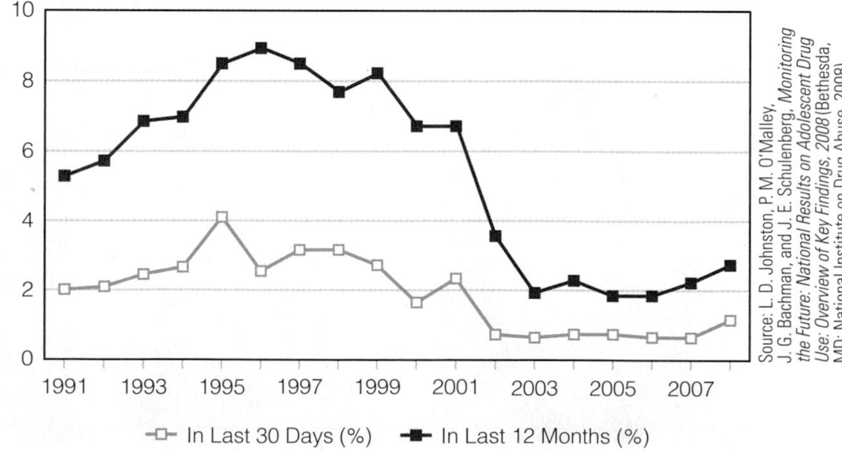

Figure 13.1 Percentages of High School Seniors Who Used LSD

Physiological Effects of LSD

- Dilation of pupils
- Increased blood pressure
- Dry mouth
- Increased salivation
- Twitching
- Dizziness
- Rapid heartbeat
- Slight tremors
- Higher body temperature
- Fatigue
- Muscle weakness
- Numbness
- Nausea
- Uterine contractions

were likely to have used other drugs as well and generally had poorer prenatal care. This does not suggest that LSD is safe but that there is not definitive proof that it is harmful.

The most significant effects of LSD are psychological, not physiological. By their nature, psychological effects are subject to interpretation. Although LSD is known to alter mood and perception, the extent to which these changes occur depends on the user's mental state, the environment in which the drug is used, previous experiences with the drug, and dosage.

Psychological changes take effect about 40 minutes after ingestion. The LSD trip consists of the following three distinct phases:

1. The first phase, lasting 1 to 2 hours, is marked by euphoria and either crying or laughing.
2. In the second stage, 2 to 3 hours after ingestion, visual illusions and hallucinations appear.
3. The third phase, 3 to 4 hours after ingestion, is characterized by distortion of time, ego disintegration, mood swings, and occasionally panic and depression.

On Campus

Although 3.3% of college students have tried LSD, individuals of the same age who are not in college are twice as likely to have used LSD. Males in college are 1½ times more likely to have used LSD than college-aged females.

Source: *Monitoring the Future: National Survey Results on Drug Use, 1975–2007.*

bufo A type of toad that produces a hallucinogenic secretion

synesthesia The hallucinogenic blending of senses (e.g., seeing sounds and hearing color)

flashbacks A phenomenon in which a person re-experiences the effects of LSD days, weeks, or months after it was last used

Synesthesia, the blending of senses in which the person hears or tastes colors and sees sounds, is one outcome of LSD. Depersonalization and disorientation are other effects. Body image may be distorted, or the user might have feelings of becoming one with the floor or whatever he or she is sitting or lying on. A user may conjure repressed memories or have a psychotic reaction lasting weeks or months. Others say that they experience mystical or religious encounters.

Although some people find changes in perception and sensation desirable, others find these changes frightening. Fear or panic can lead to a "bad trip." A person having a bad trip must be reassured that the effects are temporary and that he or she will not be left alone. A helpful person should *not* restrain this person physically. A bad trip is more likely to occur with inexperienced users and people with preexisting psychological problems. Bad trips seem to be affected by the set and setting when taking LSD. When medical intervention is necessary, major tranquilizers are administered.

Another phenomenon associated with LSD is a **flashback** in which the person reexperiences the effects of LSD days, weeks, or even months after last using it. There is no consensus on how often flashbacks occur. What causes flashbacks has not been determined conclusively, but they might be precipitated by stress or fatigue. An interesting finding is that flashbacks were less likely to occur among people who took LSD in a therapeutic or research setting rather than in a recreational setting.[30] If a flashback occurs, it tends to be brief. The frequency and duration of flashbacks are unpredictable.[31]

Possible Psychological Effects of LSD

- Time distortion
- Ego disintegration
- Depression
- Fear
- Mood swings
- Panic
- Blending of senses
- Flashbacks

Peyote

Peyote is a hallucinogen the Aztec Indians used for religious rituals. The Spanish conquerors, however, condemned it for its "satanic trickery." Peyote comes from the *Lophophora williamsii* cactus. This small, spineless cactus, measuring about 3 inches in diameter, is found in Mexico and Texas. Its psychoactive agent, **mescaline**, is named after the Mescalero Apaches. Users dry the crown of the cactus, suck it, and swallow. Chemically, mescaline produces effects similar to those of norepinephrine. An increase in norepinephrine causes excitation and increased motor activity whereas a decrease in norepinephrine causes depression. Interestingly, the alcoholic drink named Mezcal contains no mescaline.

The dried cactus is known as a "mescal button." Preparation of mescal buttons is difficult because of their foul odor, and ingesting them is unpleasant because of the rancorous taste. Users initially experience nausea, vomiting, and diarrhea, which often deter continued use. In small doses, mescaline produces euphoria. In larger doses, it generates striking hallucinations involving intense colors, tastes, and feelings.

Compared with LSD, peyote is less intense and more manageable. Peyote intoxication consists of the following two stages:

1. Contentment and sensitivity
2. Great calm, muscular sluggishness, and a shift of attention from external stimuli to introspection and meditation

Mescaline is used medically to treat patients with angina pectoris, and it is used as a respiratory stimulant for patients with pneumonia. Some scientists had promising results when they gave peyote to alcoholics.[32] Peyote may be beneficial in treating cluster headaches. This type of headache usually occurs around the same time and in the same spot on a regular basis.[33]

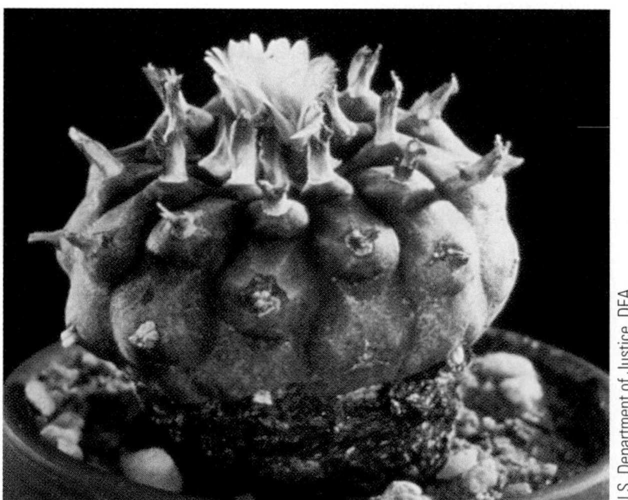

U.S. Department of Justice, DEA.

The peyote cactus is found in Mexico and in Texas.

Peyote takes effect within 30 to 90 minutes and stays in the body about 10 hours, although the hallucinations last only 2 hours. Peyote is eliminated from the body primarily in the urine. Physiological effects include dilation of the pupils, a rise in body temperature, and increases in blood pressure and heart rate. Fatalities from its use have not been documented, although a person could die from behaviors while taking the drug. Some experts believe that peyote may cause paranoid schizophrenia. Nonetheless, peyote is sold legally in Ireland.[34]

Mescaline is similar to LSD in that tolerance forms quickly, but physical dependence does not occur. There is cross-tolerance between mescaline and LSD. Synthetic mescaline can be made into a liquid, capsule, or tablet and is more palatable than natural mescaline, but synthesizing mescaline is difficult. What is sold on the streets as mescaline is commonly another drug, such as LSD.

In the early 1800s, the Apaches, Kiowas, and Commanches chewed mescal buttons and incorporated their use into their religious practices. Until 1990, members of the Native American Church, composed of several North American Indian tribes, used peyote legally in the United States for spiritual reasons. Church members considered the use of peyote a sacrament, and recreational or social use was not permitted. It is also thought that spiritual use of peyote can foster health, respect, and a sense of community.[35]

In a 6-to-3 vote, the U.S. Supreme Court ruled that individual states could forbid peyote use for religious purposes. In 2004, however, the Utah Supreme Court ruled that members of the Native American Church could use peyote without being prosecuted.[36] Other groups who claim that drugs such as peyote or marijuana are part of their religious experience have been denied legal permission to use illegal drugs.[37] With the Supreme Court decision, protection of religious freedom under the First Amendment no longer extended to sacramental use of peyote. According to Justice Antonin Scalia, "We have never held that an individual's religious beliefs excuse him from compliance with an otherwise valid law prohibiting conduct that the State is free to regulate."

Psilocybin

A drug that seems to be making a resurgence in the United States is magic mushrooms or "shrooms." The Aztecs called mushrooms containing psilocybin **teonanacatl**, which translates into "God's flesh." This drug was spiritually significant to the Aztecs, but the Spaniards tried to squelch the religious use of mushrooms after overtaking the natives.

Several species of mushrooms containing psilocybin grow in parts of the United States, Mexico, and Europe. In 1958, Albert Hofmann isolated the psychoactive ingredient. In the early 1960s, psilocybin use increased on many college campuses, but its popularity waned when LSD became more prominent.

Psilocybin is similar chemically to LSD, although its effects are shorter and are not as intense. Psilocybin can be consumed orally in the form of dried mushrooms, by drinking a beverage containing the mushrooms, or in tablet form. Also, it can be ground up and added to foods. After psilocybin is ingested, a stomach enzyme converts it into **psilocin**.

Psilocybin is more potent than mescaline but less toxic. As with mescaline and LSD, no fatal overdoses from psilocybin have been recorded. A person can die from ingesting other types of mushrooms, though, and it is easy to mistake a poisonous mushroom for psilocybin.

In small doses (4 mg), psilocybin brings about feelings of euphoria and relaxation. Higher doses distort perceptions of time and space, and the user is distracted more easily and is open to suggestion. In a 2006 study at Johns Hopkins University on the effects of the hallucinogen psilocybin, individuals given this drug rated their experience very positively. Although some participants experienced anxiety, others claimed they had a mystical-type experience.[38] The hallucinations produced by psilocybin are both visual and auditory. Psilocybin also interferes with the ability to concentrate. Like peyote, psilocybin has an unpleasant taste.

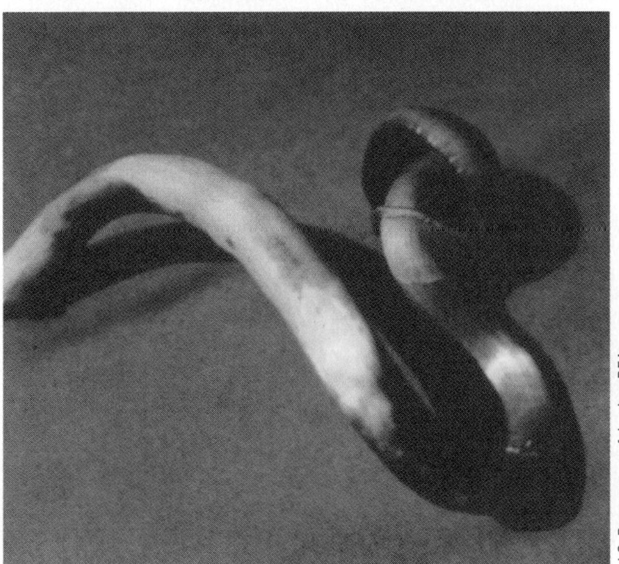

U.S. Department of Justice, DEA.

Mushrooms containing psilocybin grow in parts of the United States, Mexico, and Europe.

peyote A cactus containing the hallucinogen mescaline

mescaline A psychoactive agent or hallucinogen that is derived from the peyote cactus

teonanacatl Aztec word describing the psylocybe mushroom

psilocin The psychoactive ingredient in the psylocybe mushroom

Potential Effects of Psilocybin

- Euphoria
- Easily distracted
- Difficulty concentrating
- Elevated body temperature
- Pulse rate increases
- Wide range of emotions
- Involuntary movement of limbs
- Relaxation
- Open to suggestion
- Pupils dilate
- Blood pressure increases
- Muscle relaxation
- Hallucinations

Psilocybin dilates the pupils and raises body temperature, pulse rate, and blood pressure. Involuntary movement of arms and legs and muscle relaxation may follow use. The drug is capable of producing an array of emotional responses, ranging from uncontrolled laughter to depression. The user experiences hallucinogenic effects within 30 minutes, and these last 3 to 8 hours. Psilocybin has no current medical use, although research is being conducted into whether psilocybin can help to understand schizophrenia. Also, it has been found that psilocybin may reduce the effects of alcohol when they are taken simultaneously.

Salvinorin A

A relatively new hallucinogen is salvinorin A. Derived from the sage family, this drug has been used in traditional spiritual practices by Mazatec Indians in Oaxaca, Mexico, to produce mystical or hallucinogenic experiences. The drug, known sometimes as Salvia, is nicknamed Sally-D, Magic Mint, and Diviner's Sage.[39] Although salvinorin A is not yet illegal in the United States, it is illegal in Denmark, Australia, Belgium, and Italy. Several states such as Missouri, Delaware, North Dakota, and Illinois have banned the drug.[40]

Information about salvinorin A is spreading. There are a number of YouTube videos showing young people on the drug. Because of its increasing popularity, the Drug Enforcement Agency is studying whether to ban it, and the federal government has placed the drug on its list of drugs of concern. It is believed that an increasing number of young people are discovering this drug through the Internet and smoke shops, and an estimated 750,000 Americans ages 12 and older have tried salvinorin A in the past year.[41] A study at a public university in the southwest United States reported that 4.4% of students had tried salvinorin A at least once in the previous 12 months.[42] In Canada, a number of smoke shops sell salvinorin A, and the price ranges from $15 to $100.[43]

When smoked, salvinorin A produces a psychoactive effect that has been shown to begin within a minute and to last up to 15 minutes.[44] Like other hallucinogens, salvinorin A alters human consciousness and perception.[45] According to some individuals, its potency rivals that of LSD.[46] It is speculated that the study of salvinorin A may be beneficial in developing drugs that treat schizophrenia, Alzheimer's disease, and bipolar disorder.[47] However, research into the effects of long-term medical and recreational use of the drug is limited.[48]

Anticholinergic Hallucinogens

Plants containing **anticholinergic hallucinogens** include belladonna, datura, henbane, and mandrake. These drugs belong to the potato and tomato families and have a long, rich history involving sorcery and witchcraft. The effects of henbane are similar to those of the mandrake root. They have been used as medicines, poisons, and beauty aids. Besides producing hallucinations, these drugs can be highly toxic in large doses. In the 1970s, anticholinergic drugs were found in many over-the-counter (OTC) preparations including Sominex, Contac, Donnagel (for diarrhea), Travel-eze (for motion sickness), and Endotussin (cough syrup). Since the 1980s, anticholinergic drugs have been removed from OTC medications.

Belladonna

"Beautiful lady" in Italian, **belladonna** was used to increase the size of the pupils and produce a glassy effect on the eyes, which was considered desirable. Also known as **deadly nightshade**, it may have been used during the Middle Ages in witches' brews and satanic rituals. It consists of bluish black, soft berries called "love apples," because belladonna was believed to be an aphrodisiac. This plant is found in parts of Europe, North Africa, and Asia.

Reportedly, belladonna gives a person the feeling of flying, which explains its association with witches and broomsticks. The sensation of flying probably is derived from the irregular heartbeat and drowsiness that accompany its use. In addition to its potent hallucinogenic properties, belladonna can be extremely toxic. Consuming slightly more than a dozen berries can be fatal.

Datura

One species of **datura** plant, *Datura stramonium*, is known as **locoweed** or **Jamestown weed (jimsonweed)**. American Indians used this species in many rituals. In one peculiar use, it was thought that a person under the influence of datura would have a vision in which the person who stole an object would be revealed and the location of the object would be identified.

Also, datura was used as a rite of passage from childhood to adulthood. Algonquin Indians gave it to adolescent boys, who hallucinated for several days without recollecting the experience later.

Indications are that datura was used in China, Greece, India, and Africa. The Chinese used it for medical purposes, and in India it was included in love potions. Datura was used to treat asthma, epilepsy, delirium tremens, rheumatism, and menstrual pains. Because its side effects are potentially harmful and noxious, it seldom is used recreationally. Allegedly, in Haiti, datura is one ingredient of zombie powder, a substance that is supposed to induce a zombie-like state. Datura holds special magical and religious significance to North American and Central American Indians.

Because jimsonweed is readily available and inexpensive, its recreational use is increasing. In 2005, poison centers reported 975 incidents involving jimsonweed and other anticholinergic plants.[49] Physical effects of jimsonweed poisoning include dry mouth, burning thirst, dry skin, constipation, amnesia, dilated eyes in which bright lights are painful, inability to focus the eyes, rapid pulse, and difficulty urinating. Mental effects include restlessness, disorientation, delirium, and vivid hallucinations.[50] Symptoms appear within 30 to 60 minutes after ingestion or smoking and may last for 24 to 48 hours. The effects can be as severe as coma and death.

Mandrake

Because the root of the **mandrake** plant resembles a human body, it has been valued for its medicinal and supernatural properties and had a reputation as an aphrodisiac. The word *mandrake* means "potent male." This powerful and toxic plant grows in southern Europe, North Africa, western Asia, and the Himalayas.

Like belladonna, mandrake belongs to the nightshade family. In ancient Egypt, the mandrake plant and the water lily were used for inducing trances and in healing rituals. In Europe during the Middle Ages, its use was associated with witchcraft, sorcery, and superstition. Europeans feared and respected the mandrake. Its effects include mental confusion, increased heart rate, dilation of the pupils, dry mouth, hallucinations, and amnesia.

Two psychoactive drugs found in mandrake and other anticholinergic hallucinogens are **scopolamine** and **atropine**. In small doses, these drugs induce euphoria, feelings of sedation, disorientation, slurred speech, silly behavior, confusion, fatigue, and dreamless sleep. Other effects are vomiting, malaise, and excessive perspiration and salivation. In large amounts, mandrake can cause coma and death. Psychological and physical dependence on both drugs is uncommon.

Scopolamine formerly was given to women during childbirth. Because it causes amnesia, the medical profession thought that women would not remember labor pains. Women given scopolamine, however, often had hallucinations or delirium, so this practice was discontinued. Scopolamine has been used to treat motion sickness.[51] Atropine is used to dilate the pupils and lessen lung congestion (especially during surgery) and is an antidote for poisoning from some insecticides.

Scopolamine has been used for unscrupulous motives. Purportedly, prostitutes would slip it into the drink of a client, who then would fall into a stupor. The victim would be robbed and would have difficulty recalling what had happened.

Nutmeg and Mace

The Arabs introduced nutmeg into Europe as a medicine in the first century. It was used to treat heart disease, tuberculosis, digestive problems, kidney troubles, asthma, and fever. Though nutmeg is used without effect in food preparations, it can induce visual and auditory hallucinations if consumed in large quantities. It distorts time and space and creates a sense of detachment from reality.

Nutmeg is made from seeds of the Myristica tree, and mace comes from the fruit of the same tree. Nutmeg and mace are chemically similar to mescaline. Nutmeg is chewed or snuffed with tobacco. **Myristicin**, found in nutmeg and mace, is capable of producing an effect if 1 to 2 teaspoons are consumed, but it takes 2 to 5 hours before the effects are felt. Nutmeg and mace are not taken for hallucinogenic reasons because their unpleasant side effects include nausea, severe headache, vomiting, tachycardia, and sensory distortion, followed by an extremely noxious hangover.

Dimethyltryptamine

Dimethyltryptamine (DMT) is derived from the leaves, bark, and seeds of various plants grown in South and Central America that contain that substance. People used DMT for spiritual purposes in these regions, communicating with the spirits to cure illness. Natives using DMT would snort or blow it into each other's noses. In Brazil, DMT is found in the psychoactive beverage called ayahuasca.[52]

anticholinergic hallucinogens Substances found in datura and in Amanita muscaria mushrooms; interfere with the action of acetylcholine to produce hallucinations

belladonna (deadly nightshade) A potent hallucinogen found in Europe, North Africa, and Asia; member of the tomato and potato family

datura A hallucinogen used for sacred purposes in ancient China, Greece, India, and Africa

locoweed Another term for jimsonweed

Jamestown weed (jimsonweed) A hallucinogen derived from the datura plant; also known as locoweed

mandrake A hallucinogen derived from the nightshade family; used during the Middle Ages in connection with witchcraft and sorcery

scopolamine A psychoactive agent found in mandrake and other anticholinergic hallucinogens

atropine A psychoactive agent found in mandrake and other anticholinergic hallucinogens

myristicin Substance found in nutmeg and mace; chemically similar to mescaline and capable of producing hallucinations

dimethyltryptamine (DMT) A hallucinogen in which effects last 1 to 2 hours

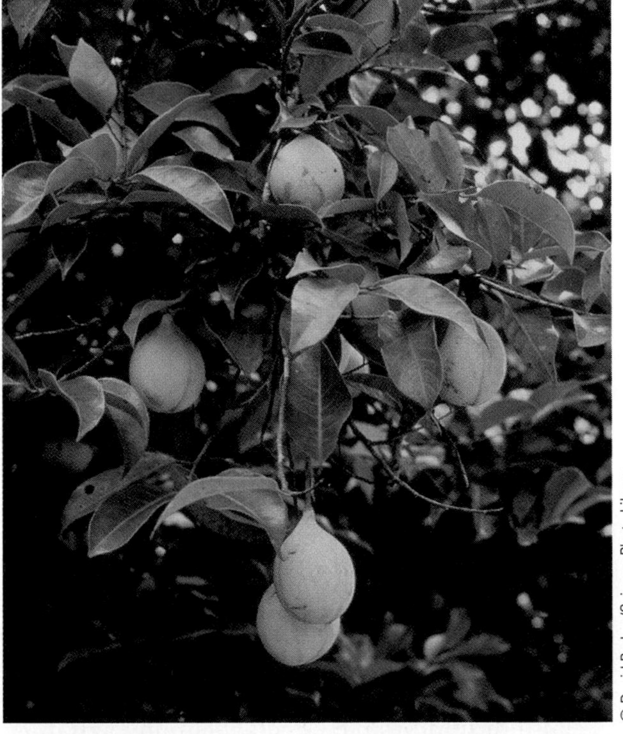

Nutmeg (the seed from the fruit of the Myristica fragrans *tree) and mace (the lacy membrane around the seed) contain small amounts of chemicals that may produce hallucinations.*

DMT was first synthesized in 1931. During the 1960s, DMT was called the "businessman's LSD," presumably because of the segment of the population that used it. The hallucinogenic effects last 1 to 2 hours. Euphoria and behavioral stimulation are associated with DMT. The drug may result in a psychotic episode, although long-term psychosis is not likely to occur when the drug is used on an occasional basis.[53] Unlike other hallucinogens, tolerance to DMT does not develop. DMT has been studied to determine whether it helps people recover from alcohol and other drug abuse, but it was not proven effective.[54]

Phencyclidine

Phencyclidine (PCP) sometimes is classified as a hallucinogen because it is capable of producing hallucinations, although the hallucinations differ from those produced by LSD. When it was developed in the 1950s, it was used as a surgical anesthetic. PCP is still used as a veterinary anesthetic outside the United States. Production of PCP in the United States became illegal in 1978.

Classifying PCP is complicated because it generates anesthetic, hallucinogenic, stimulating, or depressing effects depending on the dosage and method of administration. Some drug experts describe PCP as a **dissociative anesthetic** that causes the person to feel separated from reality.

Early Use

PCP has many nicknames, including angel dust, dust, rocket fuel, trank, and crystal. It was distributed on the West Coast in the early 1960s under the name PeaCe Pill. By the late 1960s, it was sold on the East Coast under the name "hog." When PCP first appeared in San Francisco, it was relatively popular, but its appeal declined because it induced bizarre, violent behavior.

Marketed under the name Sernyl, PCP was used originally with humans as an anesthetic. It was considered desirable for surgery, because patients remained awake yet were unable to recall their experiences because of the amnesia that PCP produced. Moreover, it had no adverse effect on circulation, heart rate, or respiration. However, it was discontinued by 1965 because of undesirable effects including agitation, delirium, and disorientation. Once the effects wore off, patients became unmanageable, confused, and disassociated from nearby surroundings. PCP later was used in veterinary medicine but has been largely replaced by similar drugs such as ketamine.

In the 1960s, when PCP was initially used on the street, it was distributed in tablet or capsule form, but it also can be injected, snorted, or smoked. When PCP was smoked, it was mixed with marijuana, tobacco, or vegetable matter. Because absorption is rapid, the effects of PCP are experienced quickly. The acute effects last 4 to 6 hours, but the user may be in a state of confusion for 8 to 24 hours. Neither tolerance nor physical dependence results, and no physical withdrawal symptoms are apparent after the person stops using the drug.

Illegal Use

Despite the unpredictable and behaviorally disruptive effects of PCP, its illegal use escalated toward the end of the 1960s and into the 1970s. Contributing to this increase was its low cost. In 1979, nearly 13% of high school seniors had tried PCP. By 1996, about 4% of seniors had tried it; in 2008, 1.8% of seniors had tried PCP.[55]

PCP frequently is used in place of other drugs such as LSD, THC, mescaline, or amphetamines. Many users view it as a desirable substitute for LSD, and it sometimes is mixed with marijuana to augment its effects. "Killer joints" and "sherms" refer to cigarettes containing PCP and marijuana.

Because PCP has a reputation for making users violent and incredibly strong, police and hospital personnel are wary of people who are using it. Media accounts have reported average-sized people breaking handcuffs, simultaneously wrestling several police officers, and being shot repeatedly before succumbing. Yet, nothing in PCP increases one's strength. Considering the fact that users are disoriented, paranoid (often the basis for violent behavior), and anesthetized, one can imagine the person failing to respond to restraints that would stop others from the same behaviors.

Effects

In small doses, PCP brings about feelings of relaxation, warmth, euphoria, and numbness; however, it interferes with concentration, distorts body image, and creates a sense of depersonalization. With increasing dosage, the user experiences confusion, poor coordination, nystagmus (irregular movement of the eyes), agitation, and impaired reaction time. With high doses, muscular rigidity, blank staring, and excessive salivation may occur. Users may have sudden mood swings and engage in repetitive actions. There is a slight increase in heart rate, blood pressure, respiration, and body temperature. In the extreme, PCP can bring about coma, seizures, and death. Dosage levels of 10 to 25 mg can be life-threatening. The synergistic effect of PCP when combined with other depressants such as alcohol and barbiturates increases its potency.

PCP can produce psychotic-like effects similar to those of schizophrenia. PCP psychosis is marked

Effects of Phencyclidine (PCP)

Small dosage

- Feelings of warmth
- Relaxation
- Poor concentration
- Depersonalization
- Nystagmus
- Agitation
- Muscle rigidity
- Sudden mood swings
- Faster heart rate
- Elevated blood pressure
- Euphoria
- Numbness
- Distorted body image
- Confusion
- Poor coordination
- Slow reaction time
- Excessive salivation
- Repetitive behavior
- Respiration
- Higher body temperature

Large dosage

- Anorexia
- Violent behavior
- Restlessness
- Suicide
- Seizures
- Paranoia
- Insomnia
- Amnesia
- Depression
- Coma
- Death

phencyclidine hydrochloride (PCP) Originally developed as an anesthetic for humans and, later, animals; also called "angel dust"

dissociative anesthetic Substance that alters the perception of pain without loss of consciousness

ketamine A drug very similar to PCP

by restlessness, memory problems, inability to eat or sleep, paranoia, and physical aggressiveness. It has been reported that recovery from PCP-induced psychosis may take 4 to 6 weeks, although current research shows that recovery may take longer.[56] PCP has been linked to suicide, drownings, and self-inflicted injuries. In recent years, treatment specialists have found that the synthetic compounds called dopamine D_3 receptor agonists may help treat PCP abusers.[57]

Ketamine

Ketamine is used in veterinary medicine in place of PCP. It is not uncommon for ketamine to be diverted from veterinarians' offices and medical supply offices.[58] Nonmedical use of ketamine, also known as Special K, K, and vitamin K, is increasing. Like PCP, ketamine is considered a dissociative anesthetic, with the user feeling separated from reality. Also, ketamine is capable of producing confusion, hallucinations, delirium, excitement, irrational behavior, muscle rigidity, tremors, respiratory depression, irregular heartbeat, loss of appetite, skin rashes, nausea, and cardiac arrest. Studies with animals demonstrate that ketamine and PCP cause significant damage to the developing fetus. In 2005, ketamine was implicated in 275 emergency room visits.[59]

Ketamine can be injected, snorted, or ingested. Its effects begin within 5 to 10 minutes and last up to an hour. Like Rohypnol and gamma-hydroxybutyrate (GHB), ketamine has been used as a date-rape drug. In combination with alcohol, it induces vomiting. Many users have reported the effects of the drug as intense and dissociative. Like cocaine, ketamine does not produce a physiological withdrawal syndrome, but some users become dependent on ketamine by demonstrating a craving for the drug.[60] In a clinical setting, ketamine is being administered to reduce the craving for heroin among addicts. Preliminary research also indicates that ketamine may be effective for treating depression.[61] So far, the drug has shown some positive results.[62]

Summary

Hallucinogens—plants capable of producing hallucinations—also have been called phantasticants, psychedelic, psychomimetic, and psychotropic. These drugs have been used for psychic purposes, to transcend boundaries of time and space, to escape from daily pressures, to communicate with a higher order, for medical reasons, and for recreation.

The FDA approved lysergic acid diethylamide (LSD) for medical use in 1953. It was used to study schizophrenia but without success. LSD also was given to alcoholics, psychiatric and terminally ill patients, and sexual deviants. Despite promising results, adverse publicity and unfounded fears that it caused brain damage brought an end to its use. Artists took LSD to enhance their creativity, but creativity is difficult to measure. The military experimented with LSD as a mind-control drug and truth serum.

On the East Coast in the 1960s, Timothy Leary popularized hallucinogens. He studied the effects of hallucinogens on personality and later formed the League of Spiritual Discovery. On the West Coast, writer Ken Kesey and his followers promoted LSD experimentation. Negative publicity caused its use to decline, and LSD was made illegal in 1965. In the last several years LSD use by high school seniors has declined further.

LSD is an extremely potent drug, capable of altering consciousness for 6 to 8 hours, though the physiological effects are short and moderate. LSD has a significant effect on mood, perception, and time. If the user experienced fear and panic, it was called a "bad trip." LSD is odorless, colorless, and tasteless. Tolerance develops rapidly, but its use is nonfatal unless the person engages in fatal behaviors while under the drug's influence. Fears of damage to chromosomes are unfounded.

Mescaline is the psychoactive ingredient in the peyote cactus. Although its effects range from euphoria to intense hallucinations lasting up to 2 hours, peyote has unpleasant side effects related to its foul odor and taste. The physiological effects are modest.

A hallucinogen gaining in popularity is psilocybin. The mushrooms that contain psylocybin are chemically similar to LSD, but their effects are shorter and less intense. Psilocybin is more powerful than mescaline. Psilocybin distorts time and space and produces feelings of euphoria, relaxation, and visual and auditory hallucinations. Some research shows that psilocybin may be effective in reducing alcohol abuse. Another hallucinogen gaining in popularity is salvinorin A.

Examples of anticholinergic hallucinogens are belladonna, datura, henbane, and mandrake. They are associated with use in sorcery and witchcraft. Belladonna, also called deadly nightshade, gives users a feeling of flying and was used to enhance beauty. Datura, better known as locoweed, was significant to North American and Central American Indians and was given to boys during rites of passage into adulthood, among other rituals. Mandrake, containing scopolamine and atropine, is said to hold special powers as an aphrodisiac. It induces euphoria, confusion, and sleep.

Nutmeg and mace are capable of producing hallucinations if they are consumed in large enough quantities. They are chemically similar to mescaline. Nutmeg is chewed or snuffed with tobacco. Because of their unpleasant side effects, however, they seldom are used recreationally.

Another hallucinogen, dimethyltryptamine (DMT), is derived from plants grown in South America and Central America. It has its origins in spiritual uses. DMT was popular briefly in the United States in the 1960s. Called the "businessman's LSD," its effects lasted just 1 to 2 hours.

Phencyclidine (PCP) can be classified as a hallucinogen, a stimulant, or a depressant because of its varying properties. PCP first was used as a human anesthetic during surgery but this was stopped as a result of undesirable effects. It later was used as an animal tranquilizer.

PCP appeared as a street drug in the 1960s but quickly fell out of favor. With small doses, users feel euphoric and relaxed, but the drug interferes with concentration, distorts body image, and can result in violent behavior. Paranoia, amnesia, restlessness, and thoughts of suicide sometimes accompany PCP use. In high doses, it can be fatal.

The effects of PCP, lasting 4 to 6 hours, are unpredictable. Many accounts describe the unusual physical strength of PCP users, but this has no scientific basis. The combination of panic and the anesthetizing effect of the drug may make PCP users difficult to control, giving the impression of incredible strength.

Ketamine, popularly known as Special K, has replaced PCP as an animal tranquilizer. Its effects are similar to those of PCP. Reportedly, ketamine has been used as a date-rape drug.

Thinking Critically

1. Currently, LSD is listed as a Schedule I drug. This means that it cannot be used for medical purposes under any circumstance. Would you support experimental use of LSD in psychotherapy? For other medical conditions? Why or why not?
2. Because LSD is nonfatal, some people consider it safe. Because it produces a powerful effect on the mind, others deem it dangerous. On what basis would you judge a drug safe or dangerous? Which is more important—physical or psychological effects? Explain.

Web Resources

Multidisciplinary Association for Psychedelic Studies (MAPS)
http://www.maps.org
This organization has been supporting psychedelic and medical marijuana research since 1986.

Substance Abuse and Mental Health Services Administration (SAMHSA)
http://www.samhsa.gov
Information regarding the trends of individuals overdosing on various drugs can be located at this site.

Partnership for a Drug-Free America
http://www.drugfree.org
This site contains extensive information on the effects of many commonly abused drugs.

Notes

1. H. E. Doweiko, *Concepts of Chemical Dependency,* 7th ed. (Pacific Grove, CA: Wadsworth, 2009).
2. D. E. Nichols, "Hallucinogens," *Pharmacology and Therapeutics,* 101 (February 2004): 131–181.
3. E. Taylor, "Psychedelics: The Second Coming," *Psychology Today* (July/August 1996): 57–591.
4. D. J. Gerber and S. Tonegawa, "Psycho-mimetic Effects of Drugs: A Common Pathway to Schizophrenia," *The New England Journal of Medicine,* 350 (2004): 1047–1048.
5. J. Duffy, "LSD Breakthrough for Mental Health Patients," *Sunday Herald,* February 24, 2008.
6. A. Hofmann, *LSD: My Problem Child* (New York: McGraw Hill, 1980), 22.
7. R. E. Schultes and A. Hofmann, *The Botany and Chemistry of Hallucinogens* (Springfield, IL: Charles C Thomas, 1973).
8. D. M. Grilly, *Drugs and Human Behavior,* 5th ed. (Boston: Allyn & Bacon, 2005).
9. J. H. Halpern, "Hallucinogens and Dissociative Agents Naturally Growing in the United States," *Pharmacology and Therapeutics,* 102 (May 2004): 131–138.
10. S. B. Karch, *The Pathology of Drug Abuse* (Boca Raton, FL: CRC Press, 2007).
11. Nichols, supra note 2.
12. J. Sigafoos, V. A. Green, C. Edrisinha, and G. E. Lancioni, "Flashback to the 1960s: LSD in the Treatment of Autism," *Developmental Neurorehabilitation,* 10 (January–March, 2007): 75–81.
13. W. L. White, *Slaying the Dragon: The History of Addiction Treatment in America* (Bloomington, IL: Chestnut Health Systems/Lighthouse Institute).
14. J. Buckman, "Theoretical Aspects of LSD Therapy," in *The Use of LSD in Psychotherapy and Alcoholism,* edited by H. Abramson (New York: Bobbs-Merrill, 1967).
15. N. Hunt, "Time to Tune in Again?" *Chemistry and Industry* (November 6, 2000): 710–721.
16. D. J. Brown, "Psychedelic Healing?" *Scientific American* (December 2007/January 2008): 67–71.
17. S. Brown, "Researchers Explore New Visions for Hallucinogens," *The Chronicle of Higher Education,* 53 (December 8, 2006): 12–15.
18. J. Cloud, "Was Timothy Leary Right? No, But New Research on Psychedelic Drugs Show Promise for Their Therapeutic Use," *Time,* 169 (April 29, 2007).
19. O. Janiger and M. Dobkin de Rios, "LSD and Creativity," *Journal of Psychoactive Drugs,* 21 (1989): 129–134.
20. Ibid.
21. S. Krippner, "Psychedelic Drugs and Creativity," *Journal of Psychoactive Drugs,* 17 (1985): 235–245.
22. L. A. Henderson, "About LSD," in *LSD: Still with Us After All These Years,* edited by L. A. Henderson and W. J. Glass (New York: Lexington Books, 1994).
23. Duffy, supra note 5.
24. Karch, supra note 10.
25. Hofmann, supra note 6.
26. J. H. Halpern and H. G. Pope, "Do Hallucinogens Cause Residual Neuropsychological Toxicity?" *Drug and Alcohol Dependence,* 53 (1999): 247–256.
27. "Hallucinogens and Dissociative Drugs," *National Institute on Drug Abuse Research Report Series* (Rockville, MD: National Institute on Drug Abuse, 2001).
28. L. D. Johnston, P. M. O'Malley, J. G. Bachman, and J. E. Schulenberg, *Monitoring the Future: National Results on Adolescent Drug Use, Overview of Key Findings, 2008* (Bethesda, MD: National Institute on Drug Abuse, 2008).
29. A. Scutro, "DoD Stops Testing Troops for LSD," *Army Times,* 68 (February 18, 2008): 26.
30. Nichols, supra note 2.
31. A. Wilde, "The Acid Test," *Cosmos,* February 2007.
32. "Study Finds No Harm in Religious Use of Peyote; Supreme Court Impact Possible," *Alcoholism and Drug Abuse Weekly,* 17 (November 14, 2005): 1–3.
33. A. Frood, "Cluster Busters," *Nature Medicine,* 13 (January 2007): 10–11.
34. F. O'Shea, "Legal! Cactus That Sends You Crazy," *The Sun* (January 9, 2007).
35. A. Frood, "Cluster Busters," *Nature Medicine,* 13 (January 2007): 10–11.
36. "Court Says Church Members May Use Peyote in Ceremonies," *Alcoholism and Drug Abuse Weekly,* 16 (July 19, 2004): 8.
37. J. Sullum, "Spiritual Highs and Legal Blows," *Reason,* 39 (June 2007): 42–54.
38. R. R. Griffiths, W. A. Richards, U. McCann, and R. Jesse, "Psilocybin Can Occasion Mystical-Type Experiences Having Substantial and Sustained Personal Meaning and Spiritual Significance," *Psychopharmacology,* 187 (2006): 268–283.
39. J. Gresko, "New Marijuana? Salvia Gains Steam," *Chicago Tribune Web Edition,* March 12, 2008.
40. S. Hoyle and A. Harris, "States Move to Ban Hallucinogen Salvia," *Stateline.org,* March 6, 2008.
41. The NSDUH Report, *Use of Specific Hallucinogens: 2006,* (Rockville, MD: Substance Abuse and Mental Health Services Administration, February 14, 2008).
42. J. E. Lange, M. B. Reed, J. M. Croff, and J. D. Clapp, "College Student Use of *Salvia Divinorum,*" *Drug and Alcohol Dependence,* 94 (April 2008): 263–266.
43. D. Hutton, "On a Magic Mint Ride; Users Say Potent—and Legal—Herb Is Safe, but Police Official Warns of All Sorts of Bad Trips," *The Toronto Sun,* February 17, 2007.
44. D. Gonzalez, J. Riba, J. C. Bouso, G. Gomez-Jarabo, and M. J. Barbanoj, "Pattern of Use and Subjective Effects of *Salvia Divinorum,*" *Drug and Alcohol Dependence,* 85 (2006): 157–162.
45. F. Yan and B. L. Roth, "Salvinorin A: A Novel and Highly Selective K-Opoid Receptor Agonist," *Life Sciences,* 75 (2004): 2615–2619.
46. C. Ketcham, "Under the Spell of the Magic Mint," *Gentlemen's Quarterly,* 77 (June 2007): 208–211, 240–242.
47. D. J. Sheffler and B. L. Roth, "Salvinorin A: The Magic Mint Hallucinogen Finds a Molecular Target in the Kappa-Opioid Receptor," *Trends in Pharmacological Sciences,* 24 (March 2003): 107–109.
48. J. Appel and D. Kim-Appel, "The Rise of a New Psychoactive Agent: *Salvia Divinorum,*" *International Journal of Mental Health and Addiction,* 5 (July 2007): 248–253.
49. D. Leinwand, "Jimson Weed Users Chase High All the Way to the Hospital," *USA Today,* November 1, 2006.
50. *Jimsonweed* (Johnstown, PA: National Drug Intelligence Center, 2003).
51. Halpern, supra note 9.
52. M. J. Barbanoj, J. Riba, S. Clos, S. Gimenez, E. Grasa, and S. Romero, "Daytime Ayahuasca Administration Modulates REM and Slow-Wave Sleep in Healthy Volunteers," *Psychopharmacology,* 196 (February 2008): 315–326.
53. R. S. Gable, "Risk Assessment of Ritual Use of Oral Dimethyltryptamine (DMT) and Harmala Alkaloids," *Addiction,* 102 (January 2007): 24–34.
54. Halpern, supra note 9.
55. Johnston et al., supra note 28.
56. K. A. Carls and V. L. Ruehter, "An Evaluation of Phencycidine (PCP) Psychosis: A Retrospective Analysis at a State Facility," *The American Journal*

of Drug and Alcohol Abuse, 32 (2006): 673–678.

57. S. Stocker, "Potential Cocaine Medications Show Effectiveness Against Psychosis Seizures," *NIDA Notes* (March 2000): 7–8.
58. J. Cloud, "Is Your Kid on K?" *Time* (October 20, 2007).
59. Substance Abuse and Mental Health Services Administration, *Drug Abuse Warning Network, 2005: National Estimates of Drug-Related Emergency Room Visits* (Rockville, MD: Office of Applied Studies, 2007).
60. K. L. R. Jansen and R. Darracot-Cankovic, "The Nonmedical Use of Ketamine, Part Two: A Review of Problem Use and Dependence," *Journal of Psychoactive Drugs,* 33 (April–June 2001): 151–157.
61. J. Cloud, "Was Timothy Leary Right?" *Time*, 169 (April, 2007).
62. E. Krupitsky, A. Burakov, T. Romanova, I. Dunaesky, R. Strassman, and A. Grinenko, "Ketamine Psychotherapy for Heroin Addiction: Immediate Effects and Two-Year Follow-Up," *Journal of Substance Abuse Treatment,* 23 (2002): 273–283.

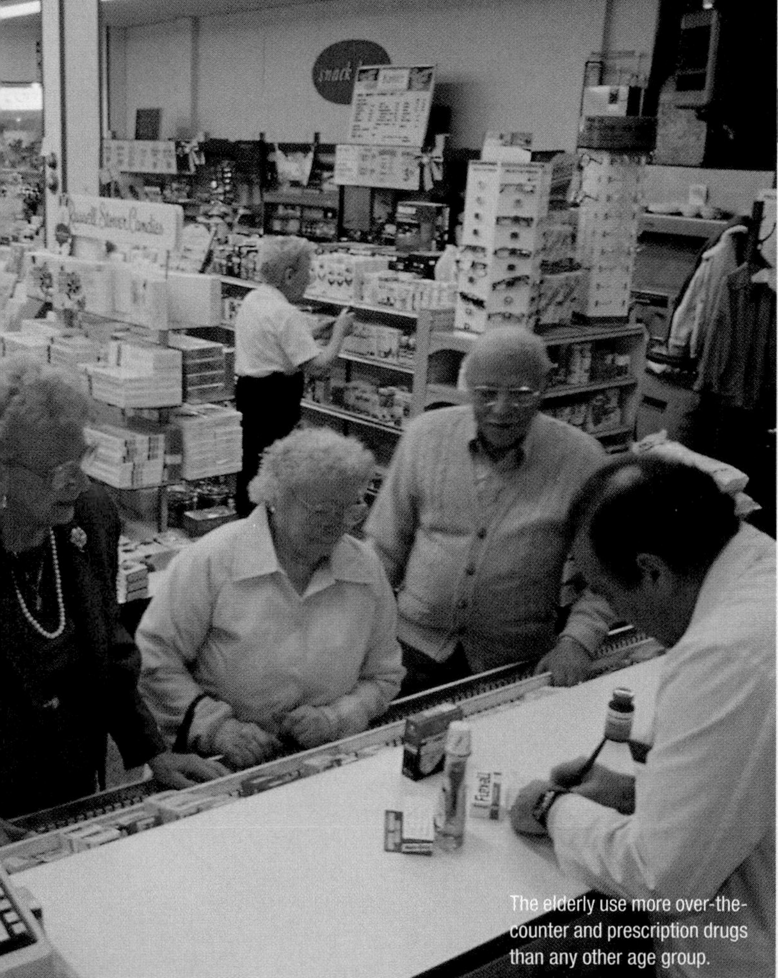
The elderly use more over-the-counter and prescription drugs than any other age group.

FACT OR FICTION?

1. About one out of every 25 eighth-grade students took cough medicine in the past year to get high.
2. A "child-resistant" container is a container that 80% of 5-year-olds need more than 5 minutes to open.
3. When it was first developed, aspirin was used to treat syphilis.
4. For preventing a heart attack, a baby aspirin is just as effective as an adult aspirin.
5. Acetaminophen accounts for more emergency room visits than aspirin.
6. Aspirin and ibuprofen are twice as effective for protecting people against heart attacks when taken together.
7. To reduce the effects of an alcohol hangover, one should take aspirin when drinking.
8. Because dextromethorphan (DMX) can have harmful side effects, individuals can buy only one bottle of DMX at a time.
9. For many people, drinking warm milk at bedtime allows them to go to sleep more easily.
10. Because of the media's attention on obesity, children today are less obese than they were 20 years ago.

Turn the page to check your answers

Chapter Objectives

After completing this chapter, the reader should be able to describe:

- The impact of the Food, Drug, and Cosmetic Act of 1938
- Differences among OTC drugs in Category I, Category II, and Category III
- Factors influencing the perception of pain
- The benefits and side effects of aspirin, acetaminophen, and ibuprofen
- How herbal drugs are regulated
- How antitussive cough suppressants and expectorants differ
- The effectiveness of OTC sleep aids
- Drawbacks related to various types of antacids
- Side effects of OTC stimulants
- The dangers of phenylpropanolamine (PPA)

14

Over-the-Counter Drugs

FACT OR FICTION?

1. **Fact:** According to data from the federal government, 3.6% of eighth-grade students took cough medicine to get high.
2. **Fact:** Child-resistant containers are containers that most 5-year-olds should not be able to open within 5 minutes, although many 5-year-olds open the containers in less than 5 minutes.
3. **Fiction:** The fact is—when it was first developed, aspirin was used to treat headaches.
4. **Fact:** A baby aspirin is as effective as an adult aspirin, without the potential for as many side effects.
5. **Fact:** Acetaminophen accounts for about four times more emergency room visits than aspirin.
6. **Fiction:** The fact is—both aspirin and ibuprofen offer cardiovascular benefit, but those benefits negate each other if both drugs are taken around the same time.
7. **Fiction:** The fact is—if alcohol and aspirin are taken at the same time, the risk of internal bleeding is increased.
8. **Fiction:** The fact is—although DMX can be harmful, there are no restrictions on its purchase.
9. **Fact:** Warm milk produces a chemical that makes falling asleep easier.
10. **Fiction:** The fact is—it is estimated that obesity is three times more common for children today than it was 20 years ago.

Billions of dollars are spent each year on over-the-counter (OTC) drugs in the United States and abroad. In the United States, four out of five adults take medicine or supplements on a weekly basis and nearly one-third take five or more daily.[1] People typically perceive OTC drugs as being relatively harmless. OTC drugs are readily accessible; moreover, a number of drugs are being switched from prescription to over-the-counter.[2] After all, if a drug does not require a prescription to be purchased, how harmful can it be?

The perception that nonprescription drugs are completely safe can have grave consequences. Not only can one become euphoric from OTC drugs, but some are known to cause hallucinations.[3] It is estimated that between 2 million and 4 million teenagers have abused OTC medicines. The most common OTC drug that is abused is dextromethorphan (DMX). Because it contains 30 mg of DMX, the drug of choice is Coricidin HBP.[4]

The federal agency that regulates prescription and over-the-counter drugs is the U.S. Food and Drug Administration (FDA), which has been in existence for more than 100 years.[5] The FDA implemented regulations requiring that more information be included on labels of OTC drugs in 2004.[6] Nonetheless, one survey of more than 4,000 adults indicated that 44% exceeded the recommended dosage of OTC drugs.[7] Because discussions of drugs often focus on illegal drugs, the potentially adverse effects of OTC drugs, as well as alcohol and tobacco, tend to be overlooked. Abuse of over-the-counter drugs by teenagers is increasing, especially abuse of decongestants, antihistamines, cough suppressants, and laxatives.[8]

One can easily understand how the use of OTC drugs has become ingrained in our society. Advertisements try to convince consumers of their need for drugs. The message is that no one has to feel pain or discomfort. Regardless of the problem, some type of medication is always available to remedy it. Advertisers prefer the term *medication* to *drug* because the former implies that the product is helpful and the latter implies that it is harmful. In 2008 legislation was introduced to give authority to the FDA to regulate advertisements for over-the-counter drugs.[9]

Over-the-Counter Drug Market

For many years OTC drugs were unregulated. People could get **patent medicines**—another term for OTC drugs—from traveling side shows or from a local pharmacist or physician. The contents of these drugs were not regulated. The Pure Food and Drug Act, passed in 1906, changed that. This law stipulated that ingredients ranging from alcohol (the most

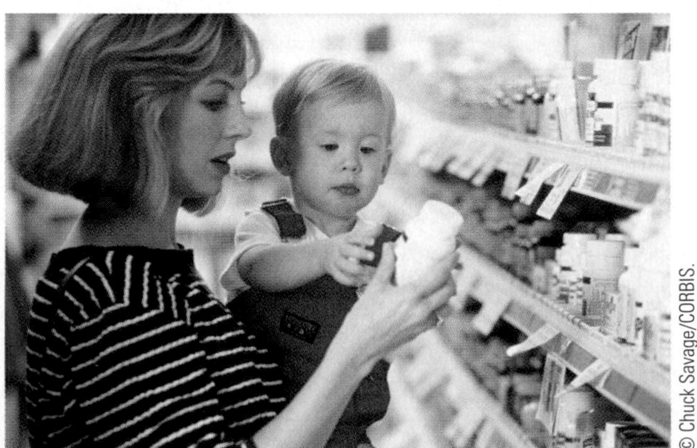

OTC products should be chosen and used wisely.

common ingredient), to opium, to cocaine, to almost anything had to be listed on labels. Despite the Pure Food and Drug Act, problems persisted. Eventually, the Food, Drug, and Cosmetic Act was enacted.

patent medicines A synonym for over-the-counter drugs

Regulating Over-the-Counter Drugs

The Food, Drug, and Cosmetic Act, passed in 1938, required that prescription drugs be proved safe and effective before being marketed. This act, however, applied only to prescribed drugs. Not until the Kefauver-Harris Amendment in 1962 did *nonprescription* drugs have to be proved safe and effective. The law stipulated that all OTC drugs had to pass this test. This task was enormous because more than 300,000 OTC preparations were on the market already.

To simplify its task, the FDA evaluated ingredients in OTC drugs rather than examining each product. The FDA identified 26 classes of OTC products and had advisory panels review the active ingredients in these classes. Existing OTC drugs could remain on the market until they were tested, a process that took many years. The FDA presented its findings in 1985. Among 348 new drugs from the largest 25 drug companies in the United States, the FDA found that 3% made important contributions to existing therapies, 13% made modest contributions, and 84% made little or no potential contribution.[10]

In 2007, the FDA proposed a new category for drugs called "behind-the-counter" drugs (BTC). Behind-the-counter drugs would be nonprescription drugs that consumers would have to ask for after consultation with their pharmacist. Behind-the-counter drugs were prescribed drugs previously. This new category for drugs would improve access to drugs for people who lack health insurance or adequate prescription drug coverage because they would not have to pay to see a physician before obtaining these drugs.[11]

Because ingredients in cold medicines can be used to make methamphetamines, President Bush signed into law the Combat Methamphetamine Epidemic Act of 2005. One provision of this bill is a ban on over-the-counter cold medicines containing pseudoephedrine, an ingredient that is frequently used to make methamphetamine. Cold medicines containing pseudoephedrine are kept behind the counter. There is a limit on the quantity of pseudoephedrine one can purchase each month and individuals are required to present photo identification to purchase products containing pseudoephedrine. Moreover, stores must maintain personal information about purchasers for at least two years.

Generic versus Brand Name Drugs

Generic drugs are copies of brand name drugs and have the same dosage, safety, strength, and quality of brand name drugs. They are also similar in how they are administered and in their intended use. The FDA requires that all drugs, whether they are generic or brand name drugs, be safe and effective. One advantage of generic drugs over brand name drugs is that they cost less.

Although generic drugs contain the same ingredients as brand name drugs, they appear different. Trademark laws in the United States require that generic drugs not look exactly like brand name drugs. Although generic drugs are less expensive than brand name drugs, not every brand name drug has a generic equivalent.[12]

Categories of Over-the-Counter Drugs

The FDA devised a three-tier system for categorizing OTC drugs.

Category I:
- a. "generally recognized as safe" (GRAS)
- b. "generally recognized as effective" (GRAE)
- c. "generally recognized as honestly labeled" (GRAHL)

Category II: Not generally recognized as safe or effective or is improperly labeled; these drugs are supposed to be removed from the shelves within 6 months unless the manufacturer demonstrates that the drug should be Category I; if research in regard to a drug's safety and effectiveness is insufficient, the drug is included in Category III.

Category III: Cannot be sold; if a drug manufacturer contests the FDA's decision, the manufacturer can request a formal hearing.

Besides reviewing OTC drugs, the FDA looks at many prescription drugs to assess their safety and effectiveness. In several instances, the FDA has ruled that a prescription drug can be marketed as an OTC drug because it is relatively safe and effective. These prescription drugs have been reformulated to be less potent. Hence, the difference between many OTC and prescription drugs is the amount of active ingredient.

Another difference between prescribed and OTC drugs is that many chemicals in prescription

Categories of OTC Drugs

Category I: Generally recognized as safe (GRAS), generally recognized as effective (GRAE), and generally recognized as honestly labeled (GRAHL)

Category II: Not generally recognized as safe or effective, or not properly labeled; removed from the shelves within 6 months

Category III: Insufficient research regarding a drug's safety and effectiveness; cannot be sold

drugs are not available for use in OTC drugs. Prescription drugs that have been switched to OTC drugs include ibuprofen (an analgesic drug sold as Nuprin, Advil, and Motrin), Dramamine (used for motion sickness), Actifed (a decongestant), Dimetapp (a cold medicine), and orlistat (alli). With the pressing need to lower health care costs, the FDA is considering making many more prescription drugs available OTC.[13]

Herbal Drugs

A largely unregulated segment of the marketplace is that of herbal drugs. Part of the problem with regulating these products is that it is unclear whether they should be classified as drugs, foods, or herbs. Herbal drugs are often marketed as food supplements. The FDA does not oversee food supplements; consequently, there is no regulation of these products. However, manufacturers of herbal drugs cannot make claims regarding their purported benefits without proof. If there are numerous complaints regarding an herbal drug, it can be removed from the market.

The use of herbal drugs in China, Indian, Rome, Greece, Egypt, and Syria dates back to 500 years ago, and today, global sales of herbal drugs are estimated at $60 billion annually.[14] Up to 20% of Americans and 41% of British people use herbal drugs.[15] While herbal drugs have evolved from fringe drugs to mainstream drugs, research into the safety and effectiveness of these drugs remains lacking.[16] One study found that nearly 20% of pediatric patients in emergency rooms had taken some type of natural health product. This information is not proof that these products cause adverse reactions, only that more research is needed.[17] There is also concern that herbal drugs will be used for euphoric or hallucinogenic purposes.[18] Table 14.1 lists selected herbal drugs and their intended uses.

Analgesics

More than 80% of Americans reported using an OTC pain reliever within the past year.[19] Advertisements constantly remind us that pain relievers are indispensable. We are told that we do not have to live with minor aches and pains that affect our daily lives. The message is clear: Pain and discomfort are nuisances that we do not have to tolerate.

The two basic types of **analgesics** are internal and external:

- *External analgesics*, such as Ben-Gay and Absorbine, are applied to the skin for sore muscles. Their benefit is more psychological than physical.
- *Internal analgesics* are taken into the body. Most analgesics are internal. Aspirin is the drug used most commonly. Americans ingest more than 10,000 *tons* of aspirin each year, which equates to 80 million aspirin or aspirin-containing tablets consumed every day.

At one time, aspirin dominated the analgesic market. Now, competitive analgesic products include acetaminophen, ibuprofen, naproxen sodium, and ketoprofen. These products effectively alleviate moderate pain, though they differ in other respects. Like aspirin, they have adverse side effects. In 2005, over 39,000 people went to emergency rooms due to acetaminophen, and over 19,000 people went to emergency rooms due to ibuprofen.[20]

Aspirin

Aspirin is the least expensive pain reliever. **Acetylsalicylic acid**, the active agent in aspirin, is similar to a chemical found in the bark of willow trees. Using willow bark for pain and fever was common among the ancient Greeks and American Indians. At one time, people in pain were given salicylic acid, but it resulted in stomach upset and nausea. By 1897, chemist Felix Hoffman of Bayer Laboratories had developed a compound combining salicylic acid and acetyl acid. This new compound, called aspirin, caused less stomach distress than salicylic acid. Aspirin works best for dull, constant pain but is ineffective for sharp pain. Aspirin is nonaddicting, it does not alter consciousness, and the senses of the user remain intact.

When a cell in the human body is injured, hormone-like chemicals called **prostaglandins** are activated. High levels of prostaglandins can cause headaches, inflammation, fever, blood clots, and menstrual cramps. These chemicals also can affect the reproductive, circulatory, and digestive systems. Aspirin inhibits the synthesis and release of prostaglandins, thereby reducing moderate pain by affecting the body's pain receptors and ameliorating inflammation and fever.

Because aspirin reduces inflammation, it is especially helpful in relieving symptoms of rheumatoid arthritis. About 21 million Americans suffer from arthritis, affecting one of six people.[21]

Aspirin acts as an **antipyretic**, or fever-reducing drug. It works on the hypothalamus, which dilates peripheral blood vessels. This increases respiration and blood flow, and the body cools down as a result. Antipyretic action is not always advantageous. Although a fever causes discomfort, it can be helpful because an elevation in body temperature destroys many bacteria and viruses. Thus, the fever-reducing effect of aspirin can be counterproductive. If the body temperature is normal, aspirin does not lower it.

Among the significant benefits attributed to aspirin is prevention of heart attacks and strokes. Taking

analgesics Drugs that relieve pain

acetylsalicylic acid The agent in aspirin that relieves pain

prostaglandins Chemicals in the body that produce pain and inflammation; aspirin alters their synthesis

antipyretic Having fever-reducing properties

TABLE 14.1 Commonly Used Herbal Supplements

Herb	Common Uses	Cautions
Chamomile	Used for GI complaints	Can cause toxicity of calcium channel blockers and antihyperlipidemics Has an additive effect when taken with alcohol or sedatives
Ginkgo	Used to improve circulation impaired by vascular disease Used to improve cognition and memory	Can increase bleeding in individuals already taking aspirin or warfarin
Melatonin	May help reestablish proper circadian rhythm	Should be taken in the early evening Can cause some stomach upset
St. John's wort	Used as an antidepressant Used as an antiviral	Can cause photosensitivity
Echinacea	Enhances the immune system Can be used as a sun protectant	Immunosuppression can occur with usage of more than 8 weeks (immunocompromised individuals should not use)
Ginseng	Used for energy	Contraindicated in individuals with blood clotting disorders Will increase blood pressure Can reduce the effectiveness of antihypertensive agents
Glucosamine	Stimulates the biosynthesis of a cartilage-building compound May also reduce inflammation	May exacerbate diabetes
Goldenseal	Used for High blood pressure Poor appetite Infections Menstrual problems Minor sciatic pain Muscle spasms Eye wash	Contraindicated in heart patients Should not be used with ear infections
Valarian	Used for its sedative action	Should not be used in children Should not be used in individuals with altered hepatic (liver) function
Kava	Used for anxiety, psychosis, and depression	Interacts with Levodopa, sedatives, central nervous system depressants, and barbiturates
Ginger	Used for motion sickness/stomach disorders	Multiple known drug interactions Can increase bleeding in individuals already taking aspirin or warfarin

half an aspirin tablet within 24 hours after a heart attack and each day for the next 30 days reduces the death rate from heart attacks by 23%.[22] It has been reported that people over age 45 who take low-dose aspirin reduce their risk of a heart attack by 25%.[23] Similarly, a study of nearly 80,000 nurses between the ages of 30 and 55 found that taking one to six aspirins weekly reduced the risk of a first heart attack in women.[24]

There are additional benefits to regular aspirin use. It has been shown that 100 mg of aspirin every other day reduced the risk of adult-onset asthma.[25] Among diabetics, aspirin use reduces the risk of retinopathy, the leading cause of blindness among people ages 20 to 65.[26] Another benefit of aspirin and other analgesic drugs is a reduction in cataracts. A study of 662,000 U.S. men and women by the American Cancer Society concluded that "regular aspirin use at low doses may reduce the risk of fatal colon cancer." Also, it has been found that aspirin may reduce the risk of breast cancer[27] as well as skin cancer.[28]

Research indicates that the cognitive functioning of elderly people who use aspirin declines more slowly than that of those who do not take aspirin.[29] However, many elderly people who take aspirin also drink alcohol—and this combination is particularly harmful because it may result in internal hemorrhaging and prolonged bleeding.[30] The risk of internal bleeding increases when aspirin is used with other anticoagulant drugs such as Warfarin.[31] Even at low dosage levels, aspirin can result in kidney damage for many elderly people.[32]

People who are allergic to aspirin develop rashes, weakness, stomach pain, breathing problems, wheezing, and asthma-like attacks that can be fatal. In other people, aspirin causes nausea, vomiting, blood loss, and iron-deficiency anemia. With as few as two to three aspirins, a person can bleed twice as long as normal. Patients having surgery and women in the late stages of pregnancy are advised not to take aspirin. Taking aspirin during pregnancy has been linked to postpartum hemorrhaging, prolonged labor, and higher perinatal mortality.

People with bleeding disorders, especially hemophilia and gastrointestinal problems, are cautioned not to use aspirin. Aspirin aggravates peptic ulcers, too.[33] To reduce stomach irritation, some people use buffered aspirin, though it does not diminish the irritation. The purpose of making an aspirin buffered is to increase sales. To minimize irritation, taking a full glass of water with aspirin helps.

Other problems related to extensive aspirin use include hepatitis, bone-marrow depression, and kidney damage. Most overdoses are seen in children. In children younger than age 5, aspirin is one of the leading causes of death by accidental poisoning. Symptoms of aspirin toxicity include perspiration, dizziness, hyperventilation, headache, thirst, ringing in the ears, and hearing loss. Unfortunately, 25% of Americans who use over-the-counter pain drugs exceed the recommended dosage.[34]

Aspirin inhibits **interferon**, a natural substance in the body that helps ward off viruses. Hence, it results in people being more susceptible to viruses, including colds.

Children with chicken pox or flulike symptoms should not be given aspirin because of the slight risk of developing Reye's syndrome. This serious condition is marked by severe personality changes, vomiting, disorientation, lethargy, and death in up to one-fourth of patients. Reye's syndrome does not occur with other analgesic drugs. In 1986, the British Committee on Safety of Medicine recommended that children under age 12 not be given aspirin without physician approval. Starting in 2003, the United Kingdom required that labels on aspirin packages state that aspirin should not be given to children younger than age 16.[35]

On Campus

Many students ingest aspirin after drinking alcohol to prevent hangovers. Aspirin does *not* prevent hangovers and may cause internal bleeding.

Source: A. D. Walling, "Risk of Gastric Hemorrhaging in Long-Term Aspirin Therapy," *American Family Physician* (May 15, 2001).

Advantages and Disadvantages of Aspirin

Advantages

- Eliminates dull pain
- Lessens inflammation
- Lowers fever
- May reduce colon, skin, and breast cancer
- May reduce risk of retinopathy and decrease cataracts
- Helps prevent heart attacks and strokes

Disadvantages

- Can cause allergic reaction
- Prolongs bleeding time
- Irritates the stomach
- Can cause kidney damage
- Can cause Reye's syndrome and possibly death

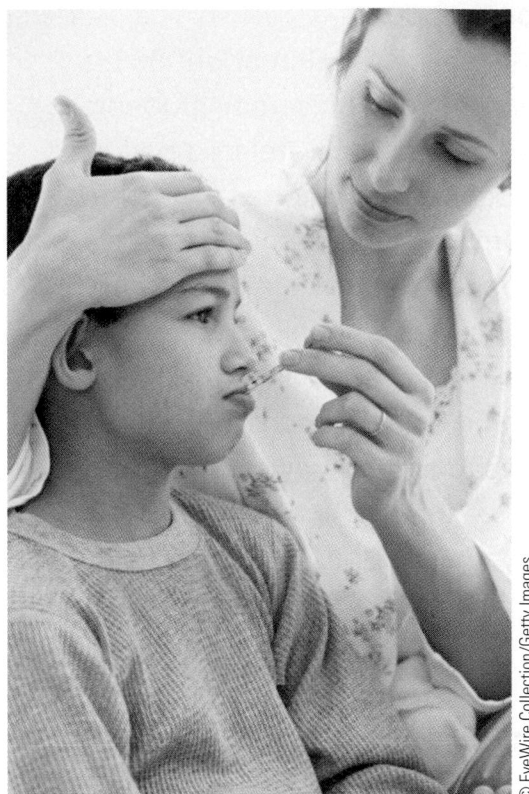
© EyeWire Collection/Getty Images.

Children with chicken pox or flulike symptoms should not be given aspirin without a doctor's approval.

interferon A natural substance in the body that wards off viral infections

phenacetin An alternative to aspirin now linked to kidney problems; its sale is prohibited

Advantages and Disadvantages of Acetaminophen

Advantages

- Lessens pain
- Reduces fever
- Irritates stomach less than aspirin
- Does not prolong bleeding

Disadvantages

- Is ineffective for inflammation
- Can cause liver damage
- Can cause diarrhea, nausea, and vomiting
- May increase risk of hypertension
- Can cause death

Acetaminophen

Because of concerns about the side effects of aspirin, many people have switched to other analgesics. One popular alternative is acetaminophen, a byproduct of **phenacetin**. Phenacetin was distributed widely in the 1940s and 1950s in combination with aspirin and caffeine. After a review, however, the FDA recommended that phenacetin use be limited to 10 days. Eventually, it was banned altogether in the United States because it was linked to kidney problems as well as heart disease, hypertension, and cancer.

First marketed in 1955, acetaminophen reduces pain and fever. Since that time, its popularity has grown immensely. OTC products with acetaminophen include Tylenol, Datril, Anacin-3, and Panadol. Acetaminophen is believed to interfere with the synthesis of prostaglandins. It is not a safe alternative to aspirin, though. According to one research group, out of every 1,000 men who took acetaminophen for arthritis, 715 will improve, 4 will go to a hospital with a bleeding ulcer, and 12 will have a heart attack.[36] Acetaminophen accounts for the second most common type of poisoning, after alcohol.[37]

Signs of overdose, which might not appear for up to 48 hours, include stomach pain, fatigue, diarrhea, nausea, and vomiting. Children have died, usually from liver failure, after taking only a few Extra-Strength Tylenol tablets. One study at the University of Texas Southwestern Medical Center found that acetaminophen was implicated in 38% of cases of acute liver failure. More cases of liver toxicity occurred after people consumed two to three times the suggested dose within a 24- to 48-hour period.[38] Also, combining acetaminophen and alcohol is especially dangerous to the liver. In addition to these detrimental effects, one study of 51,529 male health professionals found that using acetaminophen 4 to 5 times a week increased the risk of hypertension.[39]

On the other hand, two advantages of acetaminophen over aspirin are that

1. It causes less stomach irritation.
2. It does not prolong bleeding time.

Thus, it is a better alternative for people who are allergic to aspirin or who are pregnant. Also, one study of 88,142 pregnant women found that acetaminophen was not associated with congenital abnormalities.[40]

Arthritis sufferers do not receive the same anti-inflammation benefit from acetaminophen as from aspirin. Another disadvantage is that the analgesic benefit of acetaminophen is delayed if it is taken with or shortly after eating high-carbohydrate foods.

Advantages and Disadvantages of Ibuprofen

Advantages	Disadvantages
• Reduces pain • Lessens inflammation • Produces less stomach upset • May reduce risk of breast cancer and Alzheimer's disease	• Prolongs bleeding time • Can cause allergic reaction • Has numerous side effects • May increase risk of peptic ulcers and enlarged prostate • Can cause death

Ibuprofen

Another OTC drug that reduces moderate pain and inflammation is ibuprofen. It is a more potent pain reliever than aspirin and acetaminophen. One study found that people with back pain preferred ibuprofen to acetaminophen or aspirin.[41] Additionally, ibuprofen was superior to acetaminophen for relieving pain in pediatric patients.[42] When it was introduced, ibuprofen could be obtained only by prescription. In 1984, it was approved for OTC sale. Ibuprofen is less likely than aspirin to cause stomach upset, but it does prolong bleeding time. Doctors advise against using alcohol while taking ibuprofen because the combination increases the risk of stomach problems. Taking ibuprofen with food or milk helps to relieve upset stomach and mild heartburn. Analgesics with ibuprofen include Advil, Motrin-IB, and Nuprin.

Unlike acetaminophen, ibuprofen lessens inflammation. Thus, it is recommended for relieving symptoms of rheumatoid arthritis. People who are allergic to aspirin, however, might be allergic to ibuprofen also. As with aspirin and acetaminophen, individuals taking ibuprofen are cautioned against exceeding recommended dosages. Ibuprofen can impede concentration and cause drowsiness; therefore, it is not a good idea to operate equipment after taking ibuprofen.

Possible side effects from ibuprofen include vomiting, loss of hearing, nausea, elevated blood pressure, diarrhea, visual disturbances, heartburn, and congestive heart failure for people with impaired cardiac function. Its use has been linked to cataracts and death from liver failure. Ibuprofen has been implicated in the development of peptic ulcers[43] and enlarging the prostate.[44] On a positive note, ibuprofen may reduce the risk of breast cancer in women.[45] Another positive finding is that ibuprofen, as well as aspirin, might reduce the risk of developing Alzheimer's disease.[46]

On Campus

It is estimated that about 85% of American university students report backpack-related pain and discomfort. Discomfort was most common in the shoulders, lower back, upper-middle back, and neck. The findings may point to an emerging trend between pain and discomfort and time spent carrying backpacks. A loaded backpack should weigh no more than 10% to 15% of a student's body weight.

Source: Robert Preidt, *The American Occupational Therapy Association Inc., News Release,* Sept. 3, 2008.

Naproxen Sodium and Ketoprofen

Two other entries into the OTC analgesic market are **naproxen sodium** and **ketoprofen**. Aleve is a popular brand of naproxen sodium, and Orudis KT and Actron are brands containing ketoprofen. Naproxen sodium is comparable to ibuprofen in effectiveness, and its analgesic effects last up to 12 hours. Ketoprofen is as effective as ibuprofen, and it produces results in about 30 minutes. Like aspirin, acetaminophen, and ibuprofen, naproxen sodium and ketoprofen reduce fever, and like aspirin and ibuprofen, they lessen inflammation.

One advantage of naproxen sodium is its long-term pain relief. One study reported that among people who took the drug for moderate and severe headaches, 52% experienced significant pain relief when the drug was first used and 90% experienced pain relief after 3 months.[47] In a separate study of 3,000 migraine sufferers, those who were given naproxen sodium were more likely to experience relief than those individuals given placebos.[48] The majority of people taking naproxen sodium do not encounter adverse side effects.[49]

Doctors advise consumers not to drink alcohol while taking these drugs. Both drugs work best for muscle pain, arthritis, and menstrual pain. For people not taking aspirin, naproxen may protect against heart attacks.[50] In 2003, a ketoprofen patch was approved for use as treatment for joint pain.[51]

Possible side effects of both drugs are stomach upset and gastrointestinal bleeding. Asthmatics and people who are allergic to aspirin should not take these drugs. Finally, naproxen sodium can cause bloating and dizziness.

naproxen sodium An over-the-counter analgesic

ketoprofen An over-the-counter analgesic

placebo An inert substance that does not have a physical effect but may produce psychological and associated physiological reactions

histamines Chemicals that are released by the body in response to the presence of allergens

antitussives Drugs that act as cough suppressants

Cold and Allergy Drugs

OTC drugs sold to treat colds and allergies do not cure these conditions. Still, U.S. residents spend more than $2 billion each year on these drugs. What these drugs do is relieve symptoms of colds and allergies. This could be counterproductive in the long run, however. Colds are self-limiting conditions that go away notwithstanding treatment. Many people overcome colds (and other ailments) more quickly when physicians prescribe medications, even if the medications are **placebos**. A familiar adage says "A cold will end in a week with aspirin or in 7 days without anything."

The common cold has no cure. One problem with finding a cure is that a cold is far from "common" and actually is a complex condition. In addition, cough and cold remedies for children can be hazardous. One study involving 63 emergency rooms, dating from 2004 to 2005, found that 7,091 children under age 12 received treatment for adverse reactions to cough and cold medicines. The majority of children seen were between ages 2 and 5.[52] The FDA has recommended that cough and cold medicines be banned for infants.[53] The following discussion examines the types of drugs that constitute the cold and allergy market.

Antihistamines

When allergens are present, the body releases chemicals called **histamines**. Histamines protect the body from diseases by releasing antibodies that attack antigens (foreign bodies), viruses, bacteria, and chemicals in the body. In doing so, they produce runny nose and eyes, sneezing, congestion, nausea, and itching. One study found that antihistamines were effective for relieving itching[54] and for nasal imflammation.[55] Antihistamines interfere with the release of histamines and thereby provide symptomatic relief from allergies. They do not cure colds. In fact, one study found that antihistamines may actually prolong ear infections in children.[56]

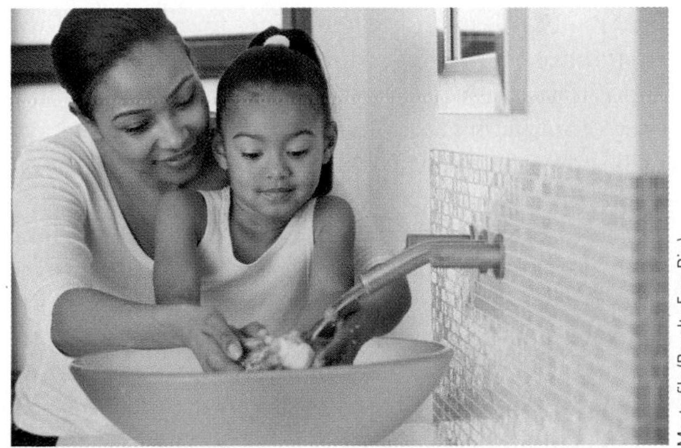

Masterfile (Royalty-Free Div.)

Washing the hands is one of the most effective means of preventing colds and other infectious diseases.

Side Effects of Antihistamines

- Dizziness
- Weakness
- Nervousness
- Poor concentration
- Headache
- Drowsiness
- Blurred vision
- Difficulty urinating
- Constipation
- Hives
- Dry mouth, nose, and throat

Antihistamines are found in cough syrups, hay fever and motion sickness preparations, and decongestants such as Contac, Dimetapp, Sudafed, and Triaminic. Antihistamines in Benadryl and similar allergy relievers make people drowsy and thereby affect driving ability. Antihistamine medications often contain alcohol, which contributes to drowsiness. Antihistamines also can produce dry mouth, nose, and throat; weakness; and constipation. An allergic reaction to antihistamines can cause blurred vision, dizziness, nervousness, headaches, hives, and an inability to urinate. Antihistamines have not been shown to increase the risk of breast cancer,[57] although some antihistamines may increase the risk of miscarriage.[58]

Cough Medicines

A cough can be productive—meaning that it produces secretions—or nonproductive. Nonproductive coughs irritate the throat. Drugs that suppress or prevent coughing are called **antitussives**. These cough suppressants act on the medulla, the brain's cough center. One study of children given antitussive cough medicines reported that 46% to 56% had satisfactory responses.[59]

Two antitussive drugs are codeine and dextromethorphan:

- **Codeine** provides relief within 15 to 30 minutes, and the effects last 4 to 6 hours after ingestion. One interesting study, however, found that chocolate was more effective than codeine in suppressing coughs.[60] Although codeine-based cough syrups do not require a prescription, their sale is regulated. Codeine causes dependency, but the risk is low compared with that for morphine. In 2007 the FDA issued a warning for nursing mothers who take codeine because there was a report of an infant who died after having been breastfed.[61]
- **Dextromethorphan (Delsym)** is nonnarcotic and does not produce dependency, although it induces drowsiness, nausea, and dizziness. In recent years, dextromethorphan has become popular among young people as a mind-altering substance because it is easy to obtain, the negative effects are not widely known, and it is socially approved. The inappropriate use of dextromethorphan is also referred to as "robo-tripping."[62]

  Dextromethorphan, also known as DMX, can be lethal. A number of deaths have resulted from DMX. It is estimated that 3 million adolescents and young adults have used nonprescription cough medicine to get high.[63] As a result, a number of congressional bills have been introduced to totally ban dextromethorphan from cough medicines.[64] At recommended doses, DMX is safe; however, at 10 times the recommended dose, it produces hallucinations.[65] Also, young people who use DMX often use alcohol and illegal drugs in conjunction with it. DMX contributes to injuries and fatalities because one's judgment is impaired.[66]

Examples of antitussive cough medicines are Pertussin 8 Hour Cough Formula, Contac Cough Formula, and Robitussin-DM.

A productive cough helps respiration by removing mucous secretions and foreign matter from the lower respiratory tract. Cough syrups that increase mucous secretions, making a cough productive, are called **expectorants**. The most common expectorant, guaifenesin, is found in Nortussin, Anti-Tuss, and Robitussin. If large amounts are consumed, expectorants produce drowsiness, nausea, and vomiting.

At least 80% of cough and cold remedies are unnecessary.[67] Several recent studies have cast doubt on the efficacy of codeine.[68] Sucking on hard candies can be just as effective in increasing mucous secretions and relieving throat irritation.

Decongestants

Decongestants constrict blood vessels of the nasal passages, improve air flow, and obstruct secretions that go to the back of the throat. Although decongestants are effective, they do have drawbacks. Some produce a **rebound effect**, in which the congestion becomes worse than it was originally. Increasing the intake of decongestants exacerbates the rebound effect. Dependency on decongestants is possible. Instructions in nasal spray packages indicate that they should not be used for more than 3 consecutive days.

Because antihistamines in decongestants shrink swollen nasal passages and relieve sinus headaches, they alleviate allergies. One decongestant is **pseudoephedrine**, the active ingredient in the OTC decongestant Sudafed. Side effects of pseudoephedrine include dry mouth, anxiety, dizziness, tremors, tachycardia, vomiting, nausea, headache, difficulty urinating, and insomnia.

Antacids

As a result of eating habits and lifestyle, stomach-related problems are prevalent. The so-called good life has wreaked havoc on our sedentary bodies. Advertisers constantly remind us that upset stomach, acid indigestion, heartburn, constipation, and diarrhea are annoyances that are easily remedied by using their products. In response, U.S. residents spend more than $1 billion annually on products such as Mylanta, Tums, Rolaids, Alka-Seltzer, and Maalox.

What causes the stomach to be irritated in the first place? The culprit is **hydrochloric acid**, which aids in digestion but also aggravates the stomach's lining. It is estimated that almost three-fourths of adults suffer from indigestion or heartburn.[69] Antacids curtail stomach acidity[70] but have many side effects. Therefore, the FDA established guidelines for antacids: They should not be used for more than 2 weeks at a time, and if a problem persists for more than 2 weeks, the user should consult a physician. Some antacids have high sodium levels, which can cause either constipation or diarrhea.

Liquid antacids are more effective than tablets. A tablet should be taken with a full glass of water. Effervescent tablets should be dissolved completely. Also, aspirin and antacids should not be taken at the same time because this combination can increase stomach upset. Although antacids are relatively safe, one concern is that they could mask symptoms of more serious underlying problems.[71] Also, some antacids impair calcium absorption, resulting in an increase in broken bones for people as they age.[72]

Suggestions for Preventing Indigestion and Heartburn

- Avoid big meals. They make the stomach work longer and harder, producing more acid.
- Eat more slowly. Eating quickly stimulates the stomach to produce extra digestive acids.
- Do not lie down right after eating. Gravity prevents food from passing through the intestines quickly.
- Avoid tight-fitting clothing. It constricts the stomach and forces stomach acid into the esophagus.
- Reduce caffeine consumption. Caffeine makes the stomach produce more acid.
- Avoid foods with high acid content. Examples are citrus fruits and tomatoes.
- Reduce alcohol and tobacco use. Both cause irritation to the stomach lining.
- Raise your head slightly while sleeping. Gravity forces digestive acids to go toward the stomach rather than the esophagus.

Source: T. Cramer, "When Do You Need an Antacid?" *FDA Consumer* (January/February 1992): 19–21.

codeine A mild narcotic that suppresses coughing; a derivative of opium

dextromethorphan (Delsym) An over-the-counter nonnarcotic drug found in cough preparations

expectorants Cough medicines that make a cough productive by increasing mucous secretions

decongestants Substances used to relieve congestion

rebound effect The side effects produced by a drug that make a condition worse than it was originally; e.g., sinuses become more congested by nasal sprays

pseudoephedrine A nasal decongestant

hydrochloric acid Acid in the stomach that can ease digestion and irritate the stomach lining

sodium bicarbonate Baking soda; an ingredient in antacids designed to neutralize excess acid in the stomach

calcium carbonate An antacid designed to relieve acid indigestion

Sodium Bicarbonate

A popular antacid used to neutralize excess stomach acid is Alka-Seltzer. A primary ingredient in Alka-Seltzer is **sodium bicarbonate**, otherwise known as baking soda. People with high blood pressure have to monitor their sodium intake. Because sodium bicarbonate can raise blood pressure, people with hypertension should know which antacids contain it. Side effects related to sodium bicarbonate are belching and flatulence. Although neither of these effects is fatal, they can be uncomfortable and embarrassing.

Calcium Carbonate

Some people with acid indigestion have switched to **calcium carbonate** because it is free of sodium. Two popular OTC drugs containing calcium carbonate are Rolaids and Tums. The benefits of calcium carbonate are temporary. In the long run, it creates more problems than it solves because it produces a rebound effect in which stomach acidity actually increases after the drug's effects wear off. Constipation can result from the use of calcium carbonate. Also, it is contraindicated for people who have severe kidney disease. On the other hand, one benefit is that it is rich in calcium.

Salts of Magnesium and Aluminum

Other ingredients frequently found in antacid medications are salts of magnesium and salts of aluminum. These counteract each other: Salts of magnesium cause constipation, and salts of aluminum bring about diarrhea. People with intestinal disorders such as irritable bowel syndrome are cautioned against using these products.

To relieve diarrhea, some people use products such as Kaopectate, a mixture of kaolin and pectate that decreases the fluid content in the stool. Antidiarrheal drugs can cause abdominal cramps, nausea, and vomiting, as well as dependence. An old standby to relieve constipation is castor oil, which stimulates contractions of the smooth muscles of the intestine. Table 14.2 identifies drawbacks of various types of antacids.

H2 Blockers and PPIs

Newer remedies include histamine (H2) blockers and proton pump inhibitors (PPIs). Both types of drugs effectively treat heartburn, although they may produce side effects such as diarrhea, constipation, and headache. In less severe cases of heartburn, H2

TABLE 14.2 Drawbacks of Various Types of Antacids

Antacid	Side Effects
Sodium bicarbonate	Increased blood pressure Belching Gas
Calcium carbonate	Rebound effect Constipation Kidney damage
Salts of magnesium/ salts of aluminum	Bowel irritation Vomiting Abdominal cramps

blockers are effective. Examples of H2 blockers are Tagamet HB and Zantac. The American College of Gastroenterology recommends PPIs because they are more effective, although one problem with PPIs is the increased risk of hip fractures in people ages 50 and older.[73] Examples of PPIs include Prilosec OTC and the prescription drug Nexium.

Sleep Aids and Sedatives

Stress, tension, and anxiety are epidemic in contemporary society, and many people depend on OTC drugs for relief. One manifestation, insomnia, affects more than one-third of adults within any given year.[74] Insomnia results in irritability, restlessness, ineffectiveness at work, lethargy, and moodiness. To overcome insomnia, some individuals take an OTC medication or sedative. The primary ingredient in many OTC sedatives and sleep aids is some type of antihistamine.[75]

Antihistamines produce drowsiness, and the sedating effects of antihistamines increase greatly in conjunction with alcohol. Therefore, taking alcohol and antihistamines at the same time is not prudent. Also, a person should not drive an automobile or engage in potentially hazardous activities while taking antihistamines. In addition, anyone who is planning to take an allergy skin test should not take antihistamines.

The benefits of antihistamines as sedatives and sleep agents are limited. Nytol, Sominex, and Sleep-Eze are advertised as OTC sleep aids, and Compoz is advertised as an OTC sedative. These products are essentially the same.

Over-the-Counter Stimulants

Just as some people have difficulty going to sleep, others have trouble staying awake. To combat fatigue and drowsiness, OTC stimulants have been designed to help people stay awake and alert. The primary ingredient in these drugs is caffeine.

Although some people use OTC stimulants in an attempt to reverse alcohol intoxication, they do not work. Giving caffeine to an intoxicated person results in a wide-awake drunk. OTC stimulants such as Vivarin and No Doz are common on many campuses. Since March 1989, the only drug that has been allowed in OTC stimulants is caffeine.

The amount of caffeine in a recommended dose of OTC stimulants is equal to 2 to 3 cups of coffee. Labels on the packages of OTC stimulants caution consumers against taking other caffeine-containing beverages—such as tea, coffee, and soft drinks—at the same time.

One consequence of excessive caffeine consumption is **caffeinism**, a condition marked by nervousness, anxiety, tachycardia, sweating, and panic in some instances. As reported in Chapter 2, "look-alike" and "sound-alike" stimulants are promoted through mail-order advertisements. These typically include nothing more than caffeine.

Weight-Loss Aids

Many people are obsessed with dieting. In the United States, an estimated $30 billion annually is spent on dietary supplements, books, foods, and related services.[76] Books on dieting are among the top sellers year after year. Magazines are replete with articles on weight loss. Many Internet Web sites promote herbal weight-loss supplements. However, despite the disclaimer statements posted on each of these Web sites, only a few mention potential drug interactions or adverse reactions.[77]

Society constantly reminds us that "thin is in" and help is available for anyone who wants to achieve that desired state. Too often, thinness is equated with attractiveness. Television shows and other media have popular actors and actresses leading viewers through aerobic exercises. Advertisements for health clubs abound in the media.

Ironically, most of the people leading the aerobic activities and appearing in the health club advertisements are thin in the first place and do not need weight-loss products. And, the same magazines that feature articles about how to lose weight include articles with recipes that would kill any diet. Many companies tout their products as helping with (in some cases guaranteeing) the loss of excess pounds with little effort. If all else fails, fat can be suctioned out through liposuction.

One drug used for weight loss is ephedrine (ephedra). When combined with other stimulants such as caffeine, ephedrine can be fatal.[78] Metabolite, a popular weight-loss product, contains this dangerous combination of ephedra and caffeine. Metabolite was responsible for 18 heart attacks, 26 strokes, 43 seizures, and 5 deaths between 1997 and 2002.[79] The FDA banned the sale of ephedrine in April 2004.[80]

Orlistat

One of the more effective weight-loss drugs is orlistat, also known as **alli**. It is the only FDA-approved weight-loss product available to adults without a prescription. Until June 2007, orlistat was available only by prescription. The prescribed version of this drug is known as Xenical. The only difference between alli and Xenical is that alli comes in 60 mg capsules and Xenical comes in 120 mg capsules.

Orlistat works by blocking the absorption of about 25% of the fat in the foods that people consume.[81] Various studies show that the average weight loss ranges from 8.8 to 11 pounds. The side effects of orlistat are not especially adverse. They include abdominal pain, liquid stool, nausea, vomiting, and flatulence. Most of the side effects are mild to moderate and seldom persist after the first four weeks.[82]

caffeinism Excessive caffeine consumption resulting in caffeine dependency

alli A weight-loss drug that blocks the absorption of fat

phenylpropanolamine (PPA) A decongestant also used as an appetite suppressant

benzocaine A topical anesthetic put into candies or chewing gum to diminish appetite

Phenylpropanolamine and Benzocaine

At one time the FDA permitted OTC sales of **phenylpropanolamine (PPA)**, caffeine, and benzocaine for purposes of weight loss. It is believed that stimulants such as caffeine suppress appetite, but no long-term research is available to support this hypothesis. PPA is a frequently used appetite suppressant. It is structurally similar to amphetamines but does not produce euphoria unless it is taken in large doses. PPA seems to affect appetite over a short time, but long-term effectiveness has not been demonstrated. Despite concerns regarding the safety and effectiveness of PPA, an FDA advisory panel approved it as a supplement for weight reduction for up to 12 weeks.

Side effects of PPA include headache, rapid heartbeat, anxiety, higher blood sugar levels, nausea, insomnia, and hypertension. It is contraindicated for clinically depressed and hypertensive individuals. The most commonly encountered problems with PPA are psychotic episodes, seizures, and stroke. In 2000, the FDA issued a strong warning against the use of PPA, stating that PPA may be responsible for 200 to 500 hemorrhagic strokes (bleeding in the brain) each year in U.S. adults younger than age 50.[83] In response, many manufacturers have voluntarily removed PPA from their products. An example of a product that used to include PPA (but no longer does) is Dexatrim. Because it acts as a decongestant, PPA also is found in OTC cold and allergy preparations.

Another purported weight-reducing drug is **benzocaine**, a topical anesthetic that is put into chewing gum and candy. When one eats candies or chews gum containing benzocaine, the tongue and palate become numb. As numbness sets in, the desire for food diminishes. The effectiveness of benzocaine as an appetite suppressant has not been determined, although it might work under the same principle that one does not usually feel like eating after visiting the dentist and receiving an anesthetic!

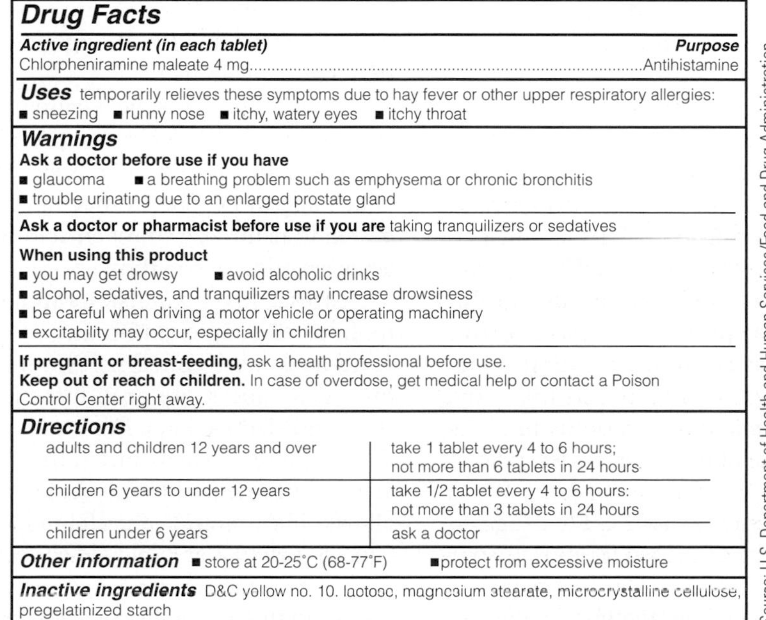

Drug Facts

Active ingredient (in each tablet)	**Purpose**
Chlorpheniramine maleate 4 mg	Antihistamine

Uses temporarily relieves these symptoms due to hay fever or other upper respiratory allergies:
■ sneezing ■ runny nose ■ itchy, watery eyes ■ itchy throat

Warnings

Ask a doctor before use if you have
■ glaucoma ■ a breathing problem such as emphysema or chronic bronchitis
■ trouble urinating due to an enlarged prostate gland

Ask a doctor or pharmacist before use if you are taking tranquilizers or sedatives

When using this product
■ you may get drowsy ■ avoid alcoholic drinks
■ alcohol, sedatives, and tranquilizers may increase drowsiness
■ be careful when driving a motor vehicle or operating machinery
■ excitability may occur, especially in children

If pregnant or breast-feeding, ask a health professional before use.
Keep out of reach of children. In case of overdose, get medical help or contact a Poison Control Center right away.

Directions

adults and children 12 years and over	take 1 tablet every 4 to 6 hours; not more than 6 tablets in 24 hours
children 6 years to under 12 years	take 1/2 tablet every 4 to 6 hours: not more than 3 tablets in 24 hours
children under 6 years	ask a doctor

Other information ■ store at 20-25˚C (68-77˚F) ■ protect from excessive moisture

Inactive ingredients D&C yellow no. 10, lactose, magnesium stearate, microcrystalline cellulose, pregelatinized starch

Source: U.S. Department of Health and Human Services/Food and Drug Administration. *Medicines in My Home: Information for Adults on Using Over-the-Counter Medicines Safely,* Publication No. (FDA) 07-1907, updated 25 October 2007.

Figure 14.1 The Drug Facts Label

Being a Smart Consumer

Because of the escalating costs of health care, many people are turning to self-care and self-medication. Visiting the doctor every time a minor ache or ailment arises is time-consuming and costly. At the same time, many advertisements for OTC drugs make claims about their benefits. Consumers must look at these advertisements carefully because, though advertisers legally cannot make false claims, they may give inaccurate impressions.

Information on labels of OTC medicines includes a list of active ingredients, directions for use, recommended dosage, warnings, and date of expiration (see Figure 14.1). Being a prudent consumer requires reading labels.

Another concern regarding self-medication is that OTC drugs often provide relief of symptoms only. Ameliorating the symptoms of an illness can encourage the ill person to minimize the seriousness of the illness or disregard its cause. This is potentially hazardous because the person might not seek additional or more appropriate treatment. *Relieving the symptoms of an illness is not the same as curing the illness.* Furthermore, some OTC drugs—such as stimulants, nasal sprays, sedatives, eye drops, cough syrups, and laxatives—can result in dependency. In short, consumers should not assume that OTC drugs are harmless.

Summary

The over-the-counter (OTC) drug market is a multibillion-dollar business. People are taking health care into their own hands, and advertisers are trying to convince consumers of the need for their products. Consumers are told that a product is available to address almost every problem. Just because nonprescribed drugs are readily accessible, this is no guarantee that they are safe and effective. A growing problem is the lack of regulation of herbal drugs.

The first attempt to regulate OTC drugs came with the Pure Food and Drug Act of 1906, but persistent problems led to enactment of the Food, Drug, and Cosmetic Act in 1938. This law stipulated that prescribed drugs had to be proven safe and effective. By 1962, the legislation was expanded to include OTC drugs. An FDA advisory panel reviewed the active ingredients in OTC drugs and, based on its findings, drugs were placed into one of three categories, relating to their OTC status.

Among the most commonly used OTC drugs are analgesics. External analgesics are used for muscle soreness. Internal analgesics reduce dull, constant pain.

The active agent in aspirin is acetylsalicylic acid, which alleviates pain, fever, and inflammation. Aspirin can help prevent heart attacks and strokes. Aspirin also has drawbacks. It prolongs internal bleeding, and some people are allergic to it.

Aspirin is a leading cause of accidental poisoning deaths in children younger than 5 years of age. Aspirin use is not advised in children up to age 18 with chicken pox or flulike symptoms because of an increased risk, though slight, of Reye's syndrome, a potentially deadly disease.

Alternatives to aspirin are acetaminophen, ibuprofen, naproxen sodium, and ketoprofen. Acetaminophen reduces pain and fever but does not alleviate inflammation; thus, it is not recommended for arthritis. Although many people switched from aspirin to acetaminophen because it causes less stomach upset and does not prolong bleeding time, it is not safer. Acetaminophen has been implicated in a number of liver-related problems. More people have gone to hospital emergency rooms from acetaminophen use than from aspirin use, and it accounts for more deaths than aspirin.

Ibuprofen lessens inflammation and pain. Although it extends bleeding time, it causes less stomach upset than aspirin. Ibuprofen use can be fatal in certain circumstances. Both naproxen sodium and ketoprofen are alternatives for reducing fever and inflammation. Naproxen sodium is as effective as ibuprofen, and its effects last up to 12 hours. Ketoprofen works as well as ibuprofen and produces results in about 30 minutes.

Cold and allergy medications provide symptomatic relief but do not cure colds and allergies. Their primary agents are antihistamines. A common side effect is drowsiness. Two types of cough medicines are antitussive cough syrups, which suppress coughing, and expectorants, which increase coughing and remove mucous secretions. Decongestants are used to constrict blood vessels in the nasal passages. A rebound effect can arise, though, causing more congestion and dependence.

Because of our typical eating habits and lifestyles, stomach-related disorders are prevalent. Many stomach problems are caused by excessive hydrochloric acid, which aggravates the stomach lining. Antacids are ingested to neutralize stomach acidity. Two types of antacids are sodium bicarbonate and calcium carbonate.

Stress, anxiety, tension, and sleeplessness affect millions of people, and many products are available to address these concerns. Antihistamines, which induce drowsiness, are prominent in many OTC sedatives and sleep agents. For some people the problem is not going to sleep but rather staying awake and alert. Caffeine is the only OTC stimulant the FDA allows. The amount of caffeine in OTC stimulants is equal to that in 2 or 3 cups of coffee. Too much caffeine causes nervousness and anxiety.

With the availability of OTC products and the desire to assume more responsibility for our own health care, people have to be wise consumers. Most OTC products relieve symptoms but do not offer cures. Therefore, consumers might think their health is improving when they actually are getting worse. People would be wise to become more informed about drugs. Being a smart consumer, at a minimum, means reading labels and following directions.

Thinking Critically

1. Although pain is a common experience, individuals have different thresholds. Some people reach for a pain reliever almost instantly when they feel discomfort. Others resist any type of medication as long as they can. How would you describe your threshold level? How soon after getting a headache do you take medicine for it?
2. The incidence of Reye's syndrome after aspirin use is very low. Should warnings regarding Reye's syndrome be included on aspirin containers? Why or why not?
3. Though many people realize that cold remedies do not cure colds, they continue to buy them. If you are one of these people, what motivates you to purchase these drugs?
4. Some experts are advocating a tax on food products that promote obesity. *Healthy People 2010* contains goals for recommended weight. The federal government has produced the MyPyramid.gov Web site and *Dietary Guidelines for Americans* to promote good eating habits. How far do you think the government should go in promoting weight loss?

Web Resources

DrKoop.com
http://www.drkoop.com
Spearheaded by former Surgeon General C. Everett Koop, this site provides information about numerous medical conditions as well as prescription and nonprescription drugs used to treat various ailments.

U.S. Food and Drug Administration, Center for Drug Evaluation and Research: Over-the-Counter (OTC) Drugs
http://www.fda.gov/cder/offices/otc/default.htm
This site features current information regarding over-the-counter drugs.

Notes

1. "America's Best Drugstores," *Consumer Reports*, June 2008: 12–17.
2. T. Gaudio, "From Behind the Wall to Over the Counter," *NJBIZ*, 20 (June 18, 2007): 19–20.
3. "Over-the-Counter Drug Abuse," *Dermatology Nursing*, 19 (February 2007): 94, 101.
4. D. T. Feinberg, "Managed Care: The Cost of Over-the-Counter Substance Abuse," *Journal of Child and Adolescent Psychopharmacology*, 16 (November 2006): 801–802.
5. A. T. Borchers, F. Hagie, C. L. Keen, and E. Gershwin, "The History and Contemporary Challenges of the US Food and Drug Administration," *Clinical Therapeutics*, 29 (January 2007): 1–16.
6. "New Rules Increase the Safety of OTC Ingredients," *FDA Consumer*, 38 (July–August 2004): 2.
7. J. W. Wooten, "Medicine Cabinet Staples Are Not Without Risk," *RN*, 66 (April 2003): 96.
8. K. Louden, "Patient Care Update: Over-the-Counter Drug Abuse," *Dermatology Nursing*, 19 (February 2007): 94–101.
9. I. Teinowitz, "Spotlight May Move to OTC Drugs," *Advertising Age*, 79 (January 21, 2008): 33.
10. A. Chetley, *Problem Drugs* (Amsterdam: Health Action International, 1995).
11. A. Lyles, "The Prescribing Continuum: Between Prescription and Over-the-Counter Drugs," *Clinical Therapeutics*, 29 (November 10, 2007): 2244–2245.
12. U. S. Food and Drug Administration, *Generic Drugs: Questions and Answers* (Washington: Department of Health and Human Services, 2007).
13. "Some Therapeutic Classes Poised for Rx-to-OTC Switches," *Medical Letter on the CDC and FDA* (March 9, 2003): 7–8.
14. N. Inamdar, S. Edalat, V. Kotwal, and S. Pawar, "Herbal Drugs in Milieu of Modern Drugs," *International Journal of Green Pharmacy*, 2 (January–March 2008): 2–10.
15. J. Ali, "Complementary Prescriptions," *Chemistry and Industry* (January 19, 2004): 18–19.
16. Inamdar et al., supra note 14.
17. R. D. Goldman, A. L. Rogovik, D. Lai, and S. Vohra, "Potential Interactions of Drug-Natural Health Products and Natural Health Products-Natural Health Products among Children," *Journal of Pediatrics*, 152 (2008): 521–526.
18. W. H. Richardson, C. M. Slone, and J. E. Michels, "Herbal Drugs of Abuse: An Emerging Problem," *Emergency Medicine Clinics of North America*, 25 (May 2007): 435–457.
19. "Consumers Still Taking Risks with OTC Painkillers," *Drug Utilization Review*, 19 (March 2003): 23.
20. Substance Abuse and Mental Health Services Administration, *Drug Abuse Warning Network, 2005: National Estimates of Drug-Related Emergency Room Visits* (Rockville, MD: Office of Applied Studies, 2007).
21. J. Adler, "Arthritis: What It Is, Why You Get It and How to Stop the Pain," *Newsweek* (September 3, 2001): 38–46.
22. S. Begley, "Jagged Little Pill: Aspirin, 100 Years Old, Still Gets No Respect," *Newsweek* (August 18, 1997): 64.
23. A. Agatston, "Turn Down the Heat," *Prevention*, 60 (April 2008): 35–36.
24. T. Nordberg, "An Aspirin a Day . . . Just Another Cliche?" *FDA Consumer* (March 1999): 14.

25. I. Kurth, A. G. Barr, J. M. Gaziano, and J. E. Buring, "Randomised Aspirin Assignment and Risk of Adult-Onset Asthma in the Woman's Health Study," *Thorax*, 63 (June 2008): 514–518.
26. J. Vekasi et al., "The Effect of Aspirin on Hemorheological Parameters of Patients with Diabetic Retinopathy," *Clinical Hemorheology and Microcirculation*, 39 (2008): 385–389.
27. "Aspirin and Breast Cancer," *Nutrition Action Newsletter*, 31 (July–August 2004): 7.
28. J. Edgar, "Simple Ways to Help Stave Off Skin Cancer," *Self*, 30 (May 2008): 202.
29. T. Sturmer, R. Glynn, T. Field, J. Taylor, and C. H. Hennekens, "Aspirin Use and Cognitive Function in the Elderly," *American Journal of Epidemiology*, 143 (1996): 683–691.
30. W. L. Adams, "Interactions Between Alcohol and Other Drugs," in *Older Adults' Misuse of Alcohol, Medicines, and Other Drugs*, edited by A. M. Gurnack (New York: Springer, 1997).
31. S. G. Johnson, K. Rogers, T. Delate, and D. M. Witt, "Outcomes Associated with Combined Antiplatelet and Anticoagulation Therapy," *Chest*, 133 (2008): 948–954.
32. R. Segal et al., "Early and Late Effects of Low-Dose Aspirin on Renal Function in Elderly Patients," *American Journal of Medicine*, 115 (2003): 462–466.
33. L. A. G. Rodriguez and S. Hernandez-Diaz, "Risk of Uncomplicated Peptic Ulcer Among Users of Aspirin and Nonaspirin Nonsteroidal Antiinflammatory Drugs," *American Journal of Epidemiology*, 159 (2004): 23–31.
34. "America's Best Drugstores," supra note 1.
35. "Aspirin Law for Under-16s," *Chemist and Druggist* (July 5, 2003): 6.
36. "Weighing Risks and Benefits of Arthritis Painkillers," *Health Facts* (November 2007): 4.
37. W. Cayley and B. S. Alper, "Acetaminophen Poisoning," *Cortlandt Forum* (May 2007): 63–64.
38. D. Ian, "The Tylenol Scare: Too Many Americans Gobble Acetaminophen Tablets Like So Many M&Ms. What Are the Risks?" *Time* (April 9, 2000): 44–49.
39. J. P. Forman, E. B. Rimm, and G. C. Curham, "Frequency of Analgesic Use and Risk of Hypertension among Men," *Archives of Internal Medicine*, 167 (2007): 394–399.
40. C. Rebordosa et al., "Acetaminophen Use During Pregnancy: Effects on Risk for Congenital Abnormalities," *American Journal of Obstetrics and Gynecology*, 198 (February 2008): 178.
41. "Survey: Ibuprofen Tops OTC Pain Meds," *Drug Store News*, 30 (May 19, 2008): 27.
42. "Ibuprofen Demonstrated to Be Superior Pain Relief for Pediatric Musculoskeletal Injuries," *Formulary*, 42 (June 2007): 394.
43. "Peptic Ulcers: What You Should Know," *American Family Physician*, 76 (October 1, 2007): 1013.
44. "NSAIDS May Worsen Enlarged Prostate Symptoms," *Urology Times*, 35 (November 2007): 20.
45. "Ibuprofen, Aspirin May Reduce Woman's Risk," *Clinical Oncology Week* (August 4, 2003): 12.
46. A. D. Walling, "Do NSAIDS Protect Patients Against Alzheimer's Disease?" *American Family Physician*, 69 (2004): 943–944.
47. "Naproxen Sodium/Sumatriptan Effective for Migraines, Improves QOL," *PharmacoEconomics and Outcome News*, 532 (July 14, 2007): 9.
48. "Health Wire: Help for Headaches," *Consumer Reports on Health* (June 2007): 2.
49. P. Winner et al., "Twelve-Month Tolerability and Safety of Sumatritian—Naproxen Sodium for the Treatment of Acute Migraine," *Mayo Clinic Proceedings*, 82 (January 2007): 61–68.
50. W. T. Elliott, "NSAIDs for Myocardial Infarction," *Travel Medicine Advisor* 12 (2004): 552.
51. "Ketoprofen Patch Agreement Signed for Joint Pain Treatment," *Manufacturing Chemist*, 74 (May 2003): 15.
52. M. K. Schaefer, N. Shehab, A. L. Cohen, and D. S. Budnitz, "Adverse Events from Cough and Cold Medications in Children," *Pediatrics*, 121 (April 2008): 783–787.
53. B. M. Kuehn, "Citing Serious Risks, FDA Recommends No Cold and Cough Medicines for Infants," *JAMA: Journal of the American Medical Association*, 299 (February 27, 2008): 887–888.
54. C. Guttman, "Antihistamine Relieves," *Dermatology Times*, 29 (May 2008): 56–57.
55. M. A. Kaliner, "A Novel and Effective Approach to Treating Rhinitis with Nasal Antihistamines," *Annals of Allergy, Asthma and Immunology*, 99 (November 2007): 383–393.
56. "Antihistamines May Prolong Infection," *USA Today Magazine*, 132 (February 2004): 10.
57. V. Nadalin, M. Cotterchio, and N. Krieger, "Antihistamine Use and Breast Cancer Risk," *International Journal of Cancer*, 106 (2003): 566–568.
58. O. Diav-Citrin, S. Schechtman, A. Aharonovich, et al., "Pregnancy Outcome After Gestational Exposure to Loratadine or Antihistamines: A Prospective Controlled Cohort Study," *Journal of Allergy and Clinical Immunology*, 111 (2003): 1239–1243.
59. S. M. Smith, K. Schroeder, and T. Fahey, "Over-the-Counter Medications for Acute Cough in Children and Adults in Ambulatory Settings," *Cochrane Database of Systematic Reviews* (2008).
60. "Chocolate Helps Suppress Coughs," *Professional Candy Buyer*, 11 (January–February 2003): 52.
61. D. S. Aschenbrenner, "A New Warning About Codeine," *American Journal of Nursing*, 107 (December 2007): 28–29.
62. "Robo-Tripping," *New Scientist*, 193 (February 3, 2007): 48.
63. "DMX Still Under Fire as Teen Misuse Studied," *Drug Store News*, 30 (March 3, 2008): 68.
64. "Congress Looks to Restrict DMX Distribution Due to Abuse," *Drug Store News*, 29 (November 12, 2007): 58.
65. M. O. Gorman, "Drugstore Dangers: Even 10-Year-Olds Are 'Robotripping' on Cough Medicines," *Prevention*, 56 (July 2004): 127.
66. Dextromethorphan (Washington, DC: National Highway Traffic Safety Administration, 2004).
67. D. A. Levine, "Pharming: The Abuse of Prescription and Over-the-Counter Drugs in Teens," *Current Opinion in Pediatrics*, 19 (June 2007): 270–274.
68. J. M. Berger, "Codeine Blues," *Family Practice News*, 30 (December 15, 2000): 23.
69. "Pharmacy Forum: Heartburn and Indigestion," *Chemist and Druggist* (October 9, 2004): 16.
70. D. S. Stricklnad, "Review: Over-the-Counter Medications Are Effective for Gastro-Oesophageal Reflux Disease," *Evidence-Based Nursing*, 10 (2007): 76.
71. L. Rolita and M. Freedman, "Over-the-Counter Medication Use in Older Adults," *Journal of Gerontological Nursing*, 34 (2008): 8–17.
72. "Antacids May Contribute to Hip Fractures," *Better Nutrition*, 69 (April 2007): 10.
73. J. Guirguis-Blake, "Medical Treatments in the Short-Term Management of Reflux Esophagitis," *American Family Physician*, 77 (March 1, 2008): 620.
74. K. Ramakrishnan and D. C. Scheid, "Treatment

Options for Insomnia," *American Family Physician*, 76 (August 15, 2007): 517–528.

75. "OTC: And So to Bed," *Chemist and Druggist* (July 31, 2004): 22.

76. M. A. Jordan and T. Haywood, "Evaluation of Internet Websites Marketing Herbal Weight-Loss Supplements to Consumers," *The Journal of Alternative and Complementary Medicine*, 13 (November 9, 2007): 1035–1043.

77. Ibid.

78. S. M. Wolfe, "Ephedra—Scientific Evidence Versus Money/Politics," *Science*, 300 (2003): 437.

79. S. Hettena, "Health Complaints Disregarded as Pill Firm Execs Grew Rich, Prosecutors Say," *Cortland Standard* (October 21, 2004): 17.

80. J. Beall, "Over-the-Counter Products for Weight Management," *The Alabama Nurse* (September, October, November 2007): 11.

81. "Weight Loss; Two Million Consumers Commit to Healthier Weight-Loss Approach with Alli," *Medical Letter on the CDC and FDA* (November 11, 2007): 130.

82. H. R. Wyatt, V. A. Catenacci, and J. O. Hill, "Over the Counter Orlistat: What Will Your Patients Want to Know?" *Obesity Management*, (October 2007): 204–209.

83. K. Sack and A. Mundy, "A Dose of Denial," *Los Angeles Times* (March 28, 2004): A11.

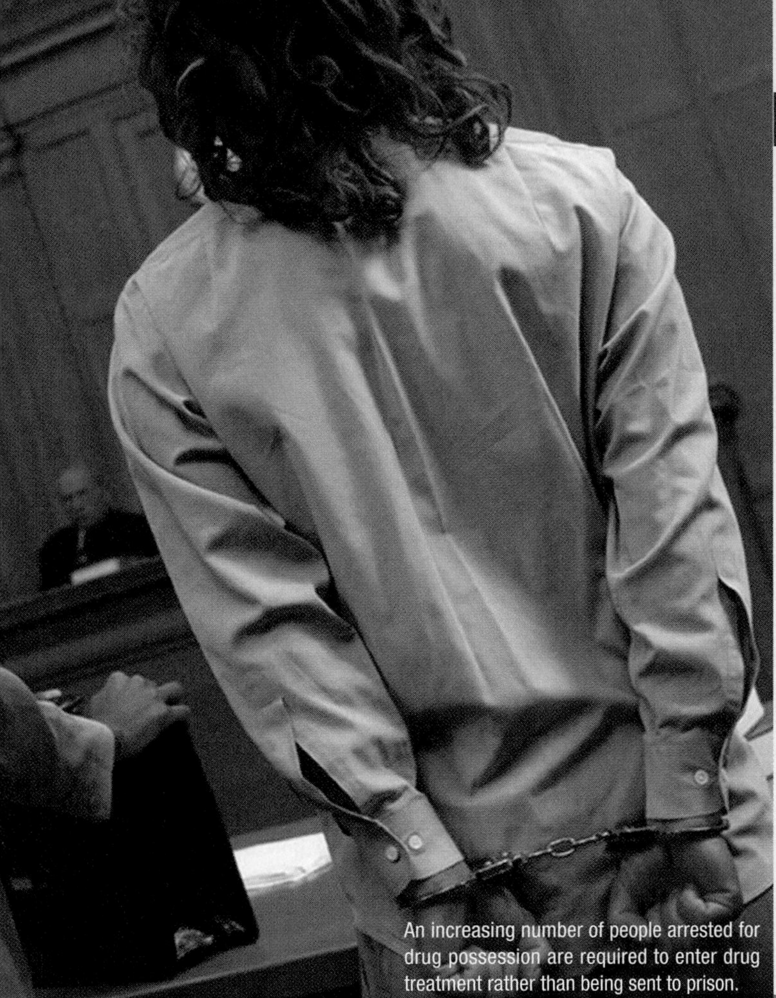
An increasing number of people arrested for drug possession are required to enter drug treatment rather than being sent to prison.

FACT OR FICTION?

1. The most common reason for not receiving drug abuse treatment is the stigma associated with receiving treatment.
2. Adults who use illicit drugs are more than twice as likely to have serious mental illness as adults who do not use an illicit drug.
3. In the early 1900s, drug addiction was viewed as a public health problem rather than as a legal problem.
4. The drug that accounts for the largest percentage of people in treatment is cocaine.
5. Although twice as many men as women enter drug treatment, the number of adolescent boys is nearly the same as the number of adolescent girls.
6. Drug addicts who enter into drug abuse treatment voluntarily have higher success rates than drug addicts who are required to go into treatment.
7. The rate at which people can stop using cocaine is about the same as the rate at which people stop smoking cigarettes.
8. More juveniles are in drug treatment for marijuana than for any other drug.
9. The majority of people who attend Alcoholics Anonymous (AA) meetings are likely to abstain from alcohol until they die.
10. Women are more likely than men to seek treatment for alcohol abuse.

Turn the page to check your answers

15 Substance Abuse Treatment

Chapter Objectives

After completing this chapter, the reader should be able to describe:

- How perceptions of the causes of substance abuse influence treatment
- Whether substance abuse treatment is more cost-effective than drug enforcement
- Factors that contribute to relapse by addicts in treatment
- Reasons people resist receiving substance abuse treatment
- The advantages and disadvantages of methadone maintenance programs
- The approach taken by therapeutic communities
- Advantages of outpatient treatment over various forms of treatment
- Features of the 12-step model
- Effectiveness of Alcoholics Anonymous

FACT OR FICTION?

1. **Fiction:** The fact is—although many people perceive a stigma to receiving drug abuse treatment, the most common reason was that abusers were not ready to receive treatment.
2. **Fact:** There is a high relationship between illicit drug use and mental illness.
3. **Fact:** Drug addiction was originally seen as a public health or medical problem. It was not until drugs were made illegal that addiction was viewed as a legal problem.
4. **Fiction:** The fact is—alcohol accounts for the highest percentage of individuals seeking substance abuse treatment.
5. **Fact:** According to data from the federal government, the numbers of adolescent males and females entering drug treatment are very comparable.
6. **Fiction:** The fact is—individuals who enter treatment voluntarily leave more quickly. The longer one stays in treatment, the more effective it is.
7. **Fact:** Numerous studies show that it is as difficult to stop cocaine use as it is to stop smoking cigarettes.
8. **Fact:** More than half of juveniles in drug treatment are there because of problems with marijuana.
9. **Fiction:** The fact is—some studies show that about one-third of AA members remain abstinent throughout their lifetimes.
10. **Fiction:** The fact is—because women are more stigmatized than men for seeking treatment for alcohol abuse, women are less likely to go into alcohol treatment.

The economic cost of illicit drug abuse for society amounts to $181 billion annually.[1] The federal government estimates that 23.6 million persons ages 12 and older need treatment for either an illicit drug or alcohol; yet, only 10.8% of those individuals receive treatment from a specialized facility.[2] Ninety-six percent of all admissions to state substance abuse agencies can be attributed to five drugs: alcohol (40%), opiates (18%), marijuana/hashish (16%), cocaine (14%), and stimulants (9%).[3] Socially, economically, and interpersonally, drug abuse is expensive. The federal government has allocated nearly $3.4 billion for drug-abuse treatment.[4] The need to prevent substance abuse is indisputable, and treatment is essential for people who require it. Despite the fact that the federal government allocates more than two-thirds of its drug-control budget to domestic law enforcement and interdiction efforts, the majority of Americans support treatment over enforcement.[5]

Underlying Causes of Drug Abuse

A national study found that people in treatment for substance abuse had problems that extended beyond drug abuse.[6] Compared with the general population, they were disadvantaged in education and employment. Proportionately, people in treatment were more likely to be male, Caucasian, ages 25 to 45, and unemployed or out of the workforce, and have less than a high school education.[7] Two groups that are showing an increasing trend in substance abuse problems are veterans and the elderly. Veterans account for 65,000 admissions at publicly funded treatment facilities.[8] Approximately 10% of all substance abusers in treatment are age 50 or older. Moreover, the number of older Americans who will require substance abuse treatment is expected to reach 1.7 million by 2020.[9] Among Americans ages 65 and older, it is estimated that 40 million will need substance abuse treatment by 2010. The primary substance of abuse is alcohol.[10]

How effective is treatment? What type of treatment is best? Also, the goals of a treatment program differ, depending on whether drug abuse is seen as a medical problem, as a breakdown in society, or as a personality weakness. If the cause of drug abuse is medical, some type of drug therapy might be in order. If the cause is social, the abuser might be taught how to deal with society. If the cause is seen as a personality defect, therapy would consist of restructuring the abuser's personality.

How substance abuse treatment is funded reflects society's view of the cause of substance abuse. Should tax dollars be used to treat people who could have prevented their substance abuse by not starting to use the substance? On the other hand, if substance abuse is the result of heredity, people have no control over their abuse of a substance. Though the immediate problem for many people might be drugs themselves, most professionals believe treatment must address the underlying causes of drug abuse, which could include poverty, inadequate health care, hunger, ethnic discrimination, and an inefficient educational system.

Should drug abusers receive treatment or incarceration, and is misuse of a substance a cause or a result of their behavior? Of prison inmates who had used heroin, methadone, cocaine, PCP, or LSD, half did not use these drugs until *after* their first arrest. Moreover, 15.8% of convicted inmates committed crimes to support their drug use.[11] If substance abusers are viewed as deviant, they are not seen in the same way as if they were seen as ill: The public sees the deviant person as one who should be locked up and the sick person as one who needs treatment.

relapse Failure to maintain a course of action, such as returning to drug abuse after initiating a treatment program

Drug Courts

One avenue for helping substance abusers is through drug courts. Because there is a strong relationship between substance abuse and criminal behavior, there is a need for the criminal justice system and substance abuse treatment programs to work with each other to curtail this problem. According to the publication *What Works: Effective Public Health Responses to Drug Use*:

> For nonviolent drug offenders whose underlying problem is substance use, drug treatment courts combine the power of the justice system with effective treatment services to break the cycle of criminal behavior, alcohol and drug use, child abuse and neglect, and incarceration.[12]

Although the first drug court was established in 1989, there are currently over 2,000 in the United States, and 10 other countries have adopted this model also. Offenders who complete substance abuse programs may be rewarded by having their sentences dismissed or reduced. The benefits of drug courts are supported by research. Fewer people are rearrested and convicted. In the first year after graduation from drug court, 16.4% of individuals were rearrested compared to 43.5% who did not go through drug courts. A study in Washington State indicated that $4,767 was saved in terms of reduced crime and taxpayer expenses. A California study found that drug courts cost $3,000 per client but saved $11,000 per client in the long run.[13] One downside is that the more intensive one's criminal background, the less likely that treatment will be effective.[14] Also, many treatment programs are underfunded.[15]

Profile of the Drug Abuser

Most people in drug treatment are Caucasian males, and the average age at admission is 34.[16] A substantial portion of drug-abusing patients have mental health problems, especially depression, psychotic and mood disorders, and antisocial personality disorders.[17] Moreover, as many as 30% to 40% of the homeless population consists of substance abusers.

Most people in treatment use more than one drug. This is especially true of individuals who have been admitted in a drug treatment program five or more times.[18] Multiple drug abuse seems to be dictated by drug availability rather than by desire for effects from a particular drug. To be drug-dependent does not mean necessarily that a person uses drugs daily. To support their behavior, drug abusers often resort to selling drugs, theft, and prostitution.

People in treatment are more likely to be unemployed and to have a low family income, and are less likely to be college graduates. Table 15.1 shows admission rates to drug treatment based on employment status and education.

History of Treatment

Using drugs to treat drug abuse was common in early treatment programs. To help abusers overcome their dependency on opiates, Freud experimented with cocaine as a substitute. Opium was also used to treat alcohol problems. When drug abuse treatment was initiated in the United States, therapy focused primarily on addiction to opiates. Until the Harrison Act of 1914, treatment was administered by private doctors who addressed opiate addiction as a medical problem.

The U.S. Public Health Service established two hospitals to serve the growing number of addicts in federal prisons. The first hospital was opened in Lexington, Kentucky, in 1935 and the second in Fort Worth, Texas, in 1938. Besides treating drug addicts who were prisoners, the hospitals treated voluntary patients. The goals of treatment were to gradually withdraw opiates from the addict, offer a drug-free environment, and provide psychotherapy. Originally, the recommended length of stay was 6 months, but later it was reduced to 4 months.

This treatment was considered ineffective. The **relapse** rate of people released in the 1940s through the early 1960s ranged between 87% and 96%.[19] Relapse usually occurred within 6 to 12 months after patients left treatment. Based on the high relapse rate of opiate addicts, this addiction was thought to be incurable; however, the high relapse rate occurred among patients who left the hospitals before completing treatment.

Current Treatment Options

In the 1960s, drug abuse treatment services expanded greatly. One type of program was the therapeutic community, a residential facility staffed by former drug addicts. The emphasis in these communities is on restructuring the addict's personality and maintaining an abstinent lifestyle.

TABLE 15.1 Admissions to Treatment by Primary Substance of Abuse, According to Employment Status (Ages 16 and Over) and Education (Ages 18 and Over): TEDS 2006*

Employment Status (Ages 16 and Over) and Education (Ages 18 and Over)	Primary Substance at Admission															
		Alcohol		Opiates		Cocaine			Stimulants							
	All Admissions	Alcohol Only	With Secondary Drug	Heroin	Other Opiates	Smoked Cocaine	Other Route	Marijuana/ Hashish	Methamphetamine/ Amphetamine	Other Stimulants	Tranquilizers	Sedatives	Hallucinogens	PCP	Inhalants	Other/ None Specified
Total admissions ages 16 and over	1,744,761	389,417	314,162	245,719	74,334	177,920	70,860	254,029	153,702	747	7,864	3,741	1,394	2,757	730	47,385
Employment status																
Employed	29.6	42.8	30.2	16.6	29.3	16.1	29.6	31.7	27.0	24.3	21.4	22.2	26.1	23.5	20.6	34.2
Full time	22.0	34.2	22.7	11.7	21.9	11.5	22.7	21.4	18.7	16.6	15.2	16.3	17.0	16.2	13.4	26.0
Part time	7.6	8.6	7.5	4.9	7.4	4.6	6.9	10.4	8.3	7.6	6.2	5.9	9.1	7.2	7.3	8.1
Unemployed	32.0	28.0	29.2	34.8	36.9	38.9	33.2	29.4	35.1	36.8	36.4	32.4	33.7	33.5	33.6	35.6
Not in labor force	38.5	29.2	40.7	48.6	33.8	45.0	37.1	38.8	37.9	39.0	42.1	45.4	40.2	43.0	45.7	30.2
Total	100.0	100.0	100.0	100.0	100.0	100.0	100.0	100.0	100.0	100.0	100.0	100.0	100.0	100.0	100.0	100.0
Admissions ages 18 and over	1,720,550	384,178	311,172	241,897	73,331	175,703	69,921	251,629	152,984	734	7,738	3,667	1,362	2,691	717	42,826
Total admissions ages 18 and over	1,659,805	382,890	302,908	244,725	73,373	177,010	68,783	199,647	149,510	672	7,634	3,574	1,199	2,688	584	44,608
Highest school grade completed																
0 to 8	6.1	6.3	5.3	7.2	4.6	5.7	6.1	5.2	5.7	7.2	6.0	3.9	5.5	6.7	9.1	12.3
9 to 11	26.8	18.1	26.6	29.1	20.3	28.8	26.8	37.3	32.5	23.9	23.1	20.9	31.5	41.1	29.1	24.6
12 (or GED)	44.2	44.6	44.4	45.7	44.9	43.4	43.3	42.8	44.8	39.4	41.0	41.5	42.9	41.4	42.9	38.5
More than 12	23.0	31.1	23.7	18.0	30.2	22.1	23.8	14.6	17.0	29.4	30.0	33.6	20.1	10.9	18.9	24.6
Total	100.0	100.0	100.0	100.0	100.0	100.0	100.0	100.0	100.0	100.0	100.0	100.0	100.0	100.0	100.0	100.0
Admissions ages 18 and over	1,639,488	376,867	300,253	242,417	72,555	175,547	68,041	197,695	148,227	852	7,501	3,634	1,182	2,665	581	41,771

*Based on administrative data reported to TEDS by all reporting states and jurisdictions.

Source: Office of Applied Studies, Substance Abuse and Mental Health Services Administration, Treatment Episode Data Set (TEDS). Data received through 10/9/07.

methadone maintenance program A type of therapy used in the treatment of heroin addiction

detoxification Eliminating drugs from the body; usually the initial step in treatment of alcohol and other drugs

Methadone maintenance programs, initiated in the 1960s, are outpatient programs in which opiate addicts receive methadone daily. Methadone eliminates the withdrawal symptoms from opiates and prevents addicts from getting high. Before entering treatment, addicts go through **detoxification**, a medically supervised program to withdraw gradually from the drugs on which they are physically dependent.

In essence, detoxification allows the body to adjust to the absence of drugs. According to the Center for Substance Abuse Treatment, three immediate goals of detoxification are the following:

1. To provide safe withdrawal from drugs
2. To provide withdrawal that is humane and protects the person's dignity
3. To prepare the person for ongoing treatment

Methadone, naltrexone, or buprenorphine is used in lieu of heroin to enable the addict to function normally, not just to alleviate withdrawal symptoms. Moreover, treatment programs address psychological and behavioral factors that contributed to drug addiction in the first place. Drug abusers can be treated in short-term or long-term residential facilities. Long-term residential programs are geared to individuals with severe dependency problems.

Sometimes drugs other than methadone are used to help an addict who is in withdrawal, because abuse of multiple drugs has become the norm. Drugs such as methadone will not help an opiate addict who also abuses cocaine or alcohol. Determining which drug or drugs to use in treatment is difficult because of these variables.

Self-help programs are growing in popularity. These programs are based on the principles of Alcoholics Anonymous.

Benefits of Treatment

Regardless of the type of treatment, treatment is desirable. The benefits are summed up as follows:

- Less expensive than incarceration
- Reduced use of illicit drugs
- Decline in criminal activity
- More stable employment
- Reduced transmission of AIDS

If the costs of drug abuse treatment are compared with the alternative costs of continued drug abuse, associated criminal activity, and medical treatment of AIDS, there is no question that the social benefits are worth the expense of drug abuse treatment.[20]

Not only do many people benefit from substance abuse treatment, but society benefits economically as well.[21] An older study of drug treatment in California noted that \$7 was saved for every \$1 that went into treatment and that the level of crime engaged in by these individuals declined by two-thirds in the year after treatment.[22] More current research reveals that there is a \$4 to \$7 reduction in the cost of drug-related crimes for every dollar spent on substance abuse treatment.[23]

Treating substance abuse is expensive, but treatment is less costly than imprisonment. The cost of incarceration ranges from \$44,860 per prisoner in Rhode Island to \$13,009 in Louisiana. Between 2007 and 2011 it is estimated that prisons will need an additional \$27.5 billion.[24] Incarcerating people has little impact on drug use. In November 2000, California voters passed an initiative that resulted in treatment rather than incarceration for tens of thousands of nonviolent drug possession offenders.[25] In many counties in California the number of people, especially employed males, who went into treatment increased.[26]

A review of drug abuse research spanning 25 years concluded that intensive and appropriate drug treatment reduces both drug use and crime.[27] A report from California found that cocaine treatment was more effective in reducing the demand for cocaine than high-profile police and military action.[28] However, a 2008 report noted that funding in California for treatment programs is inadequate.[29]

A comprehensive study of the benefits of treatment conducted in the 1990s, the National Treatment Improvement Evaluation Study, reported that after treatment, drug selling declined by 78%, shoplifting went down 82%, and arrests declined 64%.[30] Crime-related economic costs to society went from \$15,262 annually per client before treatment to \$14,089 annually per client after treatment. The amount of money that drug abusers spent on drugs declined from \$6,854 per year before treatment to \$2,687 in the year after treatment.[31] Similarly, cocaine addicts had a 69% decline in illegal activity and a 77% increase in employment in the year after treatment. Table 15.2 shows the impact of drug treatment on crime.

Of the 4,411 people in the National Treatment Improvement Evaluation Study, drug use declined from 73% before treatment to 38% 1 year after treatment. Cocaine use went from 40% before

TABLE 15.2 Drug Treatment and Criminal Activity: Percentage of Clients Engaged in Criminal Activity in 12 Months Before Versus 12 Months After Treatment Exit (N = 4,411)

	Before	After	Percent Difference*
Selling Drugs	64.0	13.9	278.3
Shoplifting	63.7	11.7	281.6
Beating Someone Up	49.3	11.0	277.7
Arrested for Any Crime	48.2	17.2	64.3
Most Support Illegal	17.4	9	48.3

*Before/after difference is statistically significant at 0.05 level.
Source: National Treatment Improvement Evaluation Study (SAMHSA, 1997).

treatment to 18% 1 year after treatment. Heroin use declined from 24% before treatment to 13% within 1 year after treatment. Other benefits included the following[32]:

- An increase in employment from 51% to 60%
- A decline in clients receiving welfare from 40% to 35%
- A drop in homelessness from 19% to 11%
- A 53% decline in substance-related medical visits
- A 56% reduction in people exchanging sex for money or drugs
- A 51% drop in people having sex with an intravenous drug user

Another area in which treatment is beneficial is in curbing AIDS. Many drug users who inject drugs share syringes. According to the Centers for Disease Control and Prevention (CDC), injected drug use is the second most frequent behavior reported by individuals with AIDS. Through its drug treatment services, the U.S. Public Health Service initiated AIDS outreach education projects, educating clients about high-risk behaviors that lead to transmission of HIV. Figure 15.1 shows the percentages of people with HIV/AIDS who contracted the disease through several of these behaviors.

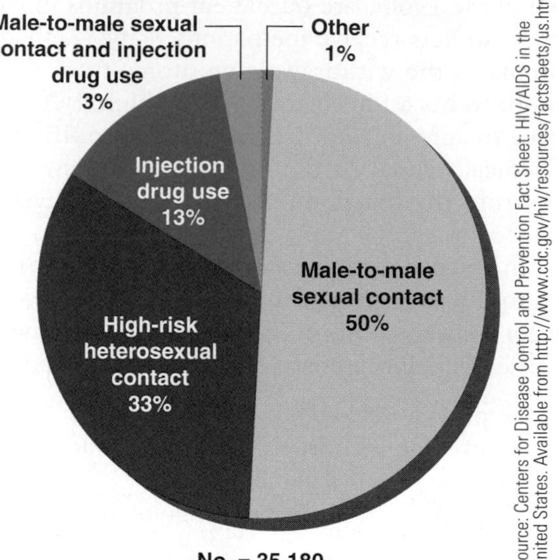

Figure 15.1 Transmission Categories of Adults and Adolescents with HIV/AIDS Diagnosed during 2006 (All Adults and Adolescents)

Treatment Issues

Funding substance abuse treatment has economic and political ramifications. Many people question the efficacy of funding treatment programs; therefore, funding is under constant public scrutiny. An important question is: What is the most effective use for the money being allocated? The treatment programs that are most cost-effective are more likely to be funded. Four pertinent issues in treating drug abuse are (1) determining whether voluntary or compulsory treatment is better, (2) matching the patients to the treatment that works best for them, (3) determining whether treatment programs designed for adults would be equally effective with adolescent substance abusers, and (4) designing programs to address the special circumstances of female addicts.

Voluntary versus Compulsory Treatment

Many drug users enter treatment under their own volition. Others are compelled to do so; prisoners, for instance, often are required to enter treatment programs. Sometimes a drug offender is given a choice between prison or treatment. A relevant question is whether compulsory participation is as effective as voluntary participation. Early studies of institutionalized clients in drug treatment in the Public Health Service hospitals in Lexington and Fort Worth showed that volunteers fared better than those required to be in treatment.[33] Other studies, however, indicate that clients who are required to receive treatment make as much progress, as measured by relapse and recidivism, as those who enter voluntarily.[34]

The key issue could be how long the person stays in treatment. Individuals who complete treatment are more likely to maintain employment and not relapse.

Nonetheless, individuals such as prisoners need follow-up care after treatment because the probability of relapse increases without this care.[35]

Matching Patients and Treatments

Because individuals have different learning styles, we can logically assume that individuals respond to different modalities for treating substance abuse. No single type of treatment applies to everyone. Many drug abusers drop out of treatment because the specific program they have attempted is poorly defined in terms of content, goals, approach, and duration.[36] Increasing evidence suggests that matching clients to specific treatments increases effectiveness of the treatment. For example, one study of cocaine abusers found that those with high abstract reasoning ability and low religious belief responded better to cognitive-behavioral therapy than to a 12-step approach. Likewise, those with low abstract reasoning ability and high religious belief fared better in a 12-step program.[37]

Matching clients to treatment is not a new concept. Before one matches clients to treatment, several questions have to be addressed:

- Which treatment produces the best outcomes for a specific group or person?
- Do members of certain ethnic or socioeconomic groups respond similarly to certain types of treatment?
- Is the effectiveness of a specific program linked to age of participants?
- Do females and males differ in their responses to treatment?

Matching treatment to gender, culture, ethnicity, language, and sexual orientation improves the likelihood of positive outcomes. Patients with severe psychiatric problems and patients from lower socioeconomic backgrounds tend not to benefit from most types of treatment, especially outpatient treatment. Also, the majority of patients with co-occurring psychiatric disorders abuse more than one substance.[38] Individuals from supportive social and economic backgrounds and with few psychiatric problems tend to respond positively to treatment. Many professionals believe that poor matching between clients and treatment approaches accounts for poor results.

Treating Adolescent Drug Abusers

In 2006, in the United States, 211,247 individuals ages 19 and younger were admitted to a drug treatment facility, and the primary drug of abuse was marijuana.[39] Among adolescents admitted into treatment, 31% are female.[40] Even though the physical, emotional, intellectual, and social consequences of adolescent drug use are well documented, few studies have looked at the effectiveness of treatment programs for adolescents. Moreover, there are inconsistencies in how the results of treatment are reported.[41] The few available studies suggest that treatment is more likely to be successful if some type of social support is in place. Also, among adolescents in treatment for marijuana, more intensive, longer programs (three months) are more effective than short (two session) programs.[42] One study examined the relative effectiveness of various modalities of treatment and found that group treatment was more effective and less expensive than family-based or individual treatment.[43]

One positive outcome of treatment is that teens who enter treatment do better academically than teens who do not receive treatment. However, the younger a person is when drug abuse starts, the less likely treatment will be successful.[44] About half of those younger than age 18 successfully complete treatment.[45] Adolescents develop different patterns and problems of drug abuse than adults. Therefore, treatment programs have to be designed specifically for adolescents.

Women and Treatment

In 1974, The National Institute on Drug Abuse's Program for Women's Concerns expanded treatment options for drug-addicted women. Nevertheless, treatment programs for women are scarce. According to one estimate, of the 7.4 million women ages 18 or older who need substance abuse treatment, only 11.2% receive it.[46] Even when treatment is available, many women are reluctant to enter a program because they are not ready to stop their drug use, the cost dissuades them from receiving treatment, or they feel stigmatized. Figure 15.2 shows the reasons that women do not enter treatment.

Among women entering treatment for the first time, the highest percentage were never married (44%), followed by formerly married women (37%), followed by currently married women.[47] Many women feel discouraged from entering treatment because the quality of treatment is questionable and the wait to get into a program is long. Also, many addicted mothers feel a sense of guilt and fear losing custody of their children.[48]

To address prenatal drug use, the emphasis is on punishing the pregnant drug user rather than on treating her. Paradoxically, many women seek treatment to reduce drug-related harm to their children. Women are more likely to stay in treatment if they attend with their children.[49] Many treatment

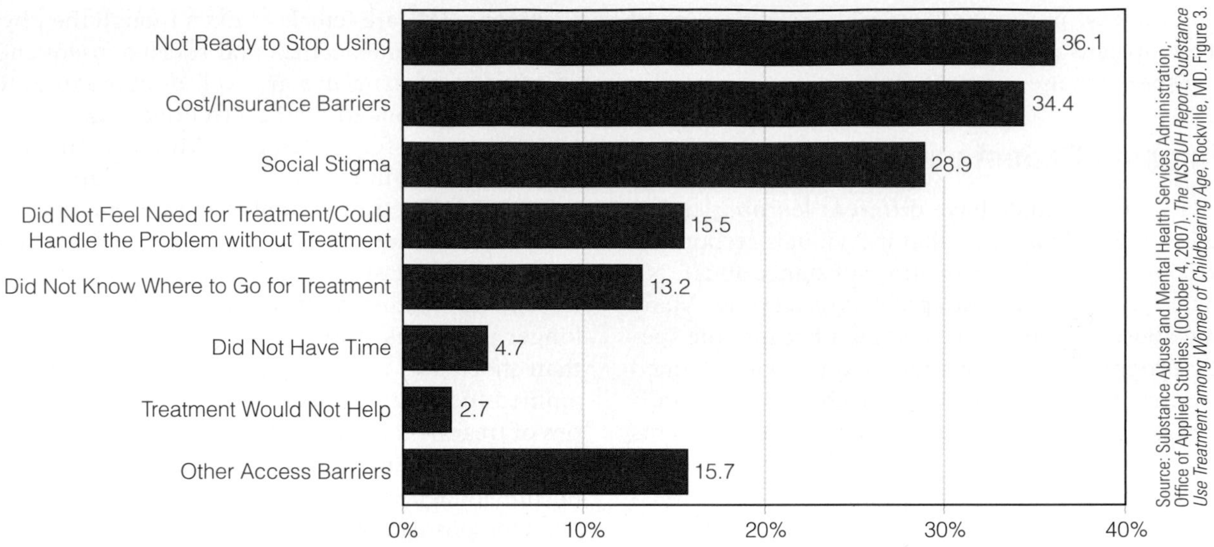

Figure 15.2 Percentages of Reasons* for Not Receiving Substance Use Treatment in the Past Year among Women Aged 18 to 49 Who Needed Treatment and Who Perceived a Need for It: 2004–2006

*Respondents could indicate multiple reasons; thus, these response categories are not mutually exclusive.
Cost/insurance barriers include "no health coverage and could not afford cost," "had health coverage but it did not cover treatment or did not cover cost," and other-specify responses of "could not afford cost; health coverage not indicated." Social stigma includes "might cause neighbors/community to have negative opinion," "might have negative effect on job," "did not want others to find out," and other-specify responses of "ashamed/embarrassed/afraid" and "afraid would have trouble with the police/social services." Did not feel need for treatment/could handle the problem without treatment includes "did not feel need for treatment," "could handle the problem without treatment," and other-specify responses of "could do it with support of family/friends/others" and "could do it through religion/spirituality." Other access barriers include "no transportation/inconvenient," "no program having type of treatment," "no openings in a program," and other-specify responses of "no program had counselors/doctors with whom you were comfortable," "services desired were unavailable or you were currently ineligible," and "attempted to get treatment but encountered delays."

programs fail to recognize that women in treatment often have concomitant problems such as divorce, family violence, psychiatric problems, and other family members with substance abuse problems. It has been shown that women in female-only drug abuse treatment centers are more likely to benefit from treatment compared to women in mixed-gender programs.[50] The majority of women in treatment have a history of rape, aggravated assault, or post-traumatic stress syndrome. Women in treatment also have significantly higher rates of eating disorders than women in general.

Problems Associated with Treatment

Treatment poses several problems. One is retention of clients and counselors. The client dropout rate is high, with a majority of people who enter treatment dropping out within the first month. Another problem arises when people resist having treatment facilities located near their home, school, or workplace. And always problematic is the rate of relapse; a high percentage of clients return to drug use.

Client Resistance to Treatment

One factor that prevents individuals from receiving treatment is cost. Of persons ages 18 or older, 31.2% indicated that the lack of health insurance and the cost of treatment precluded them from receiving treatment.[51] Gender is another factor in whether one seeks treatment. Twice as many men as women have alcohol-related problems, but men are four times more likely to get treatment. A double standard exists in that women are more stigmatized than men for having a problem with alcohol or other drugs. Age also influences whether one gets treatment. A study of cocaine dependency found that younger patients and high school dropouts were less likely to stay in treatment and keep their appointments.[52]

Several factors account for the reluctance to seek treatment:

- Many treatment facilities are not readily available or accessible.
- A large percentage of clients lack insurance and cannot afford the cost of treatment.
- The policies and philosophies of some facilities deter drug abusers from pursuing help.
- For some drug abusers the benefits of using drugs outweigh the disadvantages.

- Some clients think that legal authorities will be made aware of their drug-taking behavior if they enter treatment.

The likelihood of an individual receiving treatment improves when a family member, friend, coworker, or clergy member contacts the treatment agency for an appointment.

NIMBY (not in my back yard) A term describing how some people feel about having a controversial facility located in their neighborhoods

Community Resistance

In general, people are in favor of treatment for drug abusers but do not want drug treatment centers in their neighborhoods. Although many communities do not like treatment centers located near them, one of the most important reasons people drop out of treatment is that they do not live near the treatment facility.[53] Residents living near sites designated for drug treatment are concerned about more crime, more traffic, exposure of children to bad influences, and lower property values. The **NIMBY (not in my backyard)** syndrome should prompt treatment staffs to make concerted efforts to dispel the misgivings surrounding treatment centers.

Continuing Drug Use

Despite the benefits of treatment, rates of illicit drug use by clients remain high. The goal of abstinence is often not being realized. To determine whether the high rate of continuing illicit drug use by clients reflects a failure on the part of the treatment process or clients' underlying problems is difficult. Nonetheless, one factor that is important in reducing drug use is the duration of treatment. Treatment of at least 6 months seems to be necessary to reduce drug use significantly. One study of adolescents in treatment reported that drug usage declined somewhat but remained high nonetheless. In this study, marijuana use 1 year after treatment declined from 80.4% to 43.8%, heavy drinking went from 33.8% to 20.3%, and use of illicit drugs dropped from 48.0% to 42.2%.[54]

Relapse

Although no single cause accounts for relapse during or after drug abuse treatment, the person's surrounding environment plays an important role. Because of financial restraints, clients receive little follow-up care once they leave treatment. One study that looked at relapse among alcoholics noted that follow-up care did not reduce the rate of relapse.[55] Treatment clients usually return to the environments from which they came and, when confronted with high-risk situations, many of them relapse to unhealthy patterns of drug use because they lack the necessary coping skills or social support system. Also, if the drug abuser's spouse uses drugs, the likelihood of relapse increases.[56]

Relapse is not inevitable, though. One study found that 19% of clients remained abstinent over a 6-year period.[57] Further, an anger management program helped reduce relapse rates among cocaine abusers. Similarly, homeless veterans who engaged in healthy lifestyle behaviors while in a residential rehabilitation program were less likely to relapse.[58] In essence, the drug is not what causes the relapse but, rather, events associated with taking the drug.

Even when a person completes drug rehabilitation successfully, the compulsion to use drugs often reappears. A former addict is conditioned to experience withdrawal symptoms even after long periods of abstinence.

Sometimes objects trigger the desire for drugs. For example, white sugar or talcum powder might be a trigger for a former cocaine addict. Certain people, places, or odors—or even talking about drugs—could evoke the urge. Former cigarette smokers testify to the propensity for relapse. Mark Twain, a smoker, commented that it was easy to stop smoking—he'd stopped hundreds of times! An all-too-familiar scenario illustrating the paradox of using drugs against one's better judgment is related in the following:

The patient has been through a rehabilitation program; he has returned to his job; he is re-united with his family; and he can present an apparently genuine and logical argument that he never intends to touch the drug again. And then, as one patient said recently, "I bumped into a guy that I used to do coke with, and my heart started pounding and I started shaking. Then I went on automatic pilot."[59]

Three factors contribute to relapse among alcoholics:

1. Negative emotional states such as frustration, anxiety, depression, anger, or boredom
2. Interpersonal conflicts with a spouse, family member, friend, or employer
3. Social pressure from a person or group of people

Relapse comes sooner for problem drinkers who were depressed at the time they entered treatment.[60] Also, former alcoholics who experience severe stress are more likely to relapse.[61] Cocaine abusers are more likely to relapse if they continue using alcohol after treatment, although people who were formerly dependent on alcohol did not have higher rates of relapse.[62]

Alcoholics who remain abstinent for 5 years are unlikely to relapse, and relapse is less likely if addicts are married, have been employed for at least 4 years, and are reared in the same cultural setting as their parents.[63] Four factors related to recovery are compulsory supervision, new relationships, a substitute dependency, and membership in an inspirational group.

Personnel Recruitment and Retention

Recruiting and retaining staff members in treatment programs are difficult because of the intense demands on the staff. According to the National Institute on Drug Abuse, treatment facilities are operating at more than 90% capacity, and personnel feel overworked because of the heavy caseloads. The quality and quantity of services at many facilities have been curtailed severely. Also, the high relapse rate of clients is discouraging. Because of these reasons, plus inadequate wages and poor working conditions, personnel often seek other employment.

The New York State Division of Substance Abuse Services found that the largest obstacles for attracting and retaining staff were inadequate fringe benefits and low wages. In a vicious cycle, low staff retention causes poor morale. Additional factors that hamper staff recruitment and retention include the following:

- Reluctance to work with drug abusers
- Undesirable locations of facilities
- Inadequate supply of applicants with professional experiences and qualifications
- Fear of contracting AIDS

Treatment Programs

The range of treatment programs available complicates the decision as to which treatment program to choose. Treatment programs have different philosophies and practices and different degrees of effectiveness. To assess effectiveness is not easy, either, because effectiveness means different things to different people. To some, effectiveness means a reduction in criminal activity or drug use. To others, nothing less than total abstinence from crime or drug use indicates effectiveness. Some require abstinence for a period of 1, 2, or 5 years to denote success. People seeking treatment often have different goals as well. One study in Great Britain found that 72% wanted to stop using drugs altogether while 12% wanted to stop using particulars drugs and 12% wanted to reduce their drug use.[64]

Some people go into **spontaneous remission**. They stop taking drugs without undergoing any kind of formal treatment. Some people stop substance abuse regardless of treatment. In a study of 841 drug abusers spanning 25 years, it was found that spontaneous remission was the rule and not the exception.[65]

The forms of treatment discussed here include methadone maintenance, therapeutic communities, outpatient treatment, inpatient treatment, and self-help groups. Alcohol treatment programs are discussed separately.

Methadone Maintenance

A program of giving methadone to heroin addicts started in New York City in the early 1960s. Federal guidelines define a methadone maintenance program as any form of treatment that involves the dispensing of methadone for opiate addiction for more than 30 days. Methadone is a synthetic drug that eliminates withdrawal symptoms from opiates and prevents an opiate addict from experiencing euphoria. It is given orally and is effective for 24 hours.

Methadone is effective only for heroin and not other drugs to which a person might be addicted. To be admitted into a methadone maintenance program, addicts must have been dependent for at least 1 year. An estimated 115,000 heroin addicts are enrolled in methadone maintenance programs. However, the number of treatment slots is woefully inadequate.[66]

Patients come for the dose of methadone daily, although many clients administer the methadone to themselves at home. The demand for methadone maintenance is high, with waiting lists up to 1 year. Many clinics offer medical, psychiatric, and vocational services. These services vary considerably from one clinic to another. These additional services fulfill a critical need. For example, it has been demonstrated that drug-using men enrolled in methadone maintenance programs have poorer parenting skills than no-drug-using men.[67]

Psychotherapy in conjunction with methadone yields the best results.[68] Also, success rates are higher when patients come daily for methadone, as opposed to two to three times per week.[69] When patients attend methadone clinics, personnel counsel them about AIDS and the risks of needle sharing.

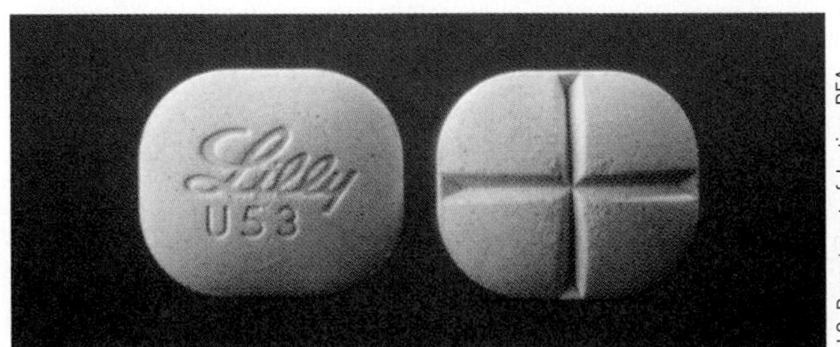

U.S. Department of Justice, DEA.

Methadone provides one treatment option for heroin addiction.

spontaneous remission Cessation of drug abuse without any type of formal treatment

levo-alpha-acetylmethadol (LAAM) An experimental drug that prevents narcotic withdrawal symptoms for about 3 days

cold turkey Elimination of a negative behavior all at once, as opposed to gradually (with or without a substitute)

therapeutic community (TC) A residential drug treatment center that utilizes confrontation techniques

A growing problem is the number of patients with the hepatitis C virus (HCV), which, like HIV, is bloodborne. It is estimated that 60% to 90% of patients in methadone maintenance programs are infected with the hepatitis C virus.[70] In the United States, the average cost to support a patient taking methadone is $3,500 annually, whereas a residential treatment program costs $12,000 per year and incarceration costs $39,600 per year.[71] One study that looked at providing methadone maintenance in the workplace found that the cost was $362 a week, considerably less than other types of treatment.[72]

The longer patients stay in treatment, the greater the benefit. Crime reduction and relapse rates improve dramatically as duration of treatment lengthens. Also, after patients leave treatment, they are less likely to engage in high-risk behaviors.[73] Likewise, prisoners who initiate methadone maintenance just prior to their release or just after their release are less likely to use heroin six months later.[74] Relapse is less likely if a strong emphasis is placed on abstinence, although the use of other drugs, such as marijuana, increases the rate of relapse.[75] Patients who drop out of treatment or who are unfavorably discharged are more likely to die from a drug overdose within 1 year after discharge.[76]

The success of methadone maintenance is noteworthy because people in these programs have a history of substance abuse that is longer and more serious than is found in patients who enter outpatient centers or inpatient therapeutic communities (discussed later). Despite its effectiveness, methadone is not a panacea. A review of 15 different studies found that methadone maintenance had no affect on alcohol use.[77]

Methadone treatment does not eliminate poverty, psychological problems, homelessness, illegal drug use, or crime. One concern is whether breastfeeding women in methadone maintenance transmit methadone in breast milk; however, the level of methadone found in breast milk poses no risk to the child.[78] Clients are required to come for treatment daily, and critics charge that the daily routine perpetuates dependency. Clients' acceptance of methadone maintenance is widespread, and fewer people drop out of methadone maintenance than other forms of treatment. Nonetheless, methadone maintenance programs have come under criticism due to reports of fatal overdoses.[79]

To address concerns over the daily use of methadone, an alternative drug, **levo-alpha-acetylmethadol (LAAM)**, received U.S. Food and Drug Administration (FDA) approval in 1993. Because of health concerns related to LAAM, the FDA requires additional warnings on LAAM labels.[80] Methadone blocks the withdrawal symptoms of heroin for a day, but LAAM works for 3 days. In contrast to methadone, addicts given LAAM were more likely to remain in treatment and less likely to get arrested.[81] Side effects of LAAM include muscle aches, difficulty breathing, impaired circulation, dizziness, vomiting, sweating, and diarrhea.

Other drugs that block the effects of opiates are naltrexone, naloxone, clonidine, and buprenorphine. Countries including Switzerland, Australia, Germany, and the Netherlands are experimenting with giving heroin to addicts. Until 1968, the British government allowed physicians to prescribe heroin. However, this program was abandoned because many unnecessary prescriptions were being filled, increasing the number of heroin addicts.[82] In a study in Switzerland in which heroin addicts were given either heroin or methadone, the addicts preferred heroin because they reported fewer side effects.[83] Another study in Germany found that addicts given heroin had improved physical and mental health while in treatment.[84]

The use of buprenorphine as a treatment for heroin addiction has increased. Because most addicts go untreated, having doctor's offices provide buprenorphine may increase the number of addicts who receive treatment.[85] An advantage of buprenorphine is that it is less addicting than other narcotic antagonists. Thus, it is easier for heroin addicts to stop buprenorphine treatment.[86] When compared to methadone maintenance, buprenorphine is less effective.[87]

Some narcotic addicts say that methadone withdrawal is worse than going **cold turkey**. Several studies indicate that 70% to 80% of patients resume use of narcotics within 1 or 2 years after treatment, and between 15% and 20% continue to use cocaine intravenously. Side effects include increased perspiration, chronic constipation, sexual dysfunction, and difficulty sleeping. These effects tend to subside within the first 6 months of treatment. Concerns remain about the long-term effects of using methadone, although nothing points to any serious negative outcomes.

Therapeutic Communities

Therapeutic communities (TCs) are drug-free residential settings where abusers reside for 1 or 2 years. They differ widely. The philosophy of therapeutic communities is that drug abuse is incurable, but it is a behavioral problem that can benefit from behavioral intervention. According to this view, drug abuse is not the core problem; a character disorder within the person is the problem.[88]

Whereas individual therapy is the focus of many treatment approaches, TCs stress group intervention techniques, especially **encounter groups**. The emphasis is on "community," as the name suggests. Residents are given chores. If they accept responsibility, they are given more responsibilities and more privileges. Residents must abstain from drugs. TCs are headed by one or two professionals, and the remainder of the staff typically consists mainly of former drug addicts.

TCs teach socially acceptable and adaptive skills. Most clients in TCs have serious social adjustment problems that are worsened by years of severe addiction. Most of the residents are opiate users. TCs provide vocational and educational assistance and improve the self-esteem and self-confidence of their residents. A stay of 3 to 12 months tends to eliminate or reduce their drug use and involvement in crime, and it increases employment rates and school attendance. The effectiveness of TCs, however, may relate more to the temperament and character of the residents. Some personality types fare better in TCs than others.[89]

Those who complete their residency do have the highest success rate. The biggest problem for TCs has been the high dropout rate. Most of the residents leave within the first 3 months of treatment—especially within the first 30 days. Clients who leave in the early stages of treatment tend to do so for personal reasons such as family or work pressures or the desire to continue getting high. Some clients believe they no longer need treatment. An equal number of clients leave TCs simply because they do not like the regimentation of the program or the program staff. TCs seem to be best suited for people with an extensive history of drug abuse problems.[90] It was found that female prisoners in a therapeutic community while in prison are significantly better in terms of mental health, criminal behavior, and HIV-risk behavior 6 months after their release.[91]

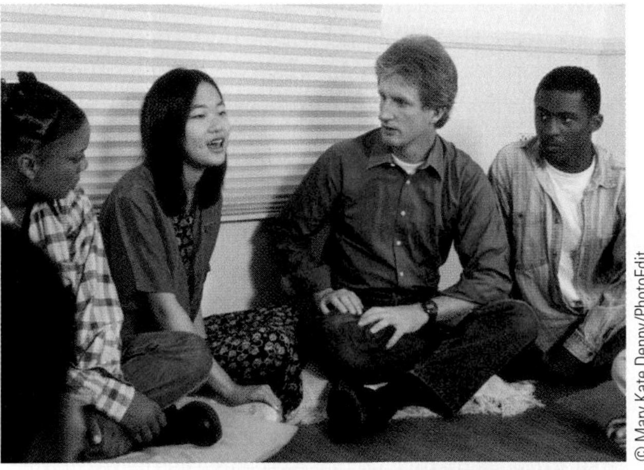

© Mary Kate Denny/PhotoEdit.

The longer drug abusers stay in treatment, the more effective the treatment.

Outpatient Treatment

The most common form of community drug abuse treatment is **outpatient treatment**. Outpatient programs are popular because they are readily available, less disruptive and stigmatizing than inpatient treatment for abusers with jobs and families, and less expensive. Treatment might involve family therapy or psychotherapy.

Outpatient treatment ranges from counseling centers to halfway houses to community centers. Many outpatient programs are identified as intensive, meaning that clients attend group therapy three times a week for 2 to 3 hours per session. Traditional outpatient programs provide social, vocational, and educational services. Outpatient therapy frequently is used after a client leaves methadone maintenance, although outpatient treatment is used in conjunction with abuse of any drug, not just narcotics.

Evaluations of outpatient programs reveal limited effectiveness. One study found that clients who travel shorter distances to receive substance abuse treatment are more likely to complete the treatment.[92] Another study reported that outpatient treatment effectively reduces criminality while improving employment.[93] One problem is that clients attending outpatient treatment centers often go back to the environments that contributed to their drug abuse initially. Outpatient treatment can be more costly for the client than inpatient treatment because insurance programs pay less for outpatient care than for inpatient care.

Inpatient Treatment

Typically, **inpatient treatment** programs are hospital based. Because this form of treatment is based on a hospital model, it is expensive. The number of inpatient treatment programs grew rapidly because of financial support from insurance companies and businesses, which now are reexamining their position on financing inpatient treatment. Inpatient treatment has been found to be no more effective than intensive outpatient treatment. Therefore, the financial concerns of businesses and insurance companies might be justified.

Of people admitted into short-term residential programs, 61% complete the program. The average length of stay is 26 days.[94] These programs tend to be highly structured, and patients are expected to abide

TABLE 15.3 Costs Associated with Four Treatment Modalities

	Average Length of Stay (Weeks)	Economic Price per Treatment Episode
Long-term Residential	20	$16,448
Short-term Residential	3	$3,287
Outpatient Methadone	99	$8,609
Outpatient Drug-Free	17	$3,557

Source: Roebuck, French and McClellan gathered information on 53 outpatient and 32 residential (inpatient) programs between 1993 and 2002.

Table copied from: A. S. Bhati, J.R. Roman, and A. Chalfin. *To Treat or Not to Treat: Evidence on the Prospects of Expanding Treatment to Drug-Involved Offenders*. Washington, DC: Justice Policy Center, The Urban Institute (April 2008).

encounter groups A type of confrontational treatment frequently used at therapeutic communities

outpatient treatment A nonresidential drug treatment program; least expensive form of treatment

inpatient treatment A residential drug treatment program based on a hospital model

by regimented schedules and rules of conduct. On admission, patients are asked about their drug-taking history and are given tests to evaluate their physical and psychological status. Group therapy and drug education are stressed in many inpatient programs. Table 15.3 shows the average length of stay in various treatment programs and their respective costs.[95]

Self-Help Groups

In recent years, the public has grown skeptical of the health care system, and many people are assuming responsibility for their own health needs. Consequently, self-help groups have proliferated as a grassroots response to perceived inadequacies within the health care system. Members of self-help groups are bound by a common denominator such as alcohol, gambling, food, shopping, or sex.

The largest self-help group is Alcoholics Anonymous (AA), based on a 12-step model, which has been incorporated into many professionally sponsored treatment programs for alcoholism (see "Alcohol Treatment" below). This model has been applied as well for other self-help groups including Narcotics Anonymous, Cocaine Anonymous, Gamblers Anonymous, Overeaters Anonymous, and Sexaholics Anonymous.

Not only do self-help groups offer fellowship and support, but they also are used in lieu of traditional therapies or after a person stops other therapies. Self-help groups complement other types of treatment. They are seen as cost-effective for maintaining changes that clients undertake and for preventing relapse. Participants in self-help groups give and receive help for their problems. Not everyone is well suited for self-help groups, though. To benefit from them, clients have to be motivated.

Narcotics Anonymous (NA)

Narcotics Anonymous emanated from the Alcoholics Anonymous Program. The first meetings were held in Los Angeles in the early 1950s. In 1983, NA published its self-titled Basic Text book, contributing to tremendous growth of the organization with chapters in Australia, Brazil, Colombia, Germany, India, Ireland, Japan, New Zealand, United Kingdom, eastern Europe, and Africa.

NA is open to all drug addicts, regardless of the particular drug or combination of drugs with which one has a problem. Membership is not restricted by social class, religion, economic status, race, ethnicity, nationality, or gender. Membership is free, although members often contribute small sums to help cover the expenses of meetings.

Critical to NA's success is the therapeutic value of addicts working with other addicts. Successes and challenges in overcoming active addiction and living drug-free, productive lives resulting from the principles contained within the Twelve Steps and Twelve Traditions of NA are shared by members. The principles of the NA recovery program include

- admitting there is a problem;
- seeking help;
- engaging in a thorough self-examination;
- confidential self-disclosure;
- making amends for harm done; and
- helping other drug addicts who want to recover.

Narcotics Anonymous emphasizes the practice of spiritual principles. NA itself is nonreligious, and each member is encouraged to cultivate an individual understanding—religious or not—of this "spiritual awakening." NA is not affiliated with other organizations, including other 12-step programs, treatment centers, or correctional facilities. NA does not employ professional counselors or therapists nor does it have residential facilities or clinics or vocational, legal, financial, psychiatric, or medical services.

NA's one mission is to provide a setting in which addicts can help one another stop using drugs and find a new way to live. NA encourages its members to abstain completely from all drugs including alcohol, although the use of psychiatric medication and other medically indicated drugs prescribed by a physician and taken under medical supervision is not seen as compromising a person's recovery in NA. Meetings are led by individual members while other members take part by sharing in turn about their experiences in recovering from drug addiction.

NA does not express positive or negative opinions on civil, social, medical, legal, or religious issues. In addition, it does not profess positions on addiction-related issues such as criminality, law enforcement, drug legalization or penalties, prostitution, HIV/HCV infection, or syringe programs.

NA membership is voluntary and no attendance records are kept. Thus, it is difficult to provide comprehensive information about its members. However, the following demographic information was revealed in a survey returned by almost half of the 13,000 attendees at the 2003 NA World Convention held in San Diego, California[96]:

- Gender: 55% male, 45% female
- Age: 3% 20 years old and under, 12% 21–30 years old, 31% 31–40 years old, 40% 41–50 years old, 13% over age 51, 1% did not answer
- Ethnicity: 70% Caucasian, 11% African American, 11% Hispanic, 8% other
- Employment status: 72% employed full-time, 9% employed part-time, 7% unemployed, 3% retired, 3% homemakers, 5% students, 1% did not answer
- Continuous abstinence/recovery: ranged from less than one year up to 40 years
- The growth of NA is reflected in the following data[97]:
  In 1983, more than a dozen countries had 2,966 meetings.
  In 1993, 60 countries had over 13,000 groups holding over 19,000 meetings.
  In 2002, 108 countries had 20,000 groups holding over 30,000 meetings.
  In 2005, 116 countries had over 21,500 groups holding over 33,500 weekly meetings.
  In 2007, there are over 25,065 groups holding over 43,900 weekly meetings in 127 countries.

Alcohol Treatment

In the United States, it is estimated that 17 million people are heavy drinkers and 57 million engaged in binge drinking in the previous month.[98] Over 700,000 Americans receive treatment for alcohol or alcohol in combination with a secondary drug.[99] Much debate surrounds the most effective treatment for alcoholics. Some cures for alcoholism, dating between 1860 and 1930, were most unusual. The Hay-Litchfield antidote promised to eliminate the desire for alcohol by creating feelings of disgust and nausea at the sight of alcohol; some ingredients included codfish, milk, eelskin, cow's urine, and alcohol. Another product was the White Star Secret Liquor Cure, which sold for 94 cents for a box of 30 capsules. The main ingredient in the capsules was erthroxylon coca—cocaine. Other peculiar therapies included inducing convulsions and psychosurgery in which part of the brain was surgically removed.

Of the various modalities for treating alcohol abuse today, none rivals the popularity of AA. A key feature of AA is total abstinence, a view that is not universally accepted. Some treatment personnel advocate a **controlled drinking approach** in which the patient learns to drink in a nonabusive manner. Drug therapy in the form of **Antabuse (disulfiram)** has been used as well.

Most people who recover from an alcohol problem for at least 1 year do so without help or treatment.[100] Also, alcoholics who attribute positive treatment outcomes to their own efforts are more likely to be successful.[101] In terms of long-term remission, those individuals who are most likely to succeed are female, those who initiated alcohol abuse later in life, and those who had friends who were less approving of drinking.[102] Motivation and having the support of family, therapists, self-help groups, or friends are instrumental in overcoming alcohol abuse regardless of treatment.

Alcoholics Anonymous

During Prohibition, many facilities were available to help alcoholics. After Prohibition, however, these facilities closed, except for those that treated wealthy individuals. The absence of treatment for alcoholics set the stage for AA. Started in 1935 by an alcoholic surgeon (Dr. Bob) and an alcoholic stockbroker (Bill W.) helping each other achieve sobriety, AA is the oldest self-help group. At its inception, AA was not a formal treatment program.

The only requirement for membership in AA is the desire to stop drinking. Its goals are sobriety and spiritual renewal. AA groups have been established in more than 100 countries.

AA membership consists of about twice as many males as females, although there is less disparity among younger members. AA employs no professional counselors, but some members emerge as leaders. AA is based on the premise that alcoholism is a disease over which the person has no control. Clients often participate in AA after having been discharged

On Campus

Twenty-one percent of full-time college students and 15% of part-time college students meet the criteria for alcohol use disorders. However, less than 10% of those students utilize alcohol-related treatment and counseling services.

Source: L.-T. Wu, D. J. Pilowsky, W. E. Schlenger, and D. Hasin. "Alcohol Use Disorders and the Use of Treatment Services Among College-Age Young Adults," *Psychiatry Services*, 58 (2007): 192–200.

controlled drinking approach Alcohol treatment based on behavior modification, in which the person learns to drink in a nonabusive manner

Antabuse (disulfiram) A drug that interferes with the metabolization of alcohol, making the drinker violently ill

from other treatment programs. Additional groups, such as Alanon and Alateen, were derived from AA. Alanon is geared to helping mates and others close to the alcoholic, and Alateen assists teenage children of alcoholics.

12 Steps of Alcoholics Anonymous

1. We admitted we were powerless over alcohol—that our lives had become unmanageable.
2. Came to believe that a Power greater than ourselves could restore us to sanity.
3. Made a decision to turn our will and our lives over to the care of God as we understood Him.
4. Made a searching and fearless moral inventory of ourselves.
5. Admitted to God, to ourselves, and to another human being the exact nature of our wrongs.
6. Were entirely ready to have God remove all these defects of character.
7. Humbly asked Him to remove our shortcomings.
8. Made a list of all persons we had harmed, and became willing to make amends to them all.
9. Made direct amends to such people wherever possible, except when to do so would injure them or others.
10. Continued to take personal inventory and when we were wrong promptly admitted it.
11. Sought through prayer and meditation to improve our conscious contact with God as we understood Him, praying only for knowledge of His will for us and the power to carry that out.
12. Having had a spiritual awakening as the result of these steps, we tried to carry this message to alcoholics and to practice these principles in all our affairs.

Central to the mission of AA is its 12 steps. Among these, the person must admit to having no control over alcohol. The person is seen as powerless over alcohol and cannot overcome alcoholism until coming to this realization. Religious conviction is important. No specific religion is promoted, but the member has to believe in a higher power for help in surmounting personal shortcomings and achieving recovery.

AA promotes character traits including honesty, humility, and patience. Two other features of the 12 steps are self-examination leading to behavior change in the way members treat themselves and others. AA considers alcoholism a disease but takes a nonmedical approach regarding its treatment.

AA meetings might be open or closed. Open meetings allow partners, friends, and other interested people to attend. Closed meetings are restricted to members. During meetings, members recount their own histories of alcohol abuse, enabling others to identify with them. In this way, new members benefit from others' experiences.

Meetings provide opportunities for members to develop alcohol-free social relationships. Learning to socialize without alcohol is part of the recovery process. Also, members learn to rely on people rather than on alcohol.

Sponsorship is another vital component. This involves a relationship between a member who has been sober for some time and one who has not been sober as long. During times when maintaining sobriety is difficult, members can turn to their sponsors for help. The sponsor program is therapeutic for the person assuming the role of sponsor *and* for the person being sponsored. Either person can terminate the relationship.

Determining the effectiveness of AA is difficult because of the standard of anonymity for its members. In general, 12-step programs have high dropout rates.[103] A Brazilian study found that only 20% of alcoholics were involved with AA after six months.[104] Despite the obstacles in evaluating AA, research has shown that 38% of patients who went from residential treatment to AA or NA were still involved with the self-help groups two years later. Also, 81% remained abstinent for a 6-month period as compared to 26% who did not attend a 12-step program.[105]

Criticisms of AA include the following[106]:

- AA treats the underlying *symptoms* of alcoholism but not its underlying causes.
- People who become dependent on AA are substituting one dependency (AA meetings) for another (alcohol).
- AA advocates that alcoholism is a disease, a position that undermines personal responsibility for behavior.
- AA ignores environmental factors that can contribute to alcoholism, such as advertising, poverty, and racism.
- AA is rigid in its beliefs.

Because AA strongly emphasizes belief in a higher power, it does not meet the needs of people who are not religious. The New York State Court of Appeals ruled that prisoners cannot be required to participate in AA because of its religious orientation.

An AA Poem

We drank for happiness
  and became unhappy.
We drank for joy
  and became miserable.
We drank for sociability
  and became argumentative.
We drank for friendship
  and made enemies.
We drank for sleep
  and awakened without rest.
We drank for strength
  and felt weak.
We drank "medicinally"
  and acquired health problems.
We drank for relaxation
  and got the shakes.
We drank for bravery
  and became afraid.
We drank to make conversation easier
  and slurred our speech.
We drank to feel heavenly
  and ended up feeling like hell.
We drank to forget
  and were forever haunted.
We drank for freedom
  and became slaves.
We drank to erase problems
  and saw them multiply.
We drank to cope with life
  and invited death.

—Author Unknown

Two self-help groups for alcoholics that do not refer to God or a higher power are Secular Organizations for Sobriety (SOS) and Rational Recovery (RR). SOS does not practice anonymity of its members. RR maintains that alcoholism is not a disease but, rather, a behavioral disorder that can be overcome by rational thinking. SOS and RR both believe that alcoholics should credit themselves if they abstain. They emphasize that sobriety is a matter of accepting personal responsibility, and they promote self-reliance and self-confidence in their members.

Moderate Drinking

For many alcoholics, abstinence is the only viable treatment. For others, the idea of lifetime sobriety dissuades them from stopping their abuse. A controlled drinking approach might be more suitable for them. In this approach, drinkers are taught to cope with peer pressure and situations that tempt them to drink excessively. The controlled drinking model is based on behavior modification.

Controlled drinking is more viable if the drinker has a stable job and marriage and *no* family history of alcoholism. The longer a person has been an alcoholic, the less likely it is that he or she can return to social drinking.

One advantage of programs emphasizing controlled drinking is that more people with severe drinking problems are likely to seek help from them to reduce their alcohol use. One dilemma is determining what is "moderate." Moreover, many alcoholics justify their continued drinking by labeling it "controlled drinking."

The controlled drinking model is contrary to the disease model. The phrase "one drink is too much and a thousand is not enough" typifies the idea that alcoholism is a disease and argues against the controlled drinking approach. The controlled drinking model has its critics, too. Can alcoholics realistically learn to drink moderately? Can cigarette smokers be satisfied with two or three cigarettes a day? Furthermore, what criteria determine who can drink moderately?

For people with a liver disease, a controlled drinking approach is not recommended. Likewise, people who lack self-control and decision-making skills are not good candidates. Moreover, the greater one's alcohol dependence, the less likely one can adopt a moderate approach to drinking.[107] AA rejects the controlled drinking approach. If a person can learn to consume alcohol moderately, claims AA, he or she was not an alcoholic in the first place. Despite AA's reservations, moderate drinking programs have been adopted in Europe, Britain, Australia, and Canada.

Moderation Management (MM) was started for problem drinkers who want to drink moderately.

Questions Pertinent to Alcoholism Treatment

- Is alcoholism a disease or a behavioral disorder?
- How effective is Alcoholics Anonymous?
- Do alcoholics have no control over their alcohol use?
- Do alcoholics need to abstain from alcohol use forever?
- Can an alcoholic recover without formal treatment?

Like other controlled drinking models, MM is based on behavioral self-management. It offers a supportive environment for those who want to come together to reduce their alcohol use and change their lifestyle. MM rejects the idea that alcoholism is a disease. MM contends that calling alcoholism a disease reinforces the notion that the abuser lacks control, which exacerbates drinking problems for those who continue to drink. Moderation-oriented programs are common in many countries including Great Britain, Sweden, Denmark, Germany, Australia, and New Zealand.

It has been shown that many people who do not seek alcohol treatment may gravitate to a moderation model. Many of these same people eventually change their goal to abstinence.[108] Not all research supports a moderate drinking approach. One study found that a moderate drinking approach was effective initially but that it was ineffective three years later.[109]

In an older study in which alcoholics were provided with behavioral self-control training, 14 of 29 alcoholics achieved moderate alcohol use and 23 were abstinent.[110] A critical factor was their alcohol use in the first 12 months after treatment. Clients were more successful if they set their own goals.[111] Controlled drinking was found to be possible with less dependence if the alcoholic believes controlled drinking is possible.[112]

Medications

Disulfiram (Antabuse)

Disulfiram, better known as Antabuse, is a medication that acts as an aversive agent by interacting with alcohol in such a way that the drinker becomes violently ill. It helps drinkers who do not think they can control their impulsive use of alcohol. Disulfiram interferes with the metabolism of alcohol and increases the level of acetaldehyde in the blood, which produces many undesirable effects including nausea, dizziness, drowsiness, excessive perspiration, fatigue, skin flush, restlessness, lowered blood pressure, blurred vision, pounding in the head and chest, and difficulty breathing.[113] The disulfiram-alcohol reaction can continue for up to 14 days after stopping disulfiram. Because of its adverse side effects and its questionable effectiveness, disulfiram is not the first pharmacological choice for treating alcoholism.[114]

The severity of effects of Antabuse depends on the amount of alcohol consumed. Both alcohol and disulfiram have to be present simultaneously in the body for the effects to occur. One limitation is the necessity of getting alcoholics to take the drugs. Another problem is that some alcoholics continue to drink despite disulfiram's noxious effects. It was found that one in three individuals who were court-ordered to take disulfiram as part of their treatment program continued to drink alcohol.[115]

Naltrexone

Naltrexone was approved by the FDA in 1994 to treat alcoholism although it is used primarily to block the effects of opiates.[116] A number of studies have found it to be beneficial for treating alcohol dependence. The FDA approved naltrexone as a treatment adjunct to reduce the risk of relapse. It does not seem to prevent alcoholics from taking just one drink, but alcoholics are less likely to binge drink while they are taking it.

Naltrexone may be most helpful after detoxification. A number of alcoholics relapse, but naltrexone reduces that number. In a study at the University of Pennsylvania, 23% of naltrexone-treated alcoholics relapsed within 12 weeks of treatment, in contrast to 54% who were given a placebo.[117] It was also noted that alcoholics with the Asp40 allele (a variant form of a particular gene) respond better to naltrexone.[118]

Besides reducing the craving for alcohol, naltrexone is a safe drug that many alcoholics find acceptable.[119] Its side effects, which last 1 to 2 weeks, include agitation, anxiety, nausea, light-headedness, sweating, and dysphoria. In addition to its use with alcoholics, naltrexone has been tested with smokers wanting to quit. Naltrexone did not affect smoking behavior but slightly reduced the withdrawal symptoms, including the craving, during abstinence.[120] Another potential benefit of naltrexone is that it may reduce pathological gambling.[121]

Acamprosate

A third type of pharmacological drug approved by the FDA for treating alcoholism is acamprosate. Approved in 2004, this drug inhibits the craving for alcohol and food.[122] It has been found that acamprosate helps to maintain abstinence if the patient is abstinent at the time acamprosate is initiated.[123] Because acamprosate is absorbed poorly when taken orally, it is desirable that the drug be administered several times daily. Also, the drug is excreted primarily through the kidneys. Thus, it should not be used with patients who have kidney problems.[124]

Summary

Although drug abuse treatment is costly, the expense of not treating it is even greater. Even though funding for drug treatment programs has increased, only a small proportion of drug abusers receive treatment. Most Americans support spending more money for treatment. Most drug abusers are socially disadvantaged young males with histories of criminal activity and psychological problems. Drug abuse treatment reduces illicit drug use and criminal activity.

In the 1930s, the Public Health Service opened two hospitals to treat drug abusers. Relapse among patients who left the program before they completed it exceeded 90%. In the 1960s, treatment services expanded greatly, resulting in issues such as determining the most cost-effective treatment, matching clients with treatment, and weighing the benefits of voluntary versus compulsory attendance. Regardless of the type of treatment, people from supportive social and economic backgrounds respond best to treatment.

Retaining personnel in treatment facilities is difficult because of poor wages and difficult working conditions. Communities object to having facilities located nearby because they fear increased crime, more traffic, lower property values, and bad influences on their children.

Drug use by those in treatment remains high. Many clients resist treatment because of the stigma. Others simply do not want to be treated. The relapse rate is high and usually stems from factors in the person's environment. The longer clients stay in treatment, the more effective it is.

One of the more successful programs for treating opiate addicts is methadone maintenance. Methadone eliminates withdrawal symptoms and blocks euphoria. During treatment, clients are given medical, vocational, and psychiatric services. Two drawbacks are that clients must come daily for treatment and that methadone causes its own dependency. Drugs such as naloxone and naltrexone have been used in place of methadone because they prevent withdrawal symptoms and euphoria for a longer time.

Another form of treatment, therapeutic communities (TCs), places a strong emphasis on group counseling, especially confrontational encounters, and on building self-esteem and self-confidence. Residents are given certain tasks, and, as they demonstrate responsibility, they are allowed more privileges. Although TCs are effective with residents who complete their stay, the vast majority of clients drop out. In recent years, retention rates have improved.

Other types of treatment are outpatient programs, inpatient programs, and self-help groups. Outpatient treatment is more popular than inpatient treatment because of easier access and lower cost; it also is less disruptive and stigmatized. Self-help groups were developed in response to traditional health care that was seen as unresponsive to meeting people's needs. Self-help groups are cost-effective and are used mainly as aftercare. People in self-help groups learn to give and receive support from others. These groups are best suited for self-motivated individuals.

The most popular treatment for alcoholism is Alcoholics Anonymous (AA). AA holds that alcoholism is a disease over which one has no control. Central to AA is its 12-step model, which emphasizes spirituality and self-examination. During meetings, members tell their personal histories and form alcohol-free social relationships. Sponsorship is an important component of AA. Members turn to their sponsors during difficult times, and both the sponsor and the person being sponsored profit from this relationship. Because AA stresses anonymity, evaluation of its effectiveness is difficult. Because AA does not meet the needs of alcoholics who are not religious, other groups emphasizing personal responsibility have developed.

An alternative to total sobriety is a controlled or moderate drinking model, based on principles of behavior modification. The person learns to drink alcohol in a nonabusive manner. The results of moderate or controlled drinking programs are mixed.

Another treatment involves taking the drug disulfiram (Antabuse), which interacts with alcohol to make the drinker ill. These effects set in if one drinks alcohol within 2 to 3 days of taking disulfiram. This treatment works while the drinker is in treatment. After treatment ends, the relapse rate is high. Two other drugs approved by the FDA to treat alcoholism are naltrexone and acamprosate.

Thinking Critically

1. Drug abuse can be viewed as a personality weakness, as a medical problem, or as a consequence of society. What do you think is the cause for drug abuse? Is it a flaw in personality, a medical issue, or the result of society?
2. Clients in treatment for drug abuse often demonstrate other psychological problems. Do you think drug abuse is a symptom or a cause of psychological problems?
3. Methadone maintenance clinics are being met with community resistance. How would you feel about having a clinic located near you? Why?
4. Inpatient treatment can be expensive. Should expense be a factor in deciding whether one should receive help in overcoming drug addiction? How should this mode of treatment be financed?

Web Resources

Office of National Drug Control Policy: Media Campaign
http://www.mediacampaign.org
This site contains information regarding the federal government's antidrug media campaign.

Indiana Prevention Resource Center
http://www.drugs.indiana.edu
This site from the University of Indiana is a clearinghouse for prevention, technical assistance, and information about various drugs including alcohol and tobacco.

Alcoholics Anonymous
http://www.aa.org
The home page for AA provides information on this organization's history and current activities and a link to the online version of *Alcoholics Anonymous: The Big Book.*

Narcotics Anonymous
http://www.na.org
In addition to basic information about this organization, the NA World Services site provides links to NA literature, including *The NA Way* magazine and handbooks, and information about events, help lines, and more.

Notes

1. NIDA Info Facts, *Treatment Approaches for Drug Addiction* (Bethesda, MD: National Institute of Drug Abuse, 2008).
2. Ibid.
3. Substance Abuse and Mental Health Services Administration, *Treatment Episode Data Set (TEDS). Highlights—2006. National Admission to Substance Abuse Treatment Services* (Rockville, MD: SAMHSA, Office of Applied Studies, 2008).
4. Office of National Drug Control Policy, *National Drug Control Strategy, 2009* (Rockville, MD: Office of ONDCP, 2008).
5. "Survey Finds Public Support for Treatment over Interdiction," *Alcoholism and Drug Abuse Weekly,* 12 (July 24, 2000): 3–5.
6. B. Ray, R. Thoreson, L. Henderson, and M. Toce, *National Admissions to Substance Abuse Treatment Services: The Treatment Episode Data Set (TEDS) 1992–1995* (Advance Report 12) (Rockville, MD: Substance Abuse and Mental Health Services Administration, 1997).
7. Substance Abuse and Mental Health Services Administration, *Treatment Episode Data Set (TEDS). Highlights—2005. National Admission to Substance Abuse Treatment Services* (Rockville, MD: SAMHSA, Office of Applied Studies, 2007).
8. W. Merrill, "Clinical Considerations in the Treatment of Veterans with Substance Abuse Disorders," *Resource Links,* 3 (Summer 2004): 5–8.
9. Substance Abuse and Mental Health Services Administration, *The DASIS Report: Older Adults in Substance Abuse Treatment: 2005* (Rockville, MD: Office of Applied Studies, November 8, 2007).
10. Substance Abuse and Mental Health Services Administration, *The DASIS Report: Adults Aged 65 or Older in Substance Abuse Treatment: 2005* (Rockville, MD: Office of Applied Studies, May 31, 2007).
11. *Survey of Inmates in Local Jails,* Bureau of Justice Statistics, Executive Office of the President, Office of National Drug Control Policy, Drug Policy Information Clearinghouse, April 1999.
12. Office of National Drug Control Policy, *What Works: Effective Public Health Responses to Drug Use* (Rockville, MD: Office of ONDCP, March 2008).
13. Ibid.
14. D. Best et al., "Treatment Retention in the Drug Intervention Programme: Do Primary Drug Users Fare Better Than Primary Offenders?" *Drugs: Education, Prevention and Policy,* 15 (April 2008): 201–209.
15. C. Kalb, T. Peng, and K. Springen, "And Now, Back to the Real World," *Newsweek,* 151 (March 3, 2008).
16. "Reasons for Not Receiving Substance Abuse Treatment," *The NSDUH Report,* November 7, 2003.
17. "22 Million Americans Suffer from Substance Dependence or Abuse," *SAMHSA News,* 11 (2003): 16–17.
18. Substance Abuse and Mental Health Services Administration, *The DASIS Report: Admission with Five or More Prior Episodes: 2005* (Rockville, MD: Office of Applied Studies, June 28, 2007).
19. J. F. Maddux, "Clinical Experience with Civil Commitment," in *Compulsory Treatment of Drug Abuse,* edited by C. G. Leukefeld and F. M. Timms (NIDA Research Monograph 86) (Washington, DC: Government Printing Office, 1988).
20. R. W. Pickens and B. W. Fletcher, "Overview of Treatment Issues," in *Improving Drug Abuse Treatment,* edited by R. W. Pickens, C. G. Leukefeld, and C. R. Schuster (NIDA Research Monograph 106) (Washington, DC: Government Printing Office, 1991).
21. J. W. Langenbacher, "Socioeconomic Analysis of Addictions Treatment," *Public Health Reports,* 111 (1996): 135–137.
22. D. C. Lewis, "More Evidence That Treatment Works," *Brown University Digest of Addiction Theory and Application,* 13 (1994): 12.
23. NIDA Info Facts, *Treatment Approaches for Drug Addiction,* supra note 1.
24. *Public Safety, Public Spending: Forecasting America's Prison Population 2007–2011* (Washington, DC: The Pew Charitable Trusts, 2007).
25. E. Nadelmann, "Rising Chorus Against the War on Drugs," *Drug Policy Newsletter,* 49 (Winter 2001): 5–7.
26. "Study Finds Admission Increase in Post-Prop 36 California," *Alcoholism and Drug Abuse Weekly,* 15 (October 20, 2003): 3.
27. M. D. Anglin and B. Perrochet, "Drug Use and Crime: A Historical Review of Research Conducted by the UCLA Drug Abuse Research Center," *Substance Use and Misuse,* 33 (1998): 1871–1914.
28. D. Rohde, "Why Drugs Keep Flowing: Too Little Emphasis on Treating Heavy Users," *Christian Science Monitor* (July 20, 1994): 8.
29. "Observers of California Treatment System Lament Lack of Progress in

Reform," *Alcoholism and Drug Abuse Weekly*, 20 (June 2, 2008): 1–3.

30. *National Treatment Improvement Evaluation Study* (Rockville, MD: Center for Substance Abuse Treatment, Substance Abuse and Mental Health Services Administration, 1997).
31. S. G. Craddock, P. M. Flynn, R. L. Hubbard, and B. W. Fletcher, "Psychosocial Outcomes of Drug Abuse Treatment Among Clients Entering Four Treatment Modalities," in *Problems of Drug Dependence, 1996*, edited by L. S. Harris (Proceedings of the 58th Annual Scientific Meeting, NIDA Research Monograph 174) (Rockville, MD: National Institute on Drug Abuse, 1997).
32. *National Treatment Improvement Evaluation Study* (Rockville, MD: Center for Substance Abuse Treatment, Substance Abuse and Mental Health Services Administration, 1997).
33. Maddux, supra note 19.
34. United Nations Office on Drugs and Crime, *Investing in Drug Abuse Treatment* (New York: United Nations, 2003).
35. "Modern Treatment for Prisoners," *Addiction*, 103 (August 2008): 1343.
36. K. M. Carroll, "Enhancing Retention in Clinical Trials of Psychosocial Treatments: Practical Strategies," in *Beyond the Therapeutic Alliance: Keeping the Drug-Dependent Individual in Treatment*, edited by L. S. Onken, J. D. Blaine, and J. J. Boren (NIDA Research Monograph 165) (Washington, DC: U.S. Department of Health and Human Services, 1997).
37. H. D. Holder, R. A. Cisler, and R. Longabaugh, "Alcoholism Treatment and Medical Care Costs from Project MATCH," *Addiction*, 95 (2000): 999–1013.
38. Substance Abuse and Mental Health Services Administration, *The DASIS Report: Male Admission with Co-occurring Psychiatric and Substance Use Disorders: 2005* (Rockville, MD: Office of Applied Studies, December 13, 2007).
39. Substance Abuse and Mental Health Services Administration, *Treatment Episode Data Set (TEDS). Highlights—2006. National Admission to Substance Abuse Treatment Services* (Rockville, MD: SAMHSA, Office of Applied Studies, 2008).
40. Substance Abuse and Mental Health Services Administration, *The DASIS Report: Adolescent Treatment Admissions by Gender: 2005* (Rockville, MD: Office of Applied Studies, March 24, 2007).
41. K. M. Harris, B. A. Griffin, D. F. McCaffrey, and A. R. Morral, "Inconsistencies in Self-Reported Drug Use by Adolescents in Substance Abuse Treatment: Implications for Outcome and Performance Measurements," *Journal of Substance Abuse Treatment*, 34 (April 2008): 347–355.
42. G. Martin and J. Copeland, "The Adolescent Cannabis Check-up: Randomized Trial of Brief Intervention for Young Cannabis Users," *Journal of Substance Abuse Treatment*, 34 (June 2008): 407–414.
43. M. T. French, et al., "The Cost-Effectiveness Analysis of Four Interventions for Adolescents with a Substance Abuse Disorder," *Journal of Substance Abuse Treatment*, 34 (April 2008): 272–281.
44. "NIDA Launches Initiatives to Combat Club Drugs," *NIDA Notes* (Bethesda, MD: National Institute on Drug Abuse, March 2000).
45. "Treatment Completion in the Treatment Episode Data Set (TEDS)," *The DASIS Report*, January 30, 2003.
46. Substance Abuse and Mental Health Services Administration, *The NSDUH Report: Substance Use Treatment among Women of Childrearing Age* (Rockville, MD: Office of Applied Studies, October 4, 2007).
47. "Marital Status of Women Aged 25–44; 2002," *The DASIS Report*, July 16, 2004.
48. H. L. Surratt and J. A. Inciardi, *Cocaine, Crack, and the Criminalization of Pregnancy* (Los Angeles: Roxbury Publishing, 1998).
49. R. R. Szuster, L. L. Rich, A. Chung, and S.W. Bisconer, "Treatment Retention in Women's Residential Chemical Dependency Treatment: The Effect of Admission with Children," *Substance Use and Misuse*, 31 (June 1996): 1001–1013.
50. N. Niv and Y. Hser, "Women-Only and Mixed-Gender Drug Abuse Treatment Programs: Service Needs, Utilization and Outcomes," *Drug and Alcohol Dependence*, 87 (March 2007): 194–201.
51. Substance Abuse and Mental Health Services Administration, *The NSDUH Report: Health Insurance and Substance Use Treatment Need* (Rockville, MD: Office of Applied Studies, February 23, 2007).
52. L. Siqueland, F. A. Crits-Cristoph, A. Frank, D. Daley, R. Weiss, J. Chittams, J. Blaine, and L. Luborsky, "Predictors of Dropout from Psychosocial Treatment of Cocaine Dependence," *Drug and Alcohol Dependence*, 52 (1998): 1–13.
53. J. O. Jacobson, "Place and Attrition from Substance Abuse Treatment," *Journal of Drug Issues*, 34 (Winter 2004): 23–51.
54. Y. Hser, C. E. Grella, R. L. Hubbard, S. C. Hsieh, B. W. Fletcher, B. S. Brown, and M. D. Anglin, "An Evaluation of Drug Treatment for Adolescents in Four U.S. Cities," *Archives of General Psychiatry*, 58 (2001): 689–695.
55. S. Petitjean, J. Boening, and G. A. Wiesbeck, "The Impact of Self-Help Group Attendance on Relapse Rates After Alcohol Detoxification in a Controlled Study," *Alcohol and Alcoholism*, 42 (March/April 2007): 108–112.
56. W. Fals-Stewart, G. R. Birchler, and T. J. O'Farrell, "Drug-Abusing Patients and Their Intimate Partners: Dyadic Adjustment, Relationship Stability, and Substance Use," *Journal of Abnormal Psychology*, 108 (1999): 11–23.
57. B. S. Brown, "Drug Use—Chronic and Relapsing or a Treatable Condition?" *Substance Use and Misuse*, 31 (1998): 2515–2520.
58. J. P. Lepage and E. A. Garcia-Rea, "The Association between Healthy Lifestyle Behaviors and Relapse Rates in Homeless Veterans," *American Journal of Drug and Alcohol Abuse*, 34 (February 2008): 171–176.
59. C. P. O'Brien, A. R. Childress, and A. T. McLellan, "Conditioning Factors May Help to Understand and Prevent Relapse in Patients Who Are Recovering from Drug Dependence," in *Improving Drug Abuse Treatment*, edited by R. W. Pickens, C. G. Leukefeld, and C. R. Schuster (NIDA Research Monograph 106) (Washington, DC: Government Printing Office, 1991).
60. S. F. Greenfield, R. D. Weiss, L. R. Muenz, L. M. Vagge, J. F. Kelly, L. R. Bello, and J. Michael, "The Effect of Depression on Return to Drinking," *Archives of General Psychiatry*, 55 (1998): 259–265.
61. H. C. Fox, K. L. Bergquist, K. I. Hong, and R. Sinha, "Stress-Induced and Alcohol Cue-Induced Craving in Recently Abstinent Alcohol-Dependent Individual," *Alcoholism: Clinical and Experimental Research*, 31 (March 2007): 395–403.
62. J. R. McKay, A. I. Alterman, M. J. Rutherford, J. S. Cacciola, and T. McLelan, "The Relationship of Alcohol Use to Cocaine Relapse in Cocaine Dependent Patients in an Aftercare Study," *Journal of Studies

on Alcohol, 60 (1999): 176–180.

63. G. E. Vaillant, "A Long-Term Follow-Up of Male Alcohol Abuse," *Archives of General Psychiatry,* 53 (1996): 243–249.
64. A. Jones, et al., *The Drug Treatment Outcomes Research Study* (Home Office: The Research, Development and Statistics Directorate, 2007).
65. R. K. Price, N. K. Risk, and E. L. Spitznagel, "Remission from Drug Abuse over a 25-Year Period: Patterns of Remission and Treatment Use," *American Journal of Public Health,* 91 (2001): 1107–1113.
66. E. Nadelmann, "Commonsense Drug Policy," *Foreign Affairs,* 77 (1998): 111–126.
67. T. J. McMahon, J. D. Winkel, and B. J. Rounsaville, "Drug Abuse and Responsible Fathering: A Comparative Study of Men Enrolled in Methadone Maintenance Treatment," *Addiction,* 103 (February 2008): 269–283.
68. C. P. O'Brien, G. E. Woody, and A. T. McLellan, "Enhancing the Effectiveness of Methadone Using Psychotherapeutic Interventions," in *Integrating Behavioral Therapies with Medications in the Treatment of Drug Dependence,* edited by L. S. Onken, J. D. Blaine, and J. J. Boren (NIDA Research Monograph 150) (Washington, DC: Government Printing Office, 1995).
69. G. Gerra, M. Ferri, E. Polidori, G. Santoro, A. Zaimovic, and E. Sternieri, "Long-Term Methadone Maintenance Effectiveness: Psychosocial and Pharmacological Variables," *Journal of Substance Abuse Treatment,* 25 (July 2003): 1–9.
70. C. E. Munoz-Plaza, et al., "Exploring Drug Users' Attitudes and Decisions Regarding Hepatitis C (HCV) Treatment in the U.S.," *International Journal of Drug Policy,* 19 (February 2008): 71–78.
71. United Nations Office on Drugs and Crime, supra note 34.
72. T. W. Knealing, M. C. Roebuck, C. J. Wong, and K. Silverman, "Economic Cost of the Therapeutic Workplace Intervention Added to Methadone Maintenance," *Journal of Substance Abuse Treatment,* 34 (April 2008): 326–332.
73. "Injection Drug Users in Methadone Treatment More Likely to Reduce Risk Behaviors," *AIDS Weekly,* December 4, 2000.
74. M. S. Gordon, T. W. Kinlock, R. P. Schwartz, and K. E. O'Grady, "A Randomized Clinical Trial of Methadone Maintenance for Prisoners: Findings at 6 Months Post-Release," *Addiction,* 103 (August 2008): 1333–1342.
75. D. A. Wasserman, M. G. Weinstein, B. E. Havassy, and S. M. Hall, "Factors Associated with Lapses to Heroin Use During Methadone Maintenance," *Drug and Alcohol Dependence,* 52 (1998): 183–192.
76. D. A. Zanis and G. E. Woody, "One-Year Mortality Rates Following Methadone Treatment Discharge," *Drug and Alcohol Dependence,* 52 (1998): 257–260.
77. A. Srivastava, M. Kahan, and S. Ross, "The Effect of Methadone Maintenance on Alcohol Consumption: A Systematic Review," *Journal of Substance Abuse Treatment,* 34 (March 2008): 215–223.
78. "Methadone and Breastfeeding," *Pediatrics for Parents,* 23 (December 2007): 2.
79. "What Makes For a Good Methadone Program?" *Alcoholism and Drug Abuse Weekly,* 19 (March 19, 2007): 1–7.
80. J. H. Jaffe, "Can LAAM, Like Lazarus, Come Back from the Dead?" *Addiction,* 102 (September 2007): 1342–1343.
81. M. D. Anglin, B. T. Conner, J. Annon, and D. Longshore, "Levo-alpha-acetylmethadol Versus Methadone Maintenance: 1-Year Treatment Retention, Outcomes and Status," *Addiction,* 102 (September 2007); 1432–1442.
82. J. Q. Wilson, "A New Strategy for the War on Drugs," *Wall Street Journal,* April 13, 2000.
83. R. B. Haemmig and W. Tschacher, "Effects of High-Dose Heroin Versus Morphine in Intravenous Drug Users: A Randomised Double-Blind Crossover Study," *Journal of Psychoactive Drugs,* 33 (April–June 2001): 105–111.
84. U. Verthein, et al., "Long-Term Effects of Heroin-Assisted Treatment in Germany," *Addiction,* 103 (June 2008): 960–966.
85. L. E. Sullivan and D. A. Fiellin, "Narrative Review: Buprenorphine for Opioid-Dependent Patients in Office Practice," *Annals of Internal Medicine,* 148 (May 6, 2008): 662–672.
86. ONDCP Drug Policy Information Clearinghouse Fact Sheet, *Heroin* (Rockville, MD: Office of National Drug Control Policy, June 2003).
87. R. P. Mattick, J. Kimber, C. Breen, and M. Davoli, "Buprenorphine Maintenance Versus Placebo or Methadone Maintenance for Opioid Dependence," *Cochrane Database of Systematic Reviews* (2008).
88. W. L. White, *Slaying the Dragon: The History of Addiction Treatment in America* (Bloomington, IL: Chestnut Health Systems/Lighthouse Institute, 1998).
89. A. Bruno, et al., "Temperament and Character Dimensions in Opiate Addicts: Comparing Subjects Who Completed Inpatient Treatment in Therapeutic Communities Vs. Incompleters," *American Journal of Drug and Alcohol Abuse,* 33 (September 2007): 707–715.
90. R. Hanser, "Drug Treatment Programs," *Crime and Justice International* (June 2002): 7–8, 25.
91. J. Sacks, et al., "Prison Therapeutic Community Treatment for Female Offenders: Profiles and Preliminary Findings for Mental Health and Other Variables (Crime, Substance Use and HIV Risk)," *Journal of Offender Rehabilitation,* 46 (2008): 233–261.
92. K. Beardsley, E. Wish, D. Fitzelle, K. O'Grady, and A. Arria, "Distance Traveled to Outpatient Drug Treatment and Client Retention," *Journal of Substance Abuse Treatment,* 25 (2003): 279–285.
93. S. Nsinmba, "Outpatient Treatment Programs: A Review Article on Substances of Abuse Outpatients Treatment Outcomes in the United States," *Addictive Disorders and Their Treatment,* 6 (September 2007): 91–99.
94. "Discharges from Short-Term Residential Treatment: 2000," *The DASIS Report,* January 9, 2004.
95. A. S. Bhati, J. K. Roman, and A. Chalfin. *To Treat or Not to Treat: Evidence on the Prospects of Expanding Treatment to Drug-Involved Offenders* (Washington, D.C.: Justice Policy Center, The Urban Institute, April 2008).
96. NA World Services, Inc., "Information about NA" (Item No. ZPR0001002) (Van Nuys, CA: NA World Services, 2007).
97. Ibid.
98. Substance Abuse and Mental Health Services Administration, supra note 3.
99. Substance Abuse and Mental Health Services Administration, supra note 3.
100. L. C. Sobell, J. A. Cunningham, and M. B. Sobell, "Recovery from Alcohol Problems with and without Treatment: Prevalence in Two Population Surveys," *American Journal of Public Health,* 86 (1996): 966–972.
101. C. G. Long, C. R. Hollin, and M. J. Williams, "Self-Efficacy, Outcome Expectations, and Fantasies as Predictors of Alcoholics' Posttreatment Drinking," *Substance Use and Misuse,* 33 (1998): 2383–2402.

102. K. K. Schutte, F. E. Byrne, P. L. Brennan, and R. H. Moos, "Successful Remission of Late-Life Drinking Problems: A 10-Year Follow-Up," *Journal of Studies of Alcohol,* 62 (2001): 322–334.
103. R. N. Cloud, N. Rowan, D. Wulff, and S. Golder, "Posttreatment 12-Step Program Affiliation and Dropout: Theoretical Model of Qualitative Exploration," *Journal of Social Work Practice in the Addictions,* 7 (2007): 49–74.
104. M. B. Terra, et al., "Do Alcoholics Anonymous Groups Really Work? Factors of Adherence in a Brazilian Sample of Hospitalized Alcohol Dependents," *American Journal on Addictions,* 17 (January–February 2008): 48–53.
105. "How Alcoholics Anonymous Works," *Harvard Mental Health Letter* (July 2007): 4–6.
106. White, supra note 88.
107. K. Witkiewitz, "Lapses Following Alcohol Treatment: Modeling the Falls from the Wagon," *Journal of Studies on Alcohol and Drugs,* 69 (July 2008): 594–604.
108. K. Witkiewitz and G. A. Marlatt, "Overview of Harm Reduction Treatments for Alcohol Problems," *The International Journal of Drug Policy,* 17 (2006): 285–294.
109. S. A. Maisto, P. R. Clifford, R. L. Stout, and C. M. Davis, "Drinking in the Year After Treatment as a Predictor of Three-Year Drinking Outcomes," *Journal of Studies on Alcohol,* 67 (November 2006): 823–832.
110. W. R. Miller, A. L. Leckman, H. D. Delaney, and M. Tinkcom, "Long-Term Follow-Up of Behavioral Self-Control Training," *Journal of Studies on Alcohol,* 53 (1992): 249–261.
111. M. B. Sobell, L. C. Sobell, J. Z. Bogardis, G. I. Leo, and W. Skinner, "Problem Drinkers' Perceptions of Whether Treatment Goals Should Be Self-Selected or Therapist-Selected," *Behavior Therapy,* 23 (1992): 43–52.
112. H. Rosenberg, "Prediction of Controlled Drinking by Alcoholics and Problem Drinkers," *Psychological Bulletin,* 113 (1993): 129–139.
113. "Antabuse: A Snapshot of How It Works," *Behavioral Healthcare Tomorrow,* 13 (August 2004): 12–13.
114. M. Angelini and Y. Brahmbhatt, "A Review of the Pharmacological Options for the Treatment of Alcohol Dependence," *Formulary,* 42 (January 2007): 14–16.
115. S. Mustard, D. C. May, and D. W. Phillips, "Prevalence and Predictors of Cheating on Antabuse: Is Antabuse a Cure or Merely an Obstacle?" *American Journal of Criminal Justice,* 31 (Fall 2006): 51–63.
116. G. Miller, "Tackling Alcoholism with Drugs," *Science,* 320 (April 11, 2008): 168–170.
117. Stephanie O'Malley, *Naltrexone and Alcoholism Treatment,* (Treatment Improvement Protocol, TIP Series 28) (Rockville, MD: U.S. Department of Health and Human Services, 1998).
118. "Predicting Naltrexone Response," *JAMA: Journal of the American Medical Association,* 299 (March 26, 2008): 1417.
119. N. MacReady, "Acamprosate and Naltrexone May Hold Promise for Alcoholics: Regimen Safe and Effective," *Family Practice News,* 34 (February 15, 2004): 22.
120. E. J. Houtsmuller, P. A. Clemmey, L. A. Sigler, and M. L. Stitzer, in *Problems of Drug Dependence, 1996,* edited by L. S. Harris (Proceedings of the 58th Annual Scientific Meeting, NIDA Research Monograph 174) (Rockville, MD: National Institute on Drug Abuse, 1997).
121. "Study of Naltrexone Buoys Hopes for Viable Gambling Treatments," *Alcoholism and Drug Abuse Weekly,* 20 (June 16, 2008): 1–7.
122. D. H. Han, I. K. Lyool, Y. H. Sung, S. H. Lee, and P. F. Renshaw. "The Effect of Acamprosate on Alcohol and Food Craving in Patients with Alcohol Dependence," *Drug and Alcohol Dependence,* 93 (March 1, 2008): 279–283.
123. H. R. Kranzler and A. Gage, "Acamprosate Efficacy in Alcohol-Dependent Patients: Summary of Results from Three Pivotal Trials," *American Journal on Addictions,* 17 (January–February 2008): 70–76.
124. R. Swift, "Emerging Approaches to Managing Alcohol Dependence," *American Journal of Health-System Pharmacy,* 64 (March 1, 2007): S12–22, S30–32.

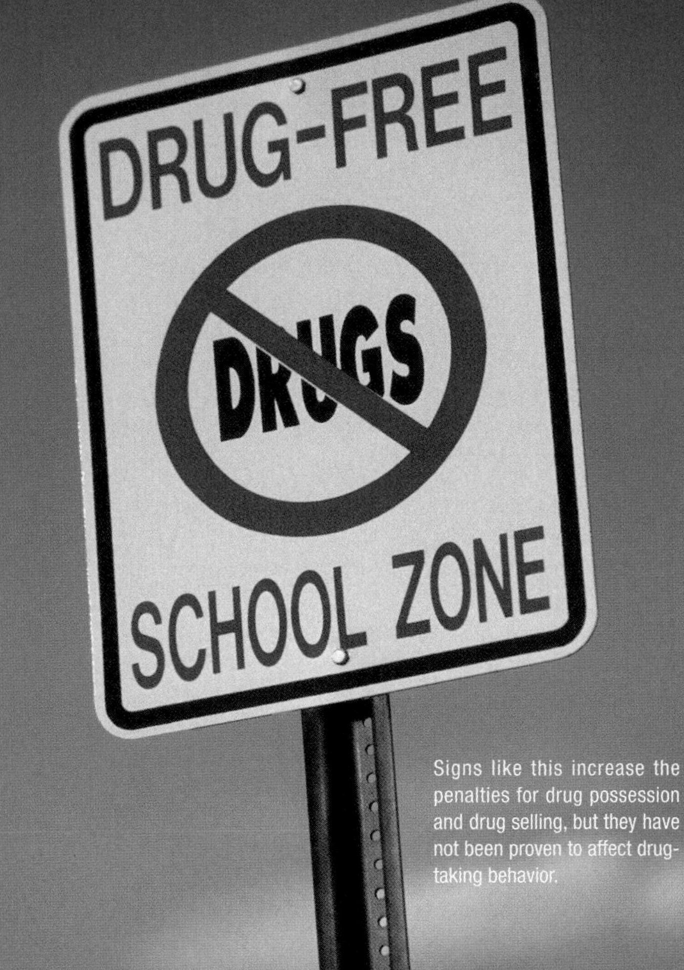

Signs like this increase the penalties for drug possession and drug selling, but they have not been proven to affect drug-taking behavior.

© Roy Morsch/CORBIS.

FACT OR FICTION?

1. Teens are six times more likely to commit violent crimes between 3:00 P.M. and 7:00 P.M. than during the 10:00 P.M. to 6:00 A.M. time period.
2. The more knowledge one has about drugs, the less likely one is to use drugs.
3. Higher cigarette taxes result in fewer teens smoking.
4. Adolescents who attend religious services frequently are less likely to use drugs than adolescents who do not attend religious services.
5. High school students who plan to go to college have higher rates of alcohol use but lower rates of cigarette use than noncollege-bound high school students.
6. Those who used alcohol before age 15 are five times more likely to abuse or become dependent on alcohol compared with those people who first used alcohol at or after age 21.
7. Unsupervised children are more likely to use drugs than supervised children.
8. Teens are less likely to use illegal drugs if their parents strongly disapprove of drug use.
9. Overall, there is more drug use among youths in urban areas than in rural areas.
10. The most widely adopted drug prevention program in the United States is DARE.

Turn the page to check your answers

Chapter Objectives

After completing this chapter, the reader should be able to describe:

- Factors hindering drug prevention efforts
- The effectiveness of drug prevention programs
- Challenges in evaluating drug prevention programs
- How families, peers, and the community affect drug use
- How high-risk youths are identified
- Characteristics of resilient children
- Factors that contribute to and prevent high-risk behaviors
- Current goals for drug education
- Educational approaches to drug education
- The impact of peer programs on the reduction of drug use

16 Drug Prevention and Education

FACT OR FICTION?

1. **Fact:** The rate of violent acts is six times greater in the hours after school than between late evening and early morning.
2. **Fiction:** The fact is—it has been found that adolescents who use drugs often know more about drugs than nonusers.
3. **Fact:** Cigarette smoking, especially among middle-class and economically disadvantaged youths, decreases significantly as cigarette taxes increase.
4. **Fact:** Young people who attend religious services frequently (at least 25 times per year) have significantly lower levels of drug use.
5. **Fiction:** The fact is—noncollege-bound students have higher rates of alcohol *and* tobacco use than college-bound students.
6. **Fact:** Sixteen percent of people who consumed alcohol by age 15 were likely to abuse or become dependent on alcohol, compared with 3% of those who used alcohol for the first time at or after age 21.
7. **Fact:** Numerous studies point out that young people who are unsupervised are more likely to experiment with drugs.
8. **Fact:** Teens do listen to parents and are less likely to use drugs if parents demonstrate strong disapproval of drug use.
9. **Fiction:** The fact is—although cocaine and crack are more likely to be used in urban areas, overall drug use among youths is as great or greater in rural areas.
10. **Fact:** Even though DARE's effectiveness is questionable, it is the most widely used drug prevention program in the United States.

Prevention is vital to keeping new drug users from becoming chronic, hardcore users.[1] Parents, schools, and communities have been shown to make a difference in reducing drug use by young people. For every $1 spent on school-based drug prevention, there are cost-savings of $5.60 from less frequent use of drugs.[2] Efforts to prevent drug abuse started more than 200 years ago, when the first surgeon general of the United States, Dr. Benjamin Rush, initiated an educational campaign to address the detrimental effects of alcohol. At the start of the 20th century, public health workers successfully conquered tuberculosis, malaria, and smallpox. Although successful strategies to prevent drug abuse have been elusive, some signs are encouraging.

Among the reasons for persistent drug use is the fact that millions of people derive satisfaction from using drugs, particularly alcohol and tobacco. Also, many drugs provide immediate gratification, a quality that has become ingrained in American culture. The immediate impact of drugs is analogous to the immediate impact that credit cards provide, in that using credit cards is comparable to buying goods without waiting. The worry of paying for goods is delayed until the bills arrive. Moreover, Americans do not like being told what to do, as evidenced during Prohibition.

The adage "An ounce of prevention is worth a pound of cure" is trite but apropos. Various approaches have been used to stem drug abuse, raising several important questions:

- What should be the goals of drug education and prevention?
- When should drug education and prevention efforts be initiated?
- What education and prevention efforts are effective?
- Who should be responsible for drug education and prevention?

Funding Drug Prevention

In the United States, most funds for drug prevention come from the federal government. In the 2009 National Drug Control Budget, $218 million was requested for the Department of Education, out of a total budget of $1.5 billion.[3] Despite the success of drug education programs, the federal government allocated less money to fight drugs by reducing the demand for drugs and increased funding for the interdiction of drugs. In a survey of community leaders, most favor spending a larger portion on reducing the demand for drugs rather than the supply of drugs.[4]

The national agency overseeing drug prevention is the Substance Abuse and Mental Health Services Administration (SAMHSA). It is responsible for the Center for Substance Abuse Prevention (CSAP), the National Institute on Alcohol Abuse and Alcoholism (NIAAA), the National Institute on Drug Abuse (NIDA), the Office of Treatment Improvement, and the National Institute of Mental Health (NIMH). Private groups involved in drug prevention include the National Council on Alcoholism and Drug Dependence, the American Public Health Association, Mothers Against Drunk Driving (MADD), and the Center for Science in the Public Interest.

Drug Abuse Prevention

Drug prevention programs in the United States have changed significantly in the last two decades. This is not surprising, considering how society has changed.

We have new and improved inventions such as cell phones, iPods, mp3 players, books on CDs, e-books, Internet dating services, satellite antennas, virtual reality, and Wi-Fi. With so many changes in society, reexamining efforts designed to prevent drug abuse is certainly reasonable. Using the same approaches today that were used in the 1970s might not be appropriate.

Drug Prevention in Retrospect

The primary focus of drug prevention in the 1970s was to reduce the supply of drugs by stopping their importation, sale, and manufacture. **Interdiction** remains a popular preventive strategy but now is complemented by other measures. Logically, if drugs are not available, they cannot be abused. The problem is that the supply of drugs entering the United States can be curtailed but not stopped completely. If one drug is unavailable, people will use other drugs in its place. Thus, the absence of drugs does not diminish the public's appetite for drugs.

Beginning in the 1980s, the focus on stopping drug abuse in the United States shifted. Some drug experts began to contend that prevention should not be directed toward prosecuting drug users or halting the flow of drugs but, rather, toward the underlying factors that contribute to drug abuse. Representative Charles Rangel, chairman of the Congressional Select Committee on Narcotic Abuse and Control, proposed that prevention focus on social and economic problems that lead to drug abuse.[5] He said that until federal politicians confront issues of poor education, inadequate health care, homelessness, unemployment, and poverty, efforts to abate drug abuse will fall short. Many inner-city youths turn to street-level drug sales because of high unemployment.[6]

Society was concerned primarily with **hard drugs** such as heroin, LSD, cocaine, and PCP. Drugs such as alcohol, tobacco, and marijuana were perceived as **soft drugs**. Though alcohol and tobacco are not desirable drugs, they are *legal*, and many honest, law-abiding, hardworking citizens smoke and drink. Alcohol, tobacco, and marijuana are known as **gateway drugs**. "Gateway" implies that these drugs are used as an introduction to other drugs. Some believe that if young people do not use gateway drugs, they will not try drugs that have more serious consequences.

High school students who use tobacco—whether in the form of cigarettes or smokeless tobacco—are more likely to binge-drink, as well as use marijuana and cocaine, than are students who do not use tobacco. Inhalants and cocaine act as gateway drugs in some groups and communities. Crack is considered a gateway drug in some poor, urban centers. The primary strategy of CSAP is to keep young people from experimenting with drugs at all.

interdiction Intervention

hard drugs Drugs that are perceived to be dangerous, such as heroin, cocaine, and LSD

soft drugs Drugs perceived to be less harmful than hard drugs; include marijuana, tobacco, and alcohol

gateway drugs Substances that are used before use of more dangerous drugs; alcohol, marijuana, tobacco, and inhalants are considered gateway drugs

Effectiveness of Prevention Programs

Determining the effectiveness of drug prevention programs is difficult. Problems in assessing the effectiveness of prevention programs include the absence of control groups, poor data collection, groups that are too small, and inappropriate statistics.[7] Another problem has been that some prevention programs do not differentiate drug use and abuse. Last, many prevention programs were not followed up to determine how long any change in drug use persisted. It is also believed that drug use during adolescence should be expected because this time of life is characterized by increased freedom and independence.[8]

A number of school-based programs reduce drug use and promote positive behaviors.[9] These projects consist of a social-behavioral curriculum, parental involvement/education, peer leadership, and communitywide task force activities. Unfortunately, very few middle schools use drug prevention programs that have been shown to work.[10] In Shin's review of effective drug education programs, five criteria were found to be essential: (1) an adequate number of hours of curricula, over at least 3 years; (2) peer involvement; (3) an emphasis on social influences, life skills, and peer resistance; (4) a change in perceived norms; and (5) involvement of parents, peers, and the community in changing norms.[11]

Goals of Drug Prevention

When discussing drug prevention, three questions require consideration:

1. What does prevention actually mean?
2. Should the goals of drug prevention be different for a person who has never used drugs than for a person who uses drugs occasionally or daily?
3. Should drug prevention be defined as a delay in the onset of drug use, the complete elimination of drug-related problems, or a significant decline in drug use?

A major limitation of drug prevention programs is that they do not clearly establish the goals they are

Selected Goals for Drug Prevention

- To prevent the individual from beginning drug use
- To minimize the risks of drugs to the user
- To reduce the risks of drug use to society
- To prevent drug dependency
- To teach responsible drug use
- To stop drug use after patterns have been established
- To delay the onset of drug use

Types of Drug Prevention

- **Primary prevention:** Aims to avert drug use from starting or from going beyond experimental use
- **Secondary prevention:** Consists of early intervention to forestall escalation of drug use
- **Tertiary prevention:** Seeks to help drug abusers after treatment has been implemented

striving to achieve. When goals are identified, a broad perspective might be helpful. Rather than identifying one goal, identifying several goals might be more useful. Goals could be geared to individuals with different levels of drug involvement. Drug prevention goals for nonusers might not be the same as those for occasional or heavy users. Also, drug prevention efforts should take cultural differences into account.

The goals of drug prevention do not have to be mutually exclusive. Goals can be written to try to reduce the individual risk of drugs as well as minimize costs to society. They can also be written to try to delay the onset of drug use with the intent of preventing drug use altogether. The latter is a sound approach because the longer people delay using drugs, the less likely they will be to use drugs. The goals of drug prevention programs often are dictated by the individuals being served or by the community and according to whether the drug is legal or illegal. With alcohol, the goal could be to reduce excessive use, whereas the goal regarding illegal drugs might be complete abstinence.

Levels of Drug Prevention

According to the Institute of Medicine, the term *prevention* is reserved for interventions that take place before the initial onset of disorder.[12] This is a simple definition. The term is confounded because of the different levels of prevention:

1. **Primary prevention:** Strives to reach people before their use of alcohol, tobacco, or other drugs. It should be initiated at a young age because most children already have tried drugs, especially alcohol, by the time they get to high school.
2. **Secondary prevention:** Attempts to minimize the potential damage resulting from drug use by targeting people who have some experience with drugs. Secondary prevention is considered an early intervention stage.
3. **Tertiary prevention:** Geared to heavy drug users and those whose patterns of drug use are well established. Basically, tertiary prevention refers to drug treatment.

Primary Prevention

Primary prevention can be aimed at reducing the demand for drugs or at curtailing the supply of drugs. Drug education is the principal approach for reducing the demand for drugs. Other strategies include mass media campaigns, community-oriented programs sponsored by service groups, drug testing, and legislation aimed at drug users. The mass media can play a significant role. For example, it has been shown

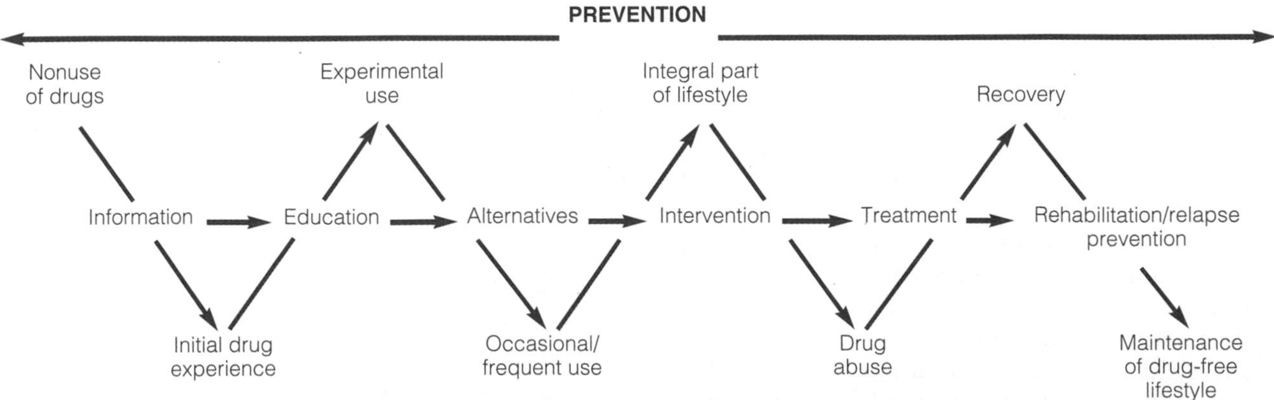

Figure 16.1 Drug Prevention Continuum

Source: W. J. Bukoski, "A Framework for Drug Abuse Prevention Research," in *Drug Abuse Prevention Intervention Research: Methodological Issues*, edited by C. G. Leukefeld and W. J. Bukoski (NIDA Research Monograph 107) (Washington, D.C.: Government Printing Office, 1991).

that adolescents who are exposed to smoking in movies are more likely to take up smoking.[13]

Secondary Prevention

Secondary prevention is geared to those who do not use drugs abusively. Again, drug education is an important component. If people are drinking alcohol legally, the goal might not be to prevent alcohol use but, rather, to encourage them to consume alcohol in a responsible way. Some argue that "responsible use" of alcohol by young people is a contradiction because it is against the law for minors to use alcohol.

The main goals of secondary prevention are to alter drug-related attitudes and behaviors, to provide alternatives to drugs, and to stress a healthy lifestyle and physical fitness. As fitness improves, drug use tends to decline. Moreover, self-concept improves as fitness levels improve. The more activities young people participate in, the less likely it is that they will use drugs.[14]

Tertiary Prevention

Because tertiary prevention involves treatment, it is beyond the scope of educational institutions. Nevertheless, schools can perform an important function by referring students who abuse drugs to appropriate facilities. In addition, schools can implement prevention programs after students have gone through intensive treatment, in order to prevent them from relapsing. As illustrated in Figure 16.1, prevention occurs at many points on a continuum.

primary prevention Preventing drug use before it begins

secondary prevention Early intervention to block more serious problems; halts escalation of drug use

tertiary prevention Treatment that seeks to help individuals after they have misused drugs

Identifying High-Risk Youths

High-risk behavior refers not only to drug abuse but also to delinquent behavior, self-destructive behavior, dropping out of school, and unprotected intercourse. Among adolescents, antisocial behaviors, delinquency, and illicit drug use are strongly correlated.[15] This does not mean that substance abuse directly causes delinquent behavior or that delinquency directly causes the use of alcohol and other drugs.[16] Nonetheless, adolescents who belong to a gang have higher rates of drug use and violent activity than their peers.[17] Some children succumb to the pressures of their circumstances and surroundings, and others rise above their situation. Others inherit a propensity for drug misuse and abuse. Psychological factors also play a role. Figure 16.2 illustrates the relationship between drug use and various types of delinquent behavior.

Resilient Children

Children from high-risk backgrounds often surmount their circumstances and avoid the temptation to turn to drugs. Many children from impoverished

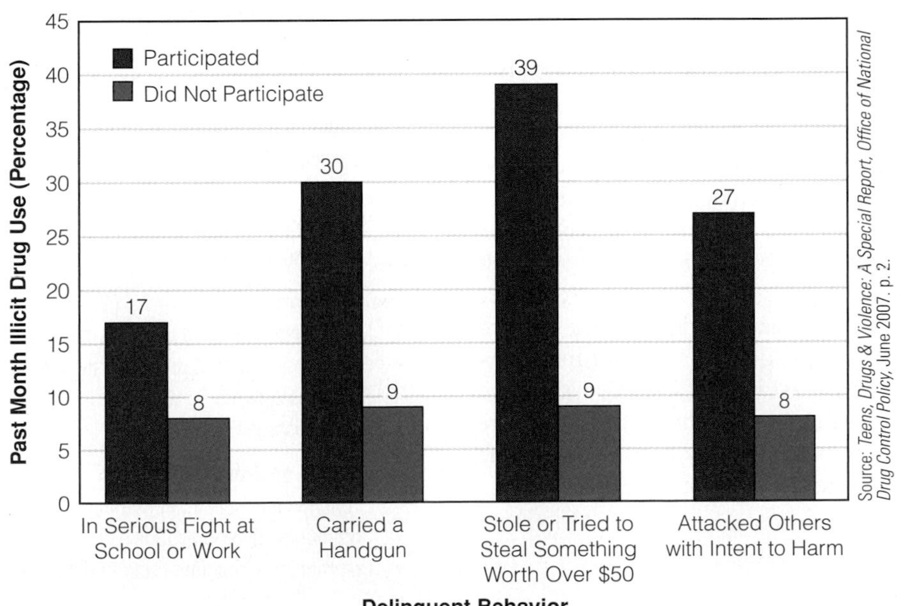

Figure 16.2 Past Month Illicit Drug Use among Youths (12–17) by Participation in Fighting and Delinquent Behavior

Characteristics of Resilient Children

- Responsive
- Flexible
- Form positive relationships
- Caring
- Skillful problem-solvers
- Educationally motivated
- Disengaged from family environment
- Active
- Adaptable
- Good sense of humor
- Empathetic
- Success oriented
- Persistent

On Campus

College students who work 20 hours or more per week are more likely to binge drink, sleep less, and do worse academically than students working less than 20 hours a week.

Source: Miller, K., Danner, F., & Staten, R. (2008). "Relationship of work hours with selected health behaviors and academic progress among a college student cohort." *Journal of American College Health*, 56: 675–679.

backgrounds become healthy, competent young adults. They display **resiliency**, suggesting that they can sustain competent functioning despite the presence of major life stressors.

Resilient children have many noteworthy characteristics. They are flexible, responsive, adaptable, and active. They have positive relationships with others and maintain a sense of humor. They are empathetic, caring, persistent, competent problem-solvers, success oriented, and educationally motivated. Somehow they are able to disengage or distance themselves from dysfunctional family environments. Although they are able to see their parents' problems, they view themselves as different and recognize that they have control over their environments. Resilient children do not avoid stress but, instead, learn to master it, to use it to their advantage. Boys and girls differ in that boys tend to be more resilient in adolescence whereas girls display more resilience during early childhood. Resilient children tend to form a strong bond with at least one person (not necessarily a parent) during the first year of life. Also, children who are given responsibilities and chores become more resilient, presumably because they contribute to the family and feel important to its functioning.

At-Risk Factors

Many young people are not resilient. A number of variables predispose young people to abuse alcohol and other drugs. These can be broadly grouped as hereditary and familial factors, peer influence, psychosocial factors, biological factors, and community factors.

Hereditary and Familial Factors

Regardless of whether the cause is environmental or genetic, the sons of men with alcohol-related problems are more likely to have alcohol-related problems. Further, rates of alcohol, cocaine, marijuana, and tobacco dependence are greater if siblings are dependent on these drugs.[18] Several studies note that older siblings have a greater influence on the drug use of younger siblings than parents.[19] Sons and daughters of parents with drinking problems have poor coping skills and personality problems and are more likely to be involved with alcohol. The attachment of males 12 to 14 years of age to their natural father in an intact family is significant as to whether young males resist abusing drugs, especially in neighborhoods where drug abuse prevalent.[20]

Drug prevention has to address the factors contributing to drug abuse in the first place. Many drug-dependent families have higher stress levels, fewer

Risk Factors for Drug Use by Adolescents and Children

Individual behavioral factors
- Academic failure
- Early antisocial behavior
- Early drug experimentation
- Early drug use

Individual attitudinal factors
- Rebelliousness against authority
- Lack of commitment to school
- Attraction to deviance
- Unfavorable attitudes toward adult behavior

Individual psychosocial factors
- Low self-esteem
- Low self-efficacy
- Sensation seeking
- Lack of social skills

Family factors
- Family history of drug use or antisocial behavior
- Family management problems (inadequate parenting skills)
- Parental tolerance for deviance
- Family disorganization

Community environment factors
- Economic and social deprivation
- Community disorganization
- Community norms favorable to deviance
- Availability of drugs
- Friends/peers who use drugs

friends, more family conflict, parental depression, and less involvement in recreational, social, religious, and cultural activities.[21] Substance-abusing parents spend half as much time with their children as nonabusing parents. There are more than 3 million reported cases of child abuse and neglect each year. Adults with a history of abuse and neglect as children are at high risk of developing substance abuse disorders. Moreover, these adults are at risk of abusing their own children.[22]

This research suggests that more emphasis should be placed on strengthening the family. Positive family influence may be protective. Parents who expect their children not to use drugs have children who are less likely to use drugs.[23] There is a strong relationship between family dinners and substance use. Teens who eat dinner with their families at least five times a week have significantly lower rates of smoking, alcohol use, the use of illegal drugs, and prescription drug abuse than teens who have dinner with their families three or fewer times a week.[24] The influence of families also is affected by culture. For example, drug use by Mexican American adolescents was more affected by family factors than drug use by adolescents in other groups.[25]

A family history of antisocial behavior or criminality increases the risk of drug problems. Also, lack of supervision of children after school is related to drug use. In a study of middle school and junior high school students, those who were home alone two or more days per week were more likely to get drunk, smoke cigarettes, use inhalants, and use marijuana.[26] The federal government reports that marijuana users are more likely to engage in delinquent behavior, and those behaviors increase as marijuana use increases.[27]

Peer Influence

Various studies point out that the influence of peers is not consistent. For example, one study on adolescent smoking behavior found that one's choice of friends may be more instrumental than peers actually pressuring one to smoke.[28] Among preteen-age children, peer influence was a smaller factor in drinking than boredom and the pleasure derived from the effects of alcohol.[29] The issue might not be peer pressure as much as peer approval, and young people crave approval from their friends. A study of students in Italy found that drugs were more likely to be used if the students believed that significant others approved of drug use.[30]

Psychosocial Factors

Many psychosocial factors are related to drug use by teens. Among these are rebelliousness and alienation from adults, school failure, lack of interest in school, antisocial behavior at an early age, and lack of aspirations regarding adult achievement.[31] Additional manifestations are frequent lying, indifference to punishment, lack of empathy toward others, and a desire for immediate gratification rather than delayed gratification. Moreover, these young people are not likely to have positive bonds with adults, nor are they likely to respond to messages about the possible hazards of drugs.

resiliency A person's ability to overcome obstacles, such as resisting drug use despite a background that increases the likelihood of drug use

Biological Factors

Some people are genetically more predisposed than others to drug dependence. Relatedly, some individuals derive more pleasure from drugs than others. The more pleasurable the drug experience is, the more likely it is that a person will be at risk for drug dependency. It has also been noted that the more self-control one has, the less likely one is to engage in drug abuse.[32]

Community Factors

Drug use is more prevalent in communities where people move often. Also, drug use is more common when children grow up in extreme poverty and deprivation. Drug taking is more prevalent in communities that lack stability because social support and controls regulating behaviors, including drug use, are not in place. In response to this knowledge, early-intervention programs are tied to treatment services in many communities.

Preventing High-Risk Behavior

Two factors associated with high-risk behavior—heredity and biology—cannot be changed. Other high-risk factors, however, can be modified. In this section we will explore strategies that can reduce the likelihood of individuals engaging in high-risk behaviors connected with drug use.

Education

Poor school performance and low expectations for school are strong predictors of drug use. Therefore, a good argument can be made for changes within the educational system as well as for developing more preschool programs such as Head Start. Many schools are implementing programs with emphases on team teaching, school-based planning, individual tutoring, and cooperative learning. School performance

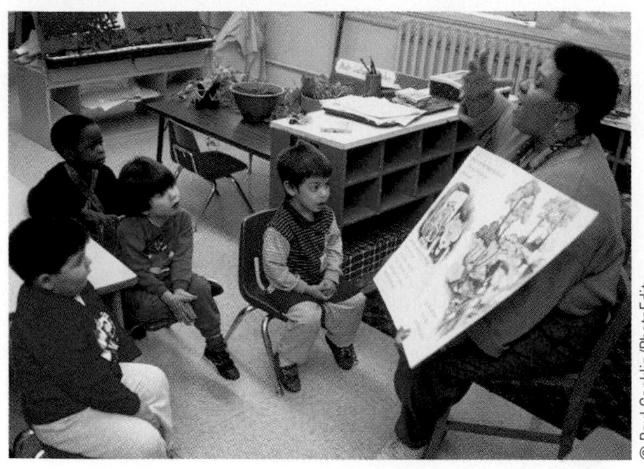

© Paul Conklin/PhotoEdit.

Head Start is a successful program of preschool education. Health screening and nutrition education are provided for at-risk children in this government-sponsored program.

improves and high-risk behaviors are reduced particularly through *experiential* education, including community service and part-time employment.

Schools often serve as the focal point for community programs. School facilities have been used to provide health care, recreational activities, after-school programs, and counseling. School alternative programs focusing on community and recreational activities, physical activities, and job training have helped youths at risk to stay off drugs. In essence, the school environment is an important component in whether students engage in drug use.[33]

Moreover, schools that maintain high expectations for students while providing support have seen academic failure decline. The consensus among experts is that children need responsible adults who are responsive to their needs. Outside of the family, a favorite teacher may be the most important role model for helping children to develop resilience.

Role of Parents

The role of parents should not be underestimated. Parental drug use greatly increases the likelihood of children's drug use, especially if there is a strong bond between the children and their parents.[34] Children growing up in a household with much discord have many difficulties, although many children in families marked by a pathologic environment and poverty do *not* develop drug problems. In contrast, parents who have high expectations for their children foster their academic success and resilience. According to the NIAAA, "Parents can have a major impact on their children's drinking, especially during the preteen and early teen years."[35]

Adolescent drug users are more likely than nonusing adolescents to perceive their parents as distant, uninvolved, mistrusting, and punitive. Thus, parents need to be more supportive of their children. In a study conducted by the National Center on Addiction and Substance Abuse (CASA), it was found that parents who take a "hands-off" approach have children who are four times more likely to use alcohol, tobacco, and illegal drugs. A program in Iowa in which parents were taught how to be better parents and how to manage family conflict showed that the onset of drug use by children was delayed.[36] One nationwide program for helping parents to dissuade their children from drug use is Parents' Resource Institute for Drug Education (PRIDE). Parental involvement in schools also helps to reduce their children's high-risk behaviors.

Community Efforts

Collaboration among schools, communities, social agencies, religious organizations, businesses, and the media is vital. However, before community efforts can reduce drug use, community leaders as well as retailers, parents, and school personnel need to be ready to mobilize their efforts.[37] Spiritual/religious involvement is a particularly important protective factor against substance abuse.[38]

Drug use is more prevalent in impoverished, urban neighborhoods. Neighborhoods marked by disorganization, violent crime, and illegal drug activity spawn drug use.[39] Young people growing up in disadvantaged neighborhoods face many environmental barriers. They lack amenities such as supermarkets, libraries, health care facilities, adequate housing, and social institutions. At the same time, they have an inordinate number of bars. Jobs have been shown to help curb drug use, yet employment opportunities for young people are in short supply. Too often the services in urban areas are fragmented because no lead agency takes charge.

According to Pentz, there are several barriers to institutionalizing community prevention efforts.

Factors That Protect Against Drug Abuse

- Small family with little conflict
- High intelligence
- Being a firstborn child
- Commitment to education
- Regular church attendance
- Belief in the expectations, values, and norms of society
- High achiever

Source: W. L. Callison, N. R. Colocino, and D. A. Vasquez, *Substance Abuse Prevention Handbook* (Lancaster, PA: Technomic Publishing, 1995).

These barriers are (1) community leaders' lack of perceived empowerment to continue prevention work, (2) communities' insufficient preparation for adopting programs that have been successful, (3) public resistance to spending more money on drug prevention programs after much money has already been spent on ineffective programs, and (4) the notion that every community is unique, and thus programs that are effective in one community will not necessarily work in other communities.[40]

values clarification A teaching strategy in which individuals are asked to express and support their values

Drug Education

Society often turns to schools to resolve social problems, whether they be teenage pregnancy, apathy, violence, racial or sexual discrimination, or drug abuse. Schools are logical places for dealing with drug problems because they have the potential to reach all children.

The Evolution in Drug Education

In the 1970s, the thrust of drug education was to provide information about the dangers of drugs, under the assumption that the more knowledge young people had about drugs, the less likely they would be to use them. Another assumption was that if young people feared drugs because of their potential harm, they would resist them. These are faulty assumptions. Knowledge does not lead to behavior change. For drug education to have any impact, emphasis has to be placed on the immediate effects of drugs. Harmful effects that take years to develop, such as emphysema and cirrhosis, have less relevance to teenagers than the effects of drugs on their breath or social standing.

The scare tactics and horror stories used in the 1970s did not prevent experimentation with drugs.[41] In some drug education programs, former addicts described how drugs ruined their lives, researchers demonstrated the effects of drugs on laboratory animals, and police warned young people about the criminal penalties for drug use. Unfortunately, these types of activities have *not* been shown to reduce drug use. Some teachers warned students that marijuana use will lead to heroin use and that once one uses heroin, one is addicted forever. Based on their own experiences, many students know this information is inaccurate or exaggerated. In addition, it has been shown that many young people are skeptical about information they are given about drugs.[42]

Values Clarification

By the mid-1970s, drug education programs were stressing **values clarification** and affective education. The focus was not on drugs but, instead, on the underlying values contributing to drug use. It was thought that improving self-esteem and interpersonal skills was essential. The belief was that, if young people were to understand and articulate their values (assuming these are life-affirming values), they would recognize the potential destructiveness of drugs.

The values clarification approach was ineffective in changing students' behavior because drug use is often consistent with their values. They do not view drug use in a negative light. Students indicated that they valued the feelings that drugs gave them and that drug use helped them to be accepted by friends. Many teens find that drugs help them cope with stress.[43] In some instances, drugs increased their confidence. Others used values clarification as an excuse or a rationalization for using drugs. Also, some political and religious groups oppose values clarification on the basis that parents and churches, not schools, should teach values.

Alternatives Approach

One approach to drug education that was popular and that is still promoted by many drug educators is the alternatives approach. The rationale is that, for any reason for using drugs, an alternative is available to satisfy the reason. If a person takes drugs to get high, drug-free activities can provide natural highs. To relax, a person can do relaxation exercises. To cope with stress, an individual can learn stress-reducing activities. People who want to alter their consciousness can meditate. Those who have a compulsive need to take drugs can substitute a positive addiction for the negative addiction. To be effective, the alternatives must be more desirable than the drugs.

A Change in Direction

In 1974, Robert DuPont, former director of NIDA, reported that most students and teachers believed that drug education programs should be abolished. In the previous year, the U.S. Special Action Office on Drug Abuse Prevention recommended a 6-month moratorium on prevention materials, prevention activities, and the implementation of prevention programs. What evolved was more emphasis on health in general and less emphasis on the pharmacology of drugs.

Current Programs

Today, drug education emphasizes developing resiliency skills, learning peer-refusal techniques, and gaining life skills. Students have to be taught how to apply the knowledge they learn in the classroom to the decisions they are required to make every day. A sound drug education program teaches young people the negative effects of drugs and how to resist pressure from others to use drugs. Unfortunately, many programs are not evaluated or are poorly evaluated.[44]

Limitations of Drug Education

Rather than dissuade students from trying drugs, many early programs stimulated curiosity, which contributed to more drug use initially, although most young people did not continue to use drugs. One way to get people to do something they should not do is to tell them they are not allowed to do it. This is analogous to the idea that forbidden fruit is sweeter.

Teachers, researchers, and drug program specialists indicate that honesty, communication, trust, and respect are the most desirable attributes of a drug education teacher. A continuing problem with drug education has been the credibility of the teacher. Some teachers distort or exaggerate the physical, psychological, and social effects of drugs. Moreover, providing false or inaccurate information can be harmful to young people.[45]

Others take a moral stance in which they preach about the evils of drugs, creating an atmosphere of distrust. Students with a drug problem will probably hesitate to talk to a teacher who moralizes, for fear of being scolded rather than helped. Teachers should not glamorize drugs, but they have to be nonjudgmental and honest. Teachers can best help a student if they neither condemn nor condone the behavior.

Many students know more (or think they know more) about drugs than their teachers. The knowledge that students have might come from their *experience* with drugs, not from their *understanding* of drugs. Experience does not translate into knowledge, although some teachers who have had experience with alcohol and tobacco believe they can help their students by relating their own experiences.

Teachers do not have to have used drugs to be credible, but they do have to be informed. States such as New York require everyone receiving teacher certification to have coursework covering drugs. Because of the constant flow of new information, every teacher has to keep abreast of the field, and schools must provide staff development.

Problems with Drug Education

- Teachers often do not keep up with the latest information.
- Students sometimes know more about drugs than the teachers do.
- Some teachers are judgmental or moralistic.
- The goals of drug education are often unclear.
- The goals of drug education are often unrealistic.

Goals of Drug Education

Drug education can have a number of possible goals. One might be to impart knowledge. This has some value, as many young people are misinformed about drugs. Presumably, if students are armed with information, they can decide for themselves whether to use drugs. This approach, however, assumes that information leads to abstinence. In reality, no link between drug knowledge and behavior has been demonstrated. When asked if a lack of knowledge was a factor in their students using drugs, teachers indicated it was not.[46]

Other goals include reducing drug abuse or dependency, preventing or delaying first-time drug use, curtailing students' drug use, and teaching responsible drug use. With young people who have experimented with or used drugs already, moderate use might be a more realistic goal. Goals for drug education are not mutually exclusive. For example, a program can delay initial drug use and also encourage drug users to explore alternatives.[47]

One-Size-Fits-All Drug Education

Drug education programs should be tailored to the students' ages and to the needs of the students and the community. Students come from diverse cultures and drug education should reflect those differing cultures.[48] To expect that techniques for first-grade students would be the same as those for high school seniors is unreasonable. Elementary students do not have the aptitude of high school students to think conceptually, and their decision-making and problem-solving abilities are less developed; they understand literal messages and respond to direct instruction. Nonetheless, because many young people experiment with drugs by ages 11 and 12, it has been recommended that drug education begin by age 10.[49]

What Works: Schools without Drugs

Objectives

1. Valuing and maintaining sound personal health and understanding the effects of drugs on health
2. Respecting laws and rules that prohibit drug use
3. Recognizing and resisting pressure to engage in drug-taking behavior
4. Promoting activities that reinforce a positive, drug-free lifestyle

Source: U.S. Department of Education.

In its 1989 publication *What Works: Schools without Drugs,* the U.S. Department of Education developed a model for drug education. The message is clear: *abstinence*. Topics for elementary students include responsible decision-making, handling feelings, and the proper use of medicines. The secondary school model emphasizes the actual effects of drugs and the role of advertising.

self-efficacy Personal success based on one's own efforts

skills training A drug prevention program in which one learns skills to prevent drug use

resistance skills training Instruction in which students are taught to recognize, manage, and elude situations involving drugs; includes dealing with peer pressure and media messages

Current Approaches to Drug Education

The primary foci of drug education today are resiliency skills, personal development, refusal skills, decision-making, and coping skills. Information about drugs and alternatives to drug use are included in many programs. Developing personal competence is believed to be more important than pharmacology in helping young people decide about drug use. Young people who rate high in **self-efficacy**—the belief that one is in charge of oneself—are more likely to avoid harmful patterns of drug use.

Personal and Social Skills Training

The premise of personal and social **skills training** is that drug-taking behavior is *learned* through modeling and reinforcement. Drug use results from the interplay of social and personal factors. This model is derived from Bandura's social learning theory[50] and Jessor and Jessor's problem behavior theory.[51] The skills training model is comprehensive, not limited to drugs. It teaches personal and social skills applicable to various situations. Included are skills for resisting media and interpersonal influences, problem-solving and decision-making, relieving stress and anxiety, relaxation, self-control, self-esteem, interpersonal relations, and assertiveness.

Drug abuse prevention programs that focus on social influences have been shown to be more effective than other prevention efforts with young adolescents.[52] Students who feel personally competent are less likely to consume alcohol.[53] Project Northland, a substance abuse program based in Minnesota, has been shown to reduce the use of alcohol, tobacco, and other drugs significantly. Project Northland focuses on three particular domains: *environmental factors*—aspects of the environment that support, permit, or discourage alcohol use by adolescents, including such things as influential role models, social support, specific opportunities or barriers to drink, and community norms and standards related to adolescent drinking; *intrapersonal factors*—personality characteristics and ways of thinking that increase or decrease the likelihood of an adolescent using alcohol, including an adolescent's level of knowledge about alcohol use consequences, personal values, attitudes, and self-efficacy; and *behavioral factors*—these include past alcohol, cigarette, and other drug use, intentions to drink in the future, and skills to resist offers to use alcohol. Project Northland has expanded and has been shown to work in Croatia.[54]

Resistance Skills Training

Young people are exposed to drugs in many situations. Perhaps they are at a party where drugs are passed around or involved romantically with a partner who encourages drug use. In **resistance skills training**, students are taught how to recognize, manage, and avoid situations that could involve drug use. Students are instructed in how to refuse drugs *effectively*, often through role-playing. Peer educators are included in many of these programs because students perceive their peers as more credible than adults.

Resistance skills training also teaches students how to counter mass media messages that encourage drug use, especially tobacco and alcohol. One difference between resistance skills training and personal and social skills training is that the former focuses on specific problems whereas the latter teaches general skills for coping with life.

Drug Prevention Programs

Two drug prevention programs grounded in social learning, which have met with some success, are Project ALERT and Life Skills Training (LST). Project ALERT has been shown to reduce weekly alcohol and marijuana use, at-risk drinking, and alcohol use resulting in negative consequences, as well as attitudes and perceptions conducive to drug use.[55]

In LST, students are taught how to avoid being persuaded by others, to manage anxiety, to communicate more accurately, to be assertive, and to enhance their self-esteem. A 5½-year study of 1,677 students found that this program significantly reduced cigarette smoking and frequency of drunkenness and marijuana use.[56]

In a study of approximately 2,000 students in grades 6 through 10, teaching refusal skills resulted in significantly reduced alcohol misuse.[57] A review of smoking prevention programs found that seventh- to ninth-grade students who were taught to identify social influences promoting tobacco use and skills to resist tobacco use were less likely to smoke, and that this resistance persisted for 1 to 4 years.[58] The effectiveness of these programs, however, lessened over time. One factor that strengthened the effectiveness of school-based programs was community involvement, especially by parents, youth groups, community organizations, and the mass media.

Drug Abuse Resistance Education (DARE)

One popular drug education program is Drug Abuse Resistance Education (DARE), which began as a joint program between the Los Angeles Police Department and the Los Angeles School District. Police officers go to classrooms and teach elementary students about drugs and personal safety. Students are asked to write essays critical of drug use and to publicly pledge their opposition to drug use. To illustrate its popularity, President George Bush proclaimed April 10, 2008, to be National D.A.R.E. Day.[59]

Despite the hundreds of millions of dollars going to the DARE program, studies of DARE's effectiveness are not encouraging. Over a short period, DARE may reduce drug use, but 1 year after the program ends, there is no difference in drug use.[60] Suffolk County, one of the largest counties in New York, discontinued its DARE program after 20 years because it was found to be ineffective.[61]

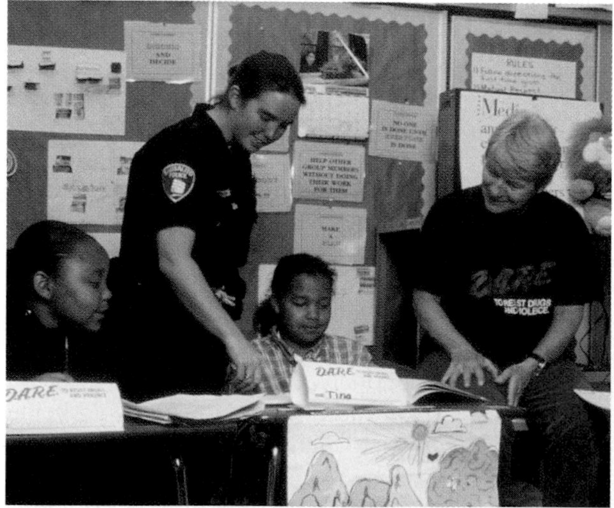

The most widely used drug prevention program in the United States is DARE (Drug Abuse Resistance Education).

In its review of numerous studies, the Government Accounting Office found that DARE had little impact on drug use.[62] Despite the fact that DARE has not been shown to work, it continues to be used because it is believed that it improves the relationships between police, children, and schools.[63]

To counter some of its critics, DARE officials are developing a new curriculum geared to seventh- and eighth-grade students. The new curriculum involves partnerships with community agencies[64] and will emphasize social norms because students tend to overestimate the drinking and drug-using habits of their peers.[65]

Just Say No!

During the Reagan administration beginning in 1980, First Lady Nancy Reagan promoted the "Just Say No" campaign. The concept is simple: Tell young people that if someone tries to persuade or encourage them to use drugs, they should refuse the drugs and walk away. For many youngsters this approach is adequate, but for others it is not, as some students do not recognize peer pressure or have the skills to refuse drugs.

Effectiveness of Drug Education

Although many drug education programs have increased knowledge and produced significant attitude changes, traditional drug education programs have not proved to be effective. Information alone does not alter behavior. For example, seven-year-old children are aware of the health hazards of smoking, yet many children smoke despite this knowledge. Students who most benefit from drug education may be those who least need it. In addition, many teachers do not have the skills and knowledge to teach about drugs in an effective way.[66] Working with disadvantaged sixth-grade schoolchildren, an alcohol prevention program was effective in reducing alcohol use up to 1 month after the program, but a 1-year follow-up demonstrated no long-term benefit.[67]

Before addressing the effectiveness of current drug education programs, criteria to determine effectiveness have to be identified. Should a drug education program be judged effective if students are better informed about drugs, if they espouse negative attitudes about drugs, if their drug use declines, or if the number of drug-related problems (such as emergency room visits from drugs) goes down? Is drug education successful if students switch from illegal drugs to alcohol and tobacco?

Sometimes drug education has the opposite effect on behavior because it stimulates curiosity and drug use may go up initially. If students experiment with drugs, though, they might do so more safely. Adolescence is a time for experimentation, and a certain amount of drug use should be expected. Rather than attempting to totally eliminate drug use, some contend, educators should work toward *reducing* drug use and misuse. The research findings are contradictory, although results of programs dealing with resistance training seem to be somewhat encouraging.

To influence drug use, *social norms* have to be changed. Although schools have an important role in drug prevention, they are just one piece of this mosaic. Students are under much pressure from sources outside of school to use illegal drugs, alcohol, and tobacco. Participation by the media, parents, and the community is essential. Also, programs emphasizing personal skills and psychosocial approaches can effectively reduce the use of alcohol and other drugs.

Effective programs include the following components[68]:

- The curricula are based on an understanding of the theory and research in drug abuse prevention.
- Information is developmentally appropriate; short-term, negative social consequences are emphasized.
- The curricula emphasize social resistance skills training as part of comprehensive health education that incorporates personal and social skills training.
- The program includes normative education, in which adolescents are taught that most people do not use drugs.
- Teachers use interactive teaching techniques such as role-playing, discussions, and small-group activities.
- Teachers receive training and support.
- The amount of time devoted to drug abuse prevention is sufficient and continued.
- Programs are culturally sensitive.
- School-based programs include the family, the community, and the media.
- Evaluation is necessary to determine effectiveness.

Health Education

In the 1800s, students were taught about the dangers of alcohol, tobacco, and other drugs. Today, drug education at the secondary level typically is taught in health education classes, and its impact is encouraging. The School Health Education Evaluation showed that sequential health education from kindergarten through 12th grade had a positive effect on knowledge, attitudes, *and* behaviors. Administrative support and teacher training are important to the success of health education.

Peer Programs

Various peer programs have been incorporated into drug prevention programs. Not all peer programs are alike. In some, peers serve as tutors; that is, older students teach younger students about drugs. In other programs peers facilitate discussions about drugs with others of the same age, or peers counsel peers. Peer programs typically function under the auspices of adults but sometimes operate without adult supervision.

Choosing appropriate peers is paramount. Administrators and teachers might identify one student as desirable whereas students identify someone else. Unconventional but responsible peer leaders seem to be best. Besides acting as role models, peer leaders have to be able to communicate effectively.

Results from peer-oriented programs are encouraging. In five approaches—knowledge only, affective only, peer programs, knowledge plus affective, and alternatives—peer programs were the most effective with the average student; for at-risk students, alternative programs were most effective.[69] A peer education program at Stanford University showed that students were less likely to engage in harmful drug use after participating in the program.[70]

Summary

Preventing drug abuse has been unsuccessful because millions of people derive pleasure from drugs, special interest groups hinder prevention efforts, and Americans do not like being told what to do. In the past, drug prevention was directed mainly at heroin, cocaine, and LSD. Now the attention has shifted to tobacco, alcohol, and marijuana—sometimes called gateway drugs. Rather than focus on drugs, some drug experts believe the causes underlying drug abuse—poverty, homelessness, poor education, and inadequate health care—should be addressed.

Evaluating prevention programs is difficult because the goals vary and "prevention" has no standard definition. Drug prevention occurs along a continuum of primary, secondary, and tertiary objectives. Primary prevention is aimed at people who have no experience with drugs; it attempts to reduce the demand for and supply of drugs. Secondary prevention is designed for people who have some experience with drugs; it tries to minimize the dangers of drug use by altering attitudes and behaviors and by stressing a healthy lifestyle. Tertiary prevention basically refers to treatment of those who are using drugs already.

Children from impoverished backgrounds tend to be designated as high-risk youths. Yet many rise above their circumstances and exhibit a resiliency to high-risk behaviors. Resilient children are characterized by a sense of humor, empathy, good relations with others, responsiveness, adaptability, problem-solving abilities, persistence, flexibility, and motivation. Also, they are able to distance themselves from their dysfunctional environments, master stress, and control their environments.

High-risk youths often grow up in households in which drugs are used, good parenting skills are lacking, and supervision is minimal. Children who are abused are at greater risk of becoming substance abusers as adults. Communities in which high-risk youths live are marked by high mobility, deprivation, population density, poverty, and disorganization. Educational programs in which students experience success, are exposed to alternative programs, and are involved in their learning have been shown to reduce high-risk behavior. Nurturing, supportive parents who give their children responsibilities are less likely to have children who use drugs. Communities can reduce drug use by providing jobs, better housing, and adequate health care.

When drug education was initiated, the emphasis was on information and scare tactics, under the incorrect assumption that knowledge and fear of the dangers of drugs would deter drug use. Drug education later promoted values clarification and affective education. These approaches were not effective, and evaluations of early drug education programs revealed that drug use actually went up, probably in part because of curiosity and the permission to explore values.

Drug education has been marked by numerous problems, such as teachers' lack of credibility and moralistic and judgmental attitudes. The goals of drug education have been unclear. Variously, they include imparting knowledge, delaying or preventing the initiation of drug use, reducing drug use, minimizing hazards associated with drug use, and instilling responsible drug use. In the "Just Say No" program, young people are told simply to walk away from drugs. Young people, however, do not always know when they are being pressured and, because of their need for peer approval, many have difficulty saying no.

The focus today is on developing resiliency, refusal skills, decision-making ability, coping skills, and personal and social skills. Students are taught how to recognize, avoid, and manage instances that place them at risk of using drugs. Peer programs have been particularly successful in curtailing drug use.

Thinking Critically

1. If you were hired to teach at a high school and were asked to develop a drug prevention program, what goals would you strive to achieve?
2. Elementary school students have different needs and problems than secondary students. How would your goals for drug education differ for elementary and secondary students? Would different drugs be addressed for each group?
3. Children growing up with parents who abuse drugs are more likely to use drugs than children whose parents do not abuse drugs. Should children of parents who abuse drugs be removed from their parents?
4. Parental attitudes regarding drugs are a strong factor in drug use by their children. If young people use drugs, should their parents be held accountable for their children's law-breaking behavior? To what extent do parents influence children's behaviors?

Web Resources

Drug Abuse Resistance Education (DARE)
http://www.dare-america.com
This site contains information regarding the DARE curriculum for kids, educators, parents, students, and others.

CASA: The National Center on Addiction and Substance Abuse at Columbia University
http://www.casacolumbia.org/
This organization publishes reports that assess what works in prevention, treatment, and law.

Notes

1. Office of National Drug Control Policy, *National Drug Control Strategy, 2009* (Rockville, MD: Office of ONDCP, 2008).
2. J. P. Caulkins, R. Liccardo Pacula, S. Paddock, and J. Chiesna, "What We Can—and Cannot—Expect from School-Based Drug Prevention," *Drug and Alcohol Review,* 23 (2004): 79–87.
3. *National Drug Control Strategy,* supra note 1.
4. *Results of the Fourth National Survey on Community Efforts to Reduce Substance Abuse and Gun Violence* (Boston: Join Together, 1999).
5. C. Rangel, "War on Drugs Must Begin on the Poverty Front" (letter to the editor), *New York Times* (December 26, 1989): A18.
6. T. Duster, "Pattern, Purpose, and Race in the Drug War: The Crisis of Credibility in Criminal Justice," in *Crack in America: Demon Drugs and Social Justice,* edited by C. Reinarman and H. G. Levine (Berkeley: University of California Press, 1997).

7. R. Midford, "Is This the Path to Effective Prevention?" *Addiction,* 103 (2008): 1169–1170.
8. G. J. Botvin, "School-Based Programmes to Prevent Alcohol, Tobacco and Other Drug Use," *International Review of Psychiatry,* 19 (December 2007): 607–615.
9. S. Farrer, "School-Based Program Promotes Positive Behavior, Reduces Risk Factors for Drug Use, Other Problems," *NIDA Notes,* 18 (February 2004): 1–6, 10.
10. P. Zickler, "Few Middle Schools Use Proven Prevention Programs," *NIDA Notes,* 17 (March 2003): 7, 14.
11. H. S. Shin, "A Review of School-Based Drug Prevention Program Evaluations in the 1990s," *American Journal of Health Education,* 32 (May/June 2001): 139–147.
12. P. J. Mrazek and R. J. Haggerty, *Reducing Risks for Mental Disorders: Frontiers for Preventive Intervention Research* (Washington, DC: Institute of Medicine, 1994).
13. K. E. Miller, "Adolescent Exposure to Smoking Depicted in Movies," *American Family Physician,* 69 (February 1, 2004): 641.
14. Substance Abuse and Mental Health Services Administration, *The NSDUH Report: Youth Activities, Substance Use, and Family Income* (Rockville, MD: Office of Applied Studies, April 19, 2007).
15. E. E. Doherty, K. M. Green, and M. E. Ensminger, "Investigating the Long-Term Influence of Adolescent Delinquency on Drug Use," *Drug and Alcohol Dependence,* 93 (January 11, 2008): 72–84.
16. Office of National Drug Control Policy, *Juveniles and Drugs: Facts and Figures* (Washington, DC: ONDCP, 2008).
17. Office of National Drug Control Policy, *Teens, Drugs and Violence: A Special Report* (Washington, DC: ONDCP, June 2007).
18. L. J. Bierut, S. H. Dinwiddie, H. Begleiter, R. R. Crowe, V. Hesselbrock, J. I. Nurnberer, B. Porjesz, M. A. Schuckit, and T. Reich, "Familial Transmission of Substance Dependence: Alcohol, Marijuana, Cocaine, and Habitual Smoking," *Archives of General Psychiatry,* 55 (1998): 982–988.
19. M. Fisher, I. Crome, J. Macleod, R. Bloor, and M. Hickman, *Predictive Factors for Illicit Drug Use among Young People: A Literature Review* (Great Britain: Home Office Online Report, 2007).
20. J. C. Ball, D. N. Nurco, R. R. Clayton, M. Lerner, T. A. Hagan, and G. A. Groves, "Etiology, Epidemiology and Natural History of Heroin Addiction: A Social Science Approach," in *Problems of Drug Dependence,* edited by L. S. Harris (Proceedings of the 56th Annual Scientific Meeting, NIDA Research Monograph 152) (Rockville, MD: National Institute on Drug Abuse, 1995).
21. D. Wright and M. Pemberton, *Risk and Protective Factors for Adolescent Drug Use: Findings from the 1999 National Household Survey on Drug Abuse* (Rockville, MD: Substance Abuse and Mental Health Services Administration, Office of Applied Studies, 2004).
22. J. Howard, *Substance Abuse Treatment for Persons with Child Abuse and Neglect Issues* (Rockville, MD: Center for Substance Abuse Treatment, 2000).
23. *National Survey of American Attitudes on Substance Abuse XII: Teens and Parents* (New York: The National Center on Addiction and Substance Abuse at Columbia University, August 2007).
24. *The Importance of Family Dinners* (New York: The National Center on Addiction and Substance Abuse at Columbia University, September 2007).
25. P. L. Ellickson, R. L. Collins, and R. B. Bell, "Adolescent Use of Illicit Drugs Other Than Marijuana: How Important Is Social Bonding and for Which Ethnic Groups?" *Substance Use and Misuse,* 34 (1999): 317–346.
26. P. F. Mulhall, D. Stone, and B. Stone, "Home Alone: Is It a Risk Factor for Middle School Youth and Drug Use?" *Journal of Drug Education,* 26 (1996): 39–48.
27. "Marijuana Use and Delinquent Behaviors Among Youths," *The NSDUH Report,* January 9, 2004.
28. J. J. Arnett, "The Myth of Peer Influence in Adolescent Smoking Initiation," *Health Education and Behavior,* 34 (August 2007): 594–607.
29. J. McIntosh and F. MacDonald, "Pre-teenage Children's Experiences with Alcohol," *Children and Society,* 22 (January 2008): 3–15.
30. F. Lucidi, A. Zelli, L. Mallia, C. Grano, P. M. Russo, and C. Violani, "The Social-Cognitive Mechanisms Regulating Adolescents' Use of Doping Substances," *Journal of Sports Sciences,* 26 (March 2008): 447–456.
31. *Community Monitoring Systems: Tracking and Improving the Well-Being of America's Children and Adolescents* (Rockville, MD: National Institute on Drug Abuse, September 2007).
32. R. E. Tarter, L. Kirisa, A. Mezzich, J. R. Cornelius, K. Pajer, M. Vanyakov, W. Gardner, T. Blackson, and D. Clark, "Neurobehavioral Disinhibition in Childhood Predicts Early Age at Onset of Substance Use Disorder," *American Journal of Psychiatry,* 160 (2003): 1078–1085.
33. A. Fletcher, C. Bonnell, and J. Hargreaves, "School Effects on Young People's Drug Use: A Systematic Review of Intervention and Observational Studies," *Journal of Adolescent Health,* 42 (March 2008): 209–220.
34. L. A. Drapela and C. Mosher, "The Conditional Effect of Parental Attachment and Adolescent Drug Use: Social Control and Social Development Model Perspectives," *Journal of Child and Adolescent Substance Abuse,* 16 (2007): 63–87.
35. *Make a Difference: Talk to Your Child about Alcohol* (Rockville, MD: National Institute on Alcohol Abuse and Alcoholism, 2000).
36. R. Mathias, "Shortened Family Prevention Programs Yield Long-Lasting Reductions in Adolescent Drug Abuse," *NIDA Notes,* 17 (May 2002): 8–10.
37. K. A. Ogilvie and R. S. Moore, "Changing Community Readiness to Prevent the Abuse of Inhalants and Other Harmful Legal Products in Alaska," *Journal of Community Health,* 33 (August 2008): 248–258.
38. "Religious Involvement and Substance Use among Adults," *The NSDUH Report,* March 23, 2007.
39. R. Martinez, R. Rosenfeld, and D. Mares, "Social Disorganization, Drug Market Activity, and Neighborhood Violent Crime," *Urban Affairs Review,* 43 (July 2008): 846–874.
40. M. A. Pentz, "Institutionalizing Community-Based Prevention through Policy Change," *Journal of Community Psychology,* 28 (May 2000): 257–270.
41. W. DeJong, "Scare Tactics," *Prevention Pipeline,* 13 (January/February 2000): 11.
42. "Teens Skeptical About Drug Advice: Research Suggests Current Drug Education Has Little Effect on Young People's Choices," *Nursing Standard,* 18 (March 17, 2004): 28.
43. *The Partnership Attitude Tracking Study (PATS): Teens 2007 Report.* Partnership for a Drug-Free America, August 2008.
44. "The Role of Schools in Combating Illicit Substance Abuse," *Pediatrics,* 120 (December 2007): 1379–1384.
45. K. W. Tupper, "Teaching Teachers to Just Say 'Know': Reflections on Drug Education," *Teaching and Teacher*

Education, 24 (February 2008): 356–367.
46. S. Norland, A. DiChiara, and A. Hendershott, "Teachers' Use of and Perceptions of a Drug Curriculum," *Journal of Alcohol and Drug Education* (Winter 1995): 100–109.
47. S. Sussman and D. S. Black, "Substitute Addiction: A Concern for Researchers and Practitioners," *Journal of Drug Education*, 38 (2008): 167–180.
48. L. H. Steiker, "Making Drug and Alcohol Prevention Relevant," *Family and Community Health*, 31 (March 2008): S52–S60.
49. S. Baldauf, "Protective Measures," *U.S. News and World Report*, 144 (March 17, 2008): 57.
50. A. Bandura, *Social Learning Theory* (Englewood Cliffs, NJ: Prentice-Hall, 1976).
51. R. Jessor and S. L. Jessor, *Problem Behavior and Psychosocial Development: A Longitudinal Study of Youth* (New York: Academic Press, 1977).
52. P. L. Lantz, P. D. Jacobson, and K. E. Warner, "Youth Smoking Prevention: What Works?" *Prevention Researcher*, 8 (April 2000): 1–6.
53. "Anti-drug Programs Worth Evaluating (Grades K–12)," *Curriculum Review*, 43 (December 2003): 11.
54. B. West, et al., "Project Northland in Croatia: Results and Lessons Learned," *Journal of Drug Education*, 38 (2008): 55–70.
55. D. Longshore, P. L. Ellickson, D. F. McCaffrey, and P. A. St. Clair, "School-Based Drug Prevention among At-Risk Adolescents: Effects of ALERT," *Health Education and Behavior*, 34 (August 2007): 651–668.
56. R. L. Spoth, G. K. Randall, L. Trudeau, C. Shin, and C. Redmond, "Substance Use Outcomes 5 1/2 Years Past Baseline for Partnership-Based, Family-School Preventive Interventions," *Drug and Alcohol Dependence*, 96 (2008): 57–68.
57. S. R. Wynn, J. Schulenberg, D. D. Kloska, and V. B. Laez, "The Mediating Influence of Refusal Skills in Preventing Adolescent Alcohol Misuse," *Journal of School Health*, 67 (1997): 390–394.
58. B. S. Lynch and R. J. Bonnie, *Growing Up Tobacco Free: Preventing Addiction in Children and Youth* (Washington, DC: National Academy Press, 1994).
59. G. Bush, "Proclamation 8235—National D.A.R.E. Day, 2008," *Federal Register*, April 11, 2008.
60. "The Truth about DARE," *Consumers' Research Magazine*, 86 (March 2003): 40–41.
61. "DARE to Say Goodbye," *District Administration*, January 2008: 18.
62. *Youth Illicit Drug Use Prevention: DARE Long-Term Evaluations and Federal Efforts to Identify Effective Programs* (Washington, DC: Government Accounting Office, 2003).
63. D. P. Rosenbaum, "Just Say No to D.A.R.E.," *Criminology and Public Policy*, 6 (November 2007): 815–824.
64. C. L. Perry, K. A. Komro, S. Veblen-Mortenson, L. Bosma, K. Munson, M. Stigler, L. A. Lytle, J. L. Forster, and S. L. Welles, "The Minnesota DARE Plus Project: Creating Community Partnerships to Prevent Drug Use and Violence," *Journal of School Health*, 70 (March 2000): 84–99.
65. "DARE to Revamp Program Approach, Focus on Social-Norms Strategy," *Alcoholism and Drug Abuse Weekly*, 13 (February 26, 2001): 1–4.
66. T. Wragg, "Just Say No to Drugs Push," *Times Educational Supplement* (March 13, 2004): 32.
67. C. E. Werch, D. M. Pappas, J. M. Carlson, and C. C. DiClemente, "Short- and Long-Term Effects of a Pilot Prevention Program to Reduce Alcohol Consumption," *Substance Use and Misuse*, 33 (1998): 2303–2321.
68. *Preventing Drug Use Among Children and Adolescents: A Research-Based Guide for Parents, Educators, and Community Leaders* (Rockville, MD: National Institute on Drug Abuse, 2003).
69. N. S. Tobler, "Meta-Analysis of 143 Adolescent Drug Prevention Programs: Quantitative Outcome Results of Program Participants Compared to a Control or Comparison Group," *Journal of Drug Issues*, 16 (1986): 537–567.
70. R. J. Castro and B. D. Foy, "Harm Reduction: A Promising Approach for College Health," *The Journal of American College Health* (September 2002): 89–91.

BIBLIOGRAPHY

Angell, Marcia. *The Truth about the Drug Companies.* New York: Random House, 2004.

Barondes, Samuel H. *Better than Prozac: Creating the Next Generation of Psychiatric Drugs.* New York: Oxford University Press, 2003.

Bennett, Joel B., and Wayne E. K. Lehman, editors. *Preventing Workplace Substance Abuse: Beyond Drug Testing to Wellness.* Washington, DC: American Psychological Association, 2003.

Booth, Martin. *Cannabis: A History.* New York: Thomas Dunne Books/St. Martin's Press, 2003.

Burns, Eric. *The Spirits of America: A Social History of Alcohol.* Philadelphia: Temple University Press, 2004.

Collins, Tony, and Wray Vamplew. *Mud, Sweat, and Beers: A Cultural History of Sport and Alcohol.* New York: Oxford, 2002.

Courtwright, David T. *Forces of Habit: Drugs and the Making of the Modern World.* Cambridge, MA: Harvard University Press, 2001.

Davenport-Hines, Richard. *The Pursuit of Oblivion: A Global History of Narcotics.* New York: Norton, 2002.

Earleywine, Mitchell. *Understanding Marijuana: A New Look at the Scientific Evidence.* New York: Oxford University Press, 2002.

Goldberg, Raymond, editor. *Taking Sides: Clashing Views on Controversial Issues in Drugs and Society.* Guilford, CT: McGraw-Hill/Dushkin, 2008.

Haustein, Knut-Olaf. *Tobacco or Health?: Physiological and Social Damages Caused by Tobacco Smoking.* New York: Springer, 2003.

Healy, David. *The Creation of Psychopharmacology.* Cambridge, MA: Harvard University Press, 2002.

Inciardi, James A., and Karen McElrath, editors. *The American Drug Scene.* Los Angeles, Roxbury Publishing, 2004.

Monroe, Judy. *Steroids, Sports, and Body Image.* Berkeley Heights, NJ: Enslow Publishers, 2004.

National Drug Control Strategy. Washington, DC: Office of National Drug Control Policy, 2009.

National Drug Threat Assessment 2008. Johnstown, PA: National Drug Intelligence Center, 2008.

Schlosser, Eric. *Reefer Madness: Sex, Drugs, and Cheap Labor in the American Black Market.* Boston: Houghton Mifflin, 2003.

Silverman, Harold M. *The Pill Book.* New York: Bantam Books, 2004.

United States Senate Committee on the Judiciary. *Narco-terrorism: International Drug Trafficking and Terrorism, a Dangerous Mix: Hearing Before the Committee on the Judiciary, United States Senate, One Hundred Eighth Congress, First Session, May 20, 2003.* Washington, DC: U.S. Government Printing Office, 2003.

GLOSSARY

acculturation The adaptation and acceptance of cultural and social norms of a new environment

acetaldehyde Product of metabolism of alcohol by the liver; also found in tobacco smoke

acetylcholine (ACH) A neurotransmitter synthesized from a molecule of choline and from acetyl CoA

acetylsalicylic acid The agent in aspirin that relieves pain

action potential The procedure by which the nerve impulse is sent down the axon

acute Describes a condition that arises abruptly and is not long lasting

acute dyskinesia Inappropriate motor movements as a side effect of antipsychotic drugs

adenosine A neurotransmitter for which caffeine acts as an antagonist

adrenaline A hormone secreted by the adrenal gland in the fight-flight-fright response; another name for epinephrine

akathesia Jerky, uncontrollable constant motion, motor restlessness, occasional protruding tongue, and facial grimace

alcohol abuse A state characterized by physical, social, intellectual, emotional, or financial problems resulting from the use of alcohol

alcohol dependence Condition in which one's body requires alcohol or else withdrawal symptoms will occur; also marked by tolerance

alcoholism Condition in which an individual loses control over intake of alcohol

alcopops Malt, distilled alcohol–containing, or wine-containing beverages that have been flavored with fruit juices or other added ingredients; an example is Mike's Hard Lemonade

alkuhl An Arabic word meaning "the essence," from which the word *alcohol* is derived

alli A weight-loss drug that blocks the absorption of fat

Amanita muscaria One of the oldest and most common hallucinogens; derived from the fly agaric mushroom

amotivational syndrome A condition characterized by apathy, an inability to concentrate, and little achievement orientation

amphetamines Powerful central nervous system stimulants

amyl nitrite An inhalant used to treat angina pectoris and congestive heart failure

anabolic steroids Substances used to increase muscle mass; related to male sex hormones

analgesics Drugs that relieve pain

analog A synthetic derivative of an existing drug

anaphylactic shock A condition caused by an allergic reaction to contaminants such as quinine, which are used to cut or dilute heroin

androstenedione Food supplement used for muscle development

Antabuse (disulfiram) A drug that interferes with the metabolization of alcohol, making the drinker violently ill

antagonists Drugs that occupy receptor sites and inhibit narcotic activity

anticholinergic hallucinogens Substances found in datura and in *Amanita muscaria* mushrooms; interfere with the action of acetylcholine to produce hallucinations

anti-emetic A drug that reduces nausea and vomiting; an example is marijuana

antipyretic Having fever-reducing properties

antitussives Drugs that act as cough suppressants

anxiolytic Refers to anxiety-reducing drugs

aphrodisiac Any substance that increases sexual desire and performance

aqua vitae Literally means "water of life"; another expression for alcohol

atropine A psychoactive agent found in mandrake and other anticholinergic hallucinogens

attention deficit/hyperactivity disorder (ADHD) A condition in which the individual is hyperactive and easily distracted, which inhibits learning

autonomic nervous system (ANS) Part of the peripheral nervous system that is automatic and involuntary

autoreceptors Units that alter the synthesis of neurotransmitters after they are released by the nerve cells

axons Parts of the neuron that send nerve impulses away from the nerve's cell body

barbital A sedative-hypnotic drug used to treat anxiety and nervousness; the original barbiturate

barbiturate (barbituric acid) A member of a class of drugs that have depressant effects

basal ganglia Part of the central nervous system

behavioral tolerance Adjustment or behaviors learned by an individual to compensate for the presence of drugs

belladonna (deadly nightshade) A potent hallucinogen found in Europe, North Africa, and Asia; member of the tomato and potato family

Benzedrine An amphetamine used to treat nasal congestion and asthma

benzocaine A topical anesthetic put into candies or chewing gum to diminish appetite

benzodiazepines A type of minor tranquilizer; examples are Librium and Valium

benzopyrene Carcinogenic compound found in marijuana and tobacco

bhang Lower leaves, stems, and seeds of the cannabis plant

bidis Flavored cigarettes from India that have considerably higher concentrations of nicotine than regular cigarettes

binge drinking Consuming five or more drinks (men) or four (women) in a short period of time

biphetamine A powerful stimulant

bipolar affective disorder A mental condition characterized by alternating moods of depression and mania; formerly called manic-depression

blackouts A common symptom of problem drinking; characterized by temporary memory loss

blood alcohol concentration (BAC)/blood alcohol level (BAL) Percentage of alcohol in the bloodstream

blunt A marijuana-containing cigar; to create a blunt, tobacco is removed from a regular cigar and marijuana is inserted

bradykinesia Motor movements that are slow and limited

bromides Nonbarbiturate sedatives used to treat epileptic convulsions

Brompton's cocktail A combination of heroin and cocaine sometimes used to treat terminally ill patients

bufo A type of toad that produces a hallucinogenic secretion

Buprenorphine A semisynthetic opiate that has an analgesic effect and is used to treat opioid addiction

butyl nitrite An inhalant no longer used for medical purposes but found in products such as perfume and antifreeze

caffeine A mild stimulant found in coffee, tea, soda pop, and chocolate

caffeinism Excessive caffeine consumption resulting in caffeine dependency

calcium carbonate An antacid designed to relieve acid indigestion

cannabinoids Chemicals found in marijuana plants

cannabis A genus of plant that is also known as marijuana

carbon monoxide Gas in cigarette smoke that interferes with oxygen-carrying capacity of blood

catecholamines A group of neurotransmitters that includes epinephrine, dopamine, and norepinephrine

Category I drugs Drugs determined to be safe, effective, and properly labeled

Category II drugs Drugs generally recognized as unsafe and ineffective or as mislabeled; must be removed from medications within 6 months after the FDA issues its final regulations

Category III drugs Drugs for which data are insufficient to determine general recognition of safety and effectiveness

central nervous system (CNS) The brain and spinal cord

cerebral cortex Part of the brain involved in intellectual functioning; affects speech, motor movement, sensory perception, hearing, vision, sensory discrimination, memory, language, reasoning, abstract reasoning, and personality

cerebrum Part of the brain that contains the cerebral cortex

charas A potent form of marijuana also known as hashish

China white A synthetic analgesic drug derived from fentanyl that mimics heroin but is considerably more potent

chippers Nickname for individuals who use narcotics occasionally or on weekends

chloral hydrate A nonbarbiturate sedative; also called "knockout drops" or Mickey Finns; induces sleep

chlorpromazine An antipsychotic drug

cholinesterase An enzyme necessary for the metabolism of acetylcholine

chronic drug use The habitual use of drugs

circumstantial-situational drug use Short-term drug use to contend with immediate distress or pressure

clove cigarettes Cigarettes made from tobacco and cloves; contain more tar, nicotine, and carbon monoxide than commercial cigarettes

codeine A mild narcotic that suppresses coughing; a derivative of opium

cold turkey Elimination of a negative behavior all at once, as opposed to gradually (with or without a substitute)

compulsive drug use Obsessive drug use without regard for society

congeners The nonalcoholic ingredients in some forms of alcohol, such as flavoring agents or other residual substances

controlled drinking approach Alcohol treatment based on behavior modification, in which the person learns to drink in a nonabusive manner

crack cocaine A variation of cocaine made by heating cocaine after mixing it with baking soda and water

crank A term for methamphetamines

creatine monohydrate Natural substance used to increase strength and short-term speed

cross-tolerance Transference of tolerance to a drug to chemically similar drugs

crystal meth A variation of methamphetamine; one example is ice

datura A hallucinogen used for sacred purposes in ancient China, Greece, India, and Africa

deadly nightshade See *belladonna*

decongestants Substances used to relieve congestion

decriminalization The reduction or elimination of penalties for illegal activities

delta-9-tetrahydrocannabinol (THC) The psychoactive agent in marijuana

dendrites Parts of the neuron that allow nerve impulses to be transmitted to the nerve's cell body

depression Dejection characterized by withdrawal or lack of response to stimulation

designer drugs Synthetic substances that are chemically similar to existing drugs

detoxification Eliminating drugs from the body; usually the initial step in treatment of the effects of alcohol and other drugs

dextromethorphan (Delsym) An over-the-counter nonnarcotic drug found in cough preparations

diacetylmorphine See *heroin*

diethyl glycol A chemical solvent

dimethyltryptamine (DMT) A hallucinogen in which effects last 1 to 2 hours

dissociative anesthetic Substance that alters the perception of pain without loss of consciousness

distillation A heating process that increases alcohol content

distilled spirits Beverages such as whiskey, rum, gin, and vodka that are produced by boiling various solutions

disulfiram See *Antabuse*

dopamine A neurotransmitter that affects emotional, mental, and motor functions

dose-response curve Graphic representation of the effects of drugs at various levels

drug Any substance that alters one's ability to function emotionally, physically, intellectually, financially, or socially

drug abuse The intentional and inappropriate use of a drug resulting in physical, emotional, financial, intellectual, or social consequences for the user

drug addiction Continuing desire for drugs based on a physical need

drug dependency Recurring desire for drugs based on a psychic or a physical need

drug misuse The unintentional or inappropriate use of prescribed or over-the-counter drugs

drug paraphernalia Items that are aids to using drugs

dystonia A type of dyskinesia marked by involuntary and inappropriate postures and muscle tones

Ecstasy See *MDMA*

effective dose (ED) The amount of drug required to produce a specific response

electroconvulsive therapy (ECT) Controlled administration of electric shock as a treatment for mental illness

elixir sulfanilamide An antibiotic that killed more than 100 people in the 1930s

employee assistance programs (EAPs) Company-sponsored programs to help employers deal with their employees who have problems, including drug use

encounter groups A type of confrontational treatment frequently used at therapeutic communities

endorphins Naturally occurring chemicals with opiate-like properties

enkaphalins Endorphins found within the brain

environmental tobacco smoke (ETS) Smoke in the air as a result of someone smoking

epinephrine A natural chemical, also called adrenaline, involved in the fight-flight-fright syndrome

Equanil The first modern drug developed to relieve anxiety

ergogenic aids Substances that provide an athletic advantage, also known as performance-enhancing drugs

ergotism A condition resulting from ingesting a fungus that grows on grains; marked by muscle tremors, burning, mania, delirium, hallucinations, and eventual gangrene

erythropoietin Hormone that enhances cardiovascular endurance by increasing red blood cell production

Erythroxylon coca Coca plant from which cocaine is derived

ether An inhalant dating back to the late 1700s

ethyl alcohol The form of alcohol that people consume

eugenol Ingredient in clove cigarettes that provides aroma and reduces coughing reflex

expectorants Cough medicines that make a cough productive by increasing mucous secretions

experimental drug use Infrequent drug use usually motivated by curiosity

extrapyramidal symptoms Neurological symptoms characterized by difficulty walking, shuffling, and inflexible joints

false negative A test that is negative for drugs even though drugs are present in the urine

false positive A test that is positive for drugs even though no drugs are present in the urine

fentanyl A synthetic narcotic that is 1,000 times more potent than heroin

fermentation The process of transforming certain yeasts, carbon, hydrogen, and oxygen of sugar and water into ethyl alcohol and carbon dioxide

fetal benzodiazepine syndrome A condition of infants caused by the mother's use of benzodiazepine during pregnancy; affected children have malformed face, poor muscle tone, tremors, poor coordination, delayed mental development, and learning disabilities

fight-flight-fright syndrome Psychological response of the body to stress, which prepares the individual to take action by stimulating the body's defense system

flashbacks A phenomenon in which a person reexperiences the effects of LSD days, weeks, or months after it was last used

fly agaric Another name for the hallucinogenic mushroom *Amanita muscaria*

fortified wines Beverages produced by adding alcohol to slightly sweetened wines

freebase A variation of cocaine in which cocaine is separated from its hydrochloride salt by heating, using a volatile chemical such as ether

Gamma-aminobutyric acid (GABA) An inhibitory neurotransmitter that regulates muscle tone in mammals

gamma-hydroxybutyrate (GHB) A type of neurotransmitter that produces relaxation and sleepiness; one of the "date rape" drugs

ganja Tops and flowers of the cannabis plant

gas chromatography/mass spectrometry A type of drug-testing procedure that is highly sophisticated and sensitive, but time-consuming and expensive

gateway drugs Substances that are used before use of more dangerous drugs; alcohol, marijuana, tobacco, and inhalants are considered gateway drugs

Halcion A drug used to induce sleep

hallucinogens A class of drugs that induce perceived distortions in time and space

hard drugs Drugs that are perceived to be dangerous, such as heroin, cocaine, and LSD

harm reduction A series of practical interventions that respond to the needs of drug users and the community where they live in an effort to reduce the harm caused by illicit drug use

hash oil Substance made by separating resin from the cannabis plant by boiling the plant in alcohol; it has a very high THC content

hashish A potent form of marijuana taken from resin of the cannabis plant

hashishiyya A group of men who, while under the influence of hashish, allegedly terrorized and killed people

hemp Marijuana plant that may be used to make rope, clothing, and paper

heroin (diacetylmorphine) A potent drug that is a derivative of opium

hippocampus Part of the brain involved with memory; altered by marijuana

histamines Chemicals that are released by the body in response to the presence of allergens

homeostasis A condition in which the body's systems are in balance

human growth hormones Hormones that stimulate protein synthesis; used by athletes to enhance performance

hydrochloric acid Acid in the stomach that can ease digestion and irritate the stomach lining

hypoglycemia A condition of low levels of sugar in the blood

hypothalamus Gland situated near the base of the brain; maintains homeostasis; affects stress, aggressiveness, heart rate, hunger, thirst, consciousness, body temperature, blood pressure, and sexual behavior

hypoxia A lack of oxygen within body tissues. Hypoxia can lead to brain damage resulting from an inadequate supply of oxygen to the brain

ibogaine A hallucinogen that is used to treat cocaine dependence

ice Crystals of methamphetamine that are smoked, inhaled, or injected

immunoassay A drug-testing procedure that tests for metabolites of drugs

inhalants Drugs that are inhaled or "sniffed"

inpatient treatment A residential drug treatment program based on a hospital model

intensified drug use Taking drugs on a steady, long-term basis to relieve a persistent problem or stressful situation

interdiction Intervention

interferon A natural substance in the body that wards off viral infections

iproniazid A monoamine oxidase inhibitor

isobutyl One type of nitrite that is used to treat angina pain; also causes vasodilation, flushing, and warmth

Jamestown weed (jimsonweed) Any hallucinogen derived from the *Datura* plant; also known as "locoweed"

ketamine A drug very similar to PCP

ketoprofen An over-the-counter analgesic

kola nut A part of a plant originally used in Coca-Cola

laudanum A drug derived from opium

lethal dose (LD) The amount of a drug required to result in death

levo-alpha-acetylmethadol (LAAM) An experimental drug that prevents narcotic withdrawal symptoms for about 3 days

limbic system Part of the central nervous system that plays a key role in memory and emotion

lithium A psychotherapeutic drug used to treat symptoms associated with mania

locoweed Another term for jimsonweed

look-alike drugs Substances that appear similar to illegal or pharmaceutical drugs

LSD (lysergic acid diethylamide) A powerful hallucinogen derived from a fungus

mainstream smoke Smoke exhaled by a smoker

major tranquilizers Antipsychotic drugs

mandrake A hallucinogen derived from the nightshade family; used during the Middle Ages in connection with witchcraft and sorcery

mania A mood disorder characterized by inappropriate elation, an irrepressible mood, and extreme cheerfulness

margin of safety The difference between a beneficial level and a harmful level of a drug

MDA A hallucinogen that is structurally similar to amphetamines

MDMA (methylenedioxymethamphetamine) A synthetic hallucinogen related to amphetamines; also called Ecstasy

medial forebrain bundle (MFB) Serves as a communication route between the limbic system and the brain stem; affects pleasure and reward

medical model The premise that a pathogen is responsible for a person's illness or disease

medulla oblongata One of two structures constituting the brain stem; helps control respiration, blood pressure, heart rate, and other vital functions

mental illness A condition caused by a mood disorder or by disorganized thinking

meperidine A synthetic derivative of morphine

meprobamate A minor tranquilizer marketed under the trade names of Miltown and Equanil; also used for treating psychosomatic conditions

mescaline A psychoactive agent, or hallucinogen, derived from the peyote cactus

methadone A drug given to heroin addicts to block withdrawal effects and euphoria

methadone maintenance program A type of therapy used in the treatment of heroin addiction

methamphetamine A more potent form of amphetamine

methaqualone A sedative-hypnotic drug that relieves tension and anxiety without barbiturate-like aftereffects

methyl alcohol Wood alcohol; not fit for human consumption

midbrain Part of the brain stem that connects the larger structures of the brain to the spinal cord

Miltown Brand name for meprobamate

minor tranquilizer Drug used primarily to relieve anxiety

monoamine oxidase inhibitor (MAO) An antidepressant drug used for acute anxiety, obsessive-compulsive behavior, and phobias

mood disorder A form of psychosis that affects the person's emotions; can be depression or mania

morphine An analgesic drug derived from opium; used medically as a painkiller

MPPP A synthetic drug that is similar to meperidine

myristicin Substance found in nutmeg and mace; chemically similar to mescaline and capable of producing hallucinations

naltrexone A narcotic antagonist that blocks the reinforcing effects of narcotics

naproxen sodium An over-the-counter analgesic

narcolepsy Condition in which the person involuntarily falls asleep; commonly called sleeping sickness

narcotic An opium-based central nervous system depressant used to relieve pain and diarrhea

negative reinforcement Relief or avoidance of pain achieved by a behavior, motivating one to repeat the behavior

neuroleptics The European term for antipsychotic drugs

neurons Messengers in the brain that transmit information via chemical and electrical processes

neurotransmitter A chemical substance manufactured in vesicles of the brain

nicotine Psychoactive component in tobacco responsible for stimulation and tobacco dependence

NIMBY (not in my back yard) A term describing how some people feel about having a controversial facility located in their neighborhoods

nitrous oxide An inhalant also known as laughing gas

norepinephrine A neurotransmitter that may help regulate appetite and reduce fatigue

normalization A term used by the Dutch for the practice of not prosecuting users of soft drugs such as marijuana

opiate A class of drugs derived from opium

opioid A family of drugs with characteristics similar to those of opium

opium The plant from which narcotics are derived

outpatient treatment A nonresidential drug treatment program; least expensive form of treatment

paraldehyde A nonbarbiturate sedative-hypnotic drug used with severely disturbed mental patients

parasympathetic nervous system Branch of the autonomic nervous system that includes acetylcholine and alters heart rate and intestinal activity

parasympathomimetics Drugs that mimic actions of the parasympathetic system, which allows the body to rest during states of emergency

parenteral drug use Drug administration by injection

Parkinsonism A form of acute dyskinesia marked by tremors, weakness in the extremities, and muscle rigidity

passive smoke Tobacco smoke present in the air from someone else's smoking and inhaled by others

patent medicines A synonym for over-the-counter drugs

pathogen Any organism that produces disease

pentothal See *thiopental*

peptides Substances linking amino acids; include

endorphins, which are naturally occurring chemicals with opiate-like properties

peripheral nervous system (PNS) Consists of the autonomic and somatic nervous systems

periventricular system Part of the central nervous system implicated with punishment or avoidance behavior

peyote A cactus containing the hallucinogen mescaline

phantasticants A term used to describe hallucinogenic drugs

pharmacological tolerance Adjustment or compensation of the body to the presence of a given drug

pharmacology The professional discipline that studies the relationships and interactions between living organisms and substances within them

phenacetin An alternative to aspirin now linked to kidney problems; its sale is prohibited

phencyclidine hydrochloride (PCP) Originally developed as an anesthetic for humans and, later, animals; also called "angel dust"

phenobarbital Second barbiturate developed; produces relaxation and relieves anxiety

phenylpropanolamine (PPA) A decongestant also used as an appetite suppressant

pituitary gland The "master gland"; responsible for controlling many bodily functions by secretion of hormones

placebo An inert substance that does not have a physical effect but may produce psychological and associated physiological reactions

polydipsia Frequent and excessive consumption of water

polyuria Frequent urination

pons One of two structures constituting the brain stem, connecting the medulla with the brain stem

positive reinforcement Pleasurable sensations associated with a behavior, motivating one to repeat the behavior

potency A drug's ability to produce an effect relative to other drugs; the less that is needed to produce a response, the more potent the drug

PPA See *phenylpropanolamine*

primary prevention Preventing drug use before it begins

primary reinforcers Stimuli that reduce physiological needs or are inherently pleasurable

proof Amount of alcohol in a beverage expressed as twice the percentage of the alcohol content

propoxyphene hydrochloride A mild narcotic that has the potential to cause dependence

proprietary drugs Drugs that can be purchased without a prescription; over-the-counter drugs

prostaglandins Chemicals in the body that produce pain and inflammation; aspirin alters their synthesis

Prozac (fluoxetine) An antidepressant drug

pseudoephedrine A nasal decongestant

psilocin The psychoactive ingredient in the psylocybe mushroom

psilocybin A hallucinogen found in certain mushrooms in Central America

psyche Refers to the mind

psychedelic A term used to describe hallucinogenic drugs; means "mind-manifesting"

psychoactive drug Any substance that has the capability of altering mood, perception, or behavior

psychoanalysis A form of talk therapy based on Freudian principles

psychosis A severe mental condition marked by loss of contact with reality

psychotogenic Refers to drugs that generate psychosis

psychotomimetic Refers to drugs that produce psychotic-like symptoms

purity Quality of a substance; state of noncontamination of a drug

Quaalude Brand name for methaqualone

rapid eye movement (REM) A stage during sleep that is needed for the sleep to be restful

rapid smoking Aversive smoking-cessation technique in which one smokes rapidly to exceed tolerance and becomes ill

rebound effect The side effects produced by a drug that make a condition worse than it was originally; e.g., sinuses become more congested by nasal sprays

rebound insomnia A side effect of sleeping pills in which falling asleep becomes more difficult rather than less difficult

recidivism Relapse

reinforcers Stimuli or events that lead to certain behaviors being repeated

relapse Failure to maintain a course of action, such as returning to drug abuse after initiating a treatment program

resiliency A person's ability to overcome obstacles, such as resisting drug use despite a background that increases the likelihood of drug use

resistance skills training Instruction in which students are taught to recognize, manage, and elude situations involving drugs; includes dealing with peer pressure and media messages

reticular activating system (RAS) Part of the central nervous system; affects sleep, attention, and arousal

reuptake A process by which a chemical is reabsorbed into the cell from which it was discharged

reverse tolerance A drug user's experiencing of the desired effects from lesser amounts of the same drug

Ritalin A mild stimulant used to treat attention deficit/hyperactivity disorder (ADHD)

Rohypnol A powerful depressant; one of the "date rape" drugs

roid rage Uncontrollable violence associated with use of anabolic steroids

salvinorin A A hallucinogen that alters perception and consciousness; effects last less than one hour

schizophrenia A type of functional psychosis; literally, "split mind"

scopolamine A psychoactive agent found in mandrake and other anticholinergic hallucinogens

secondary prevention Early intervention to block more serious problems; halts escalation of drug use

secondary reinforcers Stimuli that signal the increased probability of obtaining primary reinforcers

sedative-hypnotic Class of drugs that produce relaxing to sleep-inducing effects depending on dosage

self-efficacy Personal success based on one's own efforts

serotonin An inhibitory neurotransmitter located in the upper brain stem; plays a role in regulating sensory perception, eating, pain, sleep, and body temperature

set The psychological state, personality, and expectations of an individual while using drugs

setting The physical and social environment in which drugs are used

shooting gallery A place to buy and inject drugs

sidestream smoke Smoke that comes from the burning end of a cigarette, pipe, or cigar

sinsemilla Seedless marijuana; derived from unfertilized female cannabis plants

skills training A drug prevention program in which one learns skills to prevent drug use

snuff A form of smokeless tobacco

social-recreational drug use Taking drugs in a social environment to share pleasurable experiences among friends

sodium bicarbonate Baking soda; an ingredient in antacids designed to neutralize excess acid in the stomach

soft drugs Drugs perceived to be less harmful than hard drugs; include marijuana, tobacco, and alcohol

soldier's disease A name given to morphine dependency during the Civil War

soma From the Greek; literally means "body"

somatic nervous system Part of the nervous system that controls movement of the skeletal muscles

sound-alike drugs Substances with names that sound similar to those of illegal or prescription drugs

speed A stimulant drug; another name for methamphetamine

speedball Injectable combination of heroin and cocaine

"speed freak" Someone who uses methamphetamines over a period of time

spontaneous remission Cessation of drug abuse without any type of formal treatment

St. Anthony's fire Burning sensations caused by ergot poisoning; people during the Middle Ages would visit the shrine of St. Anthony in an attempt to cure it

stacking Ingesting or injecting several steroids at the same time

steppingstone theory Hypothesis holding that use of soft drugs such as marijuana and alcohol leads to use of harder drugs such as heroin and cocaine

sympathetic nervous system A branch of the autonomic nervous system that releases adrenaline

sympathomimetic effects An increase of blood to the brain and muscle, allowing the body to flee or fight

sympathomimetics Drugs that mimic actions of the sympathetic nervous system, which is involved with fight-flight-fright activity

synapse The space between an axon and a dendrite

synergistic effect An enhanced, unpredictable effect caused by combining two or more substances

synesthesia The hallucinogenic blending of senses (e.g., seeing sounds and hearing color)

T lymphocytes Type of white blood cells that help in fighting infections

tachycardia Faster than normal heart rate

tar A carcinogenic component of tobacco

tardive dyskinesia A side effect of antipsychotic drugs marked by involuntary repetitive facial movements and involuntary movement of the trunk and limbs

temperance Moderate alcohol use, rather than abstinence

temperance movement A social trend that developed in the United States in the 1800s when groups sought to reduce alcohol use

teonanacatl Aztec word describing the psylocybe mushroom

teratogenic Refers to substances that cause harm to the fetus

tertiary prevention Treatment that seeks to help individuals after they have misused drugs

thalidomide A sedative that was found in the 1960s to cause birth defects including missing or malformed limbs

THC See *delta-9-tetrahydrocannabinol*

theobromine A stimulant found in chocolate; chemically related to caffeine

theophylline A stimulant found in tea; in the same chemical family as caffeine

therapeutic community (TC) A residential drug treatment center that utilizes confrontation techniques

therapeutic window The amount of drug needed for therapeutic purposes

thin-layer chromatography A simple, inexpensive, urine-based drug test

thiopental (pentothal) A barbiturate that is used as a general anesthetic

Thorazine Major tranquilizer used to treat psychosis

threshold dose The smallest amount of a drug required to produce an effect

tinnitus A condition marked by constant ringing in the ears

toluene The psychoactive agent in glue

toxicity A drug's ability to disturb or nullify homeostasis

transdermal method Administration of drugs by applying them on the surface of the skin

tricyclic antidepressants Drugs that effectively remove the symptoms of acute depression

tryptophan An amino acid that affects serotonin levels, allowing one to fall asleep more easily

tyramine An amino acid that interacts with monoamine oxidase inhibitors to cause very high levels of hypertension

unipolar depression A mental disorder marked by alternating periods of depression and normalcy

Valium (diazepam) A minor tranquilizer

values clarification A teaching strategy in which individuals are asked to express and support their values

Veronal Brand name for barbital

vesicles Saclike structure at the end of the axon

Wellbutrin An antidepressant drug that is used to help people stop smoking

Whiskey Rebellion A protest by farmers in southwestern Pennsylvania against a tax on whiskey

withdrawal symptoms Physical signs that appear when drug use is stopped

xanthine A type of stimulant of which caffeine is one

INDEX

Note: Page numbers marked *t* are tables; those in italics are figures.

D

E

Commonly Abused Drugs

	Examples of *Commercial* and Street Names	DEA Schedule*/ How Administered**	*Intoxication Effects*/Potential Health Consequences
Cannabinoids			
hashish	boom, chronic, gangster, hash, hash oil, hemp	I/swallowed, smoked	*euphoria, slowed thinking and reaction time, confusion, impaired balance and coordination*/cough, frequent respiratory infections; impaired memory and learning; increased heart rate, anxiety; panic attacks; tolerance, addiction
marijuana	blunt, dope, ganja, grass, herb, joints, Mary Jane, pot, reefer, sinsemilla, skunk, weed	I/swallowed, smoked	
Depressants			
barbiturates	*Amytal, Nembutal, Seconal, Phenobarbital;* barbs, reds, red birds, phennies, tooies, yellows, yellow jackets	II, III, V/injected, swallowed	*reduced anxiety; feeling of well-being; lowered inhibitions; slowed pulse and breathing; lowered blood pressure; poor concentration*/fatigue; confusion; impaired coordination, memory, judgment; addiction; respiratory depression and arrest, death *Also, for barbiturates—sedation, drowsiness*/depression, unusual excitement, fever, irritability, poor judgment, slurred speech, dizziness, life-threatening withdrawal
benzodiazepines (other than flunitrazepam)	*Ativan, Halcion, Librium, Valium, Xanax*; candy, downers, sleeping pills, tranks	IV/swallowed, injected	*for benzodiazepines—sedation, drowsiness*/dizziness
flunitrazepam***	*Rohypnol*; forget-me pill, Mexican Valium, R2, Roche, roofies, roofinol, rope, rophies	IV/swallowed, snorted	*for flunitrazepam*—visual and gastrointestinal disturbances, urinary retention, memory loss for the time under the drug's effects
GHB***	*gamma-hydroxybutyrate*; G, Georgia home boy, grievous bodily harm, liquid ecstasy	I/swallowed	*for GHB*—drowsiness, nausea/vomiting, headache, loss of consciousness, loss of reflexes, seizures, coma, death
methaqualone	*Quaalude, Sopor, Parest*; ludes, mandrex, quad, quay	I/injected, swallowed	*for methaqualone—euphoria*/depression, poor reflexes, slurred speech, coma
Dissociative Anesthetics			
ketamine	*Ketalar SV*; cat Valiums, K, Special K, vitamin K	III/injected, snorted, smoked	*increased heart rate and blood pressure, impaired motor function*/memory loss; numbness; nausea/vomiting *Also, for ketamine—at high doses, delirium, depression, respiratory depression and arrest*
PCP and analogs	*phencyclidine;* angel dust, boat, hog, love boat, peace pill	I, II/injected, swallowed, smoked	*for PCP and analogs—possible decrease in blood pressure and heart rate, panic, aggression, violence*/loss of appetite, depression

*Schedule I and II drugs have a high potential for abuse. They require greater storage security and have a quota on manufacturing, among other restrictions. Schedule I drugs are available for research only and have no approved medical use; Schedule II drugs are available only by prescription (unrefillable) and require a form for ordering. Schedule III and IV drugs are available by prescription, may have five refills in 6 months, and may be ordered orally. Most Schedule V drugs are available over-the-counter.
**Taking drugs by injection can increase the risk of infection through needle contamination with staphylococci, HIV, hepatitis, and other organisms.
Source: National Institute on Drug Abuse, 2004. www.drugabuse.gov

(continued)

Commonly Abused Drugs—*cont'd*

	Examples of *Commercial* and Street Names	DEA Schedule*/ How Administered**	*Intoxication Effects*/Potential Health Consequences
Hallucinogens			
LSD	*lysergic acid diethyl-amide*; acid, blotter, boomers, cubes, microdot, yellow sunshines	I/swallowed, absorbed through mouth tissues	*altered states of perception and feeling; nausea*/persisting perception disorder (flashbacks) *Also, for LSD and mescaline—increased body temperature, heart rate, blood pressure; loss of appetite, sleeplessness, numbness, weakness, tremors* *for LSD—persistent mental disorders*
mescaline	buttons, cactus, mesc, peyote	I/swallowed, smoked	
psilocybin	magic mushroom, purple passion, shrooms	I/swallowed	*for psilocybin—nervousness, paranoia*
Salvia divinorum	Diviner's sage	not scheduled/chewed, smoked	*for* Salvia divinorum*—laughter, recalled memories, euphoria*
Opioids and Morphine Derivatives			
codeine	*Empirin with Codeine, Fiorinal with Codeine, Robitussin A-C, Tylenol with Codeine;* Captain Cody, Cody, schoolboy; (with glutethimide) doors & fours, loads, pancakes and syrup	II, III, IV/injected, swallowed	*pain relief, euphoria, drowsiness*/nausea, constipation, confusion, sedation, respiratory depression and arrest, tolerance, addiction, unconsciousness, coma, death *Also, for codeine—less analgesia, sedation, and respiratory depression than morphine*
fentanyl and fentanyl analogs	*Actiq, Duragesic, Sublimaze*; Apache, China girl, China white, dance fever, friend, goodfella, jackpot, murder 8, TNT, Tango and Cash	I, II/injected, smoked, snorted	
heroin	*diacetylmorphine*; brown sugar, dope, H, horse, junk, skag, skunk, smack, white horse	I/injected, smoked, snorted	*for heroin—staggering gait*
morphine	*Roxanol, Duramorph*; M, Miss Emma, monkey, white stuff	II, III/injected, swallowed, smoked	
opium	*laudanum, paregoric*; big O, black stuff, block, gum, hop	II, III, V/swallowed, smoked	
oxycodone HCL	*Oxycontin*; Oxy, O.C., killer	II/swallowed, snorted, injected	
hydrocodone bitartrate, acetaminophen	*Vicodin*; vike,Watson-387	II/swallowed	

*Schedule I and II drugs have a high potential for abuse. They require greater storage security and have a quota on manufacturing, among other restrictions. Schedule I drugs are available for research only and have no approved medical use; Schedule II drugs are available only by prescription (unrefillable) and require a form for ordering. Schedule III and IV drugs are available by prescription, may have five refills in 6 months, and may be ordered orally. Most Schedule V drugs are available over-the-counter.
**Taking drugs by injection can increase the risk of infection through needle contamination with staphylococci, HIV, hepatitis, and other organisms.
Source: National Institute on Drug Abuse, 2004. www.drugabuse.gov